Intestinal Ion Transport

Intestinal Ion Transport

Edited by J. W. L. Robinson

Département de Chirurgie Expérimentale
Hôpital Cantonal Universitaire
Lausanne

The Proceedings of the International Symposium on
Intestinal Ion Transport held at Titisee in May 1975

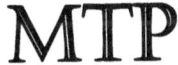

Published in UK by
MTP Press Ltd
St Leonard's House
Lancaster, Lancs.

ISBN-13: 978-94-011-6158-9   e-ISBN-13: 978-94-011-6156-5
DOI: 10.1007/978-94-011-6156-5

William Clowes & Sons Limited
London, Colchester and Beccles

Contents

CONTENTS

CONTENTS

List of Participants

ABRAMOW M.
Laboratoire de Médecine Expérimentale
Fondation Reine Elisabeth
Avenue Jean Crocq 1
BRUXELLES
Belgium

ALVARADO F.
Department of Physiology
University of Puerto Rico Medical School
P.O. Box 5067
SAN JUAN
Puerto Rico
  Present address:
  Laboratoire de Physiologie Comparée
  Faculté des Sciences
  Université de Paris-Sud
  ORSAY
  France

ARMSTRONG W. McD.
Department of Physiology
Indiana University Medical Center
1100 West Michigan Street
INDIANAPOLIS, Indiana
U.S.A.

BINDER H. J.
Department of Internal Medicine
Yale University
NEW HAVEN, Connecticut
U.S.A.

BÖHMER R.
Department für klinische Chemie
Universitätsklinik
Steinhövelstrasse 9
ULM
West Germany

CASE R. M.
Department of Physiology
University Medical School
NEWCASTLE-UPON-TYNE
England

CASPARY W. F.
Abteilung für Gastroenterologie
Medizinische Universitätsklinik
Humboldtallee
GÖTTINGEN
West Germany

DENNHARDT R.
Institut für angewandte Physiologie
Lahnberge
MARBURG/Lahn
West Germany

DESJEUX J. F.
Hôpital Hérold
7, Place Rhin-Danube
PARIS
France

DIEZI J.
Institut de Pharmacologie de l'Université
21, Rue du Bugnon
LAUSANNE
Switzerland

DOWLING R. H.
Gastroenterology Unit
Guy's Hospital
LONDON
England

EBEL H.
Institut für klinische Physiologie
Kliniken Steglitz
Hindenburgdamm 30
BERLIN
West Germany

EDMONDS C. J.
Clinical Research Centre
Watford Rd.
HARROW, Middlesex
England

ELLORY J. C.
A.R.C. Institute of Physiology
BABRAHAM, Cambridgeshire
England

FIELD M.
Department of Medicine
Beth Israel Hospital
330 Brookline Avenue
BOSTON, Massachusetts
U.S.A.

LIST OF PARTICIPANTS

FORTH W.
Institut für Pharmakologie und Toxikologie
Ruhr-Universität
Postfach 2148
BOCHUM-Querenburg
West Germany

FRIZZELL R. A.
Department of Physiology
Pittsburgh University Medical School
PITTSBURGH, Pennsylvania
U.S.A.

GILLES-BAILLIEN M.
Laboratoire de Biochimie générale et comparée
Institut Léon-Fredericq
17, Place Delcour
LIÉGE
Belgium

HIRANO T.
Ocean Research Institute
University of Tokyo
NAKANO-TOKYO
Japan

KINNE R.
Max-Planck Institut für Biophysik
Kennedy-Allee 70
FRANKFURT-am-Main
West Germany

LAHLOU B.
Laboratoire de Physiologie Comparée
Faculté des Sciences
Parc Valrose
NICE
France

LAUTERBACH F.
Institut für Pharmakologie und Toxikologie
Ruhr-Universität
Postfach 2148
BOCHUM-Querenburg
West Germany

LEVIN R. J.
Department of Physiology
Sheffield University
SHEFFIELD
England

LORENZ-MEYER H.
Medizinische Universitätsklinik
Mannkopffstrasse
MARBURG/Lahn
West Germany

LOVE A. H. G.
Department of Medicine
Queen's University
BELFAST
Northern Ireland

LUISIER A.-L.
Département de Chirurgie Expérimentale
Hôpital Cantonal Universitaire
LAUSANNE
Switzerland

MAETZ J.
Station Zoologique
VILLEFRANCHE-sur-Mer, Alpes Maritimes
France

MATUCHANSKY Cl.
Département de Gastroentérologie
Hôpital St. Lazare
Rue Fbg. St.-Denis
PARIS
France

MENGE H.
Département de Chirurgie Expérimentale
Hôpital Cantonal Universitaire
LAUSANNE
Switzerland

Permanent address:
Medizinische Universitätsklinik
Mannkopffstrasse
MARBURG/Lahn
West Germany

MIRKOVITCH V.
Département de Chirurgie Expérimentale
Hôpital Cantonal Universitaire
LAUSANNE
Switzerland

MÜLLER F.
Physiologisch-Chemisches Institut der Karl-Marx-Universität
Liebigstrasse 16
LEIPZIG
East Germany

MUNCK B. G.
Institute of Medical Physiology A
University of Copenhagen
Juliane Maries vej 28
KØBENHAVN Ø
Denmark

MUNDAY K. A.
Department of Physiology & Biochemistry
University of Southampton
SOUTHAMPTON
England

MURER H.
Max-Planck Institut für Biophysik
Kennedy-Allee 70
FRANKFURT-am-Main
West Germany

NELL G.
Institut für Pharmakologie
Universität des Saarlandes
HOMBURG/Saar
West Germany

PARSONS D. S.
Department of Biochemistry
South Parks Road
OXFORD
England

RASK-MADSEN J.
Medical Department F
Glostrup Hospital
GLOSTRUP
Denmark

   Present address:
   Blegdamshospitalet
   Epidemic Dept. M
   University Hospital
   KØBENHAVN N
   Denmark

RIECKEN E. O.
Medizinische Universitätsklinik
Mannkopffstrasse
MARBURG/Lahn
West Germany

ROBINSON J. W. L.
Département de Chirurgie Expérimentale
Hôpital Cantonal Universitaire
LAUSANNE
Switzerland

ROMMEL K.
Department für klinische Chemie
Universitätsklinik
Steinhövelstrasse 9
ULM
West Germany

RUMMEL W.
Institut für Pharmakologie
Universität des Saarlandes
HOMBURG/Saar
West Germany

SCHARRER E.
Institut für Tierphysiologie der Universität
Veterinärstrasse 13
MÜNCHEN
West Germany

SEPÚLVEDA F. V.
Département de Chirurgie Expérimentale
Hôpital Cantonal Universitaire
LAUSANNE
Switzerland

SHARP G. W. G.
Institut de Biochimie Clinique
Sentier de la Roseraie
GENÈVE
Switzerland

   Permanent address:
   Massachusetts General Hospital
   BOSTON, Massachusetts
   U.S.A.

SIMMONDS W. J.
Department of Physiology
University of Western Australia School of
Medicine
Shenton Park
PERTH, Western Australia
Australia

SKADHAUGE E.
Institute of Medical Physiology A
University of Copenhagen
Juliane Maries vej 28
KØBENHAVN Ø
Denmark

SMITH M. W.
A.R.C. Institute of Physiology
BABRAHAM, Cambridgeshire
England

TURNBERG L. A.
Hope Hospital
SALFORD, Lancs
England

WHITTEMBURY G.
Centro de Biofísica y Bioquímica
Instituto Venezolano de Investigaciones
Científicas
Apartado 1827
CARACAS
Venezuela

WINGATE D. L.
Department of Physiology
The London Hospital Medical College
LONDON
England

WINNE D.
Pharmakologisches Institut der Universität
Wilhelmstrasse 56
TÜBINGEN
West Germany

WRIGHT E. M.
Max-Planck Institut für Biophysik
Kennedy-Allee 70
FRANKFURT-am-Main
West Germany

Permanent address:
Department of Physiology
University of California Medical Center
LOS ANGELES, California
U.S.A.

Foreword

This is the fourth Falk Symposium devoted to the study of intestinal absorption. As in the case of its predecessors[1-3], I hope that the relaxed atmosphere will enable the participants from all corners of the world to exchange views, not only in this room, but also at less formal moments in the cellar, on the lake, or in the buses that transport us to different parts of the Schwarzwald. We are all eternally grateful to Dr Herbert Falk for undertaking to sponsor this meeting, and to him and his staff for the impeccable organisation which will permit us to work in such a pleasant environment.

In the organisation of the programme, one or two innovations have been introduced which are perhaps foreign to routine gastroenterological meetings. First, the average age in this room is rather lower than at most gatherings of this nature, which means that those who carry out the experiments will be responsible for their presentation; they are after all the ones who have made the relevant small observations which lead to the advancement of knowledge. Secondly, there is a smattering of nephrologists and comparative physiologists among us. I have invited nephrologists in fields in which I consider that they have advanced further than their gastroenterological counterparts, whilst the inclusion of the comparative gentlemen, who often use the same techniques as conventional gastroenterologists but thereby discover interesting new mechanisms when studying, for instance, the adaptation of fish to sea water, might hopefully act as a stimulus in the planning of new work, which is the main purpose of the meeting. Lastly, the concept of the "discussion paper" immediately following one of the 23 main presentations has been introduced. I had naively hoped that the discussion papers would all be directly related to their preceding main paper, but in some cases, despite relevance to the principal topic of the meeting, they only bear a vague connection with the preceding presentation. Nevertheless, in this volume, the general discussions are published as they were held, namely immediately after the discussion paper.

Finally, it is my pleasure to thank my colleagues in Lausanne for their encouragement during the past year, and in particular my secretary, Miss Winefred Happee, for all her excellent work in the course of the organisation of the scientific programme.

J. W. L. Robinson

1. Rommel, K. und Clodi, P. H. (eds) (1970) *Biochemische und klinische Aspekte der Zuckerabsorption*. (Stuttgart/New York: Schattauer-Verlag).
2. Rommel, K. and Goebell, H. (eds) (1973) *Biochemical and clinical aspects of peptide and amino acid absorption*. (Stuttgart/New York: Schattauer-Verlag).
3. Dowling, R. H. and Riecken, E. O. (eds) (1974) *Intestinal adaptation*. (Stuttgart/New York: Schattauer-Verlag).

1
Dual Sodium Pumps in the Kidney

G. WHITTEMBURY
and F. PROVERBIO

Centro de Biofísica y Bioquímica,
Instituto Venezolano de Investigaciones Científicas (IVIC),
Caracas

In the kidney, as in other epithelia, sodium absorption is not linked to potassium secretion. Therefore no close relationship between transepithelial sodium and potassium movements can be established. In order to test the possibility that the postulated sodium-for-potassium exchange pump is responsible for sodium reabsorption, one requires direct information about unidirecttional sodium and potassium movements across the peritubular membrane in order to relate them to sodium reabsorption. This is at present technically difficult. One approximation has consisted of trying to correlate net sodium reabsorption with peritubular potassium concentration in proximal tubules perfused via the lumen and the peritubular capillaries. Sodium reabsorption has been shown in this case to be related to the peritubular potassium concentration[1]. A similar relationship has been found to hold in the perfused amphibian kidney. Furthermore, net sodium reabsorption has been shown to maintain a close relationship with peritubular potassium influx[2].

To gain further insight into the Na^+ pump mechanisms, kidney slices and isolated tubules have been employed. In these preparations, inhibitors at high concentrations can be used, and drastic changes in the cellular and bathing fluid ionic concentrations can be induced so that the normal function can be altered. The effects of these perturbations can be correlated with the observed ionic distribution and movements. With these experimental techniques, several lines of evidence have been obtained showing that the sodium pump exchanges sodium for potassium:

(1) Sodium and potassium move in opposite directions across tubular cell membranes. Thus, in slices of renal tissue, (a) cell sodium decreases when cell potassium increases; that is, a clear relationship can be established between net movements of sodium from the cell to the extracellular space and net entry of potassium into the cells, and vice versa[3–10]; (b) net sodium extrusion depends on the potassium concentration in the extracellular medium[6–8]; (c) net potassium entry depends on the intracellular sodium concentration[6].

(2) Ouabain inhibits both extrusion of sodium and uptake of potassium such that the magnitude of the net sodium extrusion inhibited is equivalent to the net potassium entry inhibited[6,8,9].

(3) Cells of kidney slices can also extrude sodium in the presence of rubidium or caesium instead of potassium in the extracellular fluid. These ionic movements are partially inhibited by ouabain. The magnitude of the net

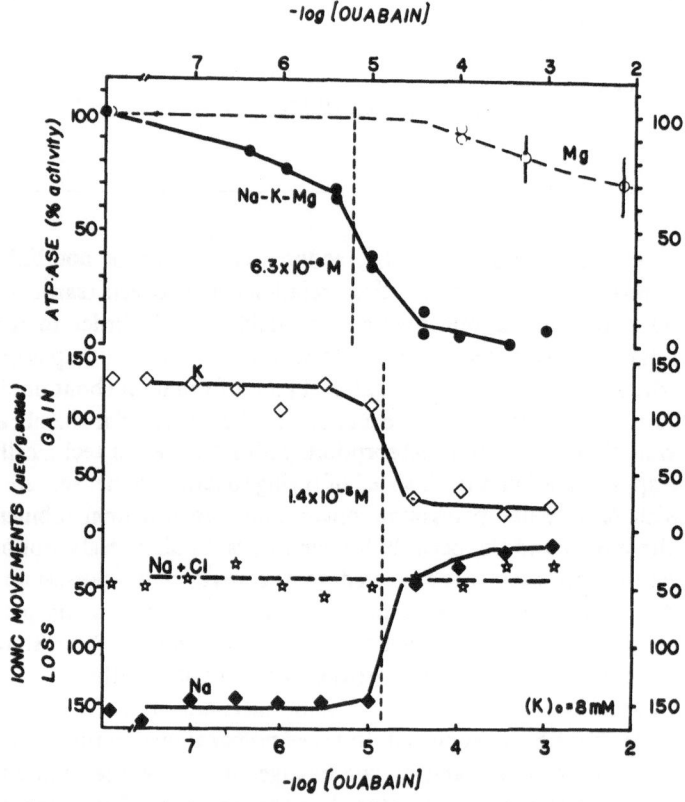

Figure 1.1 Dose–response curves of $(Na^+ + K^+)$-ATPase and Mg^{++}-ATPase activity (top) of a kidney cortex microsomal preparation, and ionic movements (exchange of Na^+ for K^+ and extrusion of Na^+ with Cl^-) observed in guinea-pig kidney cortex slices bathed in a medium containing 8 mM K^+ (bottom), both as functions of the ouabain concentration (taken from reference 12)

rubidium or caesium entry inhibited is stoichiometrically equivalent to the magnitude of the net efflux of sodium inhibited by ouabain[11].

(4) Finally, as illustrated in Figure 1.1, the dose–response curves of the inhibitory action of ouabain on the sodium–for–potassium exchange, just described, is closely paralleled by its inhibitory action on the $Na^+ + K^+$-stimulated ATPase activity of a cell membrane preparation for the same tissue[6,12,13].

There are further reasons to link the $Na^+ + K^+$-stimulated ATPase with sodium–potassium transport in the kidney: The sodium–potassium pump requires renewed synthesis of ATP since it is inhibited by DNP and anoxia. The $Na^+ + K^+$-stimulated ATPase is found in very high concentrations in the kidney, and it seems to be situated in the expected cytological location in the cell[14]. The ATPase activity increases when animals have been adapted to conditions in which the sodium pump activity should be enhanced, because the kidney needs to reabsorb more sodium (on administration of adrenal steroids, unilateral nephrectomy, high protein diet) or to excrete more potassium (chronic potassium loading)[15]. The ATPase activity decreases when the sodium–potassium pump is expected to be idle, for instance after adrenalectomy[15] and extracellular volume expansion[15(a)] (conditions which diminish sodium reabsorption in the kidney) and in post-obstructive diuresis in the rat[16].

These observations agree well with the view that the energy for the function of the sodium pump comes from hydrolysis of ATP at the level of the cell membrane, a reaction that is stimulated by sodium from the inside and by potassium from the outside, and is sensitive to the cardiac glycoside, ouabain. However, there are some limitations to the existing observations to complete the link of sodium-extruding mechanisms to ATP hydrolysis. For example, it has not been possible in the kidney — as it has in the red cell and in the axon — to test whether the transport system shows vectorial aspects[17], or whether ATP can be synthesised when the sodium-potassium pump is run backwards.

There are also a number of puzzling findings that have resulted in suggestions that the classical scheme of the sodium–potassium pump should be modified.

Some observations arise from kidney slice studies *in vitro* and some from work with perfused kidney.

(1) If there was only one system to effect sodium reabsorption, complete inhibition of the energy supply to the system (that is, inhibition of the $Na^+ + K^+$-stimulated ATPase activity by ouabain) should block all sodium reabsorption by the kidney. However, about one-half to one-third of the filtered sodium (and chloride) continues to be reabsorbed when the $Na^+ + K^+$-stimulated ATPase activity is 100% inhibited. The remaining reabsorption can be blocked with cyanide and iodoacetate. Thus the ouabain-resistant sodium reabsorption

is also dependent on metabolic energy. It must be concluded, therefore, that other reabsorptive mechanisms may be in operation[15,18].

(2) Although, as mentioned above, in the perfused amphibian kidney sodium reabsorption correlates well with peritubular potassium uptake under control conditions, this relationship can be markedly altered by different experimental manoeuvres, so that sometimes near normal sodium reabsorption is accompanied by very low potassium uptake whilst, under other conditions, negligible sodium and chloride reabsorption with normal potassium uptake occurs[2].

(3) In mammalian kidney slices, it has been observed that sodium can be extruded with chloride, even in the presence of ouabain concentrations that completely inhibit the exchange of sodium for potassium[3,8,9,12]. From these observations, the description of the two modes of sodium extrusion has emerged: (A) *Sodium can be expelled in exchange for potassium* and this mode of sodium extrusion is very sensitive to ouabain and seems little affected by ethacrynic acid[8,9,12], furosemide and triflocin[19]; (B) *sodium can be expelled with chloride and water*. This mode of sodium extrusion which is paramount to volume regulation proceeds in the absence of external potassium and in the presence of ouabain at a concentration which clearly inhibits sodium–for–potassium exchange. Mode (B) is curtailed by ethacrynic acid[8,9,12,25], furosemide[26], and triflocin[19]. It is stimulated (even in the presence of ouabain) by angiotensin[20]. Both modes of sodium extrusion are inhibited if ouabain is added together with either ethacrynic acid[8,9], furosemide or triflocin[19]. It may be concluded that hydrolysis of ATP is the source of energy for both modes of sodium extrusion since both are inhibited by dinitrophenol and anoxia[8,9].

Three main types of explanation, which have in common the proposal for mechanisms working in parallel, have been offered to account for such observations. Kleinzeller's excellent review should be consulted[3].

(1) The cryptic pump hypothesis considers that there is a difference in the accessibility of the external bathing solutions to the sodium pumps situated on the surface of the kidney continuous with the basement membrane, which would be easily accessible and inhibitable by ouabain, and those pumps situated deep in the crypts that exist in the peritubular membrane of kidney cells. Sodium extrusion in a medium without potassium can be accounted for because the cellular potassium that is lost in the crypts is readily rebound by the sodium pump, so that the potassium concentration is not really 0 in the crypts[10,21]. This allows sodium to be expelled from the cells even in the presence of a nominal potassium concentration of 0 in the external medium. Ouabain would not reach these 'cryptic' sodium pumps[10]. Thus sodium extrusion can continue in the presence of ouabain. This view has received recent support from work in isolated tubules. It was found that in the usual preparation, both modes of Na^+ extrusion could be described and, in the

4

presence of ouabain, extrusion of sodium with chloride could be observed: but if the tubules were dialysed in order to lower their potassium concentration, no extrusion of sodium could be observed in the presence of ouabain[5]. Although this possibility had been previously considered[10], it was rejected[8,9] since it is difficult to understand how the cardiac glycoside cannot have access to the crypts, thus leaving a fraction of the sodium pumps uninhibited, although exchange of sodium for potassium can be maximally inhibited at ouabain concentrations several orders of magnitude lower than those that leave the extrusion of sodium with chloride unaffected. One of the limitations of the experiments with isolated tubules is that the failure to observe extrusion of sodium with chloride and water only occurs under conditions in which the intracellular ionic composition is severely distorted. Under these circumstances, the supply of metabolic energy for the ouabain-resistant mode of extrusion of sodium might be upset.

(2) Kleinzeller[3] has provided evidence for the existence of a mechanochemical (contractile) mechanism with physical properties determined by calcium and ATP metabolism which may counterbalance a major hydrostatic pressure gradient in kidney cells. This mechanism can qualitatively explain most of the present observations, namely extrusion of sodium or lithium with chloride and water, the relationship between calcium, ATP and volume regulation, the finding of a calcium ATPase and the presence of filamentous contractile structures at the basal aspects of the cells[3].

(3) Finally, the existence of a second sodium pump[8,9,12,20,24,26] or a volume regulating mechanism[22,23] which would extrude sodium has also been considered. The main arguments in its favour are (a) the observation that mode B of sodium extrusion proceeds even in the absence of potassium in the bathing medium and in the presence of ouabain; (b) the difference in the inhibitory action of ouabain on the one hand, and of ethacrynic acid, triflocin and furosemide on the other. The first inhibits mainly mode A of sodium extrusion and the latter mainly mode B of Na^+ extrusion; and (c) the observation that angiotensin stimulates mode B when mode A is inhibited by ouabain[20]. Although the cryptic pump hypothesis seems the most reasonable choice when only the action of ouabain is considered, the necessity of two pumps arises when the observation of two types of inhibitor is considered.

It seems at present that further experiments are required to settle between these possibilities. One of the limitations arises from the highly artificial conditions (of sodium-loaded cells) which need to be used to demonstrate the alternative mode of sodium extrusion, so that the relative roles of both mechanisms of sodium extrusion cannot be assessed.

A new Na^+-stimulated ATPase

In view of the possible existence of a second Na^+-extruding mechanism, which would also derive its energy from hydrolysis of ATP, we decided to look for a ouabain-insensitive, Na$^+$-stimulated ATPase in microsomal fractions of kidney tissue. Outermost slices of kidney cortex of guinea pigs were obtained as described[7]. The tissue was homogenised at 0 °C in sucrose Tris/EDTA mixture, the homogenate was centrifuged at 10 000 g, the supernatant at 100 000 g, and the sediment from the last centrifugation was suspended in the sucrose/Tris/EDTA solution. An aliquot was used for the study of the ATPase activity of the fresh preparation and the rest was submitted to an ageing process which consisted of leaving the preparation in the refrigerator at 4 °C in the same extraction medium for several days. The ATPase activity was assayed as a function of the period of storage. (The procedure is described in detail in reference 27 where the work is presented *in extenso*.)

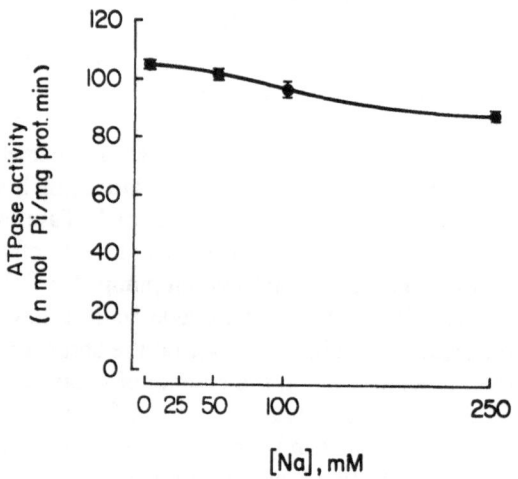

Figure 1.2 Inhibitory effect of increasing Na$^+$ concentration (Cl$^-$ salt) on the Mg^{++}-dependent ATPase activity of fresh microsomal preparation from the guinea-pig kidney cortex (from reference 27)

The fresh preparation showed the well known Mg^{++}-dependent and Na$^+$ + K$^+$-stimulated ATPase activities with a ouabain sensitivity[12] which parallels that of the Na$^+$-for-K$^+$ exchange between cells and medium in guinea pig kidney cortex slices (Figure 1.1). We decided to age the preparation by storage since ageing is known to diminish the Mg^{++}-dependent activity and to enhance the Na$^+$ + K$^+$-stimulation[28]. When experiments were performed in which only Na$^+$ was added to the fresh preparation in the hope of finding a Na$^+$-stimulated, Mg^{++}-dependent ATPase, Na$^+$ revealed an inhibitory action, in agreement with published work[29,30] (see Figure 1.2).

However, the degree of inhibition induced by Na$^+$ decreased with the period of storage, so that on about day 7–10, no inhibition by Na$^+$ remained. With further storage, a small but consistent stimulation by Na$^+$ was disclosed. This is shown in Figure 1.3. We were happy to find that this stimulation by Na$^+$

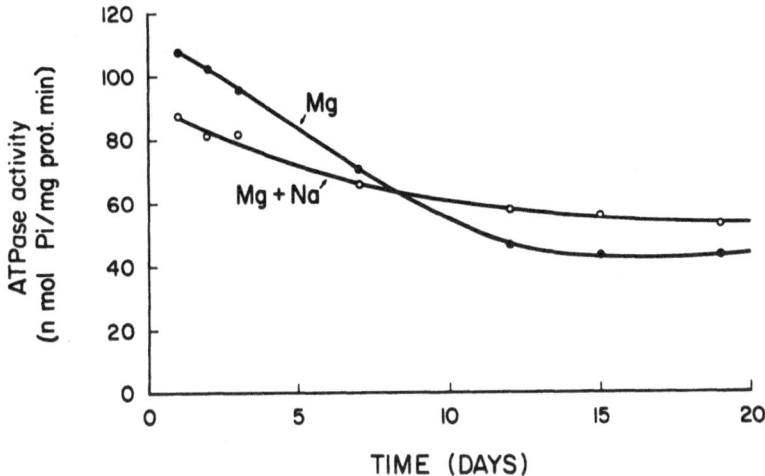

Figure 1.3 Activity of the Mg^{++}-dependent ATPase as a function of days of storage, studied in the absence (dots) and in the presence (circles) of 100 mM Na^+ (from reference 27)

was insensitive to ouabain, when concentrations of up to 10 mM were used. In all that follows, concentrations of 1 mM were always employed.

Possibilities of error

Experiments were performed to ascertain whether the Na^+-stimulation was related to a $Mg^{++} + Ca^{++}$-dependent ATPase which would be activated by endogenous calcium present in the microsomal preparations. No difference in the Na^+-stimulated activity nor in the Mg^{++}-ATPase activity was noticed between experiments in which aged microsomal preparations were incubated in the presence or absence of 0.5 mM EGTA, a strong chelator of calcium. These experiments and the different sequence of stimulation by cations of this Na^+-stimulated, Mg^{++}-dependent ATPase as compared with the Ca^{++}-ATPases described in the literature[31,32] permitted the conclusion that the ouabain-insensitive Na^+-stimulation is unrelated to the activity of a Ca^{++}-ATPase.

The possibility that the Na^+-stimulation of the Mg^{++}-dependent ATPase was due to the presence of mitochondrial Mg^{++}-ATPase activity seems remote. (a) The fresh preparations showed only a very small succinic dehydrogenase activity. (b) Its activity was not inhibited by addition of 15 μm oligomycin. (c) Its activity was not stimulated by the presence of 100 μm 2,4-DNP[33,34].

This Mg^{++}-dependent, Na^+-stimulated phosphohydrolytic activity seems specific for ATP since it is not seen when AMP is used as substrate.

A Mg^{++}-dependent, Na^+-stimulated ATPase has also been found in nerve[35], in brain and kidney[36,37], in erythrocyte ghosts[38], and in brain[39]. But this Na^+-ATPase activity was highly sensitive to cardiac glycosides, and it therefore seems unrelated to the system described by ourselves[27].

7

Characteristics of the Na⁺-stimulated, Mg⁺⁺-dependent ATPase

(1) It is stimulated by Na^+ and by Li^+, and not by other cations (Table 1.1).

(2) The Na^+-stimulation is independent of the anion accompanying Na^+.

(3) As has been stated above, it is insensitive to the presence of ouabain.

(4) It does not require K^+ for its activity.

(5) It is more sensitive to inhibition by ethacrynic acid than both the Na^+ + K^+-stimulated ATPase and the Mg^{++}-dependent ATPase (Table 1.2).

(6) It is inhibited by 1 mM triflocin which does not inhibit either the Mg^{++}-dependent or the Na^+ + K^+-stimulated ATPase (Table 1.2).

(7) It is inhibited by 10^{-5} M furosemide, a concentration that leaves the other two ATPase activities unaffected. Ethacrynic acid, triflocin and furosemide preferentially inhibit the extrusion of Na^+ with Cl^- and water, with only very little effect on the exchange of Na^+ for K^+ in the kidney[19].

(8) This Na^+-stimulated ATPase activity appears clearly after 14 days of storage of the microsomal preparation from untreated kidney tissue. The stimulation by Na^+ appears earlier (about 7 days' storage)[40] if the tissue has been treated with angiotensin II, which has been shown to increase ouabain-resistant Na^+ extrusion in the kidney[20].

(9) The pH optimum for its activity lies between 6.8 and 7.0. It seems that spontaneous acidification of the buffer (originally at pH 7.2) also accelerates the appearance of the stimulation by Na^+.

Some of the characteristics listed above accord with the conditions that should be fulfilled by the energy source of the system responsible for the proposed mode B of Na^+ extrusion. Much work remains to be performed to solve several unanswered questions. Can the yield of this new ATPase activity be increased? What is the possible physiological role of these observations? We also need to know whether this Na^+-stimulated ATPase is present *in vivo*. We have to rule out the possibility that the Na^+-stimulated ATPase activity is due

Table 1.1 Action of different monovalent cations on the Mg^{++}-ATPase activity in a 12-days aged microsomal preparation.

Incubation medium	ATPase activity (10^{-9} mol Pi/mg protein min)
Mg^{++} alone	52
Mg^{++} + Na^+	65**
Mg^{++} + Li^+	60**
Mg^{++} + K^+	55
Mg^{++} + Rb^+	53
Mg^{++} + Cs^+	56
Mg^{++} + NH_4^+	52
Mg^{++} + choline$^+$	55

5 mM Mg^{++}, 100 mM of Cl^- salt of the cations given and 10^{-3} M ouabain were used. Only the results with Na^+ and with Li^+ (**) were statistically different ($P < 0.001$) from those obtained with Mg^{++} alone[27].

Table 1.2   Inhibitors and ATPases; action of inhibitors on the Mg⁺⁺-ATPase activity and on the Na⁺-stimulated ATPase activity[19]

	Mg^{++}	Na^+	$Na^+ + K^+$
Control	69.3 ± 2.3	23.7 ± 2.4	80.7 ± 4.7
Furosemide 10^{-5} M	68.5 ± 2.5	3.4 ± 3.9	80.1 ± 4.9
Control	64.5 ± 3.0	17.1 ± 3.2	51.6 ± 3.4
Triflocin 10^{-3} M	64.1 ± 0.9	0.1 ± 1.4	51.4 ± 1.4
Control	39.0 ± 0.1	12.5 ± 1.8	47.0 ± 1.3
Ethacrynic acid 10^{-3} M	35.0 ± 0.6	2.5 ± 1.0	31.0 ± 1.6
Ethacrynic acid 2×10^{-3} M	27.5 ± 1.0	0.0 ± 0.6	28.0 ± 1.0

Na⁺-stimulated ATPase levels calculated as (Mg⁺⁺ + Na⁺)-minus Mg⁺⁺-activity, and (Na⁺ + K⁺)-stimulated ATPase activity as (Mg⁺⁺ + Na⁺ + K⁺)-minus Mg⁺⁺-activity of three preparations. Mg⁺⁺ concentration was 5 mM, Na⁺ concentration (as NaCl) 100 mM, K⁺ concentration (as KCl) 10 mM. Ouabain was present in the assay of the Mg⁺⁺ and (Mg⁺⁺ + Na⁺) activities. No ouabain was added when the (Mg⁺⁺ + Na⁺ + K⁺) activity was assayed. $N = 3–5$. Similar results with each agent were obtained when the experiment was repeated on three different lots of animals. (ATP hydrolysed is given as nmol Pi/mg protein min).

to other endoplasmic reticulum contaminants and is not present in the cell membranes. Does intracellular Na⁺ indeed activate the ATPase in the intact cell? Can changes produced in the living organism in mode B of Na⁺ extrusion be correlated with changes in the activity of the Na⁺-stimulated ATPase? Finally, if there are two Na⁺ pumps, what is their relative role in kidney function? I am afraid I am leaving you with more questions than answers.

Acknowledgements

Thanks are due to Mrs M. A. Silva and to Mr Henry Linares for excellent assistance. Part of this research was supported with a grant for Project 0296 from CONICIT and with a grant from the Regional Programme for Scientific and Technological Development from OEA.

References

1. Windhager, E. E. (1974). Some aspects of proximal tubular salt reabsorption. *Fed Proc.*, **33**, 21.
2. Giebisch, G., Sullivan, L. P. and Whittembury, G. (1973). Relationship between tubular net sodium reabsorption and peritubular potassium uptake in the perfused Necturus kidney. *J. Physiol. London.*, **230**, 51.
3. Kleinzeller, A. (1972). Cellular transport of water. In: *Metabolic Pathways*, D. M. Greenberg (ed.) Vol. 6. p. 91 (New York: Academic Press).
4. Mudge, G. H. (1951). Studies on K accumulation by rabbit kidney slices: effect of metabolic activity. *Amer. J. Physiol.*, **165**, 113.
5. Podevin, R. A. and Boumendil-Podevin, E. F. (1972). Effects of temperature, medium K, ouabain and ethacrynic acid on transport of electrolytes and water by separated renal tubules. *Biochim. Biophys. Acta*, **282**, 234.
6. Whittam, R. and Willis, J. S. (1963). Ion movements and oxygen consumption in kidney cortex slices. *J. Physiol. London.*, **168**, 158.

7. Whittembury, G. (1965). Sodium extrusion and potassium uptake in guinea-pig kidney cortex slices. *J. Gen. Physiol.*, **48**, 699.
8. Whittembury, G. (1968). Sodium and water transport in kidney proximal tubular cells. *J. Gen. Physiol.*, **51** (Suppl.), 303s.
9. Whittembury, G. and Proverbio, F. (1970). Two modes of Na extrusion in cells from guinea-pig kidney cortex slices. *Pflügers Arch.*, **316**, 1.
10. Willis, J. S. (1968). The interaction of K, ouabain and Na on the cation transport and respiration of renal cortical cells of hamster and ground squirrels. *Biochim. Biophys. Acta*, **163**, 516.
11. Proverbio, F. and Whittembury G. (1975). Effect of ouabain on Rb$^+$, Cs$^+$ and Cl$^-$ movements in kidney slices. (In preparation)
12. Proverbio, F., Robinson, J. W. L. and Whittembury, G. (1970). Sensitivities of (Na$^+$ + K$^+$)-ATPase and Na$^+$ extrusion mechanisms to ouabain and ethacrynic acid in the cortex of the guinea-pig kidney. *Biochim. Biophys. Acta*, **211**, 327
13. Whittam, R. and Wheeler, K. P. (1961). The sensitivity of a kidney ATPase to ouabain and to Na and K. *Biochim. Biophys. Acta*, **51**, 622
14. Schmidt, U., Schmid, H., Funk, B. and Dubach, U. C. (1974). The function of Na,K-ATPase in single portions of the rat nephron. *Ann. N. Y. Acad. Sci.*, **242**, 489
15. Epstein, F. H. and Silva, P. (1974). Role of Na,KATPase in renal function. *Ann. N.Y. Acad. Sci.* **242**, 519
15a. Kramer, H. J. and Comick, H. C. (1974). Effect of extracellular volume expansion on renal Na-K-ATPase and cell metabolism. *Nephron*, **12**, 281
16. Wilson, D. R., Knox, W., Hall, E. and Sen, K. (1974). Renal sodium and potassium activated adenosine triphosphatase deficiency during post-obstructive diuresis in the rat. *Can. J. Physiol. Pharmacol.*, **52**, 105
17. Whittam, R. and Ager, M. E. (1964). Vectorial aspects of adenosine–triphosphatase activity in erythrocyte membranes. *Biochem. J.*, **93**, 337
18. Ross, B., Leaf, A., Silva, P. and Epstein, F. H. (1974). Role of the Na-K-ATPase in sodium transport by the perfused rat kidney. *Amer. J. Physiol.*, **226**, 624
19. Pérez-González, M., Proverbio, F., Condrescu-Guidi, M. and Whittembury, G. (1975). Action of triflocin and furosemide on ion movements and ATPase activities kidney cortex slices. (In preparation)
20. Munday, K. A. Parsons, B. J. and Poat, J. A. (1971). The effect of angiotensin on cation transport by rat kidney cortex slices. *J. Physiol. Lond.*, **215**, 269
21. Whittembury, G. (1967). Sobre los mecanismos de absorción en el tubo proximal del riñón. *Acta Cientif. Venezolana*, **3(Supl.)**, 71
22. Macknight, A. D. C. (1968). Water and electrolyte contents of rat renal cortical slices incubated in potassium-free media and in media containing ouabain. *Biochim. Biophys. Acta*, **150**, 263
23. Macknight, A. D. C., Pilgrim, F. P. and Robinson, B. A. (1974). The regulation of cellular volume in liver slices. *J. Physiol. Lond.*, **238**, 279
24. Robinson, J. W. L. (1972). The inhibition by glycine and β-methyl glucoside transport in dog kidney cortex slices by ouabain and ethacrynic acid: contribution to the understanding of sodium-pumping mechanisms. *Comp. Gen. Pharmacol.*, **3**, 145
25. Jairala, S. W., Vieyra, A. and MacLauglin, M. (1972). Influence of ethacrynic acid and ouabain on the oxygen consumption and potassium and sodium content of the kidney external medulla of the dog. *Biochim. Biophys. Acta*, **279**, 320
26. Jairala, S. W., Saravalli, O., Palazzi, J., Gardia, A. P. and Vergara, E. (1975). Influence of furosemide, ethacrynic acid and ouabain on the oxygen consumption and electrolyte content of dog kidney cortex slices. (In preparation)
27. Proverbio, F., Condrescu-Guidi, M. C. and Whittembury, G. (1975). Ouabain-insensitive Na$^+$-stimulation of an Mg^{++}-dependent ATPase in kidney tissue. *Biochim. Biophys. Acta*, **394**, 281

28. Robinson, J. W. L. (1970). The difference in sensitivity to cardiac steroids of $(Na^+ + K^+)$-stimulated ATPase and amino acid transport in the intestinal mucosa of the rat and other species. *J. Physiol. Lond.*, **206**, 41

29. Gutman, Y., Wald, H. and Czaczkes, W. (1973). Urea and sodium: effect on microsomal ATPase in different parts of the kidney. *Pflügers Arch.*, **345**, 81

30. Cole, C. H. and Dirks, J. H. (1971). A comparison of Na^+ activation of ATPase in the red cell, renal cortex and renal medulla. *Can. J. Physiol. Pharmacol.*, **49**, 63

31. Schatzmann, H. J. and Rossi, G. L. (1971). $(Ca^{2+} + Mg^{2+})$-activated membrane ATPases in human red cells and their possible relation to cation transport. *Biochim. Biophys. Acta*, **241**, 379

32. Parkinson, D. K. and Radde, I. C. (1971). Properties of a Ca^{2+} and Mg^{2+}-activated ATP-hydrolyzing enzyme in rat kidney cortex. *Biochim. Biophys. Acta*, **242**, 238

33. Lardy, H. A., Johnson, D. and McMurray, W. C. (1958). Antibiotics as tools for metabolic studies. I. A. survey of toxic antibiotics in respiratory, phosphorylative and glycolytic systems. *Arch. Biochem. Biophys.*, **78**, 587

34. Kagawa, Y. and Racker, E. (1966). Partial resolution of the enzymes catalysing oxidative phosphorylation. VIII. Properties of a factor conferring oligomycin sensitivity on mitochondrial ATPase. *J. Biol. Chem.*, **241**, 2461

35. Skou, J. C. (1960). Further investigations on a Mg and Na activated adenosine triphosphatase, possibly related to the active, linked transport of Na and K across the nerve membrane. *Biochim. Biophys. Acta*, **42**, 6

36. Skou, J. C. (1962). Preparation from mammalian brain and kidney of the enzyme system involved in active transport of Na^+ and K^+. *Biochim. Biophys. Acta*, **58**, 314

37. Fujita, M., Nagano, K., Mizuno, N., Tashima, Y., Nakao, T. and Nakao, M. (1968). Comparison of some minor activities accompanying a preparation of sodium-plus-potassium ion-stimulated adenosine triphosphatase from pig brain. *Biochem. J.*, **106**, 113.

38. Czerwinski, A., Gitelman, H. J., and Welt, L. G. (1967). A new member of the ATPase family. *Amer. J. Physiol.* **213**, 786

39. Neufeld, A. H. and Levy, H. M. (1969). A second ouabain-sensitive sodium-dependent ATPase in brain microsomes. *J. Biol. Chem.*, **244**, 6493

40. Proverbio, F., Condrescu-Guidi, M. C. and Whittembury, G. (1975). Effect of low salt diet and angiotensin on the appearance of a Na-stimulated ouabain sensitive ATPase in kidney cortex. (In preparation)

1
Discussion Paper on

The Effects of Ion Replacements on Sodium Pump Activity and the Response of Kidney Cortex Slices to Angiotensin

K. A. Munday, B. J. Parsons and J. A. Poat

*Department of Physiology and Biochemistry,
University of Southampton*

The object of this paper is to describe recent experiments performed with the hormone angiotensin which lend further indirect support to the concept of the second sodium pump in kidney, as just described by Dr Whittembury in his paper.

It is well established that there are at least two mechanisms for the extrusion of sodium from kidney cortex slices which have been previously sodium-loaded and potassium-depleted. One process is linked to potassium uptake. The second is refractory to ouabain and independent of potassium and is generally referred to as the second sodium pump[1-4]. Using the sodium-loaded kidney slice preparation, it has been shown that the hormone angiotensin in low physiological concentrations can stimulate the loss of sodium and water via this second sodium pump[5]. This action of angiotensin *in vitro* is qualitatively similar to the action of the hormone in the kidney preparation *in vivo* where, at low infusion rates, it gives an antinatriuretic, antidiuretic response. Whether or not this action *in vivo* is due to a direct stimulation of tubular transport mechanisms or is secondary to changes in renal blood flow, is in some dispute[6,7] but in kidney slices the hormone clearly increases sodium pump activity.

Further studies on the mechanism of action of angiotensin have shown that protein synthesis inhibitors such as cycloheximide and puromycin inhibit this stimulatory response. However, in the presence of actinomycin D, at concentrations which inhibit the incorporation of [³H]uridine into RNA by some 75%, angiotensin was fully effective. These observations suggest that some protein synthesis event at the translational level is, in some way, necessary for the response[8]. These findings are in keeping with those of Davies *et al*[9]

12

using a stripped everted colon sac preparation. However, all attempts to show a stimulation of labelled amino acid incorporation into protein by angiotensin have been unsuccessful, suggesting that the protein involved in the transport process may be produced in very small quantities compared with the total synthetic capacity of the tissue. Unlike that of most polypeptide hormones, the response to angiotensin in both intestinal and kidney preparations does not appear to be mimicked by the addition of cyclic AMP or phosphodiesterase inhibitors. The possibility that angiotensin might exert its action through a lowering in cyclic AMP levels was also discounted. This paper presents recent experiments on the involvement of calcium and chloride in the angiotensin stimulated response.

Requirement for calcium

Sodium-loaded, potassium-depleted kidney slices were incubated in modified Krebs' phosphate saline[10], which was potassium-free. The results in Table 1.1 show that angiotensin stimulates potassium-independent sodium extrusion in the presence of calcium and the response is lost when calcium is chelated with 5 mM-EGTA. When the calcium content of the incubation medium is raised to 12.5 mM, the response is restored, indicating that it is the absence of calcium and not the presence of EGTA which is responsible for the loss of the response. Again these results are very similar to those obtained with the colon sac preparation *in vitro* where calcium > strontium > barium in supporting the angiotensin stimulation of fluid transport, but magnesium is ineffective[11]. The interpretation of these results poses problems. The involvement of calcium in a hormone-mediated process has often implicated cyclic AMP as a secondary messenger. However, investigation of this possibility has shown

Table 1.1 The effect of calcium on the angiotensin-stimulation of sodium loss from rat kidney cortex slices previously loaded for 12 minutes in a glucose-free potassium-free medium under anaerobic conditions. Sodium extrusion was measured after 10 minutes incubation at 25 °C in the absence of potassium and the presence of glucose and oxygen

	Sodium loss (μEq/g dry wt.)	P
2.5 mM calcium		
Control	104 ± 10 (13)	
+ 10^{-12} M angiotensin	143 ± 11 (13)	< 0.02
2.5 mM calcium + 5 mM EGTA		
Control	120 ± 10 (8)	
+ 10^{-12} M angiotensin	120 ± 7 (8)	N.S.
12.5 mM calcium + 5 mM EGTA		
Control	106 ± 4 (4)	
+ 10^{-12} M angiotensin	141 ± 13 (5)	< 0.05

Results are expressed as mean ± S.E.M. Number of observations in parentheses

that angiotensin has no effect on cyclic AMP levels in the kidney slice preparation[12] and does not affect the activity of the intestinal adenyl cyclase[13]. The possibility exists that calcium is important for the attachment of angiotensin to its receptors and indeed preliminary observations indicated that in kidney tissue, the binding of ^{3}H-angiotensin is much reduced in the absence of ionic calcium (Table *1.2*).

Table *1.2*   The effect of calcium on the binding of tritiated angiotensin to kidney cortex slices.

	^{3}H-angiotensin binding (dpm bound/100 mg tissue)	P
2.5 mM Ca^{++}	2513 ± 177 (11)	
0 mM Ca^{++} + 5 mM EGTA	1613 ± 110 (10)	< 0.001

The slices were incubated for 2 minutes at 37 °C in the presence of 2×10^{-10} M angiotensin. The values are corrected for contribution of the extracellular space but not for non-specific binding. EGTA was added to the incubation medium to ensure complete removal of calcium.

Results are expressed as a mean ± S.E.M. Number of observations in parentheses.

These results do not preclude the possibility that calcium may be important for other stages in the hormone-mediated event, although measurement of ^{45}Ca fluxes both into and out of kidney cortex slices failed to demonstrate any change following the administration of angiotensin (Munday, Parsons and Smith, unpublished observations). Furthermore there is no evidence to suggest that calcium is important in any way for the function of the second sodium pump, and indeed Whittembury at this Symposium has presented evidence that a Ca^{++}-ATPase is not involved in this process.

Requirements for chloride

The nature of the ion linked to ouabain-resistant active sodium extrusion is of great interest. Whittembury and Proverbio[13] presented evidence that this might be chloride. The conclusion is supported by the experiments reported in

Table *1.3*   The effect of substituting chloride with other anions on sodium loss and potassium uptake occurring in 10 minutes at 25 °C from slices which have been previously sodium-loaded in buffer where Cl$^-$ was replaced by the appropriate anion.

Anion replacement	Na$^+$ extrusion/K$^+$ uptake
Chloride (control)	2.22
Isethionate	1.18
Citrate	1.53
Gluconate	1.42
Acetate	1.51
Pyruvate	1.91
Succinate	1.12
Sulphate	1.50

14

Table *1.3*, in which chloride in the incubation medium was replaced with a variety of anions and the effect of such replacements on sodium extrusion and potassium uptake into kidney cortex slices was assessed.

In every experiment, the ratio of Na$^+$ extrusion/K$^+$ uptake fell as a consequence of the rate of Na$^+$ loss from the tissue being reduced and the uptake of potassium remaining unchanged. Thus chloride replacement by succinate (an anion which has a very similar mobility to chloride) caused the sodium extrusion to fall from 195 ± 15 to 93 ± 11 (16) (the number of observations in each series) μEq/g dry wt. while the potassium uptake was not significantly affected, being 88 ± 2 and 83 ± 5 (16) μEq/g dry wt. in the two cases. These observations strongly suggest that the anion linked to Na$^+$ extrusion is Cl$^-$. This contention is further supported by our observation that the carbonic anhydrase inhibitor, acetazolamide, has no effect on sodium extrusion from loaded slices by the 'second sodium pump'. Substituting bicarbonate saline for phosphate saline also failed to enhance ion movements, indicating that HCO$_3^-$ is almost certainly not the anion involved.

More recent experiments with the angiotensin-stimulated intestinal fluid transport *in vivo* led to the conclusion that in this tissue an electrically neutral process is involved[15]. This may be sodium chloride linked (see also Munday and York, this volume). Addition of angiotensin at 10^{-12} M (the concentration which normally stimulates sodium extrusion) to succinate-chloride-free-buffer has no effect on Na$^+$ loss from loaded kidney cortex slices, indicating that the angiotensin-stimulated process is dependent on the presence of the anion chloride in the incubation medium. Further support for this view comes from the observation (Munday, Parsons and Evans, unpublished observations) that the ability of angiotensin to stimulate fluid transport in the rat distal colon *in vitro* is lost when chloride ions are replaced with sulphate ions.

In summary, there is good evidence that angiotensin stimulates sodium and water transfer in kidney and intestinal tissues via a sodium chloride linked process which, at least in the intestine, is electroneutral.

Acknowledgements

The authors wish gratefully to acknowledge the experimental contributions of Mr D. J. Smith and Mrs J. Evans.

References

1. Kleinzeller, A., and Knotková, A. (1964). The effect of ouabain on the electrolyte and water transport in kidney cortex and liver slices. *J. Physiol. Lond.*, **175**, 172.
2. Macknight, A. D. C. (1968). Water and electrolyte contents of rat renal cortical slices incubated in potassium-free media containing ouabain. *Biochim. Biophys. Acta.*, **150**, 263
3. Whittembury, G. (1968). Sodium and water transport in kidney proximal tubular cells. *J. Gen. Physiol.*, **51**, 303s.

4. Willis, J. S. (1966). Characteristics of ion transport in kidney cortex of mammalian hibernators. *J. Gen. Physiol.*, **49**, 1221

5. Munday, K. A., Parsons, B. J. and Poat, J. A. (1971). The effect of angiotensin on cation transport by rat kidney cortex slices. *J. Physiol. Lond.*, **215**, 269.

6. Barraclough, M. A., Jones, N. F. and Marsden, C. D. (1967). Effect of angiotensin on renal function in the rat. *Amer. J. Physiol.*, **212**, 1153

7. Bonjour, J. P. and Malvin, R. L. (1969). Renal extraction of PAH, GFR and $U_{Na}V$ in the rat during infusion of angiotensin. *Amer. J. Physiol.*, **216**, 554

8. Munday, K. A., Parsons, B. J. and Poat, J. A. (1972). Studies on the mechanism of action of angiotensin on ion transport by kidney cortex slices. *J. Physiol. Lond.*, **224**, 195.

9. Davies, N. T., Munday, K. A. and Parsons, B. J. (1972). Studies on the mechanism of action of angiotensin on fluid transport by the mucosa of rat distal colon. *J. Endocrinol.*, **54**, 483

10. Poat, J. A. and Munday, K. A. (1971). Cation transport in kidney slices. In G. A. Kerkut, (ed.) *Experiments in Physiology and Biochemistry*, vol. 4, p. 147 (New York: Academic Press)

11. Munday, K. A., Parsons, B. J., Poat, J. A. and Smith, D. J. (1973). The effect of divalent cations on angiotensin stimulation of fluid transport by rat colon. *J. Physiol. Lond.*, **232**, 89 P

12. Munday, K. A., Parsons, B. J. and Poat, J. A. (1974). The action of angiotensin on sodium transport by rat kidney cortex *in vitro*. In Inserm colloque; *Nephron Physiology: Mechanism and Regulation*, p. 181

13. Angles d'Auriac, G., Meyer, P., Munday, K. A., Parsons, B. J. and Poat, J. A. (1975). The role of cyclic 3'5'-adenosine monophosphate in the response of the intestine and kidney to angiotensin. *J. Endocrinol.* (In press)

14. Whittembury, G. and Proverbio, F. (1970). Two modes of Na extrusion in cells from guinea-pig kidney cortex slices. *Pflügers Arch.* **316**, 1

15. Levens, N. R., Munday, K. A. and York, B. (1975). The effect of angiotensin II on fluid transport, transmural p.d. and resistance in the rat distal colon *in vivo. J. Endocrinol.* (In press)

Discussion 1

Abramow: Would Dr Whittembury care to comment about the possibility of overlapping of the functions of the two pumps he described, or to give another explanation, such as species differences, to account for the following findings (1) In separated renal tubules from the rabbit kidney, ouabain not only produces an increase in the Na^+ content and a decrease in the K^+ content of the cells, but chloride and water also get in. (2) In the isolated perfused rabbit proximal convoluted tubule, ouabain greatly inhibits, if not abolishes, net fluid absorption?

Whittembury: The conditions used to show the second mode of sodium extrusion (sodium-loaded kidney cells) are such that the real fraction of one or other mode of sodium extrusion under normal conditons cannot be evaluated. I should tend to speculate that when the classical mode is working at a slower pace, the other could take over and compensate.

Robinson: In this respect, may I comment that, using identical methods to those of Dr Whittembury, but dog kidney cortex slices, we found much more overlap between the actions of the two pumps than he did with guinea-pig tissue, though the effects of ouabain and ethacrynic acid are always additive. Thus there is a certain amount of species variation.

Smith: Would you care to comment on the fact that the presence of pump B can be demonstrated immediately, while it takes several days before you can show the presence of a Na^+-activated, ouabain-insensitive ATPase?

Whittembury: You see, we still have this difficulty. In order to show the Na^+-stimulated, ouabain-resistant ATPase, we have to age the preparation. On the other hand, it is encouraging that manoeuvres that would stimulate mode B of sodium extrusion hasten the appearance of the Na^+-stimulated ATPase. For example, a non-treated kidney tissue will show Na^+-stimulation of the ATPase by day 15–20. If the tissue has been treated with angiotensin, the sodium stimulation appears at day 2–4.

Parsons: Does the ouabain-insensitive enzyme depend upon the H^+-concentration in the same way as does the classical Na^+-K^+-ATPase?

Whittembury: The Na^+-stimulated ATPase works best at pH 7.0 or lower, while the classical Na^+-K^+-ATPase is most active at pH higher than 7.2. Your question is very important: it allows me to point out that there is a slight acidification of the medium in which the membrane fraction is suspended during the ageing procedure, so that the sodium-stimulated ATPase appears when the pH of 7.0 is reached.

Case: Is there a dose–response relationship for inhibition of your second ATPase and for transport, as you showed on an early slide for the action of ouabain on the Na^+-K^+-ATPase and ion transport?

Whittembury: We are working on this subject now in an attempt to make the correlation that you ask for; this is of great importance.

Levin: There appear to be differences in enzyme activity in the presence and absence of chloride. Is this an indication of the same chloride effect as in Dr Munday's experiments?

Whittembury: The lower rate of ATP hydrolysis that you observed on the slide corresponds to the Mg^{++}-ATPase activity. The increase in activity due to stimulation by sodium alone seems to be independent of the accompanying anion.

Case: I should like to ask Dr Munday whether the need for extracellular calcium is related to its concentration, or whether simply trace quantities of the ion in the incubation medium are necessary.

Munday: The need for extracellular Ca^{++} is not entirely dose-dependent.

Diezi: I have three questions: (1) Is angiotensin I also effective in stimulating Na^+ efflux? (2) Is there a time-lag before the effect of angiotensin II? (3) Is the effect of angiotensin II inhibited by antagonists?

Munday: Angiotensin I effect in stimulating sodium efflux has not been studied. There was a small significant time delay in the response of sodium extrusion from the loaded kidney slices to stimulation by angiotensin II. The time-course for the experiments, reported by Munday *et al.* (reference 5 page 16), show a lag of 2 minutes in the angiotensin response. The rationale for the choice of 15 minutes as the experimental period for extrusion of sodium from the loaded slices is given in this reference. Finally, we have not yet studied the effect of any angiotensin II antagonist on this sodium extrusion response.

2
Bioelectric Parameters and Sodium Transport in Bullfrog Small Intestine

W. McD. ARMSTRONG

Department of Physiology,
Indiana University School of Medicine,
Indianapolis

INTRODUCTION

This discussion is primarily concerned with some recent and continuing studies in the author's laboratory. These investigations are directed towards an analysis, in terms of current models of epithelial transport and electrophysiology, of the relationship between transepithelial Na^+ transport and bioelectric parameters in the small intestine. One of the most striking developments in epithelial physiology during recent years has been the formation of general functional principles which, *mutatis mutandis*, are applicable to all transporting epithelia[1,2]. It is hoped, therefore, that the results and conclusions presented herein, though restricted in large measure to studies with one experimental system, the isolated small intestine of the bullfrog (*Rana catesbeiana*), will be of interest within the broader context of intestinal and epithelial transport.

Na⁺ transport in isolated bullfrog small intestine

The unique role of net mucosal to serosal (m → s) Na^+ transport in relation to absorptive function and electrophysiological behaviour in the intestinal tract of mammals and amphibia has long been recognised[3,4]. In the isolated small intestine of the bullfrog, as in many other *in vitro* preparations of the small intestine[4], net m → s Na^+ transfer occurs in the absence of known chemical or electrochemical gradients[5] and is sensitive to metabolic and other inhibitors[6,7]. In brief, as discussed in detail elsewhere[5], it appears to meet the criteria in terms of which net intestinal Na^+ absorption is usually classified as active transport[4]. In normal sodium chloride Ringer solutions, active m → s transfer of Cl^-, as well as Na^+, occurs[5]. Thus, under these conditions, the relationship between Na^+ transport and the transmural electrical characteristics of the tissue, potential difference (E_{Tr}) and short-circuit current (I_{sc}), is not necessarily a simple one. When Cl^- in the bathing medium is completely replaced by SO_4^-, net Na^+ is the only ion actively transported by the tissue. As expected, when isolated sheets of bullfrog small intestine are mounted between identical sodium sulphate media, the spontaneous E_{Tr} is invariably serosal positive[5,7-10].

Further, when actively transported sugars or amino acids are added to the mucosal medium, E_{Tr} and I_{sc} are stimulated to an equivalent extent[11] and the equivalence between I_{sc} and net m → s Na^+ transport is maintained[5,12]. Thus, under these conditions, there appears to be a rather direct and explicit relationship between transepithelial Na^+ transport and the electrical parameters of bullfrog small intestine, and this relationship seems to correspond, in many respects, to the behaviour in sodium chloride media of isolated mammalian small intestine[13-16]. In addition, when mounted between sodium sulphate (or sodium chloride) Ringer solutions at 25 °C (pH 7.2), isolated bullfrog small intestine is remarkably stable with respect to its bioelectric and ion transport characteristics. This permits experimental manipulation of the tissue for periods of time up to 6–8 hours.

PATHWAYS OF TRANSEPITHELIAL Na⁺ TRANSPORT IN THE SMALL INTESTINE

The transcellular pathway

Net m → s flow of Na^+ ($\mathcal{J}_{net}$) across the epithelial cell layer of the small intestine is of course the difference between two unidirectional fluxes, a mucosal to serosal ($\mathcal{J}_{ms}$) and a serosal to mucosal ($\mathcal{J}_{sm}$) flux. Early models of transepithelial Na^+ transport in the intestine[4,14] were based on the archetypal scheme proposed by Koefoed-Johnsen and Ussing[17] for Na^+ transport by the isolated frog skin. In terms of these models, both $\mathcal{J}_{ms}$ and $\mathcal{J}_{sm}$ were assumed to proceed via a transcellular route. $\mathcal{J}_{sm}$ was assumed to be wholly passive whereas $\mathcal{J}_{ms}$ included an active component. In the small intestine, a number of observations strongly suggested that the active component of $\mathcal{J}_{ms}$ (the Na^+ pump) was restricted to the serosal or lateral–serosal border of the epithelial absorptive cells. Thus, the cardiac glycoside ouabain, a potent inhibitor of the Na^+ pump in a variety of cell species, was found to inhibit net Na^+ transport only when it was added to the medium bathing the serosal surface of isolated rat[18] or rabbit[13] small intestine. Later[7] this observation was confirmed for isolated bullfrog small intestine. In addition, thermodynamic considerations[4] indicate that the exit of Na$^+$ from the cell interior through the lateral or serosal membrane of the epithelial cell is an energy-requiring step. In media containing Na$^+$ concentrations approximating that of the blood plasma, the steady-state Na$^+$ concentration distribution *in vitro* is such that the Na$^+$ content of the epithelial cells is much lower than that of the external medium[19-22]. Further, measurement of the electrical potential profile across the epithelial cell layer of the small intestine reveals two potential steps. One of these (E_m) is the measured potential difference between the mucosal medium and the cell interior. The other (E_s) is the corresponding potential difference between the cell interior and the serosal medium. Both these steps are orientated so that the cell interior is negative with respect to the external medium[9,31,46,49]. Hence, E_{Tr} is given by the difference between E_m and E_s.

The above findings clearly indicate that sodium ions entering an epithelial cell from the mucosal medium do so down an electrochemical gradient. Thus, *sensu strictu*, net mucosal entry of Na$^+$ into the intestinal absorptive cell does not require external energy.* On the other hand, net exit of Na$^+$ across the lateral or serosal cell membrane is, in terms of the above considerations, an energy requiring process.

Recently, more direct evidence concerning the orientation and magnitude of the Na$^+$ electrochemical potential gradient ($\Delta \bar{\mu}_{Na}$) across the mucosal and serosal membranes of epithelial cells of the small intestine has emerged from the measurement, with cation-selective microelectrodes, of the intracellular Na$^+$ activity in these cells[24]. In epithelial cells of isolated bullfrog small intestine, maintained between identical sulphate Ringer solutions (pH 7.2) containing 102.4 mEq K$^+$ per litre and with mannitol added to bring the total measured osmolality to 208 $\pm$ 1 (SE) mosmol/kg water, the average intracellular Na$^+$ activity was 14.4 mM[24], whereas the mean apparent intracellular Na$^+$ concentration under the same conditions was about 35–40 mM[10,22]. Thus, in terms of the microelectrode technique, at least 50% of the apparent intracellular Na$^+$ does not appear as free osmotically active Na$^+$ in the cytoplasm. Of more immediate import in the present context is the fact that, if one combines the mean intracellular Na$^+$ activity with the average values for the mucosal and serosal membrane potentials under the same conditions[9], one obtains $\Delta \bar{\mu}_{Na}$ values of the order of 6000 J/Eq Na$^+$ across the mucosal and serosal cell membranes[25].

The idea that net absorptive Na$^+$ transport, and hence a substantial part of $\mathcal{J}_{ms}$, in the small intestine proceeds via a transcellular route and involves an obligatory uphill step at the lateral/serosal membrane of the absorptive cell is thus supported by an impressive body of evidence. An essentially similar

---

* It is important to note that this argument does not of course *exclude* the possibility of 'pumps' or energy-requiring Na$^+$ transport processes in the mucosal cell membrane which might be involved, for example, in Na$^+$ secretion under certain conditions[23].

scheme is currently postulated for other epithelia such as the isolated amphibian skin and urinary bladder, and also for the gall bladder and renal tubule of a number of animal species.[1]. This mechanism is an essential component of the standing osmotic gradient model of Diamond and Bossert[26] which has been successfully applied to the analysis of ionic transfer in a number of epithelial systems, and, in brief, appears at this time to be well established in epithelial physiology. Its existence in the small intestine of the bullfrog will be assumed for the remainder of this discussion.

The paracellular shunt pathway

Until comparatively recently, the situation with respect to $\mathcal{J}_{sm}$ in the small intestine was somewhat equivocal. Since E_{Tr} is usually a few mV serosal positive when the tissue is bathed by identical Ringer solutions, transcellular Na^+ movement from the serosal to the mucosal medium under these conditions is passive in an overall thermodynamic sense. However, certain observed characteristics of $\mathcal{J}_{sm}$ under these conditions are difficult to reconcile with a purely passive transcellular movement of Na^+. A notable example is the fact that, when active $m \rightarrow s$ Na^+ transport is completely inhibited by serosal ouabain, $\mathcal{J}_{sm}$ does not increase[13], although, under these conditions, cellular Na^+ is markedly increased[27].

An alternative to the transcellular route for transepithelial Na^+ transport originated with the proposal of Ussing and Windhager[28] that intercellular (paracellular) shunt pathways for ions such as Na^+ and K^+ exist across the isolated frog skin. Since then, the idea that paracellular shunts which are permeable to water, ions and other low molecular weight solutes exist in virtually all epithelia has received abundant support in the literature and seems now to be firmly established as a basic principle in epithelial physiology[1]. Indeed, it has become customary to categorise epithelia as 'tight' or 'leaky' depending on the relative resistances of the shunt pathway and the parallel transcellular pathway[2].

Available evidence strongly supports the idea that the shunt pathways are located in the junctional regions between the epithelial cells[1,23], though in certain cases, including the small intestine, the sites of physiological cell desquamation may also be implicated[29]. These pathways are now considered to constitute the major route of passive ionic permeation across many epithelia[2].

In the small intestine, the existence of paracellular shunt pathways which might play a significant part in the transmural transport of fluid and electrolytes, though previously suggested by Smyth and Wright[30], received its first explicit experimental support from the studies of Clarkson[29] who showed that Na^+ fluxes in the isolated rat ileum could best be explained by an active cellular pathway together with a parallel intercellular diffusive pathway. The latter exhibited the characteristics expected for Na^+ diffusion through aqueous channels bounded by fixed anionic groups.

Interest in the role of paracellular shunt pathways in intestinal ion transport was further stimulated by studies on the effect of actively transported sugars and amino acids on the bioelectric parameters of *in vitro* preparations of bullfrog[9] and rabbit[31] small intestine (see page 27). In these studies, the observed effects of these solutes on E_m and E_s appeared to require the presence of a relatively highly conducting shunt pathway through which the intrinsic electromotive forces (V_m and V_s) across the mucosal and serosal membranes of the epithelial cells are electrically coupled. In recent years, an impressive body of evidence has been assembled in support of the concept that relatively low resistance paracellular pathways are the major route for passive transepithelial movement of ions[23] and, under certain conditions, of a number of non-electrolytes[32] in the intestine.

Of particular interest in the present context are those studies which appear to establish the fact that, for Na$^+$ ions, J_{sm} occurs primarily if not solely through the shunt pathway. Frizzell and Schultz[33] and Munck and Schultz[34] examined unidirectional fluxes of Na$^+$ across the brush border of rabbit ileum and rat jejunum under conditions where the transepithelial potential (E_{Tr}) was clamped at various values over the range ± 50 mV. They concluded that extracellular shunts account for some 80% of the total ionic conductances of these tissues, and that the properties of the shunt pathway are consistent with those of neutral polar pores rather than negatively charged pores. These pores have an apparent diameter of 10–15 Å and display the cation permeability sequence $P_K > P_{Rb} > P_{Na}$. Further, these authors concluded[33,34] that all or virtually all of the serosal to mucosal flux of Na$^+$ (J_{sm}) occurs via this pathway (see also[35]). A quantitatively different but broadly similar result was obtained by Desjeux, Tai and Curran[36]. According to these authors, some 75% of J_{sm} proceeds via the shunt pathway. The remaining 25% occurs through a transcellular pathway which may be important in Na$^+$ secretion. In short, despite some discrepancies in detail, there appears to be fairly general agreement that a major fraction of J_{sm} occurs through a paracellular pathway.

Effect of actively transported solutes on J$_{ms}$ and J$_{sm}$ in isolated bullfrog small intestine

In isolated bullfrog small intestine maintained between identical sodium sulphate media[11], as in preparations of mammalian small intestine[37] *in vitro*, addition of an actively transported sugar or amino acid to the medium bathing the mucosal surface of the cells causes marked increases in E_{Tr} and I_{sc}. These increases occur in parallel — for the addition of a given amount of sugar or amino acid to the external medium, the fractional increases in E_{Tr} and I_{sc} are the same. Also, at a constant external Na$^+$ concentration, sugar and amino acid-induced increases in E_{Tr} and I_{sc} are saturable functions of the concentration of added solute and can be analysed in terms of simple Michaelis–Menten kinetics. It is, however, important to note that, despite their similarities, the increases in E_{Tr} and I_{sc} elicited by sugars and amino acids respectively appear to be due to different and largely separate mechanisms[37].

Under conditions where the I_{sc} is wholly or predominantly attributable to active m $\rightarrow$ s Na$^+$ transfer, one would predict that this parameter would also be increased by the addition of an actively transported sugar or amino acid to the mucosal medium. This prediction has been amply confirmed by direct measurement, using radiotracer techniques, of the unidirectional transepithelial fluxes J_{ms} and J_{sm}. In a number of studies[5,13–15,38–41], consistent increases in J_{net} (the *difference* between J_{ms} and J_{sm}) have been reported for preparations of small intestine *in vitro* from a variety of animal species following addition of actively transported sugars or amino acids to the mucosal bathing medium. There is, however, considerable variation in the results for the effects of these solutes on the individual fluxes, J_{ms} and J_{sm}, under short-circuit conditions. Some years ago, we reported[5] that the actively transported sugar glucose induced a statistically significant decrease in J_{sm} across isolated bullfrog small intestine without affecting J_{ms}. A similar conclusion can be drawn from the results of Schultz and Zalusky[13,14] for an *in vitro* preparation of rabbit ileum. As pointed out by Kimmich[42], these findings are not easily reconciled with current models of the interdependence between Na$^+$ fluxes and those of sugars and amino acids in the small intestine[37]. In contrast to the above mentioned data, Field, Fromm and McColl[40] reported that, in sheets of rabbit ileal mucosa stripped of their muscular layers and bathed by a medium richer in HCO$_3^-$ than that employed by Schultz and Zalusky[13,14], glucose increased J_{ms} without affecting J_{sm}. A similar stimulating effect of mucosal glucose on J_{ms} in isolated short-circuited rat jejunum was observed by Munck[41].

The issue under discussion is further complicated by the results reported for actively transported solutes other than glucose. Thus, the sugar analogue, 3-O-methyl glucose, which closely resembles glucose in its effects on E_{Tr} and I_{sc}, but which, unlike the latter, is not metabolised by the small intestine, appears to cause an increase in J_{ms} across the isolated rabbit ileum without affecting J_{sm}[14]. Also, the enhancing effect of the actively transported amino acid, alanine, on I_{sc} across the isolated rabbit ileum seems to be due mainly to a decrease in J_{sm}[15]. By contrast, in isolated bullfrog small intestine[5], valine appeared to cause an increase in J_{ms} and similar results were reported[41] for the effect of proline on the I_{sc} across the isolated rat jejunum.

Because of these complexities, we recently[12] reinvestigated the effects of the actively transported solutes, D-glucose, 3-O-methyl glucose [3-O-methyl-D-glucopyranose] and L-valine, on J_{ms} and J_{sm} across sheets of isolated bullfrog small intestine bathed by identical sodium sulphate media. In these experiments, ^{22}Na and ^{24}Na were used as tracers. Steady state J_{ms} and J_{sm} values were first determined simultaneously in the same piece of tissue under control conditions (in the absence of added solute). Then, following addition of glucose, 3-O-methyl glucose or valine to the medium and re-establishment of a steady state, the effect of each of these solutes on $\mathcal{J}_{ms}$ and $\mathcal{J}_{sm}$ were determined. The results of a representative experiment from this series are shown in Figure 2.1. It is apparent that, following addition of 3-O-methyl glucose to the medium, both $\mathcal{J}_{ms}$ and $\mathcal{J}_{sm}$ increased compared to their control values.

Table 2.1 summarises the results obtained in the complete series of experiments. It is evident from this table that all three actively transported solutes employed in this investigation induced striking increases in $\mathcal{J}_{ms}$.

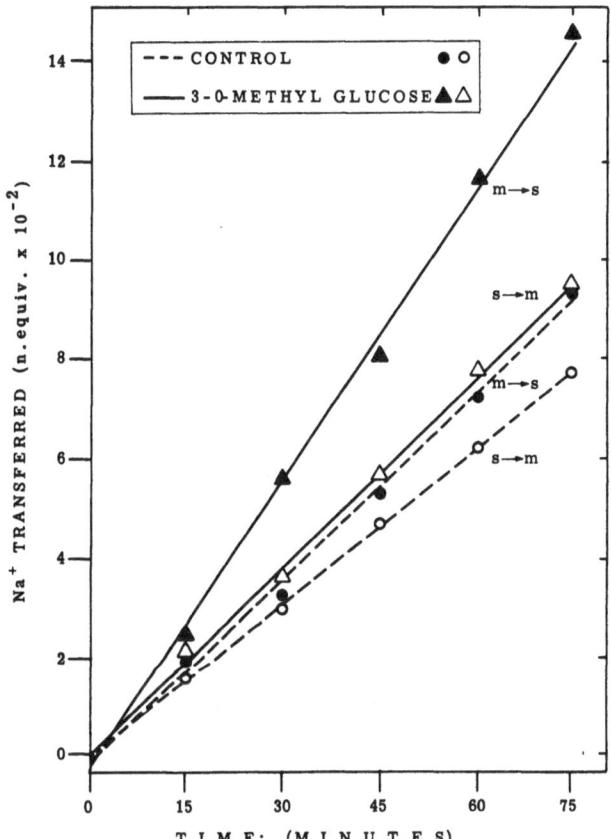

Figure 2.1 Effect of 3-O-methyl glucose on $\mathcal{J}_{ms}$ and $\mathcal{J}_{sm}$ across isolated bullfrog small intestine (see reference 12)

Statistical analysis of the data showed that this increase was significant ($P <$ 0.01) in all three cases. At the same time, all three solutes caused a statistically significant ($P < 0.05$) increase in $\mathcal{J}_{sm}$ (Table 2.1). As expected from the fact that I_{sc} is increased in the presence of these solutes[12], the increase in $\mathcal{J}_{ms}$ was, in all three cases, significantly greater than the corresponding increase in $\mathcal{J}_{sm}$.

These results are readily accounted for in terms of the mechanisms for transepithelial Na⁺ transport discussed on pages 20 and 22. One notes at the

Table 2.1 Effect of glucose, 3-O-methyl glucose, and valine in Na$^+$ fluxes in isolated bullfrog small intestine

Solute	J_{ms}	J_{sm}
None	37.4 ± 1.2 (6:30)	35.6 ± 1.6 (6:30)
Glucose (11 mM)	46.1 ± 2.0 (6:30)	38.7 ± 2.9 (6:30)
None	32.4 ± 1.5 (4:20)	22.5 ± 1.5 (9:44)
3-O-methyl glucose (35 mM)	44.0 ± 3.0 (4:20)	25.1 ± 1.8 (9:44)
None	27.9 ± 1.1 (4:20)	26.3 ± 1.7 (4:20)
Valine (20 mM)	38.4 ± 2.0 (4:20)	30.8 ± 1.1 (4.20)

Mean (±SE) flux values are given in nEq/cm^2 min. Figures in parentheses following flux values represent the number of animals used and the number of individual flux determinations for each set of conditions. (Table calculated from reference 12)

outset that, as found with other preparations of the small intestine *in vitro*[13-15,41], J_{ms} and J_{sm} across short-circuited bullfrog small intestine are large compared to the difference between them, both in the absence and in the presence of actively transported solutes (Table 2.1). Thus, it can be postulated[23] that J_{ms} as well as J_{sm} is largely due to ionic diffusion through the shunt pathway and that the difference between them (J_{net}) probably represents a relatively small active transcellular movement of Na$^+$ in the m → s direction. The increase in J_{ms} elicited by actively transported sugars and amino acids is consistent with the enhanced mucosal entry of Na$^+$ which has been observed following exposure of the luminal aspect of isolated rabbit ileum to these solutes[43,44] and can be ascribed largely to an enhancement of the active transcellular component of Na$^+$ transport. Since, as already discussed, J_{sm} appears to take place for the most part via the paracellular route, the concomitant increase in this parameter can be explained as follows: In terms of the standing osmotic gradient hypothesis[26] one can predict that, under short-circuit conditions (i.e. when E_{Tr} is zero), the major driving force for J_{sm} will be the Na$^+$ concentration gradient between the closed ends of the intercellular spaces and the mucosal medium. It seems reasonable to suppose that the enhanced J_{ms} induced by glucose, 3-O-methyl glucose and valine (Table 2.1) will increase this local Na$^+$ concentration gradient. Assuming that the diffusion coefficient for Na$^+$ in the junctional pathway is not markedly changed by these solutes, this could give rise to the increase in J_{sm} observed in the experiments*.

* It seems likely that the discrepancies between the effect of glucose on J_{ms} and J_{sm} observed in the investigation under discussion[12] and the results previously reported[5] for the effect of this solute on Na$^+$ fluxes under apparently identical conditions are due to differences in methodology. In the earlier study, Na$^+$ fluxes in the absence and in the presence of added glucose were determined in separate experiments with different groups of animals. It now appears (see reference 12 for further discussion) that the control values for J_{ms} and J_{sm} observed by Quay and Armstrong[5] were abnormally high so that the stimulating effect of glucose on these parameters was effectively masked and, in fact, there was an apparent decrease in J_{sm} in the presence of glucose.

THE SHUNT PATHWAY AND BIOELECTRIC PARAMETERS IN BULLFROG SMALL INTESTINE

Effect of actively transported sugars and amino acids on E_m and E_s

Direct measurement of the response of E_m and E_s to actively transported sugars in bullfrog[9] and rabbit[31] small intestine showed that the primary electrical event induced by these solutes is a *decrease* in E_m. This decrease (ΔE_m) was not observed in the absence of Na+ or in the presence of solutes such as D-valine, mannitol, fructose or sorbose[9,31] whose mucosal influx is Na+-independent. Further, the decrease in E_m elicited by actively transported sugars was rapidly reversed by the addition of phlorizin, a potent inhibitor of intestinal sugar uptake, to the mucosal medium. Simultaneous measurement of the *increase* in E_{Tr} (ΔE_{Tr}) induced by these solutes showed that the ratio $\Delta E_m / \Delta E_{Tr}$ was consistently greater than unity at a high level of statistical

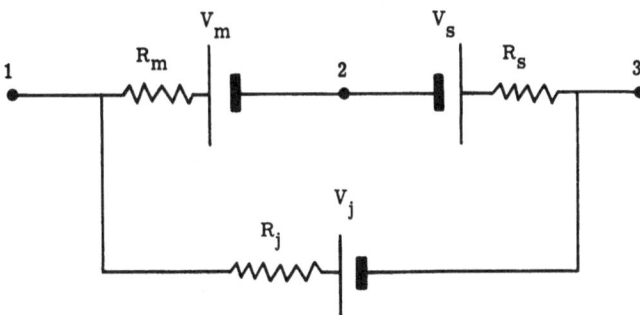

Figure 2.2 Equivalent electrical circuit for the small intestine (see reference 10)

significance, indicating that, in addition to a decrease in E_m, there was, under these conditions, a smaller but significant decrease in E_s. These results are readily explained as follows: The decrease in E_m induced by actively transported sugars and amino acids is consistent with the idea that coupled entry of Na+ and these solutes across the brush border membrane of the epithelial cells is electrogenic[23,37,45]. In the absence of coupling between E_m and E_s, and assuming no direct effect of actively transported non-electrolytes on the lateral–serosal membrane of the epithelial cells, one would predict a quantitative equivalence between ΔE_m and ΔE_{Tr}. However, if E_m and E_s are coupled via a relatively low resistance paracellular pathway, a change in E_m will induce a concomitant, though not necessarily equal, change in E_s.

Figure 2.2 shows an electrical equivalent circuit for coupling between E_m and E_s in intestinal epithelia. In this circuit, V_m and V_s are the intrinsic electromotive forces across the mucosal and lateral-serosal membranes and R_m and R_s are the corresponding membrane resistances (these may include parallel *transmembrane* shunt resistances[31]). R_j is the resistance of the shunt pathway and V_j is a diffusion potential across this pathway. V_j may be considered to arise, as a result of active solute transfer, across the tight junction between the closed ends of the lateral-serosal intercellular spaces and the mucosal medium[26]. Points 1, 2 and 3 of Figure 2.2 represent potential measuring electrodes in the mucosal medium, the cell interior, and the serosal medium respectively. Throughout the present discussion, it is assumed that point 1 is maintained at ground (zero) potential at all times.

In Figure 2.2, V_m and V_s are given the orientation which are normally found for the *measured* membrane potentials E_m and E_s in the small intestine[9,31,46-49]. The orientation assigned to V_j is based on the studies of Machen and Diamond[50] with isolated rabbit gall bladder. With the exception that V_j is considered to be finite when the mucosal and serosal sides of the tissue are bathed by identical solutions, Figure 2.2 is identical to the circuits previously proposed by White and Armstrong[9] and Rose and Schultz[31]. Analysis of Figure 2.2 for E_{Tr} and E_m gives

$$E_{Tr} = [(R_j(V_s - V_m) - V_j(R_m + R_s)]/R_t \qquad (1)$$

and

$$E_m = -[V_m(R_s + R_j) + R_m(V_s + V_j)]/R_t \qquad (2)$$

where $R_t = (R_m + R_s + R_j)$; and, for a change in V_m only

$$\Delta E_m / \Delta E_{Tr} = (R_j + R_s)/R_j \qquad (3)$$

Equation (3) indicates that, under these conditions, any finite value of R_s/R_j will result in an attenuation of Δ_{Tr} relative to ΔE_m and that the degree of attenuation will depend on R_s/R_j. Thus, equation (3) accounts qualitatively for the results obtained with bullfrog[9] and rabbit[31] small intestine and suggests that electrical coupling through a relatively low resistance shunt pathway is an essential component in the effect of actively transported organic non-electrolytes on the bioelectric parameters of this tissue. This is consistent with the fact that the onset of the increase in E_{Tr} following exposure of the mucosal surface of the small intestine to these solutes is extremely rapid[14,16,45], that the inhibition by mucosal phlorizin of sugar-induced increases in E_{Tr} is also rapid[7,14,47], and that the increases in E_{Tr} and E_m elicited by actively transported sugars and amino acids are virtually simultaneous[9,31]. Quantitatively, the relationship between ΔE_m and ΔE_{Tr} may be much more complicated than equation (3) suggests and further studies are required to elucidate the exact role played by electrical coupling between E_m and E_s in the generation of the potential changes induced by actively transported organic non-electrolytes. Among the additional factors which may contribute to the overall electrical response of the tissue to these solutes are: changes in E_s due to stimulation of an electrogenic or rheogenic lateral–serosal Na^+ pump[23,31,33] (see page 29), a change in R_j due to cell swelling[10,20,22] and the possibility of asymmetrical changes in E_m and E_s due to a decrease in intracellular K^+ activity[24].

Results similar to those reported for bullfrog[9] and rabbit[31] small intestine were found in the proximal tubule of newt kidney[51]. However, conflicting results have been reported for the jejunum of the tortoise[46,47], hamster[47] and rat[48,49] and for rat ileum[48]. In these studies ΔE_{Tr} was attributed solely to an increase in E_{s}. The possible origins of these discrepancies will not be reviewed in detail here. They have been discussed elsewhere by the author[52] and by others[23]. Suffice it to say that, in those instances where simultaneous changes in E_{Tr} and E_{m} were examined during impalement of a single epithelial cell[9,24,31], depolarisation of E_{m} was consistently observed.

Actively transported sugars and the lateral–serosal Na$^+$ pump

The increased $\mathcal{J}_{\mathrm{ms}}$, together with the enhanced mucosal entry of Na$^+$ into epithelial cells of the small intestine induced by actively transported sugars, argues strongly in favour of a stimulatory effect of these solutes on the outwardly directed lateral–serosal Na$^+$ pump, and indeed stimulation of an electrogenic Na$^+$ pump has long been considered likely as a contributing factor to the effect of actively transported non-electrolytes on E_{Tr} and I_{sc}[53]. In terms of the model shown in Figure 2.2, such an effect would tend to make ΔE_{Tr} less attenuated with respect to ΔE_{m} than equation (3) would indicate. Rose and Schultz[31] and Frizzell and Schultz[33] have presented evidence that this is probably true for isolated rabbit ileum. Further evidence that the lateral–serosal Na$^+$ pump is electrogenic or rheogenic in character is discussed in a recent review[23].

Since the stimulatory effect of mucosal sugars (and amino acids) on I_{sc} and E_{Tr} is independent of the metabolic utility of these solutes[4,42], the question of the mechanism by which this stimulus is evoked has been of considerable interest. One proposal which possessed the twin attractions of simplicity and plausibility considered the pump to be in effect a variable output device whose rate of operation (under constant metabolic conditions) is controlled primarily by the available substrate level, or the intracellular Na$^+$ concentration. In the presence of actively transported solutes, it was assumed that enhanced mucosal Na$^+$ entry increased the intracellular Na$^+$ concentration significantly with the result that the Na$^+$ pump rate was also increased. Attempts to demonstrate these expected increases by direct chemical determinations of cellular Na$^+$ in small intestinal mucosa were rather consistently unsuccessful[19,20,21]. However, it could be argued that real but significant increases in intracellular Na$^+$ might be obscured by the uncertainties inherent in chemical determinations of this parameter in a complex tissue[54]. For this reason Lee and Armstrong[24] examined, with cation selective microelectrodes, the effect of the actively transported sugar analogue, 3-O-methyl glucose, on the intracellular Na$^+$ activity (a_{Na}) of epithelial cells of isolated bullfrog small intestine maintained between identical sodium sulphate media. The results were somewhat disconcerting in that 3-O-methyl glucose induced a small but very significant ($P < 0.01$) decrease in a_{Na} compared to the control value of this parameter in the absence of added solute. There is at present considerable debate concerning the 'transport pool' (that is, the fraction of total tissue Na^+ involved in the transport process) of Na^+ in small intestine and other epithelia. Several lines of evidence indicate that this may be quite small[1]. Thus, failure to demonstrate a significant increase in a_{Na} in the presence of an actively transported solute is not, *per se*, inconsistent with a pump mechanism which is rate-limited by the available supply of Na^+ in the transport pool. However, a significant decrease in this parameter seems more difficult to explain in these terms. The model shown in Figure 2.2 and the results of White and Armstrong[9] on the electrical effects of actively transported sugars and amino acids in bullfrog small intestine suggest an alternative hypothesis for the stimulation of I_{sc} by these solutes. In terms of this hypothesis[24], the Na^+ pump is regarded as a device whose work output under the conditions of our experiments is governed primarily by the load against which it operates (this is the electrochemical potential gradient, $\Delta\bar{\mu}_{Na}$, for Na^+ between the cell interior and the serosal medium) rather than the size of the Na^+ transport pool available to it. The formal statement of the hypothesis (equation (4)) assumes that the thermodynamically active moiety of the total cellular Na^+ corresponds to the transport pool. It is not yet clear[1] whether this is so for epithelial cells, but the notion receives significant support for the elegant studies of Thomas[55] on the relationship between the rate of Na^+ pumping and a_{Na} in neuronal cells of the snail, *Helix aspera*. The hypothesis also requires that the efficiency with which metabolic energy is coupled to the pumping of Na^+ through the lateral–serosal membrane is not significantly altered by actively transported but non-metabolised organic solutes. Assuming that a_{Na} and the Na^+ transport pool in bullfrog small intestine are at least approximately equivalent, one may write for the work/unit time (W_p) performed by the lateral–serosal pump:

$$W_p = \mathcal{J}_p \cdot \Delta\bar{\mu}_{Na} = \mathcal{J}_p \cdot (RT \ln a_{Na}^0/a_{Na} + E_s F) \qquad (4)$$

where $\mathcal{J}_p$ is the pumped Na^+ flux across the lateral–serosal membrane, a_{Na}^0 is the Na^+ activity of the serosal medium and R, T and F have their usual meanings. For a constant value of W_p, a decrease in E_s permits the cell to adjust to a new steady state in which both a_{Na}^0/a_{Na} and $\mathcal{J}_p$ are maintained at higher levels than in the control situation, i.e. under these conditions a decrease in a_{Na} relative to a_{Na}^0 can be predicted. When a_{Na} is held constant[24], equation (4) is consistent with an absolute decrease in the value of a_{Na}^0 if E_s decreases, as it does in the presence of actively transported sugars and amino acids[9].

The increase in I_{sc} induced by actively transported solutes follows directly from the above line of reasoning. Short circuiting, i.e. bringing E_{Tr} to zero, means that E_s becomes equal to E_m.* Since E_{Tr}, i.e. (E_s-E_m), is greater in the presence than in the absence of actively transported non-electrolytes, the current (I_{sc}) required to bring these two parameters to equality is correspondingly increased.

This hypothesis, according to which the stimulatory effect of actively transported non-electrolytes on the lateral–serosal Na⁺ pump is an indirect one mediated by solute-induced changes in the bioelectric parameters of the tissue, offers an explanation for a puzzling phenomenon which we have frequently observed and which is illustrated in Figure 2.3 (taken from an experiment performed by Dr J. F. White in the author's laboratory). It is apparent from

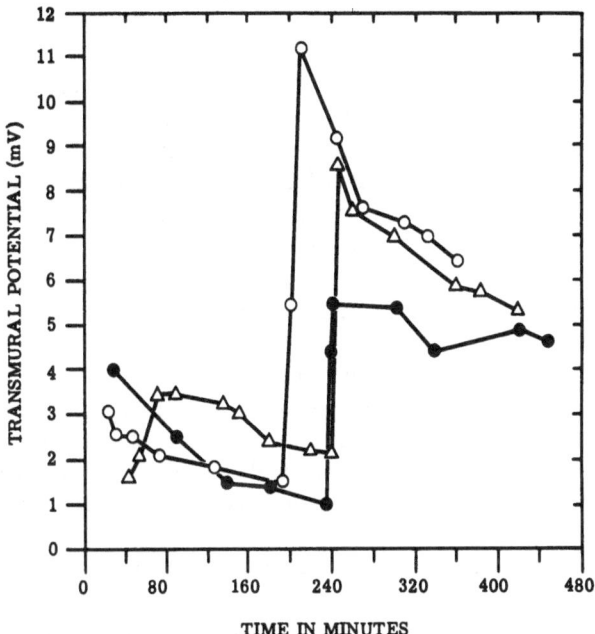

Figure 2.3 Three experiments illustrating the effect of glucose on E_{Tr} in isolated bullfrog small intestine (experiments performed by Dr J. F. White)

Figure 2.3 that, following the addition of glucose to the medium bathing the mucosal surface of the epithelial cells, E_{Tr} rose rapidly to a maximum and then declined more slowly to a steady value which was significantly greater than the initial level. In terms of equation (4) this transient component of the increase in E_{Tr} can be formulated as follows: The solute-induced decrease in E_m and the corresponding decrease in E_s are extremely rapid[9] and probably occur before there is any significant perturbation in a_{Na}. This rapid decrease in the

---

* We recently measured E_m in isolated bullfrog small intestine under short-circuit conditions (Armstrong, W. McD., Brich, D. M., and Stogsdill, D. C., unpublished observations) and found that, under these conditions, it does not differ greatly from its open circuit value.

term $E_s F$ of equation (4) without any change in the term $RT \ln a_{Na}^0 / a_{Na}$ permits W_p to increase suddenly giving rise to a greatly enhanced serosal efflux. If the latter is electrogenic, a corresponding increase in E_s due to this accelerated Na^+ efflux will be superimposed on the increase in E_{Tr} which arises from mucosal depolarization. Subsequently as a_{Na} declines (and pump efflux also declines somewhat) the system 'settles back' towards a new steady state and E_{Tr} falls to a lower value. In terms of this explanation, the biphasic response of E_{Tr} seen in experiments such as that shown in Figure 2.3 can be interpreted as further evidence for the electrogenic nature of the Na^+ pump in the small intestine.

Influence of the shunt pathway on E_{Tr} and I_{sc}

Equation (1) predicts that, in any given set of circumstances, both the magnitude and the orientation (with respect to a grounded mucosal solution) of E_{Tr} will depend on the difference between the terms $R_j(V_s - V_m)$ and $V_j(R_m + R_s)$. If $R_j(V_s - V_m) > V_j(R_m - R_s)$. Na^+ will be serosal positive and vice versa. If all the other parameters on the right hand side of equation (1) remain constant, this difference clearly depends on the magnitude of R_j. This dependence of E_{Tr} on R_j is generally considered to be one of the main reasons for the low spontaneous E_{Tr} values, relative to those observed in 'tight' epithelia such as isolated amphibian skin and urinary bladder, which are found in leaky epithelia such as the small intestine. Hence, an increase in R_j across a leaky epithelium such as the small intestine should induce an increase in E_{Tr}, when this parameter is serosal positive, and a decrease in R_j should have the opposite effect. We examined this prediction with sheets of isolated bullfrog small intestine mounted in an Ussing chamber between identical sodium sulphate Ringer solutions[10]. Since it has been reported[28,31,56] that the shunt resistances in various epithelia are inversely related to the osmolality of the bathing medium, we attempted to vary R_j in this manner. Three bathing solutions were employed. All had the same ionic composition and differed only in their total osmolality. Osmolality was adjusted by varying the amount of mannitol added to each of the three media. The medium designated 'normal' herein was, in fact, slightly hypotonic with respect to frog plasma. It had a total osmolality of 208 ± 1 (SE) mosmol/kg water. The solutions designated 'hypertonic' and 'hypotonic' had osmolalities of 259 ± 2 and 151 ± 1 (SE) mosmol/kg water respectively. Figure 2.4 shows the results of an experiment from this series, in which E_{Tr} and I_{sc} were first permitted to reach an electrical steady state in the normal medium. Subsequently, at the times indicated in the figure, both the mucosal and the serosal bathing media were replaced simultaneously by a hypertonic medium, a second aliquot of the normal medium, a hypotonic medium and finally a second moiety of the hypertonic medium. It is apparent from Figure 2.4 that both E_{Tr} and I_{sc} changed in inverse relation to the osmolality of the bathing medium, that is, in direct relationship to the presumptive changes in R_j. In addition, it is evident from Figure 2.4 that, following this rather extensive series of osmotic shocks, the tissue responded normally[11] to the addition of glucose, indicating that it was still viable. Nevertheless, in subsequent experiments of this series only the steady state values of E_{Tr} and I_{sc}, achieved following the first change from a normal

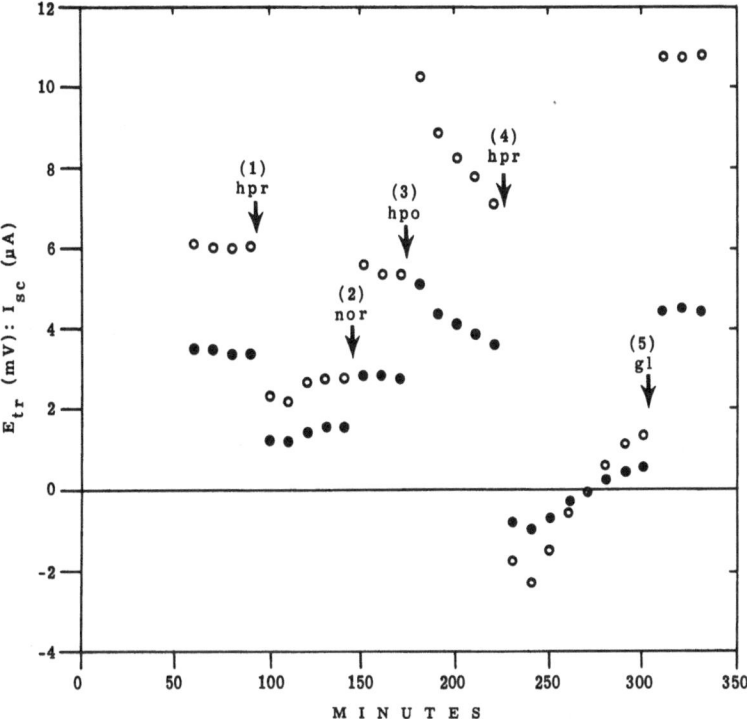

Figure 2.4 Response of E_{Tr} (●) and I_{sc} (○) across isolated bullfrog small intestine to changes in the osmolality of the bathing medium. The tissue was first allowed to attain a steady-state E_{Tr} and I_{sc} in a normal (nor) sodium sulphate Ringer solution (see text). Both the mucosal and serosal solutions were then replaced with a hypertonic (hpr) medium (arrow 1). At the time indicated by arrows 2, 3 and 4, the mucosal and serosal bathing solutions were replaced by normal, hypotonic (hpo) and hypertonic Ringer solutions respectively. Finally, glucose (gl) was added to both bathing media (arrow 5) (see reference 10)

medium to a hypertonic or hypotonic medium, were considered for quantitative purposes. In three experiments in which the tissue was first equilibrated in a normal medium and then exposed to a hypertonic medium, E_{Tr} decreased from 2.6 ± 0.4 mV to 1.3 ± 0.2 mV and I_{sc} decreased from 12.0 ± 3.4 μA/cm^2 to 6.1 ± 1.4 μA/cm^2. Similarly, in five experiments in which a normal medium was replaced by a hypotonic medium, E_{Tr} increased from 2.8 ± 0.3 to 4.0 ± 0.3 mV and I_{sc} increased from 13.1 ± 1.4 to 18.3 ± 2.5 μA/cm^2. These decreases and increases were statistically significant. A more

33

extensive set of measurements of E_{Tr} was made in a separate series of experiments (Table 2.2 and page 36), in which the effect of external osmolality on E_{Tr} was confirmed.

The dependence of E_{Tr} on external osmolality observed in this study is not unexpected in view of the widespread evidence that the shunt pathway is of paramount importance as a determinant of E_{Tr} in leaky epithelia[1,2,23]. However, the results described above underline the fact that, in such epithelia, although the activity of an electrogenic Na^+ pump may contribute to E_{Tr}, there is not necessarily a simple or explicit relationship between the two.

The osmotically induced changes in I_{sc} observed in these experiments are in a sense more intriguing than the corresponding changes in E_{Tr} since they provide some insight into the electrical characteristics of the shunt pathway. It will be evident from Figure 2.2 that a dependence of E_{Tr} on R_j can be predicted regardless of the value of V_j, that is, even if the shunt pathway is considered as a simple resistive element of the circuit shown. This is not the case for I_{sc} even though electrical shunting, through conducting junctional pathways, of the intrinsic e.m.f.s across the mucosal and serosal cell membranes means that the so-called open-circuit condition is in reality a partially short-circuited state and that, for a given set of conditions, the degree of internal 'short circuiting' in the absence of an external current supply is inversely related to the magnitude of R_j. The short-circuit current is the external current which must be supplied, when the tissue is bathed by symmetrical media, to maintain E_{Tr} at zero. Considering points 1 and 3 of Figure 2.2 to be connected to an external source of current and setting $V_j = 0$ one obtains

$$I_{sc} = (V_s - V_m)/(R_m + R_s) \qquad (5)$$

Equation (5) predicts that I_{sc} under these conditions is independent of the value of R_j. However, if V_j in Figure 2.2 has a finite value, one finds

$$I_{sc} = [(V_s - V_m)/(R_m + R_s)] - V_j/R_j \qquad (6)$$

In these circumstances, I_{sc} depends directly on R_j if all other parameters of equation (6) remain constant.

Three important consequences of equation (6) may be noted. First, a change in I_{sc} which results from a change in R_j alone indicates the existence of a finite diffusion potential in the shunt pathway. The fact that, as noted above, I_{sc} across the isolated bullfrog small intestine did vary with external osmolality in our experiments can be interpreted as indicating that this tissue, like the isolated rabbit gall bladder[50], maintains a finite diffusion potential across the junctional shunt even when the mucosal and serosal bathing media are identical. Second, E_{Tr} and I_{sc} in the intestine are, in a certain sense, coupled since both are constrained to respond in a similar fashion to a change in R_j equations (1) and (6)). Third, although I_{sc} in leaky epithelia corresponds at all times to the net rate of epithelial ion transport, it does not necessarily reflect the intrinsic rates of specific mucosal to serosal ion pumps. Hence, in such epithelia, an osmotically induced change in I_{sc} is not necessarily indicative of

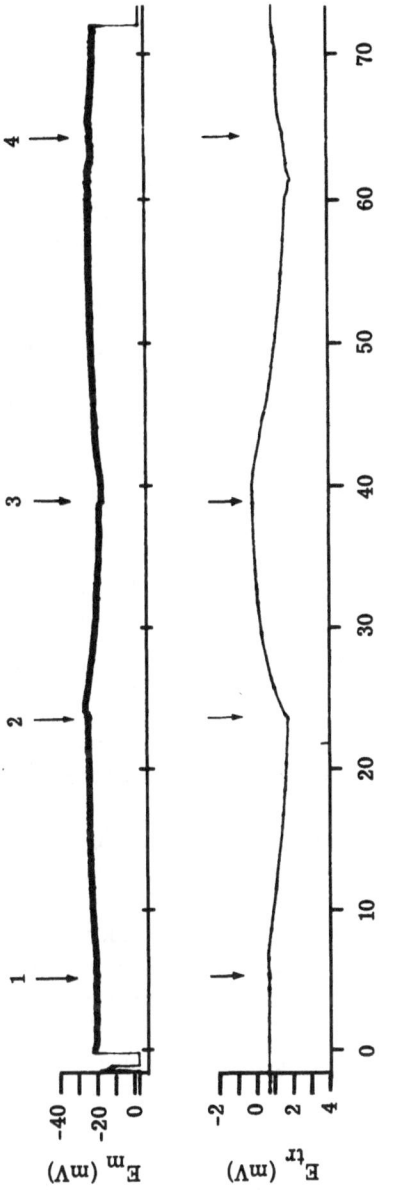

Figure 2.5 Response of E_{Tr} (lower tracing) and E_m (upper tracing) to changes in osmolality. Arrow 1, normal Ringer solution replaced by hypotonic solution; arrow 2, hypotonic solution replaced by hypertonic solution; arrow 3, hypotonic solution reintroduced; arrow 4, preparation perfused with normal medium (see reference 10)

an osmotic effect on the activity of the Na$^+$ pump[57]. Finally, it is apparent from equations (1) and (6) that, for epithelia which possess relatively low resistance shunt pathways, the ratio Na$^+$/I_{sc} does not give a valid estimate of total transepithelial resistance.

R_j and E_m — orientation of V_m

In a companion set of experiments to those discussed in the previous section, the effect of external osmolality on E_m was determined[10]. A representative experiment from this series is shown in Figure 2.5 and a summary of the results obtained (together with the data collected simultaneously from the effect of external osmolality on E_{Tr}) is given in Table 2.2. It is apparent from Figure 2.5 and Table 2.2 that there was a significant hyperpolarisation of the mucosal membrane (that is, an increase in the negativity of the cell interior with respect to the mucosal solution) in hypotonic media and a corresponding depolarisation in hypertonic media. Measurements of the effect of external

Table 2.2 Effect of medium osmolality on E_{Tr} and E_m in the isolated bullfrog small intestine

Change	n	ΔE_{Tr}*	ΔE_m*
Hyper → Hypo	15	1.7 ± 0.3	-4.2 ± 1.2
Hypo → Hyper	21	-1.8 ± 0.2	4.7 ± 0.9

* Mean values ± SE. A positive value for ΔE_{Tr} means that E_{Tr} became more positive with respect to the mucosal solution. A positive ΔE_m means that the cell interior became less negative with respect to the mucosal solution. Negative values for ΔE_{Tr} and ΔE_m have the opposite meanings. (Table calculated from reference 52)

osmolality on intracellular Na$^+$ and K$^+$ concentrations[10] indicated that changes in these parameters could not account for the observed changes in E_m under these conditions.

An analysis[10], in terms of the circuit shown in Figure 2.2, of the response of E_m to external osmolality sheds some interesting light on the question of the true orientation of V_m in the small intestine. In high resistance epithelia such an isolated frog skin[28] and toad bladder[58], E_m under open-circuit conditions is normally orientated so that the cell interior is positive with respect to the mucosal solution. Similarly, V_m in such epithelia is usually assigned the opposite orientation to that shown in Figure 2.2 for the small intestine[59]. There appears, at this time, to be fairly general agreement that the orientation of V_s for leaky as well as tight epithelia is as shown in Figure 2.2. However, in an ingenious analysis of electromotive forces in epithelial cells, Schultz[60] showed that, under certain conditions, a mucosal positive value for E_m may be consistent with an opposite orientation for V_m. Using Figure 2.2 as a basis, this conclusion can readily be confirmed as follows. If the sign of V_m (with respect to point 1) in Figure 2.2 is reversed, one obtains

$$E_m = [V_m(R_s + R_j) - R_m(V_s + V_j)]/R_t \qquad (7)$$

Equation (7) shows that $E_m > 0$ when $V_m(R_s + R_j) > R_m(V_s + V_j)$ and vice versa. Thus, in theory, a decrease in R_j without change in any other parameter on the right-hand side of equation (7) could result in an inversion of the sign of E_m. In support of this conclusion, Schultz[60] cites the observation[28] that the five to eight-fold reduction of R_j in isolated frog skin exposed on the outside to a hypertonic sodium sulphate–urea solution resulted in a reversal of the open-circuit E_m and correctly infers that, in low resistance epithelia, E_m under open-circuit conditions may not reflect the true orientation of V_m.

However, if $R_j \ll R_t$, as seems to be the case in the small intestine[33,34], so that, for a small change (ΔR_j) in R_j, R_t can be assumed to remain virtually constant, equation (7) gives

$$\Delta E_m = V_m \ (\Delta R_j)/R_t \tag{7a}$$

that is, a decrease in R_j should give rise to an increase in the absolute magnitude (hyperpolarisation) of E_m if the latter is inside negative. The opposite would hold true for an increase in R_j. On the other hand, if V_m is orientated as indicated in Figure 2.2, one finds by analogy with equations (7) and (7a),

$$E_m = - \ [V_m(R_s + R_j) + R_m(V_s + V_j)]/R_t \tag{8}$$

and

$$\Delta E_m = -V_m(\Delta R_j)/R_t \tag{8a}$$

Under these conditions a decrease in R_j would cause a depolarisation of E_m and vice versa.

It is at once apparent that the results illustrated in Figure 2.4 and Table 2.2 are the converse of those predicted by equations (7) and (7a) and are in agreement with the predictions of equations (8) and (8a). Hence, the above analysis supports the conclusion that the inside negative E_m normally observed in epithelial cells of the small intestine accurately reflects the orientation, though not the magnitude of V_m. The experiments reported in this section also suggest a method (experimental manipulation of R_j) by which the true orientation of V_m in other leaky epithelia can be inferred from measurements of E_m.

CONCLUSION

This account of work performed in the author's laboratory on the Na⁺-transporting and electrophysiological properties of isolated bullfrog small intestine seeks to show how flux studies, electrical potential measurements and intracellular ionic activity determinations combine to support the idea that low resistance paracellular shunt pathways are a major determinant of the ion transport and bioelectric properties of small intestinal epithelia. Conversely, an attempt is made to illustrate the fact that the paracellular shunt concept is an important unifying principle in epithelial physiology. Recent years have witnessed exciting progress towards a unitary theory of epithelial function. This review is offered in the hope that it may stimulate further efforts in this direction.

Acknowledgements

The author wishes to acknowledge his gratitude to his students and collaborators for their able contributions to the studies reviewed herein. These studies were supported by USPHS grants AM 12715 and HL 06308. Computer services were provided by the Research Computation Center, Indiana University, Indianapolis and supported in part by USPHS grant FR 00162.

References

1. Ussing, H. H., Erlij, D. and Lassen, U. (1974). Transport pathways in biological membranes. *Physiol. Revs.*, **36**, 17.
2. Frömter, E. and Diamond, J. M. (1972). Route of passive ion permeation in epithelia. *Nature New Biol.*, **235**, 9
3. Ussing, H. H. (1960). The alkali metal ions in isolated systems and tissues. In O. Eichler and A. Farah (eds.) *Handbuch der Experimentellen Pharmakologie*, Vol. 13, pp. 1–195. (Berlin: Springer-Verlag)
4. Schultz, S. G. and Curran, P. F. (1968). Intestinal absorption of sodium, chloride and water. In C. F. Code and W. Heidel (eds.) *Handbook of Physiology*, Section 6, Vol. III, pp. 1245–1275 (Washington, D.C.; American Physiological Society)
5. Quay, J. F. and Armstrong, W. McD. (1969). Sodium and chloride transport by isolated bullfrog small intestine. *Amer. J. Physiol.*, **217**, 694
6. Armstrong, W. McD., Suh, T.K. and Gerencser, G. A. (1972). Stimulation by anoxia of active chloride transfer in isolated bullfrog small intestinal epithelia. *Biochim. Biophys. Acta*, **255**, 647
7. Gerencser, G. A. and Armstrong, W. McD. (1972). Sodium transfer in bullfrog small intestine — stimulation by exogenous ATP. *Biochim. Biophys. Acta*, **255**, 663
8. Levin, R. J. (1966). Transmural potentials across the small and large intestine of the bullfrog *Rana catesbeiana*. *Proc. Soc. Exp. Biol. Med.*, **121**, 1033
9. White, J. F. and Armstrong, W. McD. (1971). Effect of transported solutes on membrane potentials in bullfrog small intestine. *Amer. J. Physiol.*, **221**, 194
10. Armstrong, W. McD., Byrd, B. J., Cohen, E. S., Cohen, S. J., Hamang, P. H. and Myers, C. J. (1975). Osmotically induced electrical changes in isolated bullfrog small intestine. *Biochim. Biophys. Acta* (In press)
11. Quay, J. F. and Armstrong, W. McD. (1969). Enhancement of net sodium transport in isolated bullfrog small intestine by sugars and amino acids. *Proc. Soc. Exp. Biol. Med.*, **131**, 46
12. Armstrong, W. McD. and Brich, D. M. (1975). Response of unidirectional Na^+ fluxes across isolated bullfrog small intestine to transported solutes. (In preparation)
13. Schultz, S. G. and Zalusky, R. (1964). Ion transport in isolated rabbit ileum. I. Short-circuit current and Na^+ fluxes. *J. Gen. Physiol.*, **47**, 567
14. Schultz, S. G. and Zalusky, R. (1964). Ion transport in isolated rabbit ileum. II. The interaction between active sodium and active sugar transport. *J. Gen. Physiol.*, **48**, 1043.

15. Schultz, S. G. and Zalusky, R. (1965). Interactions between active sodium transport and active amino acid transport in isolated rabbit ileum. *Nature, Lond.*, **205**, 292

16. Lyon, I. and Crane, R. K. (1966). Studies on transmural potentials *in vitro* in relation to intestinal absorption. I. Apparent Michaelis constants for Na⁺-dependent sugar transport. *Biochim. Biophys. Acta*, **112**, 278

17. Koefoed-Johnsen, V., and Ussing, H. H. (1958). The nature of the frog skin-potential. *Acta Physiol. Scand.*, **42**, 298

18. Sawada, M. and Asano, T. (1963). Effects of metabolic disturbances on potential difference across intestinal wall of rat. *Amer. J. Physiol.*, **204**, 105

19. Schultz, S. G., Fuisz, R. E. and Curran, P. F. (1966). Amino acid and sugar transport in rabbit Ileum. *J. Gen. Physiol.*, **49**, 849.

20. Csáky, T. Z. and Esposito, G. (1969). Osmotic swelling of intestinal epithelial cells during active sugar transport. *Amer. J. Physiol.*, **217**, 753

21. Koopman, W. and Schultz, S. G. (1969). The effects of sugars and amino acids on mucosal Na⁺ and K⁺ concentrations in rabbit ileum. *Biochim. Biophys. Acta*, **173**, 338

22. Armstrong, W. McD., Musselman, D. L. and Reitzug, H. C. (1970). Sodium, potassium and water content of isolated bullfrog small intestinal epithelia. *Amer. J. Physiol.*, **219**, 1023

23. Schultz, S. G. Frizzell, R. A. and Nellans, H. N. (1974). Ion transport in mammalian small intestine. *Ann. Rev. Physiol.*, **36**, 51

24. Lee, C. O. and Armstrong, W. McD. (1972). Activities of sodium and potassium ions in epithelial cells of small intestine. *Science*, **175**, 1261

25. Armstrong, W. McD., Byrd, B. J. and Hamang, P. M. (1973). The Na⁺ gradient and D-galactose accumulation in epithelial cells of bullfrog small intestine. *Biochim. Biophys. Acta*, **330**, 237

26. Diamond, J. M. and Bossert, W. H. (1967). Standing-gradient osmotic flow. A mechanism for coupling of water and solute transport in epithelia. *J. Gen. Physiol.*, **50**, 2061

27. Curran, P. F., Hajjar, J. J. and Glynn, I. M. (1970). The sodium-alanine interaction in rabbit ileum: effect of alanine on Na fluxes. *J. Gen. Physiol.*, **55**, 297

28. Ussing, H. H. and Windhager, E. E. (1964). Nature of shunt path and active transport path through frog skin epithelium. *Acta Physiol. Scand.*, **61**, 484

29. Clarkson, T. W. (1967). The transport of salt and water across isolated rat ileum: evidence for at least two distinct pathways. *J. Gen. Physiol.*, **50**, 695

30. Smyth, D. H. and Wright, E. M. (1966). Streaming potentials in the rat small intestine. *J. Physiol. Lond.*, **182**, 591

31. Rose, R. C. and Schultz, S. G. (1971). Studies on the electrical potential profile across rabbit ileum. Effects of sugars and amino acids on transmural and transmucosal electrical potential differences. *J. Gen. Physiol.*, **57**, 639

32. Csáky, T. Z. (1975). Transcellular and intercellular intestinal transport. In T. Z. Csáky (ed.). *Intestinal Absorption and Malabsorption*, pp. 177–185. (New York: Raven Press)

33. Frizzell, R. A. and Schultz, S. G. (1972). Ionic conductances of extracellular shunt-pathway in rabbit ileum. *J. Gen. Physiol.*, **59**, 318

34. Munck, B. G. and Schultz, S. G. (1974). Properties of the passive conductance pathway across *in vitro* rat jejunum. *J. Memb. Biol.*, **16**, 163

35. Nellans, H. N., Frizzell, R. A. and Schultz, S. G. (1974). Brush border processes and transepithelial Na and Cl transport by rabbit ileum. *Amer. J. Physiol.*, **226**, 1131

36. Desjeux, J. F., Tai, Y-H. and Curran, P. F. (1974). Characteristics of sodium flux from serosa to mucosa in rabbit ileum. *J. Gen. Physiol.*, **64**, 274

37. Schultz, S. G. and Curran, P. F. (1970). Coupled transport of sodium and organic solutes. *Physiol. Revs.*, **80**, 637

38. Barry, R. J. C., Smyth, D. H. and Wright, E. M. (1965). Short-circuit current and solute transfer by rat jejunum. *J. Physiol. Lond.*, **181**, 410

39. Taylor, A. E., Wright, E. M., Schultz, S. G. and Curran, P. F. (1968). Effect of sugars on ion fluxes in intestine. *Amer. J. Physiol.*, **214**, 836

40. Field, M., Fromm, D. and McColl, I. (1970). Ion transport in rabbit ileal mucosa. I. Na and Cl fluxes and short-circuit current. *Amer. J. Physiol.*, **220**, 1388

41. Munck, B. G. (1972). Effects of sugar and amino acid transport on transepithelial fluxes of sodium and chloride of short-circuited rat jejunum. *J. Physiol. Lond.*, **223**, 699

42. Kimmich, G. A. (1973). Coupling between Na^+ and sugar absorption in small intestine. *Biochim. Biophys. Acta*, **300**, 31

43. Schultz, S. G., Curran, P. F., Chez, R. A. and Fuisz, R. E. (1967). Alanine and sodium fluxes across mucosal border of rabbit ileum. *J. Gen. Physiol.*, **50**, 1241

44. Goldner, A. M., Schultz, S. G. and Curran, P. F. (1969). Sodium and sugar fluxes across the mucosal border of rabbit ileum. *J. Gen. Physiol.*, **53**, 362.

45. Hoshi, T. and Komatsu, Y. (1970). Effects of anoxia and metabolic inhibitors on the sugar-evoked potential and demonstration of sugar-outflow potential in toad intestine. *Tohoku J. Exp. Med.*, **100**, 47

46. Gilles-Baillien, M. and Schoffeniels, E. (1965). Site of action of L-alanine and D-glucose on the potential difference across the intestine. *Arch. Internat. Physiol. Biochim.*, **73**, 355

47. Wright, E. M. (1966). The origin of the glucose-dependent increase in the potential difference across the tortoise small intestine. *J. Physiol. Lond.*, **185**, 486

48. Lyon, I., and Sheerin, H. E. (1971). Studies on transmural potentials *in vitro* in relation to intestinal absorption. VI. The effect of sugars on electrical potential profiles in jejunum and ileum. *Biochim. Biophys. Acta*, **249**, 1

49. Barry, R. J. C. and Eggenton, J. (1972). Membrane potentials of epithelial cells in rat small intestine. *J. Physiol. Lond.*, **227**, 201

50. Machen, T. E. and Diamond, J. M. (1969). An estimate of the salt concentration in the lateral intercellular spaces of rabbit gall bladder during maximal fluid transport. *J. Memb. Biol.*, **1**, 194

51. Marayama, T. and Hoshi, T. (1972). The effect of D-glucose on the electrical potential profile across the proximal tubule of the newt kidney. *Biochim. Biophys. Acta*, **282**, 214

52. Armstrong, W. McD. (1975). Electrophysiology of sodium transport by epithelial cells of the small intestine. In T. Z. Csáky (ed.) *Intestinal Absorption and Malabsorption.* pp. 45–66. (New York: Raven Press)

53. Barry, R. J. C. (1967). Electrical changes in relation to transport. *Brit. Med. Bull.*, **23**, 266

54. Lev, A. A. and Armstrong, W. McD. (1975). Ionic activities in cells. In A. Kleinzeller and F. Bronner (eds.). *Current Topics in Membranes and Transport.* Vol. 6, pp. 59–123. (New York: Academic Press)

55. Thomas, R. C. (1972). Intracellular sodium activity and the sodium pump in snail neurones. *J. Physiol. Lond.*, **220**, 55

56. Windhager, E. E., Boulpaep, E. L. and Giebisch, G. (1966). Electrophysiological studies on single nephrons. In *Third International Congress on Nephrology*, Washington, D. C., Vol. I, p. 35

57. Lipton, P. (1972). Effect of changes in osmolarity on sodium transport across isolated toad bladder. *Amer. J. Physiol.*, **222**, 821

58. Frazier, H. S. (1962). The electrical potential profile of the isolated toad bladder. *J. Gen. Physiol.*, **45**, 515

59. Herrera, F. C. (1971). Frog skin and toad bladder. In E. E. Bittar (ed.) *Membranes and Transport*, Vol. 1, pp. 1–47. (New York: Wiley-Interscience)

60. Schultz, S. G. (1972). Electrical potential differences and electromotive forces in epithelial tissues. *J. Gen. Physiol.*, **59**, 794

2

Discussion Paper on
The Role of the Paracellular Route in Water Transport by Rat Jejunum *In Vitro*

B. G. Munck

Institute of Medical Physiology A, Copenhagen

Recently, Patlak and Rapoport[1] pointed out that, when net volume flow down an osmotic gradient across a heteroporous membrane is prevented by applying a hydrostatic pressure on the hyperosmotic side, a net flux to the hypo-osmotic side can be demonstrated for another solute present in equal concentrations on both sides of the membrane, even when solute–solute interactions can be disregarded.

In a preparation of rat jejunum *in vitro* with glucose-induced net water transport, the hydrostatic interstitial pressure is increased. This preparation can therefore be considered as an approximation to the model described by Patlak and Rapoport[1].

Net volume transport across epithelia is regarded as linked to a primary transport of solutes. For rat jejunum (as for other leaky epithelia), it is then of interest to know whether the transported solutes are osmotically active both across the cell membranes and across the paracellular pathway.

PEG-4000 does not enter the epithelial cells but does cross the epithelium, though with difficulty. The flux ratio of PEG-4000 for rat jejunum should therefore be sensitive to the convective effect of a net volume flow through the paracellular pathway of this epithelium. Consequently PEG-4000 should be well suited as a means of examining the direction of a net volume flow through this pathway.

Unidirectional transmural fluxes of ^{14}C-PEG-4000 across the short-circuited rat jejunum were measured at 0.5 mM PEG-4000 in media with 28 mM D-glucose or without glucose. The results are shown in Figure *2.1*, presented as the ratio J_{sm}/J_{ms}. These results indicate that in the presence of glucose, there is a net volume flow directed towards the mucosal solution

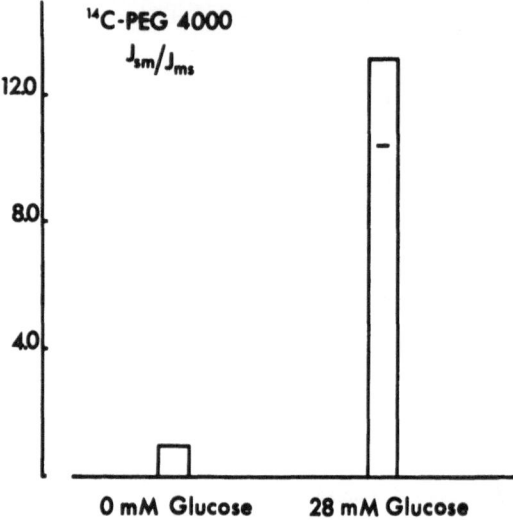

Figure *2.1* The columns represent the ratio between the unidirectional transmural fluxes of ^{14}C-PEG-4000 across short-circuited rat mid small intestine mounted in Ussing chambers and bathed with identical solutions on both sides (0.5 mM PEG-4000 in Krebs phosphate buffer). In the absence of glucose, the fluxes are too low to be very precisely measured. At 28 mM D-glucose the mucosa-to-serosa flux ($\mathcal{J}_{ms}$) is increased enough to be accurately measurable and the serosa-to-mucosa flux ($\mathcal{J}_{sm}$) is increased by a factor of 11. For this latter condition, the column represents the mean −1 SE of four paired measurements

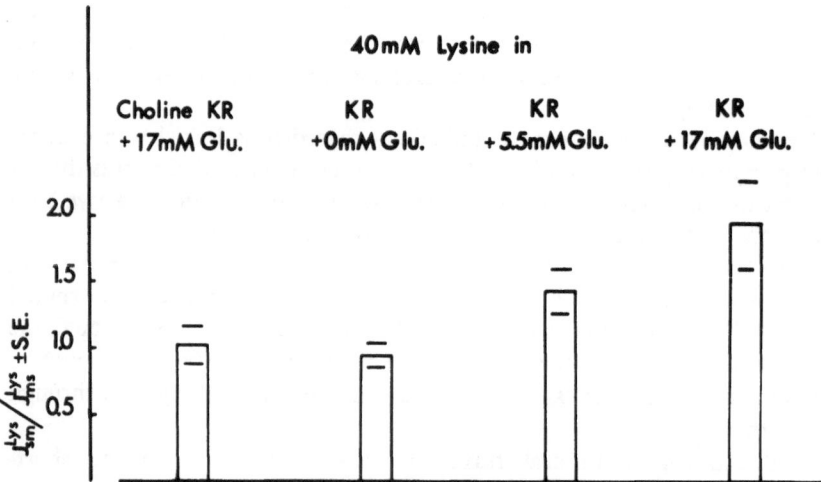

Figure *2.2* Each column represents the mean ±1 SE of the ratio between unidirectional fluxes of lysine determined with four pairs of adjacent pieces of rat mid small intestine. The measurements were made in the short-circuited state with identical solutions bathing the two sides of the preparation. The values for $\mathcal{J}_{ms}^{Lys}$ were essentially the same in all four conditions

through the paracellular shunt. This means that in leaky epithelia (like those of the small intestine, the gall bladder, and the renal proximal tubule), the reflection coefficients across the paracellular pathway are negligible, and that for the transport solutes solvent drag consequently does not contribute to lumen-to-blood movement via this pathway.

The phenomenon described here is appropriately termed a 'fluid circuit' process. Finally, I should like to demonstrate that this fluid circuit can profoundly affect transport of amino acids. This is done by the data shown in Figure 2.2 which demonstrate that with increasing concentrations of glucose, the ratio $J_{sm}^{Lys}/J_{ms}^{Lys}$ exceeds unity to a correspondingly greater extent.

Reference

1. Patlak, C. S. and Rapoport, S. I. (1971). Theoretical analysis of net tracer flux due to volume circulation in a membrane with pores of different sizes. Relation to solute drag model. *J. Gen. Physiol.*, **57**, 113

Discussion 2

Smith:	My sympathy for your approach leads me to defend it in one way and to attack it in another. First the defence. It may be said that changing fluid osmolarity as you do will produce artefactual changes in tissue conductance. I doubt this, since in our biological preparation (newborn pig ileum), we see similar correlations between short-circuit current and conductance with no change in fluid osmolarity. However, I do not think this *necessarily* means we are short circuiting a diffusion potential. Any change in sodium pumping rate will alter the amount of fluid within the intercellular spaces. This will change the intercellular pressure. If this then alters the tightness of the junctional complexes, this will produce a change in conductance as a *secondary* event, giving the reported correlation. Is there any way to distinguish between these two possibilities?
Armstrong:	First, may I turn your argument around? A major point in my discussion was that concurrent changes in E_{Tr} and I_{sc} of the kind we observed in our osmotic studies do not *necessarily* require one to invoke alterations in the rate of sodium pumping. To answer your question: I agree that a decrease in R_j as a secondary consequence of increased sodium pumping is indeed possible. If one is dealing with an electroneutral pump, this involves primarily a change in R_j alone and would seem (in terms of the equivalent circuit I discussed) to be formally equivalent to an osmotically induced change in this parameter. However, if the pump is electrogenic or rheogenic, V_s (and/or V_j) will change as well as R_j. This could, I believe, be distinguished from a change in R_j alone, particularly if quantitative values for the parameters of the circuit are available.
Wright:	In the presence of osmotic gradients across the intestine, the short-circuit current will not equal the active transport of sodium, as part of the PD is a 'steaming potential'.
Armstrong:	Since both the mucosal and the serosal bathing media were changed simultaneously, one feels that any streaming potentials generated during such a change would be transient. Transient streaming potentials could be the reason why the establishment of a new electrical steady state following a change of the medium was rather slow in our experiments. However, if the time constants for equilibration within intercellular spaces and mucosal and serosal unstirred layers in the intestine are comparable to those in, for example, the gall bladder, I think one can assume that the steady-state values we report for transmural electrical parameters are essentially free from complications due to streaming potentials.

44

3
Absorptive and Secretory Processes in Intestine

HENRY J. BINDER

Department of Internal Medicine,
Yale University,
New Haven, Connecticut,
USA

The extensive studies of cholera during the past few years have resurrected the phenomena of intestinal electrolyte secretion. In the two decades prior to 1968, study of intestinal electrolyte transport centred exclusively on absorption with little or no attention paid to secretion. During the past several years, multiple examples of net fluid and electrolyte secretion have been demonstrated[1-4]. Secretion has been observed in several diarrhoeal illnesses, induced by multiple physiological and pathological stimuli and even noted under normal conditions. Study of experimentally induced ion secretion is often complicated by the multiple effects of the potential secretogogue. Therefore, the demonstration that net water and electrolyte secretion occurs in the guinea-pig small intestine presented an unique opportunity to evaluate a natural 'secretory' process[5].

Powell *et al.* had observed net fluid and electrolyte accumulation during perfusion of the jejunum and ileum of the guinea-pig[5]. In those studies, there was no evidence to suggest that this net fluid accumulation was secondary to increased luminal osmolarity, diminished absorption, altered motility, an increase in mucosal permeability or an augmentation of hydrostatic pressure. These initial studies suggested that an active secretory process, perhaps similar to that present in cholera, might explain this phenomenon. Therefore, to determine the characteristics of absorptive and secretory processes of guinea-pig intestine, ileal mucosa was studied *in vitro* in a modified Ussing chamber[6]. This method permits determination of electrical parameters and bidirectional Na+ and Cl- fluxes under conditions in which chemical, electrical, osmotic, and hydrostatic concentration gradients are absent. These studies were performed with Don W. Powell in the laboratory of the late Peter F. Curran[7,8].

45

In preliminary studies performed under open-circuit conditions, net Na^+ secretion and net Cl^- absorption were observed. The spontaneous electrical PD was -4.5 mM. These observations are qualitatively similar to those observed *in vivo*. Under short-circuit conditions, net Na^+ absorption (0.4 μEq/ h.cm^2) and net Cl^- secretion (-1.0 μEq/h.cm^2) were present. (Positive values represent net absorption and negative ones net secretion). However, I_{sc} was 4.3 μEq/h.cm^2 and was not accounted for by the measured Na^+ and Cl^- fluxes.

Select removal of HCO_3^- resulted in little change in either I_{sc} or J_{net}^{Na}, but J_{net}^{Cl} increased significantly to -2.3 μEq/h.cm^2. A model of opposing absorptive and secretory processes was proposed to explain these observations. Further, we suggested that the secretory process had a greater affinity for HCO_3^- than for Cl^-.

Additional experiments were performed to determine the nature of the absorptive and secretory processes. If the secretory process was electrically neutral, then electrogenic Na^+ absorption would be responsible for the I_{sc} and the measured Na^+ transport would be the difference between the electrogenic absorptive process and the neutral secretory process. An alternative model would propose an electrogenic secretory process. In this situation, the measured Na^+ transport and electrogenic Na^+ absorption would be identical but I_{sc} would be the sum of the absorptive and secretory processes.

The results of ion replacement experiments in which bicarbonate-free, chloride-free sodium-free solutions were used have provided significant support for a neutral Na^+/anion ($NaHCO_3$ and/or $NaCl$) secretory process.

In the absence of HCO_3^- and Cl^-, I_{sc} was unchanged but J_{net}^{Na} increased so that it was approximately 85% of I_{sc}. In Na^+-free media both I_{sc} and J_{net}^{Cl} were abolished. These results are only compatible with the model of a neutral Na^+/anion secretion.

Further support for this model was obtained by additional experiments that were performed with ouabain, theophylline, and 3-O-methyl glucose (Table 3.1). The addition of ouabain resulted in a marked decrease in I_{sc}, in net Na^+ secretion, but without significant effect on J_{net}^{Cl}. A ouabain-sensitive electrogenic Na^+ absorptive process associated with a ouabain-insensitive neutral secretory process would explain these results.

The addition of theophylline, a phosphodiesterase inhibitor which results in increased mucosal concentrations of cyclic AMP, provoked net Na^+ secretion and an increase in net Cl^- secretion without altering I_{sc}. Cyclic AMP-stimulation of the neutral secretory process would be consistent with these

Table 3.1 A summary of some of the properties of the opposing absorptive and secretory processes observed in studies *in vitro*[7,8] of guinea-pig ileum

	Na$^+$ Absorption	Na$^+$ Secretion	Anion secretion
Increased by	3-O-methyl glucose Glucose	Theophylline Glucose	Theophylline Glucose
Decreased by	Ouabain	Anion removal	Na removal

results. Finally, 3-O-methyl glucose an actively transported but non-metabolized hexose, increased J_{net}^{Na} and I_{sc} equally; J_{net}^{Cl} remained constant. Glucose appeared to increase both Na^+ absorption and NaCl secretion.

These experiments demonstrate that in the guinea-pig intestine, ion transport can be separated into opposing absorptive and secretory processes. These results suggest the presence of a neutral Na^+/anion (NaHCO$_3$ and/or NaCl) secretory pump that has a greater affinity for bicarbonate than chloride. Additional studies by Powell on the effect of cholera enterotoxin on ion secretion in rabbit ileum are also compatible with this model of neutral secretion and suggest the possibility of a unified model of secretion[9-11]. In contrast, Field has proposed an alternative model of ion secretion with emphasis on electrogenic anion secretion and a decrease in substrate-independent Na^+ absorption[12,13]. Further, the effects of cyclic AMP on Na^+ and Cl^- transport in the large intestine are not compatible with this model of neutral transport[14]. Although a single model of ion secretion would be attractive, the available experimental evidence is conflicting and does not support such an interpretation. Additional studies of both naturally occurring and experimentally produced secretion should provide further understanding of the secretory process.

References

1. Hendrix T. R. and Bayless, T. M. (1970). Digestion: intestinal secretion. *Ann. Rev. Physiol.*, **32**, 139
2. Field, M. (1974). Intestinal secretion. *Gastroenterology*, **66**, 1063
3. Binder, H. J. (1975). Ion transport in small and large intestine. In M. H. F. Friedman (ed.), *Functions of the Stomach and Intestine*, pp. 247–258. (Baltimore: University Park Press)
4. Schultz, S. G. and Frizzell, R. A. (1972). An overview of intestinal absorptive and secretory processes. *Gastroenterology*, **63**, 161
5. Powell, D. W. and Malawar, S. J. (1968). Secretion of electrolytes and water by the guinea-pig small intestine *in vivo*. *Amer. J. Physiol.*, **215**, 1226
6. Schultz, S. G. and Zalusky, R. (1964). Ion transport in isolated rabbit ileum. I. Short-circuit current and Na fluxes. *J. Gen. Physiol.*, **47**, 567
7. Powell, D. W., Binder, H. J. and Curran, P. E. (1972). Electrolyte secretion by the guinea-pig ileum *in vitro*. *Amer. J. Physiol.*, **223**, 531
8. Binder, H. J., Powell, D. W. and Curran, P. E. (1972). Effect of hexoses on ion transport in guinea-pig ileum. *Amer. J. Physiol.*, **223**, 538
9. Powell, D. W., Binder, H. J. and Curran, P. E. (1973). Active electrolyte secretion stimulated by choleragen in rabbit ileum *in vitro*. *Amer. J. Physiol.*, **225**, 781
10. Powell, D. W. and Farris, R. K. (1974). Theophylline, cyclic AMP, choleragen, and electrolyte transport by rabbit ileum. *Amer. J. Physiol.*, **227**, 1428
11. Powell, D. W. (1974). Intestinal conductance and permselectivity changes with theophylline and choleragen. *Amer. J. Physiol.*, **227**, 1436
12. Field, M. (1971). Ion transport in rabbit ileal mucosa. II. Effects of cyclic 3′,5′-AMP. *Amer. J. Physiol.*, **221**, 992
13. Field, M. and Fromm. D. (1972). Effect of cholera enterotoxin on ion transport across isolated ileal mucosa. *J. Clin. Invest.*, **51**, 796
14. Binder, H. J. and Rawlins, C. L. (1973). Effect of conjugated dihydroxy bile salts on electrolyte transport in rat colon. *J. Clin. Invest.*, **52**, 1460

3

Discussion Paper on

Further Evidence for a Na⁺ 'Neutral' Secretory Process in Rabbit Ileum

Jehan F. Desjeux

INSERM U 83 and Department of Paediatrics, Université Paris VII, Hôpital Hérold, Paris

In rabbit ileum, the difference observed between short-circuit current, I_{sc}, and Na⁺ flux, $\mathcal{J}_{net}^{Na}$, has raised the possibility of two Na⁺ transport processes: (1) a Na⁺ absorptive process represented by I_{sc} and (2) a Na⁺ secretory process represented by the difference between I_{sc} and $\mathcal{J}_{net}^{Na}$ ($\mathcal{J}_{net}^{Na} < I_{sc}$). In order to examine the possible involvement of a secretory component in $\mathcal{J}_{net}^{Na}$, we have made use of the following approach[1]: it was assumed that the transmural unidirectional flux of Na⁺ from serosa to mucosa, $\mathcal{J}_{sm}^{Na}$, could in principle be described as the sum of a diffusional flux through the extracellular shunt, $\mathcal{J}_{dsm}^{Na}$, and a flux through a cellular pathway, $\mathcal{J}_{csm}^{Na}$. For relatively small changes in diffusional forces (PD), $\mathcal{J}_{csm}^{Na}$ would be PD-independent. The results indicate the presence of a PD-independent flux presumably $\mathcal{J}_{csm}^{Na}$. $\mathcal{J}_{csm}^{Na}$ comprises approximately 25% of $\mathcal{J}_{sm}^{Na}$ in Ringer's solution containing 10 mM glucose and 25 mM bicarbonate. It is reduced to negligible values by replacement of all chloride and bicarbonate ions by isethionate, and it is independent of the I_{sc}. This component of $\mathcal{J}_{sm}^{Na}$ has a number of characteristics consistent with involvement in a specific secretory process mediating an electrically neutral secretory transport of sodium plus anion from serosa to mucosa.

Reference

1. Desjeux, J. F., Tai, Y. H.and Curran, P. F. (1974). Characteristics of sodium flux from serosa to mucosa in rabbit ileum. *J. Gen. Physiol.*, **64**, 274

Discussion 3

Wright: Would you care to speculate on the location of the neutral NaCl pump and the nature of the coupling between solute and water secretion?

Binder: I do not know, but I can offer several possibilities. The secretory process might be located in the crypt epithelia, in the villus epithelia but not in the 'absorptive' cells, or in the same cell as the absorptive process. I do not think there are any data to permit definite conclusions. The crypt is attractive, for it might provide an area for coupling of solute and water movement as occurs in the intercellular spaces.

Field: Recent studies* indicate that adenylate cyclase in intestinal villus cells can be selectively stimulated by cholera toxin and that this selective effect is associated with a shift in fluid transport towards secretion. Thus villus cells are clearly involved in the secretory process. Whether crypt cells are also involved, and, if so, whether in the same or a different way remains to be established. With more prolonged exposure to cholera toxin, adenylate cyclase in both villus and crypt cells is stimulated and the fluid transport change is greater than when short exposure to toxin stimulates villus cell cyclase alone. With regard to the anatomical locus of coupling between secretory water and ion flow, crypts need not be postulated, although they certainly represent one possibility. The space between the microvilli is another possibility.

Love: Have you looked at potential interactions between cholera toxin and theophylline on active chloride and bicarbonate secretion? Does glucose-enhanced secretion decrease the effectiveness of the glucose-stimulated sodium absorption — particularly in view of the value of glucose in preventing the diarrhoea of cholera?

Binder: No, we have not looked at ion fluxes across epithelia treated with both cholera enterotoxin and theophylline at the same time. The studies of electrical parameters would suggest that there might not be any augmentation of the secretory response. The apparent stimulation of the neutral secretory response by glucose should not reduce the effectiveness of oral therapy in cholera, since this is an *in vitro* phenomenon and is related to the 'substrate' property of glucose and not to its 'transport' property.

Munck: May I ask Dr Desjeux whether he has observed effects of changing the transepithelial PD on the transepithelial resistance?

Desjeux: Across rabbit ileum, there is a linear relationship between the current and the PD over a range of +9 to −9 mV.

* de Jonge, *BBA*, **381**, 128, 1975.

4
Ion Fluxes in Isolated Guinea-pig Intestinal Mucosa

F. O. LAUTERBACH

Institute of Pharmacology and Toxicology,
Ruhr-University,
Bochum

INTRODUCTION

The movement of molecules across the intestinal wall has to be regarded in its most simplified form as a permeation process in a three-compartment system, which consists of the intestinal lumen, the mucosal cell and the interstitial space, separated by the luminal and basolateral membranes of the mucosal cell. For our understanding of the permeation processes, therefore, not only a knowledge of transepithelial fluxes, but furthermore a detailed analysis of influx and efflux across these two membranes is necessary. There are two main possibilities for the determination of these fluxes and their coefficients: directly from influx and efflux measurements and indirectly from the steady-state values of the transepithelial fluxes and the tissue concentrations if the substrate is administered both to the luminal and to the blood side of the epithelium.

Obviously most of the widely employed methods *in vitro* are only capable to a limited extent of contributing to the characterisation of *both* membranes of the mucosal cell, since they allow direct access only to the luminal border, whereas substrate flow at the contraluminal side is severely restricted by the additional underlying tissue layers, so the concentrations at the basal pole of the cell remain undefined. The use of an isolated mucosal epithelium as a separating membrane in a flux chamber with free access to the contraluminal cell border as well thus seems to be advantageous and highly desirable.

Therefore the topic of this paper will be the description of a preparation of isolated mucosa which is so rapid, easy and reproducible that it can be used for the large series of experiments necessary for kinetic studies, and the demonstration of some results concerning the events occurring in the two plasma membranes in different permeation processes.

THE PREPARATION OF GUINEA-PIG ISOLATED MUCOSA

Briefly, the method is as follows[1,2]: Pieces of small intestine — 1–2 cm long — are excised from guinea-pigs under ether anaesthesia, opened lengthwise along the mesenteric border and gently spread out, serosal side down, on a frosted glass plate. While the flat sheet is held down on its outer edge by a

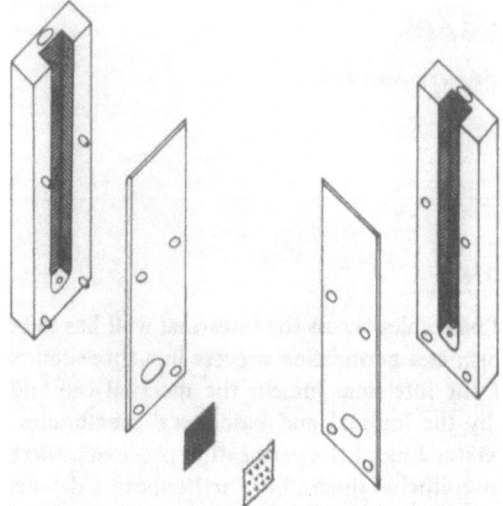

Figure 4.1 Method of the isolated mucosa. Picture shows the assembly of isolated mucosal epithelium, nylon mesh (thickness 0.15 mm, width of mesh 0.205 mm), polyvinylchloride foils (thickness 0.1 mm) with window of 5 mm diameter and four holes for insertion of fixing pins, and chambers made of acrylic glass. Outer dimensions of chambers 65 × 20 × 9 mm; chamber lumen is 6 mm in width and 4 mm in depth. All rims are slightly greased with vaseline. Routine filling volume is 0.2 ml. Composition of normal incubation solution (mM): 96.5 NaCl, 7 KCl, 3 $CaCl_2$, 1 $MgSO_4$, 0.9 sodium phosphate buffer (pH 7.4), 29.4 tris-(hydroxymethyl)-amino-methane buffer (pH 7.4), 14 glucose, 14 mannitol

microscopic glass slide, the mucosal epithelium is stripped off with an ordinary sharp razor blade, which is quickly drawn over the tissue. By this small but important modification of the method originally described by Dickens and Weil-Malherbe[3], the epithelium is neatly separated from the other tissue layers at the bases of the crypts and obtained as a continuous sheet.

Histological examination reveals that the contraluminal side of the mucosal cell is covered only with a small layer of loose connective tissue. The villous space is almost empty and opens freely to the blood side of the epithelium.

The mucosa is now floated in oxygenated saline, captured on a little piece of nylon mesh, and put between two plastic foils, where it closes a circular window of 5 mm diameter. The whole assembly is quickly clamped between two hemi-chambers which are locked together by means of a tube clamp. The chambers are simultaneously filled with 0.2 ml of the respective incubation solutions by means of two piston pipettes through drill holes in the chamber walls, which serve afterwards as inlets for moistened oxygen (Figure 4.1).

Incubation is performed in a water bath at 37 °C. Since the interval between excision of the gut piece from the animal and start of the incubation is only 2–3 min, two or even three series of 12 experiments each are easily performed by two technicians during one laboratory day. At the end of the experiment, the solutions are withdrawn and the mucosa is punched out by means of a little machine constructed for that purpose.

FLUXES OF WATER AND THIOUREA

The first process briefly to be mentioned here is permeation by diffusion, where one expects to find neither a net transport nor pumps in the membranes. Among others, [^{3}H]-water and [^{14}C]-thiourea were used as test substrates[2], whose transepithelial fluxes and tissue uptake were measured after addition either to the luminal or the blood side. Transepithelial water fluxes reached a steady-state value of 0.06 μl cm^{-2} s^{-1} after a short lag phase of approximately 1.5 minutes. No significant differences between the transepithelial fluxes in the two directions could be observed. The concentration of tritiated water in the cell water reached 46% and 41% of the [^{3}H] concentration in the incubation solution after administration from the luminal and blood side respectively. Similar results were obtained with thiourea, with transepithelial flux rates approximately 2/5 of the values measured for water.

From the four parameters obtained from these experiments — two transepithelial fluxes in both directions and two steady-state tissue concentrations after loading from both directions — the coefficients for the four fluxes across the luminal and basolateral membranes can be calculated (Table 4.1). As expected for a diffusing substrate, the influx and efflux coefficients

Table 4.1 Flux coefficients for water and thiourea

	Flux coefficients (10^{-4} cm s^{-1})			
	k_{12}	k_{21}	k_{32}	k_{23}
Water	1.30	1.53	1.17	1.29
Thiourea	0.56	0.52	0.48	0.44

Water or thiourea was administered to the isolated mucosa either from the luminal or the blood side. Flux coefficients were calculated from the steady-state fluxes and the steady-state concentrations in the cell water. Luminal, mucosal and blood side compartments are numbered 1, 2 and 3 respectively; thus k_{12} is the coefficient for the flux from luminal solution into the cell, etc. (see Figure 4.3) (from reference 2)

across a given membrane are identical within the limits of experimental error. The permeability of water 1.3×10^{-4} cm s^{-1}, is approximately 2.5 times greater than the permeability of thiourea. Furthermore — since the uptake from both sides was almost identical — we get almost identical flux coefficients for the luminal and the basolateral membranes. That means that the passive permeabilities of both membranes — calculated on the basis of uniform serosal area — are found to be the same. If one keeps in mind that the ratio of the two transepithelial fluxes in a three-compartment system with no back flux can be described by the equation

$$\frac{\mathcal{J}_{13}}{\mathcal{J}_{31}} = \frac{k_{12}/k_{21}}{k_{32}/k_{23}}$$

one realises that this is by no means a necessary condition for a diffusing substance. Any combination of passive permeabilities will yield a flux ratio of 1, since $k_{12} \equiv k_{21}$ and $k_{32} \equiv k_{23}$ (for indices refer to Figure 4.3). This result — though somewhat surprising — seems not to be restricted to small test molecules, since we obtained similar results with far larger molecules like cortisol and other drugs[1,4].

SODIUM FLUXES

Permeation and uptake in steady-state experiments

The second situation observed in permeation studies with the isolated mucosa is the existence of no net transport in spite of the existence of pumps. This is the case for sodium (Figure 4.2). Under the conditions of our experiments, there is no net flux of sodium or only a negligible one as compared to the transepithelial fluxes. The permeation rate is identical in both directions. As for water, the permeation rate becomes constant as soon as the sodium concentration in the cell water has reached its steady state. Transepithelial sodium flux then amounts to 1.8 nmol cm^{-2} s^{-1}, from which a coefficient for the transepithelial sodium flux of 0.18×10^{-4} cm s^{-1} is calculated. The ratio of water to sodium permeability of the isolated mucosa is thus 3.3, a value rather similar to that found both *in vivo* and *in vitro* for different species by other authors (Table 4.2). Likewise the absolute values of the transepithelial sodium and water permeabilities in the isolated mucosa are comparable to those reported for small rodents. In dog and man, higher permeabilities are estimated, which must be attributed, at least in part, to the higher mucosal-to-serosal area ratio in these species (see legend to Table 4.2).

Tissue uptake of ^{22}Na is a rapid process. As with water, labelling of the tissue is almost independent of the side to which the isotope is added. The concentration of ^{22}Na in the cell water approaches 23% of the initial concentration of the incubation medium after addition to the luminal side, and 20% after addition to the blood side (Figure 4.2).

A first inspection revealed that there exist no gross differences as to the sodium content and the degree of labelling of the sodium pool between different segments of the small intestine (Table 4.3).

What deserves comment is the degree of labelling of the intracellular sodium pool. Sodium concentration in cell water in these series of experiments was found to be 70–75 mM, which is in good agreement with the values

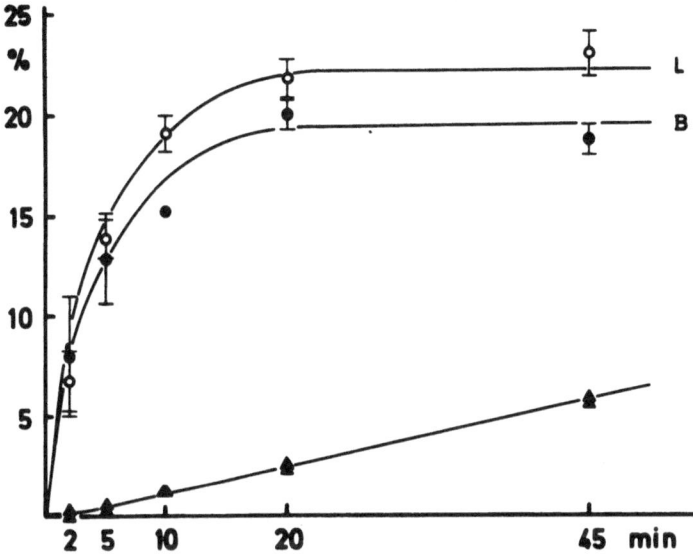

Figure 4.2 Permeation and uptake of ^{22}Na. ^{22}Na was added to the isolated mucosa either from the luminal (open symbols) or the blood side (filled symbols). *Abscissa*: incubation time; *ordinate*: permeation (triangles) and tissue uptake (dots) of ^{22}Na found in counter-compartment and cell water respectively, expressed as a percentage of ^{22}Na concentration added initially. Correction for extracellular ^{22}Na was made by adding 2.5 mM Na$^+$-sulphanilate to the incubation solution and estimation of sulphanilate space by the Bratton–Marshall method. Each dot represents the mean value ±SEM from 2 to 22 experiments; total number of experiments: 99. Errors of permeation smaller than diameter of symbols

reported for the rabbit ileum[26] and rat jejunum[27,28]. Since the system — as shown by the steady-state experiments — is almost symmetrical, half of this pool should be labelled from each side, so that a ^{22}Na concentration of approximately 35% of that of the incubation solution and a relative specific activity (specific activity of intracellular sodium/specific activity of extracellular sodium) of 0.5 is to be expected. In contrast, intracellular ^{22}Na concentration is found to be only 20% and the relative specific activity is only 0.3. Even after loading the mucosae from both sides for 45 minutes, the relative specific activity only reaches 0.65 instead of 1 (Table 4.4).

Table 4.2 Comparison of flux coefficients for transepithelial water and sodium movements in different species with that of the isolated mucosa of guinea-pig

| Species | Gut segment | Method | Flux coefficients (10^{-4} cm.s^{-1}) | | | | Ratio of flux coefficients | | Reference |
| | | | Water | | Na$^+$ | | Water/Na$^+$ | | |
			k_{13}	k_{31}	k_{13}	k_{31}	q_{13}	q_{31}	
Man	Jejunum	in vivo	4.3	3.8	2.6	1.9	1.7	2.0	5
	Ileum	" "	5.2	5.0	2.3	1.8	2.3	2.8	
Dog	Duodenum	" "	3.14	3.1	1.27	1.2	2.5	2.6	6
	Ileum	" "	4.16	3.4	1.67	1.1	2.4	3.1	7
	Ileum	" "	3.0	2.5	2.8	1.5	1.1	1.7	8
	Small intestine	" "	1.50	1.67	0.68	0.95	2.2	1.8	9
	Duodenum	" "	1.53		0.60		2.5		
	Jejunum	" "	2.85		1.20		2.4		
	Ileum	" "	5.16		2.80		1.8		
	Jejunum	" "			1.8	1.6			10
	Ileum	" "			1.3	0.9			11
	Small intestine	" "	5.16						
Rabbit	Ileum	" "			0.16	0.09			12
	Ileum	everted sac gut wall in flux chamber			0.16	0.15			13
	Jejunum				0.18	0.16			
	Ileum	" "			0.16	0.11			14
	Ileum				0.19	0.13			
Guinea-pig	Jejunum	isolated mucosa in flux chamber	0.60	0.60	0.18	0.18	3.3	3.3	2; this paper
	Caecum	gut wall in flux chamber			0.14	0.090			15

Species	Region	Method				Ref.
Rat	Jejunum ♂	*in vivo*	0.70			16
	Jejunum ♀	" "	1.42			17
	Caecum	gut wall in flux chamber	0.83			
	Ileum	*in vivo*		0.90	0.53	18
	Ileum	perfused loop *in vivo*		0.37	0.17	19
	Jejunum	gut wall in flux chamber		0.13	0.12	13
	Ileum	" "		-0.39	-0.27	
				0.22	0.18	
				-0.30	-0.22	
Tortoise (*Testudo hermanni*)	Small intestine	isolated mucosa in flux chamber		0.093	0.077	20, 21
	Colon	flux chamber		0.022	0.006	
Toad	Colon	flux chamber		0.038	0.018	15
Frog	Stomach	isolated mucosa in flux chamber	0.48			22
Marine fish (*Cottus scorpius*)	Small intestine	gut sac		0.33	0.11	23

k_{13} denotes coefficients for the fluxes from gut lumen to blood (or serosal compartment), k_{31} denotes coefficients for fluxes in the opposite direction. If necessary, literature values have been recalculated to provide fluxes across 1 cm² serosal area. The following ratios of mucosal/serosal area have been used: Man 30[5], dog 10[24], rat ileum 4[25]. For the guinea-pig a ratio of 6.7 can be calculated from measurements of villus basal diameter and villus height in histological sections, regarding the villus as a regular cone. 1 mg dry weight of rat jejunum = 0.081 cm² serosal area.

Table 4.3 Sodium concentrations in cell water of isolated mucosae of different parts of the small intestine

	Side of administration	Distance from pylorus (cm)			
		3	40	60	75
Na$^+$ (µmole/ml cell water)	Lumen	66.1	62.4	64.1	84.6
		75.3	74.1	64.3	77.8
	Blood	64.7	72.5	69.6	76.3
		63.9	73.8	57.8	65.4
^{22}Na (%)	Lumen	29.9	19.9	26.8	24.2
		21.3	23.1	23.0	19.2
	Blood	20.7	19.9	19.4	17.6
		19.0	24.0	19.3	19.6

Approximately 10 cm of intestine were used, starting at the distance from pylorus indicated. Concentration of ^{22}Na is expressed in percent of ^{22}Na concentration initially given.

Thus approximately one-third of the intracellular sodium pool seems to belong to an extremely slow exchanging pool, in agreement with the results of Armstrong[29] in the frog intestine.

Coefficients for sodium influx and efflux across the luminal and basolateral membranes of the mucosal cell can be calculated from the steady-state values of transepithelial fluxes and tissue concentrations, assuming that sodium fluxes are proportional to its concentration in the concentration range studied (Figure 4.3). The similarity of the properties of both faces of the isolated mucosa with respect to sodium fluxes is expressed by very similar influx and efflux coefficients in both membranes. Furthermore, in both membranes, efflux coefficients are 2.5 times higher than influx coefficients. Thus, assuming a negative intracellular potential with respect to both sides of the mucosal cell as shown for other animals[30,31], sodium is pumped out against

Table 4.4 Relative specific activity of intracellular sodium

Concentration in cell water	Loading from		
	Lu	Bl	Lu + Bl
Na$^+$ (mM)	76.4 ± 3.4	72.4 ± 4.1	51.2 ± 5.1
^{22}Na (%)	23.0 ± 1.1	18.8 ± 0.8	36.6 ± 3.4
Relative specific activity	0.33 ± 0.02	0.27 ± 0.02	0.65 ± 0.03
n	18	19	9

Isolated mucosa was loaded with ^{22}Na for 45 minutes from luminal side, blood side or both sides. Concentration of ^{22}Na in percent of the concentration of the incubation solution at start of experiment. Relative specific activity = spec. act. of Na$^+$ in cell water/spec. a ct. of Na$^+$ in solution. Guinea-pigs from inbred strain Madaus, Cologne, were used for series with administration on one side, animals from Fa. Rost, Witten, for experiments with administration on both sides.

an electrochemical gradient across both membranes of mucosal cells. Owing to the identity of the pump: leak ratio in both membranes, no net transport occurs in spite of the existence of two pumps. Nothing can be said of course from these experiments about the driving forces for the sodium extrusion. One model which seems compatible with the results observed is that proposed by Curran and coworkers[32] which consists of one electrogenic absorptive and one neutral secretory sodium pump.

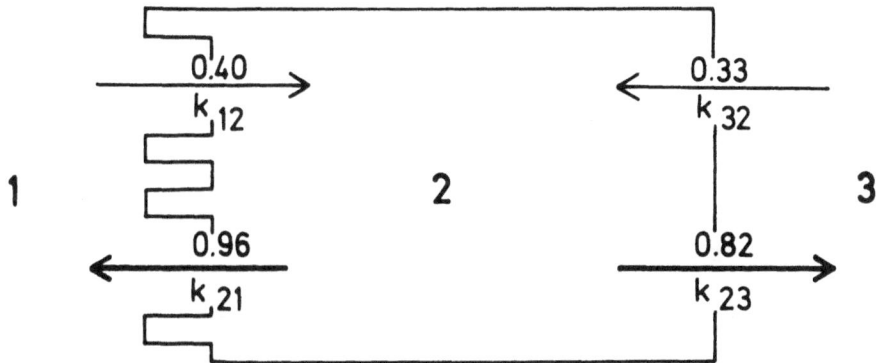

Figure 4.3 Influx and efflux coefficients for ^{22}Na. These have been estimated from steady-state experiments with the isolated mucosa. Compartments 1, 2, 3 denote respectively the luminal solution, mucosal tissue and blood side solution. All values in 10^{-4} cm s^{-1}

Influx measurements

The estimation of flux coefficients from influx and efflux experiments offers the possibility of an independent proof of the coefficients estimated from steady-state experiments. Influx of ^{22}Na proceeds linearly with time between 15 and 60 seconds from both sides of the mucosa, if an appropriate correction for the extracellular sodium is made by simultaneous estimation of inulin or

Table 4.5 Regression lines and influx coefficients for ^{22}Na from influx experiments

Marker for extracellular space	Regression line				Flux coefficients (10^{-4} cm s^{-1})	
	Lumen		Blood			
	b	a	b	a	k_{12}	k_{32}
Inulin	0.014	0.45	0.009	0.42	0.69	0.44
Sulphanilate	0.011	0.24	0.009	0.12	0.55	0.44

Table indicates slope and ordinate intercept of the regression lines ($y = bx + a$) of figure 4.4 and those of a comparable series, where sulphanilate was used instead of [^{14}C]inulin. In the two last columns, the influx coefficients calculated from the slopes of the respective regression lines, are tabulated.

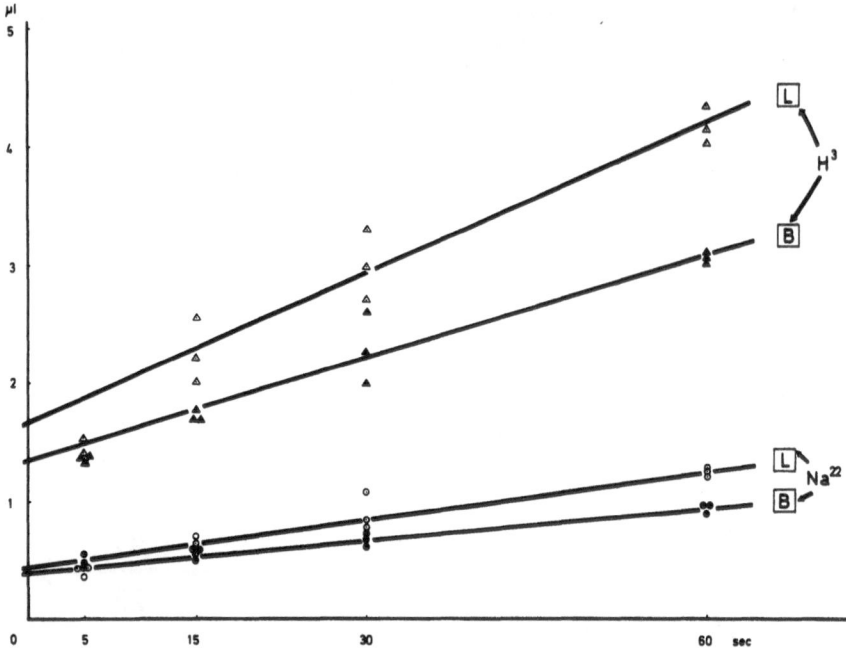

Figure 4.4 Influx of ^{22}Na and [^{3}H]water in the isolated mucosa. Mucosae were equilibrated with normal incubation solution (for composition, see legend to Figure 4.1). After 45 minutes, the solutions were withdrawn and fresh solutions, one of which contained simultaneously ^{22}Na, [^{3}H]water and [^{14}C]inulin, were added at the times indicated on the abscissa. ^{22}Na-, ^{3}H- and ^{14}C-activities in the mucosa were estimated, after extraction with 0.5 M TCA, by liquid scintillation spectrometry, using Bray's[33] scintillation fluid and a desk computer for correction of cross-counting. L and B denote influx from the luminal and blood side. For the sake of simplicity, uptake (ordinate) is expressed in μl, which means the amount of sodium contained in 1 μl incubation solution, thus 1 μl = 96.5 nmoles Na $\approx$ 3 nCi ^{22}Na

sulphanilate space (Figure 4.4). In spite of these corrections, the regression lines do not pass through the origin, which might at least partially be due to the faster filling of small extracellular interstices by the small sodium ion as compared to the marker molecules. The lower ordinate intercept found in experiments with sulphanilate instead of inulin (Table 4.5) as well as the higher ordinate intercepts found for tritiated water influx (Figure 4.4) are consistent with this explanation. As in the steady-state experiments, a somewhat higher coefficient for the influx across the luminal membrane is calculated from the slope of the regression lines. The absolute values of coefficients from influx experiments exceed those obtained under steady-state conditions by a factor of 1.3–1.7 (Table 4.5).

As a point of comparison, water influx proceeds approximately three times faster in both membranes, since for water influx coefficients of 2.1×10^{-4} cm s^{-1} and 1.5×10^{-4} cm s^{-1} were found in the same experiments.

Efflux measurements

The efflux of sodium was estimated by two different series of experiments. In
the first series, mucosae were preloaded with ^{22}Na from both sides and the
appearance of ^{22}Na in tracer-free incubation solutions was followed, the volumes of which were enlarged from 0.2 to 0.5 ml for this purpose (Figure 4.5).

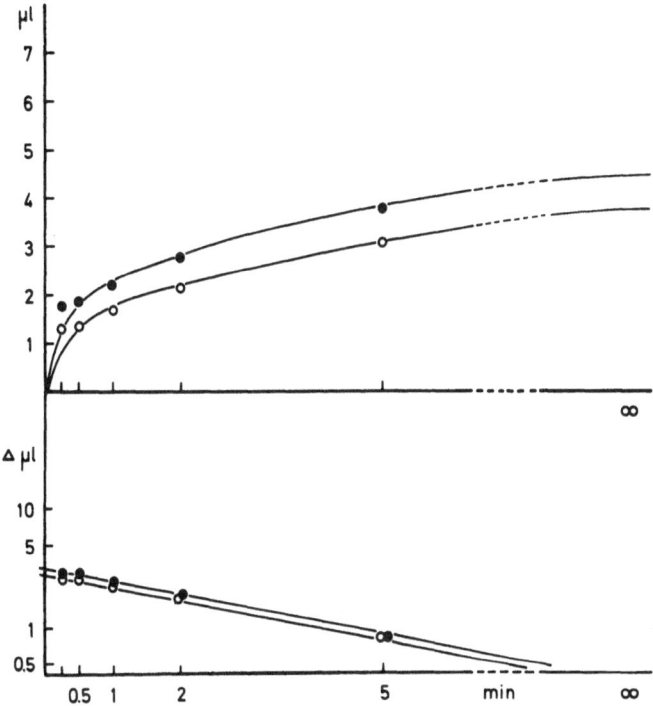

Figure 4.5 Efflux of ^{22}Na from the isolated mucosa. Mucosae were preloaded for 45 minutes
with ^{22}Na from both sides. Afterwards the chambers were rapidly flushed with icecold 0.308 M
mannitol and refilled with 0.5 ml tracer-free incubation solution. Samples were withdrawn at
the times indicated on the abscissa. Upper part of the picture gives the total amount released to
the luminal side (circles) or the blood side (dots) in μl ^{22}Na (see legend to Figure 4.4) versus time.
Lower part demonstrates a semilogarithmic plot of $\Delta\mu l = \mu l_\infty - \mu l_t$ versus time, where μl_∞ is
the total amount of ^{22}Na released to either the luminal (circle) or blood (dots) side at infinite
time; μl_∞ was calculated by distributing the remaining activity in the mucosa in proportion to
the amount released to either side

By semilogarithmic analysis of the cumulative appearance curves, two straight
lines are obtained, the slopes of which represent the sum of the efflux coefficients and the ordinate intercepts indicate the portion of the intracellular
pool which is released to the luminal and blood sides respectively (see Appendix). Two parallel lines were obtained, indicative of one single intracellular
sodium pool. Their ordinate intercepts were almost identical, so that an equal

extrusion of sodium to both sides of the mucosa has to be postulated. Efflux coefficients calculated from three such experiments are $0.89 \pm 0.07 \times 10^{-4}$ cm s^{-1} for efflux to the luminal side (k_{21}) and $0.86 \pm 0.06 \times 10^{-4}$ cm s^{-1} for efflux to the blood side (k_{23}), which agree closely with the efflux coefficients obtained from the steady-state experiments (see Figure 4.3).

For a more detailed analysis of efflux kinetics, an improved method was developed. Instead of using a supporting nylon mesh, the isolated mucosa was glued to the fenestrated polyvinyl chloride foils by means of a tissue adhesive (n-butyl-α-cyanoacrylate; Histoacryl® Braun Melsungen AG), a procedure previously described for positioning frog skin between flux chambers[34]. After preloading the mucosae with ^{22}Na for 45 minutes in the incubation chambers described above, they were washed by dipping them three times for one second in a large volume of icecold isotonic mannitol. They were then placed between

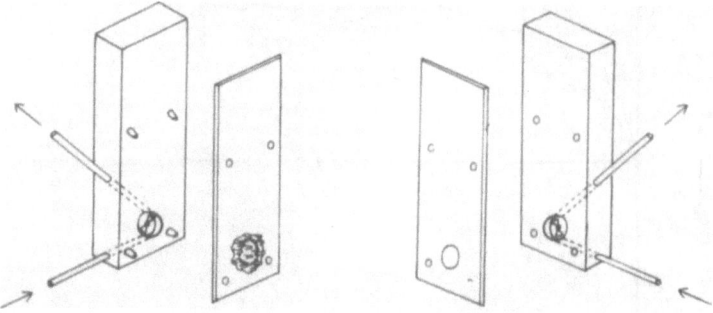

Figure 4.6 Stirred chamber for efflux experiments with the isolated mucosa. Mucosa is glued to PVC-foils by means of a tissue adhesive and placed between two chambers of 6 mm diameter and 4 mm depth, which are magnetically stirred and continuously perfused (for further details see text)

two circular flux chambers of only 0.1 ml volume, which were stirred magnetically and perfused with tracer-free medium at a rate of 0.75 ml/min (Figure 4.6). Effluents were collected at 0.5–2-minute intervals. Tightness of the mucosae was confirmed by estimation of the permeation of sulphanilic acid added at 2.5 mM concentration to the perfusion solution on one side.

By this method, efflux of ^{22}Na was measured after preloading the mucosa from both sides, from the luminal side (Figure 4.7) and from the blood side, the latter without (Figure 4.8) and with 10^{-4} M ouabain in the perfusate on the blood side (Figure 4.9). It is readily seen from the higher resolution obtained by this procedure that the ^{22}Na efflux from the isolated mucosa is a multi-exponential process. At least three compartments can be obtained from an analysis of the total efflux curves (Figures 4.7, 4.8 and 4.9). The transfer coefficients and half-times of these compartments observed under different conditions are listed in Table 4.6. Pool sizes calculated for compartments II and III are given in Table 4.7. As usual in compartmental analysis, an attribution of these formal compartments to their morphological counterparts is not easy.

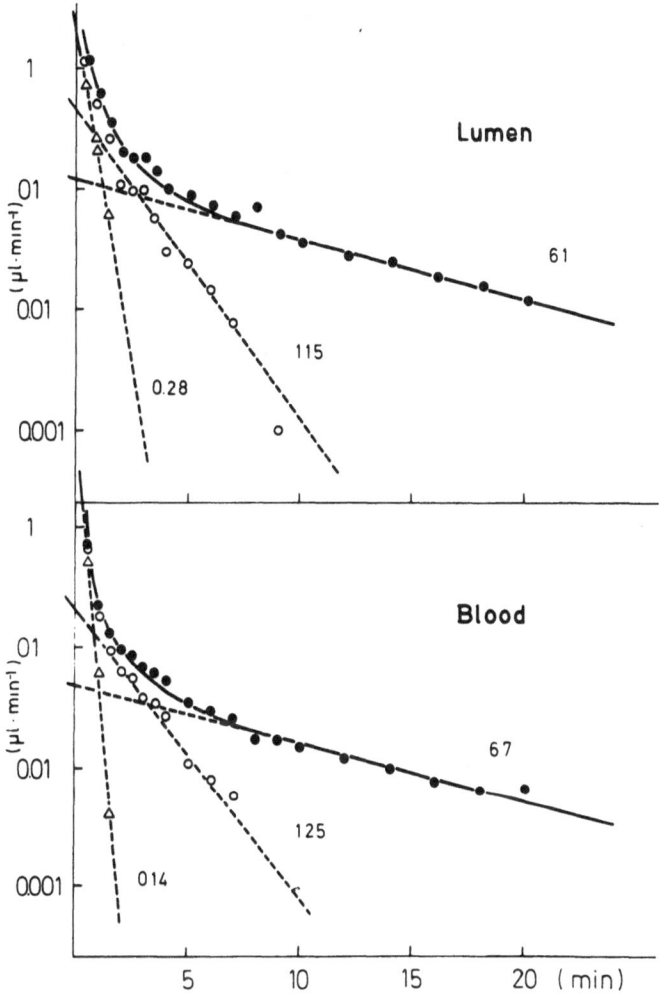

Figure 4.7 Efflux of ^{22}Na from isolated mucosa after preloading from luminal side. For experimental procedure see text. *Abscissa*: time elapsed since start of efflux period; *ordinate*: log of efflux velocity, F (μl min^{-1}), where 1 μl = amount of ^{22}Na contained in 1 μl loading solution ($\approx$3 nCi Na^{22}). Upper and lower part: Efflux to the luminal and blood side respectively. Straight lines were obtained by peeling off procedure; regression lines — log F = b · t + a — were calculated by the method of least squares. Half-times (min) are indicated beside the curves

The fastest compartment (named compartment I) has a half-time of approximately 0.3 minutes, independent of the preloading side of the mucosae and the side to which efflux is measured (Table 4.6). Theoretically, the fastest compartment should represent the chamber washout[35]. Since the chamber volume (v) is 0.1 ml and perfusion rate (f) is 0.75 ml/min, a rate coefficient (f/v) of 7.5 min^{-1} and a half-time of 0.09 min can be calculated for chamber washout under the present conditions; the latter is considerably less than the values observed. Thus, it has to be concluded that the fast compartment contains, in

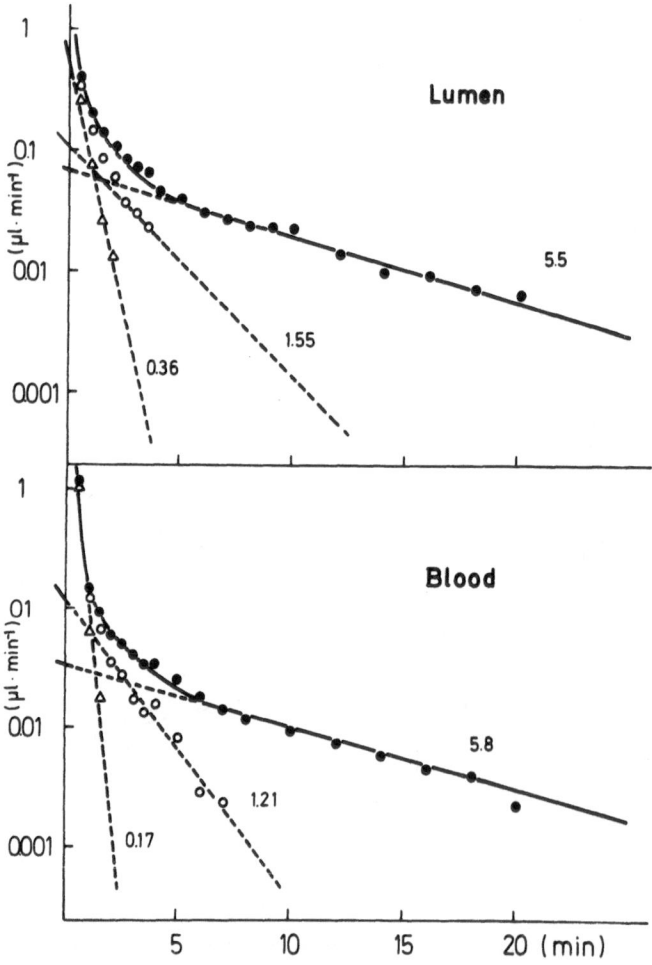

Figure 4.8 Efflux of ^{22}Na from isolated mucosa after preloading from blood side. Same procedures as in Figure 4.7

addition, tissue sodium either from extracellular or from rapidly exchanging intracellular sources. The existence of the extremely rapid phase of initial ^{22}Na influx (Figure 4.4) is in agreement with this explanation. Shorter sampling intervals during the initial phase of efflux will be necessary for a further resolution of this compartment.

Efflux from the second compartment (II) proceeds with a mean half-time of 1.25 minutes. No significant differences between the slopes of the luminal and blood side efflux curves were observed, which is indicative of efflux from one single compartment to both sides of the isolated mucosa. Furthermore, this

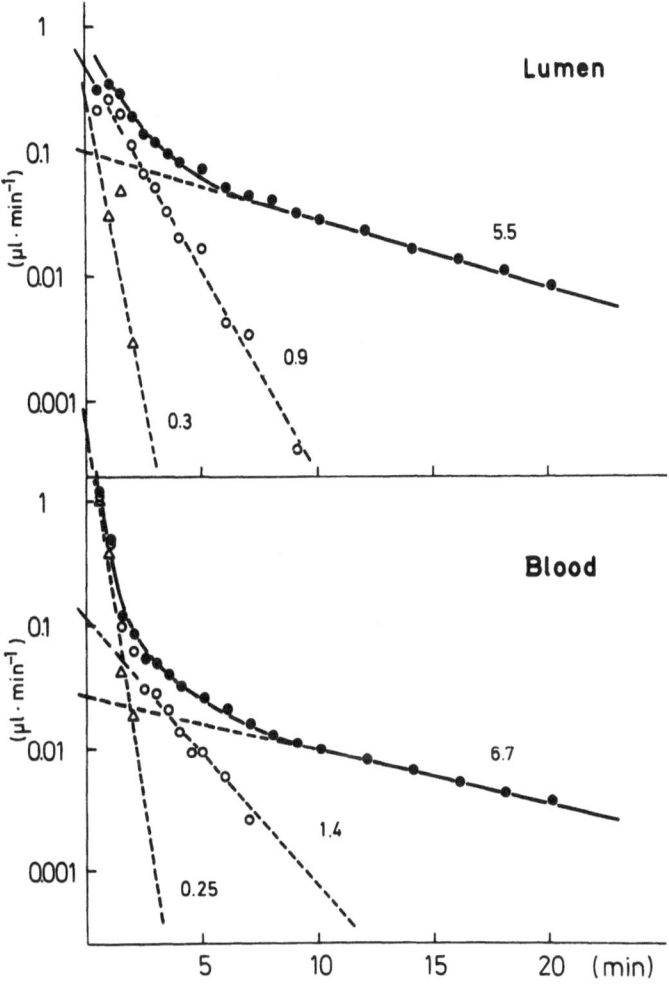

Figure 4.9 Efflux of ^{22}Na from isolated mucosa under the influence of ouabain after pre-loading from blood side. Same procedure as in Figure 4.8, but perfusate on blood side contained 10^{-4} M ouabain

half-time was found to be independent of the preloading side. Therefore it can be concluded that the same compartment is loaded with ^{22}Na from either side. Otherwise it would have to be assumed that two different compartments loaded from one side or the other have the same half-times.

Table 4.6 Transfer coefficients and half times for the efflux of ^{22}Na under different conditions

Mucosae preloaded from	Experiment number	K(min^{-1}) for compartment						$t_{1/2}$ (min) for compartment					
		I		II		III		I		II		III	
		Lu	Bl	Lu	Bl	Lu	Bl	Lu	Bl	Lu	Bl	Lu	Bl
Both sides	1	1.39	1.93	0.513	0.677	0.126	0.101	0.50	0.36	1.34	1.02	5.5	6.8
Luminal side	2	2.43	4.81	0.601	0.552	0.112	0.103	0.28	0.14	1.15	1.25	6.1	6.7
	3	2.45	2.05	0.440	0.541	0.099	0.087	0.28	0.34	1.57	1.28	6.9	7.9
Blood side	4	1.67	2.94	0.624	0.675	0.115	0.117	0.41	0.23	1.11	1.02	6.0	5.9
	5	1.93	4.07	0.447	0.573	0.124	0.118	0.36	0.17	1.55	1.21	5.5	5.8
Blood side Ouabain*	6	2.81	1.91	0.578	0.486	0.140	0.128	0.25	0.36	1.20	1.42	4.9	5.4
	7	2.32	2.81	0.755	0.507	0.125	0.101	0.30	0.25	0.91	1.37	5.5	6.7
Mean values (± SEM)		1.97 ±0.21	3.16 ±0.56	0.525 ±0.038	0.604 ±0.030	0.115 ±0.005	0.105 ±0.006	0.37 ±0.04	0.25 ±0.04	1.34 ±0.10	1.16 ±0.06	6.0 ±0.3	6.6 ±0.4
exp. 1–5		2.57 ±0.35		0.564 ±0.026		0.110 ±0.004		0.31 ±0.03		1.25 ±0.06		6.3 ±0.2	
		2.56 ±0.24	2.36 ±0.45	0.667 ±0.089	0.497 ±0.011	0.133 ±0.008	0.115 ±0.014	0.28 ±0.03	0.31 ±0.05	1.06 ±0.15	1.40 ±0.02	5.2 ±0.3	6.1 ±0.6
exp. 6–7		2.46 ±0.22		0.581 ±0.061		0.124 ±0.008		0.29 ±0.03		1.22 ±0.12		5.6 ±0.4	

For experimental procedure see text; transfer coefficients ($K = b/\log e$) are obtained from the slope of the regression lines (see Figures 4.7–4.9).
* 10^{-4} M ouabain in perfusion solution on blood side.

66

Table 4.7 Total size and distribution of ^{22}Na pools of intermediate (II) and slow (III) compartments

Mucosa preloaded from	Intracellular ^{22}Na (μl)*†	Exp. No.	^{22}Na pools (μl)*							
			Compartment II				Compartment III			
			Total	Lu	Bl	Lu/Bl	Total	Lu	Bl	Lu/Bl
Both sides	1.36 ±0.13 (2)	1	2.33	1.25	1.08	1.16	1.29	0.64	0.65	0.98
Luminal side	0.95 ±0.12 (4)	2	1.19	0.83	0.36	2.28	1.45	1.07	0.38	2.76
		3	1.17	0.96	0.22	4.36	0.83	0.52	0.31	1.69
Blood side	0.76 ±0.12 (5)	4	0.61	0.21	0.40	0.52	1.24	0.77	0.47	1.63
		5	0.44	0.22	0.22	1.0	0.80	0.55	0.25	2.16
Blood side 10^{-4} ouabain in perfusion solution on blood side		6	0.40	0.27	0.13	2.11	0.53	0.38	0.15	2.47
		7	0.96	0.78	0.18	4.17	1.14	0.90	0.24	3.77

Pool sizes per mucosa are calculated from the ordinate intercepts (initial flow rate) of the respective regression lines and the corresponding transfer coefficients. (Interference of chamber compartment with estimation of pool sizes[35] was neglected, since rate coefficient of chamber washout is high in comparison with the transfer coefficient for compartment II and III).

* μl = amount of ^{22}Na contained in 1 μl loading solution.
† Intracellular content of ^{22}Na (μl/mucosa) from control experiments for comparison. Mucosae were preloaded and washed with mannitol as in efflux experiments. Correction for extracellular space by simultaneous estimation of [^{3}H]polyethylene glycol (mol. weight 900).

Most likely this second compartment represents the sodium transport pool. The total amount of ^{22}Na found in this compartment roughly corresponds to the intracellular ^{22}Na content estimated in parallel experiments with mucosae loaded and washed under identical conditions, but not subjected to the efflux procedure (Table 4.7). (It should be kept in mind, however, that differences might arise both from small irregularities in the manually performed washing procedure and from differences in transfer time from one chamber to the other, which usually took approximately one minute). Furthermore, ouabain altered the distribution of that pool between the luminal and blood side compartment in the expected manner: Whereas after loading from the blood side without ouabain, the total ^{22}Na in this compartment is equally liberated to both sides or even preferentially released to the blood side, in experiments with 10^{-4} M ouabain in the perfusate on the blood side, ^{22}Na extrusion to the blood side is reduced, and the release to the luminal side is increased in compensation (Table 4.7). To what extent the observed small shifts in half-time (retardation of efflux to the blood side and enhancement of efflux to the luminal side) are a significant effect of ouabain has to be evaluated by further experiments.

Since compartment II seems to represent the transport compartment, an attempt should be made to estimate the efflux coefficients across the luminal and basolateral membranes of the mucosal cell from these experiments (see Appendix). The mean transfer coefficient for the efflux of the total pool across both membranes, as obtained from the slope of the regression lines, is 0.56 min^{-1}. The mean wet weight of the mucosae in these experiments was 13.3 mg, indicative of a cellular water space of 0.0062 ml. Therefore, since the area was 0.2 cm^2, for the sum of the efflux coefficients $(k_{21} + k_{23})$ we get $(0.56 \times 0.0062)/(60 \times 0.2)$ cm s^{-1} = 2.9×10^{-4} cm s^{-1}. To obtain the individual values k_{21} and k_{23}, this sum has to be divided in proportion to the amount released from the pool to the luminal and blood sides. In the present experiments, a tendency for preferential release to the preloading side is observed. Otherwise, the absolute amounts released to the countercompartment are roughly the same (see experiments 2 to 5 in Table 4.7). Therefore it seems reasonable to assume that the values on the preloading side are distorted by inclusion of some extracellular ^{22}Na from the preloading period and that intracellular ^{22}Na is approximately equally distributed to both sides.

Thus, $k_{21} \approx k_{23} \approx 1.45 \times 10^{-4}$ cm s^{-1}. As observed in the influx experiments, the absolute value is about 1.6 times higher than the value obtained from the steady-state experiments, whereas the ratio of efflux/influx coefficients is apparently independent of the method of flux coefficient determination.

The third compartment is characterised by a half-time of 6 minutes, a value clearly too low to account for the movements from the transport pool. The same half-time was found in control experiments, where the mucosa was pretreated as usual, but punched out before the efflux period started.

Therefore it seems probable that this slow compartment corresponds mainly to the rim washout. According to the estimated pool sizes in normal and control experiments, however, participation of a slow component of mucosal sodium cannot be completely ruled out at present.

FLUXES OF QUATERNARY AMMONIUM IONS

Concerning the third situation — the existence both of pumps and of a net transport process — an unusual example will be mentioned here, namely the active secretion of quaternary ammonium compounds.

Quaternary ammonium compounds are rather peculiar substances with respect to the time course and concentration dependence of their absorption. Absorption of some of them starts very fast but soon comes to a standstill in spite of high amounts of unabsorbed substance[36]. Furthermore, absorption is concentration-dependent[37] in a fashion which can be interpreted as an increase in absorption rate from a lower to a higher plateau with increasing intestinal concentration[1,38]. This behaviour led to the suggestion that a secretory mechanism for these compounds might exist in the intestine, which in fact could be demonstrated by the accumulation of tetraethylammonium bromide in the intestinal lumen after i.v. application[1,38].

Further investigation of this secretory mechanism by means of the isolated mucosa revealed that the uptake of tetraethylammonium bromide, N^1-methylnicotinamide and N-methylscopolamine from the blood side obeys saturation kinetics and permeation proceeds faster from the blood side to the luminal side than in the absorptive direction under aerobic conditions, whereas under anaerobic conditions the flux ratio is unity[39]. These and other results, which will be published elsewhere[4], indicated that the quaternary ammonium ions are transported in the intestinal epithelium by two transport systems in series, where at least that located in the luminal membrane functions as a secretory pump transporting the ion against an electrochemical gradient towards the intestinal lumen. The elucidation of this mechanism provided an explanation for the strange absorptive behaviour of the quaternary compounds, whose absorption plateau now can be understood as the establishment of an equilibrium between absorption and secretion[40], and whose increase in absorption rate with increasing dose is due to the saturation of the opposing secretory mechanism.

Thus, the preparation of the isolated mucosa proved to be a valuable tool for the study of intestinal permeation mechanisms. The simplicity with which the ratio of transepithelial fluxes can be measured has not only substantiated the secretory mechanism for quaternary ammonium compounds, but furthermore revealed the existence of intestinal secretion of cardiac glycosides[1,41,42], and of organic anions such as phenol red among others[1,43]. Moreover, the accessibility of the basolateral membranes in combination with the possibility of performing steady-state experiments as well as influx and efflux measurements in the same preparation offers an unique possibility to study the individual properties of both faces of the mucosal epithelium and to help in the illumination of the black box, which the mucosal cell has remained for a long time.

SUMMARY

The mucosal epithelium of guinea-pig small intestine was isolated in a simple and rapid fashion and used as a separating membrane between two flux chambers. Flux coefficients for influx and efflux across the luminal as well as across the basolateral membranes of the mucosal cell were estimated both from transepithelial fluxes and tissue uptake under steady-state conditions and from influx and efflux measurements.

The passive permeabilities of the luminal and contraluminal membranes, per unit of serosal area, for water, thiourea and a number of drugs are almost identical.

For the transepithelial Na^+ fluxes in both directions, no significant differences could be observed under the experimental conditions; transepithelial permeability was 1.8×10^{-4} cm s^{-1}. ^{22}Na concentration in cell water reached a steady state of 23% and 20% of extracellular ^{22}Na concentration after administration from the luminal and blood sides respectively. Absence of net Na^+ flux is thus due to identical pump:leak ratios at both faces of the mucosal epithelium. Within 45 minutes, only two-thirds of the intracellular Na^+ exchanged with extracellular ^{22}Na. Efflux of ^{22}Na proceeds from at least three compartments, which are characterised by half-times of 0.3, 1.25 and 6 minutes. These half-times are independent of the preloading side. Identical half-times are observed for efflux towards the luminal and blood side. The fastest compartment can be explained by washout of chamber volume and extracellular sodium, the slowest one at least in part by rim washout. The 1.25-minute compartment can be ascribed to the sodium transport pool in view of its pool size, its flux coefficients and the shifting of the ratio between luminal and blood side efflux towards higher values by the addition of ouabain on the blood side.

The transepithelial flux of quaternary ammonium compounds is higher from the blood side to the luminal side than vice versa, revealing an intestinal secretory mechanism for these substances. This mechanism consists of two transport systems in series in the basolateral and luminal membranes of the mucosal cell, where at least the latter functions as a pump transporting the organic cations against an electrochemical gradient into the intestinal lumen. Similar secretory systems for cardiac glycosides and organic anions were uncovered by means of the isolated mucosa.

Acknowledgements

The author wishes to thank Dr G. Nell for his suggestions concerning the use of tissue adhesives in mounting epithelia.

The skilful technical assistance of Miss D. Grün, Miss D. Nitz, Mrs K. Stein, Mrs E. Mannheim and Mrs R. Warmer in performing the experiments, and the valuable help of Mrs E. Holz in typing the manuscript were greatly appreciated.

References

1. Lauterbach, F. O. (1975). Resorption und Sekretion von Arzneistoffen durch die Mucosaepithelien des Gastrointestinaltraktes. *Arzneim. Forsch.*, **25**, 479
2. Lauterbach, F. O. (1975). A simple preparation of isolated guinea-pig intestinal mucosa: General properties and passive permeabilities of luminal and basolateral membranes. (Submitted for publication)
3. Dickens, F. and Weil-Malherbe, H. (1941). Metabolism of normal and tumour tissue. 19. The metabolism of intestinal mucous membrane. *Biochem. J.*, **35**, 7
4. Turnheim, K. and Lauterbach, F. O. (1975). Absorption and secretion of monoquaternary ammonium compounds by the isolated intestinal mucosa. (In preparation)
5. Soergel, K. H., Whalen, G. E. and Harris, J. A. (1968). Passive movement of water and sodium across the human small intestinal mucosa. *J. Appl. Physiol.*, **24**, 40
6. Code, C. F., Bass, P., McClary, G. B., Newnum, R. L. and Orvis, A. L. (1960). Absorption of water, sodium and potassium in small intestine of dogs. *Amer. J. Physiol.*, **199**, 281
7. Visscher, M. B., Fetcher, E. S. jr., Carr, C. W., Gregor, H. P., Bushey, M. S. and Erickson Bakker, D. (1944). Isotopic tracer studies on the movement of water and ions between intestinal lumen and blood. *Amer. J. Physiol.*, **142**, 550
8. Berger, E., Kanzaki, G., Homer, M. A. and Steele, J. M. (1959). Simultaneous flux of sodium into and out of the dog intestine. *Amer. J. Physiol.*, **196**, 74
9. Heaton, J. W. and Code, C. F. (1969). Sodium–glucose relationships during intestinal sorption in dogs. *Amer. J. Physiol.*, **216**, 749
10. Visscher, M. B., Varco, R. H., Carr, C. W., Dean, R. B. and Erickson, D. (1944). Sodium and ion movement between the intestinal lumen and the blood. *Amer. J. Physiol.*, **141**, 488
11. Lifson, N., Gruman, L. M. and Levitt, D. G. (1968). Diffusive-convective models for intestinal absorption of D_2O. *Amer. J. Physiol.*, **215**, 444
12. Love, A. H. G., Mitchell, T. G. and Neptune, E. M. jr. (1965). Transport of sodium and water by rabbit ileum, *in vitro* and *in vivo*. *Nature (London)*, **206**, 1158
13. Taylor, A. E., Wright, E. M., Schultz, S. G. and Curran, P. F. (1968). Effect of sugars on ion fluxes in intestine. *Amer. J. Physiol.*, **214**, 836
14. Schultz, S. G. and Zalusky, R. (1963). Transmural potential difference, short-circuit current and sodium transport in isolated rabbit ileum. *Nature (London)*, **198**, 894
15. Ussing, H. H. and Andersen, B. (1955). The relation between solvent drag and active transport of ions. *Proc. 3rd Intern. Congr. Biochem.*, p. 434 (Brussels 1956) (New York: Academic Press)
16. Winne, D. (1966). Der Einfluss einiger Pharmaka auf die Darmdurchblutung und die Resorption tritiummarkierten Wassers aus dem Dünndarm der Ratte. *Naunyn-Schmiedeberg's Arch. Pharmak. Exp. Path.*, **254**, 199

17. Berger, E. Y., Pecikyan, F. R. and Kanzaki, G. (1968). Anesthetic gases and water structure. The effect of xenon on tritiated water flux across the gut. *J. Gen. Physiol.*, **52**, 876

18. Curran, P. F. and Solomon, A. K. (1957). Ion and water fluxes in the ileum of rats. *J. Gen. Physiol.*, **41**, 143

19. Curran, P. F. (1960). Na, Cl, and water transport by rat ileum *in vitro*. *J. Gen. Physiol.*, **43**, 1137

20. Baillien, M. and Schoffeniels, E. (1961). Origine des potentiels bioélectriques de l'épithélium intestinal de la tortue grecque. *Biochim. Biophys. Acta*, **53**, 537

21. Baillien, M. and Schoffeniels, E. (1967). Fluxes of inorganic ions across the isolated intestinal epithelium of the Greek tortoise. *Arch. Int. Physiol. Biochim.*, **75**, 754

22. Durbin, R. P., Frank, H. and Solomon, A. K. (1956). Water flow through frog gastric mucosa. *J. Gen. Physiol.*, **39**, 535

23. House, C. R. and Green, K. (1965). Ion and water transport in isolated intestine of the marine teleost, *Cottus scorpius*. *J. Exp. Biol.*, **42**, 177

24. Warren, R. (1939). Serosal and mucosal dimensions at different levels of the dog's small intestine. *Anat. Rec.*, **75**, 427

25. Fisher, R. B. and Parsons, D. S. (1950). The gradient of mucosal surface area in the small intestine of the rat. *J. Anat.*, **84**, 272

26. Schultz, S. G., Fuisz, R. E. and Curran, P. F. (1966). Amino acid and sugar transport in rabbit ileum. *J. Gen. Physiol.*, **49**, 849

27. Faelli, A., Esposito, G. and Capraro, V. (1966). Intracellular concentration of sodium and glucose correlated with transport phenomena. *Arch. Sci. Biol. (Bologna)*, **50**, 234

28. Csáky, T. Z. and Ho, P. M. (1966). Effect of mucosal potassium on the intestinal glucose transport. *Pflügers Arch. Ges. Physiol.*, **291**, 63

29. Armstrong, W. McD. (1975). Electrophysiology of sodium transport by epithelial cells of the small intestine. In T. Z. Csáky (ed.). *Intestinal Absorption and Malabsorption*, p. 45. (New York: Ravens Press)

30. Schultz, S, G. and Curran, P. E. (1968). Intestinal absorption of sodium chloride and water. In: Code, C. F. (ed.). *Handbook of Physiology, Section 6: Alimentary Canal, Vol. III: Intestinal Absorption*. p. 1245. (Washington, D.C.: American Physiological Society)

31. Gilles-Baillien, M. and Schoffeniels, E. (1967). Bioelectric potentials in the intestinal epithelium of the Greek tortoise. *Comp. Biochem. Physiol.*, **23**, 95

32. Powell, D. W., Binder, H. J. and Curran, P. F. (1972). Electrolyte secretion by the guinea-pig ileum *in vitro*. *Amer. J. Physiol.*, **223**, 531

33. Bray, G. A. (1960). A simple efficient liquid scintillator for counting aqueous solutions in a liquid scintillation counter. *Analyt. Biochem.*, **1**, 279

34. Helman, S. I. and Miller, D. A. (1971). *In vitro* techniques for avoiding edge damage in studies of frog skin. *Science*, **173**, 146

35. Finn, A. L. and Rockoff, M. L. (1971). The kinetics of sodium transport in the toad bladder. I. Determination of the transport pool. *J. Gen. Physiol.*, **57**, 326

36. Levine, R. R. (1961). The influence of the intraluminal intestinal milieu on absorption of an organic cation and an anionic agent. *J. Pharmacol. Exp. Therap.*, **131**, 328

37. Levine, R. R. and Pelikan, E. W. (1961). The influence of experimental procedures and dose in the intestinal absorption of an onium compound, benzomethamine. *J. Pharmacol. Exp. Therap.*, **131**, 319

38. Lauterbach, F. O. (1970). Werden quaternäre Ammoniumverbindungen über einen enteralen Sekretionsmechanismus resorbiert? *Naunyn-Schmiedeberg's Arch. Pharmak.*, **226**, 388

39. Turnheim, K. and Lauterbach, F. O. (1971). Intestinal absorption and secretion of quaternary ammonium compounds. *Acta Pharmacol. Toxicol.*, **29** (Suppl. 4), 60

40. Turnheim, K. and Lauterbach, F. O. (1972). Intestinal transport of quaternary ammonium compounds *in vivo*. *Naunyn-Schmiedeberg's Arch. Pharmak.*, **274**, R 118

41. Lauterbach, F. O. (1970). Untersuchungen über den Mechanismus der Permeation cardiotoner Steroide durch die Mucosa des Dünndarmes — ein Beitrag zur Theorie der Resorption von Pharmaka. *Habilitationsschrift, Bochum/Essen*

42. Lauterbach, F. O. (1971). Absorption of cardiac glycosides. *Acta Pharmacol. Toxicol.*, **29** (Suppl. 4), 80

43. Sund, R. B. S. and Lauterbach, F. O. (1975). Secretion of a sulfonic acid by the isolated mucosa of guinea-pig small intestine. (In preparation)

44. Schoffeniels, E. (1957). An isolated single electroplax preparation. II. Improved preparation for studying ion flux. *Biochim. Biophys. Acta*, **26**, 585

45. Dost, F. H. (1968). *Grundlagen der Pharmakokinetik.* (Stuttgart: Georg Thieme Verlag)

Appendix

Efflux coefficients can be obtained by the following procedures (for a detailed description, see, for example[35,44,45]). Consider:

K_{ij} the transfer coeffcient (min^{-1}) from compartment i to compartment j.
$m_{2(0)}$ the amount in the (cellular) compartment 2 at start of the efflux period.
$m_{1(t)}$, $m_{1(\infty)}$ the amount in compartment 1 at t and infinite min after start of the efflux period.

Since substrate is released simultaneously from compartment 2 to compartment 1 and 3, the appearance rate (amount/unit time) in compartment 1 is

$$F_{21} = \frac{dm_1}{dt} = K_{21} \cdot m_{2(0)} \cdot e^{-(K_{21}+K_{23})t} \tag{1}$$

or

$$\log F_{21(t)} = \log (K_{21} \cdot m_{2(0)}) - 0.434 (K_{21} + K_{23})t \tag{2}$$
$$= \log F_{21(0)} - 0.434 (K_{21} + K_{23})t$$

For the amount released to compartment 1 until t one gets

$$m_{1(t)} = m_{1(\infty)} - m_{1(\infty)} \cdot e^{-(K_{21}+K_{23})t} \tag{3}$$

or

$$\log (m_{1(\infty)} - m_{1(t)}) = \log m_{1(\infty)} - 0.434 (K_{21} + K_{23})t \tag{4}$$

Similar equations, of course, are valid for efflux to compartment 3.

Thus, either by semilogarithmic plotting of the amount released per unit time or the difference between the total amount released at infinite time and time t to compartment 1 (or 3), one gets straight lines whose slopes represent the sum of the two transfer coefficients and whose ordinate intercepts give the initial appearance rate or the portion of the tissue pool released to the respective side.

Flux coefficients (k_{ij}) are obtained from the transfer coefficients by introducing the membrane area A (which is assumed to be the area of the window between both chambers — 0.2 cm^2 in the present paper) and the volume V of tissue compartment 2, thus

$$k_{ij} = K_{ij} \cdot \frac{V}{A} \qquad (5)$$

4

Discussion Paper on

Na$^+$ Compartmentation in the Jejunal Mucosa of the Tortoise

M. Gilles-Baillien

Laboratory of General and Comparative Biochemistry,
University of Liège

It was suggested in 1961 that in the jejunal mucosa of the tortoise, *Testudo hermanni hermanni* Gmelin, active transport mechanisms for Na$^+$ exist not only at the serosal border but also at the mucosal pole, both of which contribute to the maintenance of a low intracellular sodium concentration[1]. On the other hand, in an attempt to determine the extracellular space of our preparation of jejunal mucosa, Na$^+$ exchange kinetics were studied[2]. The complex exponential curve obtained by measuring the radioactivity remaining in the preparation as a function of time (when submitted to washout) can be decomposed into three simple exponentials, the fastest one corresponding to an extracellular space of a volume identical to the inulin space of this preparation. The other two exponentials are indicative of two distinct Na$^+$ pools exchanging Na$^+$ at very different rates, thus suggesting the presence of two compartments which could be representative of the two cell types of the tortoise jejunal mucosa: enterocytes and goblet cells. Moreover a 20% fraction of the total Na$^+$ of the preparation of jejunal mucosa appears to be inexchangeable[3]. Recently the following experiments have been performed: jejunal mucosa was loaded with radioactive Na$^+$ only across the mucosal surface and submitted to washout of both mucosal and serosal surfaces.

Conversely in other experiments only the serosal surface was incubated with radioactive Na$^+$ and again the mucosal and serosal effluxes were measured during the washout. Figure *4.1* shows the results of such experiments. Briefly, they indicate that Na$^+$ goes into different compartments depending on whether it comes from the mucosal or from the serosal saline. At least four compartments can be identified besides the fast exchanging extracellular ones, all four being quantitatively important. Two of them are loaded when measuring transepithelial influx, the two others being concerned only when measuring transepithelial outflux. Transfer coefficients can be better estimated by summing up the activity washed out and the activity remaining in the cell at the end of the experiment[4] as shown in Figure 4.2. Moreover a direct estimate of the amount of Na^+ in the different compartments can be obtained. The curve with open circles is a speculative summation of the two

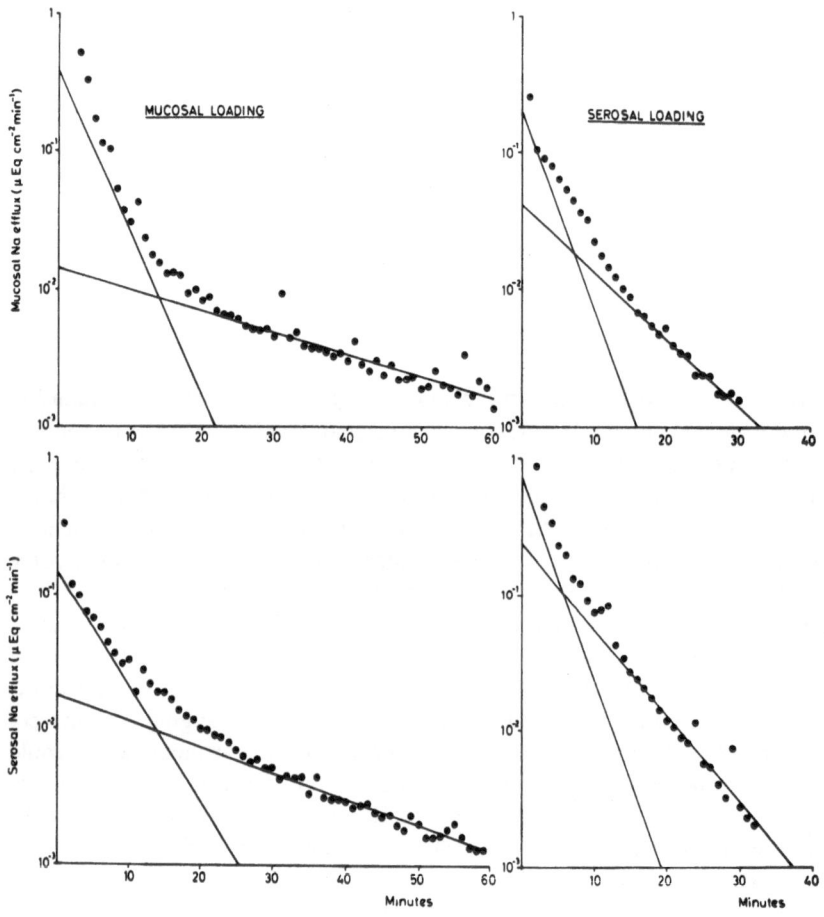

Figure 4.1 Na^+ effluxes from the jejunal mucosa of the tortoise. Washout experiments after loading with radioactive Na^+ either through the mucosal or through the serosal border

others, which causes two compartments to disappear: a slowly exchanging compartment masks a rapid one, and two compartments appear as a single one because of too similar transfer coefficients. It is also striking to note that this speculative curve reproduces fairly exactly the curves obtained previously by directly measuring the remaining activity in a preparation which has been loaded simultaneously from both sides[2]. Finally when the amounts of Na^+ found in the four compartments are pooled, they do not exceed the total intracellular exchangeable fraction of Na^+ determined independently[3], thus indicating that little overlap if any exists between the four compartments.

These results provide evidence that 'absorption' and 'secretion' of Na^+ could involve distinct pathways, passing through different cellular pools.

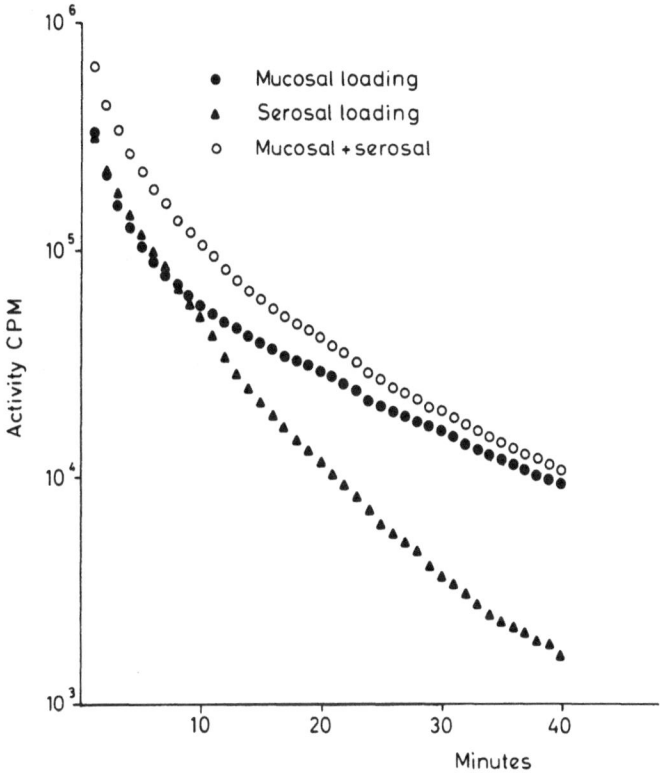

Figure 4.2   Radioactivity remaining in the jejunal mucosa during washout

References

1. Baillien, M. and Schoffeniels, E. (1961). Origine des potentiels bioélectriques de l'épithélium intestinal de la tortue grecque. *Biochim. Biophys. Acta*, **53,** 357

2. Gilles-Baillien, M. (1968). The extracellular space of the isolated intestinal epithelium of the Greek tortoise. *Arch. Int. Physiol. Biochim.*, **76,** 731.

3. Gilles-Baillien, M. (1972). Inexchangeable fraction of the cationic content in the intestinal epithelium of the tortoise *Testudo hermanni hermanni* Gmelin. *Arch. Int. Physiol. Biochim.*, **80,** 789

4. Schoffeniels, E. (1957). An isolated single electroplax preparation. II. Improved preparation for studying ion flux. *Biochim. Biophys. Acta*, **26,** 585

Discussion 4

Parsons: Have you any evidence that the size of the extracellular space available to PEG from the blood side in the guinea-pig mucosa depends upon the rate of sodium pumping? For example, it is smaller when the tissue is loaded with PEG in the presence of ouabain?

Lauterbach: This question cannot be answered from the present experiments, since ouabain was only added to the solutions during the efflux period. Furthermore, the mucosae were briefly washed with icecold mannitol after preloading.

Robinson: I should like to congratulate Dr Lauterbach on his technically brilliant work. His technique, which was first published several years ago (Lauterbach, *Naunyn-Schmiedebergs Arch. Pharmak. Exp. Pathol.*, **260**, 167, 1968), is probably more delicate than any other that we shall be hearing about at this meeting, and the results that he has shown us testify to its wide applicability in his hands. One comment that I should like to make is that he has shown, in a system that is hardly hindered by diffusion barriers and such inconveniences of cruder methodology, that the two unidirectional fluxes of sodium across guinea-pig ileum are almost identical. Many of us here have tried to measure net ion fluxes across the small intestine and have encountered the tremendous disadvantage inherent in the fact that any net flux is very small in comparison with the two unidirectional fluxes. This is why I, for one, have started to use the colon as a model for ion transport, since this disadvantage is absent in that tissue.

5
Polarity of Epithelial Cells in Relation to Transepithelial Transport in Kidney and Intestine

R. KINNE and H. MURER,

Max-Planck-Institut für Biophysik, Frankfurt/Main

INTRODUCTION

Epithelia are characterized by a morphological polarity of their cells. This polarity consists mainly of a different arrangement of the plasma membranes at the two cell poles. In the renal proximal tubule and in the small intestine, the apical plasma membrane or brush border is composed of numerous microvilli. At the basal pole of the cell, interdigitations of the cell occur to form the basal infoldings, which are more pronounced in the proximal tubule than in the small intestine.

This morphological polarity was considered relatively early to reflect a functional polarity of the epithelial cell, and it was postulated that dissimilarities in the properties of the apical and the basal–lateral plasma membranes form the basis for the vectorial transport performed by these cells.

The direct investigation of the transport properties of the apical and basal–lateral plasma membranes however was hindered to a different extent by the inaccessibility of the cell surfaces to experimental manipulations. In the intestine, studies on the properties of the brush border membrane were relatively easy to perform because the size of the lumen allowed perfusion of

Abbreviations

Carbonyl cyanide *p*-fluoromethoxy-phenylhydrazone, CF-CCP
N-2-hydroxyethylpiperazine-N-2-ethane-sulphonic acid, HEPES
Tris(hydroxymethyl)aminomethane, Tris
2(N-morpholino)-ethane-sulphonic acid, MES

the intact gut[1,2] and the use of the everted sac technique[3-5]. Moreover, in tissue preparations such as intestinal rings[3-5], the luminal surface of the cells is in direct contact with the incubation medium, and thus mainly processes taking place at the apical cell pole are studied. The approach to the contraluminal cell face was complicated because the epithelium is covered at the basal pole by various overlying cell layers. The isolation of epithelial cells after a selective inhibition of transport processes located at the luminal face, as developed by Bihler and Cybulsky[6], provided the first preparation of intact intestinal cells in which the properties of the contraluminal membrane could be studied.

In the kidney, sophisticated techniques had to be developed which make it possible to investigate separately the two cell surfaces of the tubule by microperfusion of the tubule combined with simultaneous perfusion of the peritubular capillaries[7,8]. A similar preparation was developed by Burg *et al.* where segments of the nephron are isolated from rabbit kidney and perfused *in vitro*[9]. A differentiation between luminal and contraluminal transport steps was also attempted by the multiple indicator dilution technique[10-12]. In essence, this technique consists of the comparison of renal transit time of the substance tested with that of the non-reabsorbed, non-secreted marker, inulin. In renal tissue slices and non-perfused isolated tubules, the contraluminal faces of the epithelial cells are predominantly, if not exclusively, exposed; indeed the most ideal preparation for studies of peritubular transport processes is the isolated flounder tubule which forms cyst-like structures[13].

Although the technical difficulties of approaching the luminal and contraluminal cell surfaces separately have now been overcome, several problems remained unsolved. In the cell, the relative rate of uptake of monosaccharides, for example, depends not only on the properties of the cell membrane-bound transport system but is also influenced by intracellular metabolism and by the intracellular concentration of compounds which can act as counterflow substrates for the transport system under study. Moreover, the question of the kind of energy which supports the transport, that is, whether a 'primary active' or 'secondary active' transport is involved in the transepithelial transfer, is difficult to clarify in the intact cell.

In order to obtain further insight into the molecular mechanism of transmembranal transport and to avoid the above-mentioned difficulties, methods were developed to isolate the plasma membranes of the apical and basal cell poles separately and to study their transport properties in the form of membrane vesicles. In the vesicular system, the characteristics of the membrane-bound transport systems can be studied without interference from intracellular metabolism under conditions where the compositions of both the intra- and extra-vesicular spaces are well defined.

The present contribution will deal with the isolation of brush border microvilli and basal–lateral plasma membranes from kidney and intestine and will report mainly on the role of sodium in amino acid and monosaccharide translocation across the two membranes. Thereby an attempt will be made to distinguish between the two hypotheses which have been proposed to account for the fact than Na$^+$ is a required factor in transepithelial active transport. Both Csáky[14] and Tucker and Kimmich[15] have suggested that a direct input of metabolic energy is required for Na$^+$-dependent transport, e.g. via ATP hydrolysis by means of a Na$^+$-stimulated ATPase. A second model, the Na$^+$ gradient hypothesis[3,4], envisages a mechanism whereby Na$^+$ movement down a concentration difference provides the driving force for 'secondary active' transport.

Isolation of luminal and contraluminal plasma membranes

In the pioneering work of Miller and Crane[16], two criteria were used to identify the brush border fragments during their isolation: Their morphological appearance and their high content of hydrolases such as alkaline phosphatase

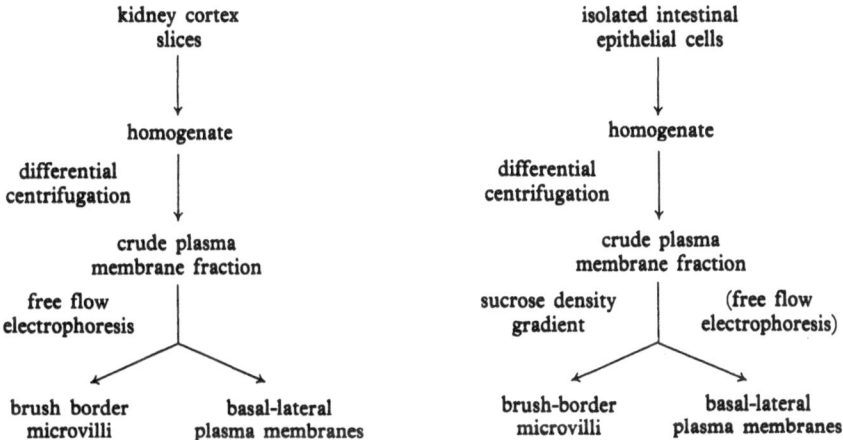

Figure 5.1 Isolation scheme for the separation of luminal (brush border-microvilli) and contraluminal (basal–lateral plasma membranes) borders of renal and intestinal epithelial cells

and sucrase. These two enzymes can be considered as markers for the microvillus membranes and were also used by other authors who isolated brush border fragments from kidney[17-25] and intestine[26-31].

Plasma membranes devoid of alkaline phosphatase but with a high specific activity of Na$^+$-K$^+$-ATPase could also be isolated from kidney[25,32–34] and intestine[27,28,30,31,35]. These membranes are most probably derived from the basal pole of the epithelial cells, since an asymmetric distribution of the Na$^+$-K$^+$-ATPase could be demonstrated in the renal proximal tubule by microdissection studies combined with quantitative histochemistry[36] and in the intestine by autoradiographic studies on ouabain binding[37].

The transport data reported below have mainly been obtained with membrane vesicles isolated from the luminal and contraluminal cell poles simultaneously under identical conditions, following the isolation scheme given in Figure 5.1. The first prerequisite in membrane isolation is to start with a cell population that is as homogeneous as possible, in order that the isolated plasma membranes are defined with respect to their cellular origin. In the kidney therefore, cortex slices which contain predominantly proximal tubular epithelial cells are used as the starting material. In the small intestine, epithelial cells are isolated prior to the homogenisation, so that, in contrast to intestinal scrapings, mucus and crypt cells are excluded from the homogenate. From the homogenate, a crude plasma membrane fraction is prepared by differential centrifugation which is characterized by a 7–10-fold increase in the specific activities of the brush border marker enzymes and by a 6–8 fold increase in those of the basal–lateral plasma membranes. The plasma membrane fraction is almost devoid of intracellular organelles such as nuclei, lysosomes, mitochondria and endoplasmic reticula. The separation of luminal

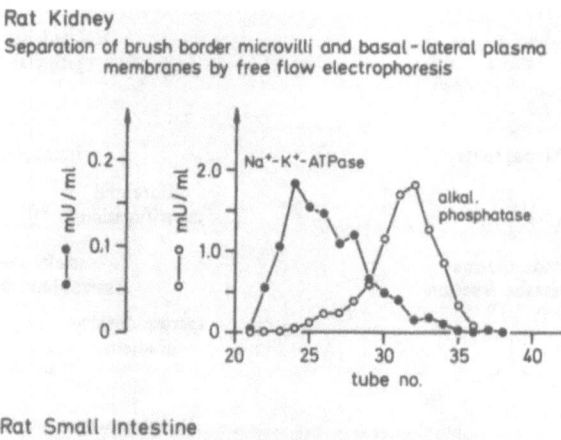

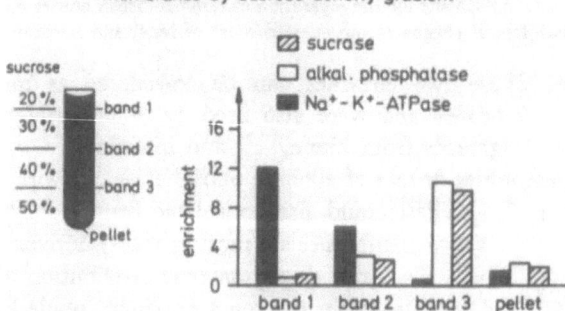

Figure 5.2 Separation of brush border microvilli and basal–lateral plasma membranes from renal cortex by free flow electrophoresis (upper part) and from intestinal epithelial cells by density gradient centrifugation. The distribution of the marker enzyme for brush border membranes (alkaline phosphatase) and for basal–lateral plasma membranes (Na^+-K^+-ATPase) is given on the figure

from contraluminal membranes is then achieved by a further purification step. In the kidney, the two membranes could so far only be separated by free flow electrophoresis[25], whereas in the intestine sucrose density gradient centrifugation also gave a good resolution of the two membranes[31]. In Figure 5.2, the distribution of alkaline phosphatase and Na^+-K^+-ATPase after free flow electrophoresis of renal plasma membranes and after sucrose density gradient centrifugation of intestinal plasma membranes is shown.

In the electrophoresis (upper part of Figure 5.2), renal as well as intestinal basal–lateral plasma membranes[30] show a higher electrophoretic mobility than the brush border microvilli. In the sucrose density gradient, the apparent buoyant density of the intestinal basal–lateral plasma membrane vesicles is lower than that of the brush border microvillous vesicles. The same is observed with renal membranes[38], but the differences were not large enough to give a satisfactory separation; it was therefore necessary to use the free flow electrophoresis.

SOLUTE TRANSPORT IN BRUSH BORDER MEMBRANES

Uptake of D-glucose and L-glucose

In principle, the sugar transport into the vesicles is measured as the uptake of labelled substrates by the isolated membranes. The transport is terminated by

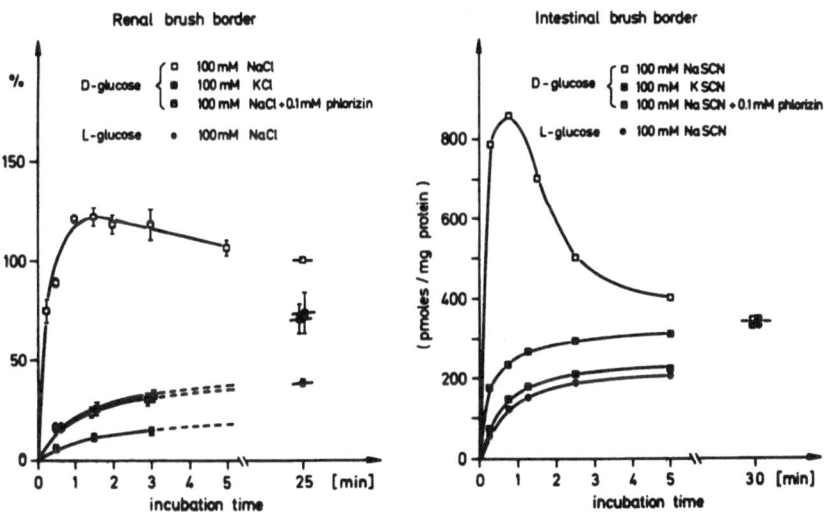

Figure 5.3 Sugar transport by brush border microvilli isolated from rat kidney cortex and intestinal epithelial cells. The incubation medium contained D-[^{3}H]glucose (1 mM), 100 mM mannitol, 1 mM HEPES–Tris (pH 7.5) and the indicated salts. For the renal brush border microvilli, the values are expressed as a percentage of the amount of D-glucose taken up in the presence of sodium chloride at equilibrium; for the intestinal brush border microvilli, the values are given in pmol/mg protein. Renal membranes were isolated by free flow electrophoresis and intestinal membranes by the method of Hopfer et al.[29]

dilution of the sample with icecold buffer and collection of the membranes by Millipore filtration[29].

The radioactivity retained by the filters is determined and considered as the amount taken up by the membranes.

When isolated brush border microvilli are incubated with the two stereoisomers of glucose, a different time-course of uptake is obtained[39,40] (Figure 5.3). D-glucose entry is more rapid than that of L-glucose, both in the renal and intestinal brush border membranes. The differentiation between the two isomers is especially pronounced when sodium is present in the incubation medium. Phlorizin inhibits the initial rate of uptake of D-glucose but does not markedly influence the equilibrium value. Stereospecificity, phlorizin sensitivity and sodium dependence are properties observed for transepithelial sugar transport in the kidney[7] and the intestine[4]. Therefore it can be concluded that the glucose transport system found in isolated brush border microvilli is identical with the glucose transport system operating *in vivo* in the luminal cell membrane.

Distinction between binding of sugar to the membrane and sugar transport into an intravesicular space

Figure 5.4 shows the equilibrium uptake of labelled D-glucose by aliquots of the same membrane preparation suspended in media with different

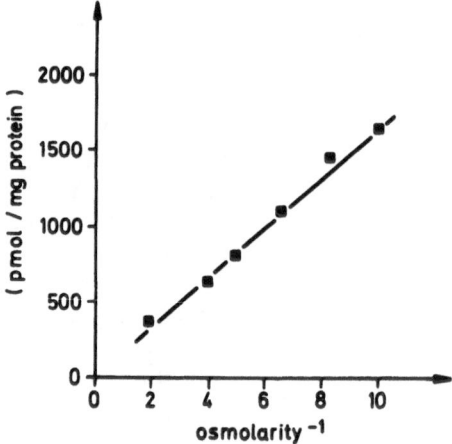

Figure 5.4 Effect of medium osmolarity on D-glucose uptake by isolated brush border microvilli (intestine). Preparation of membranes (in 100 mM cellobiose, 1 mM HEPES adjusted with Tris to pH 7.5, and 0.1 mM MgSO$_4$) as described by Hopfer *et al*.[29]. Uptake of D-glucose was measured in aliquots of the same membrane preparation from media with the following final composition: NaSCN (25 mM), HEPES–Tris (1mM), MgSO$_4$ (0.1 mM), D-(^{3}H)-glucose (1 mM) and cellobiose to give the indicated osmolarity (shown as inverse osmolarity). Length of incubation: 10 minutes

osmolarities. The change in the osmolarity is achieved by increasing concentrations of the impermeable solute cellobiose. This experiment demonstrates that glucose uptake is inversely proportional to the medium osmolarity. On extrapolation to infinity (zero on the inverse osmolarity scale), no uptake is observed. Thus, the membrane vesicles behave as predicted from osmotic considerations. Therefore, under the conditions of these experiments, the measured substrate uptake can be accounted for completely by transport into an osmotically reactive space and does not represent binding to the membranes. Other permeant sugars or neutral amino acids show identical behaviour.

Cation requirements of glucose transport

Table 5.1 demonstrates the effect of various cations on glucose transport by intestinal and renal brush border membranes. Sodium stimulates D-glucose uptake maximally. Among the other cations, only lithium has a limited ability to

Table 5.1 Effect of cations on glucose transport by brush-border microvilli

Cation	Renal brush border	Intestinal brush border
Na$^+$	100	100
K$^+$	31	42
Li$^+$	26	67
Rb$^+$	21	—
Cs$^+$	30	—
Choline	23	39
Tris	16	41

The medium contained D-[^{3}H]glucose (1 mM), 100 mM mannitol and 100 mM of the chloride salts of the indicated cations. Length of incubation was one minute for renal brush border and ten seconds for intestinal brush border. The values are expressed as percent of the transport observed in the presence of 100 mM NaCl.

replace sodium. This effect of lithium is smaller in the renal brush border membranes than in those of the intestinal brush border. Similar results have been obtained with galactose and alanine in intestinal brush border vesicles[41,42] and with phenylalanine in renal brush border membranes[43]. Since replacement of potassium, rubidium, caesium and choline by iso-osmotic mannitol gave identical results, it can be concluded that only sodium and to a small extent lithium can stimulate glucose and neutral amino acid transport by isolated brush border vesicles.

Effect of the sodium gradient

It is known that sodium increases the affinity of sugar and amino acid transport systems[4,7,8] for their substrates and that the intracellular accumulation of these compounds is dependent on the presence of a sodium gradient[4,44].

In isolated membrane vesicles, the uptake can be studied separately under gradient conditions and under conditions where all ions are in equilibrium. As shown in Figure 5.5, the uptake of D-glucose is enhanced even in the absence of a sodium gradient indicating a direct interaction of sodium and the glucose transport system. The presence of a sodium gradient across the membranes stimulates the initial rate of D-glucose uptake and leads in addition to a transient accumulation of D-glucose inside the brush border vesicles. The overshooting non-electrolyte uptake in this experiment was obtained in the absence of ATP as an energy source and in membrane vesicles which are virtually free of Na^+-K^+-ATPase. These results are therefore not consistent with

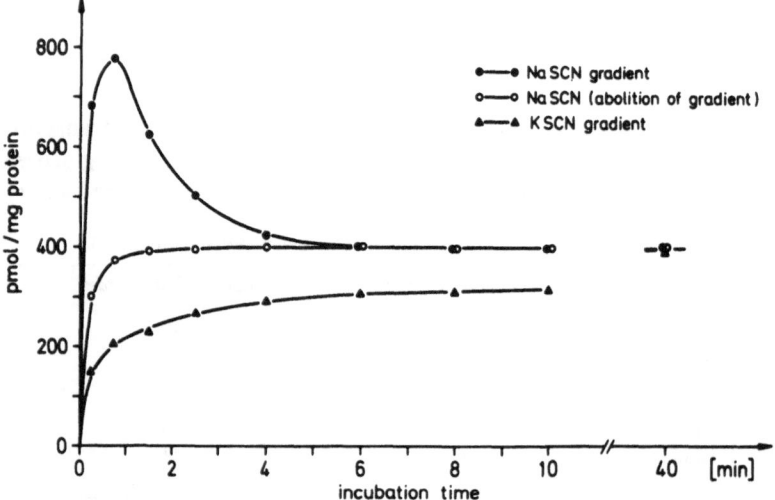

Figure 5.5 Effect of a sodium gradient on D-glucose uptake by isolated brush border microvilli. The membranes were prepared, as described by Hopfer *et al.*[29], in a buffer containing 100 mM D-mannitol, 0.1 mM $MgSO_4$ and 1 mM HEPES–Tris (pH 7.5). D-glucose uptake was initiated by the addition of the membranes to the incubation medium which had the following final compositions: 1 mM D-[U-14C]glucose, 100 mM D-mannitol, 0.1 mM $MgSO_4$, and 1 mM HEPES–Tris (pH 7.5) with either 100 mM NaSCN or 100 mM KSCN. The NaSCN gradient was abolished by preincubation of the membranes with 100 mM NaSCN for 10 minutes at 25 °C; D-glucose uptake was initiated subsequently in 100 mM NaSCN as indicated above

any hypothesis assuming a direct input of metabolic energy into active sodium dependent D-glucose transport[14,15] and are in agreement with the sodium gradient hypothesis[4].

Influence of membrane potential on sodium-dependent glucose and amino acid transport

Cotransport of a non-electrolyte with sodium is *per se* an electrogenic transport except when it is coupled to the stoichiometric movement of an anion in the same direction or of a cation in the opposite direction. Such electrogenicity can either be demonstrated directly by electrical measurements or indirectly by studying the influence of the membrane potential on the transport of the non-electrolyte. Three approaches were chosen in the following experiments to alter the membrane potential[45]. Firstly, the effect of anions on glucose uptake was studied. Replacement of chloride by the relatively impermeable anion sulphate should decrease or even reverse the membrane potential of the vesicles which in the presence of a sodium chloride gradient, is most probably inside negative. Replacement of chloride by the lipophilic anion thiocyanate should increase the membrane potential. As shown in Table 5.2, the initial rate of D-glucose uptake is greatest in the presence of a sodium thiocyanate gradient and

Table 5.2 Effect of anions on glucose transport by brush border microvilli

Salt		Renal brush border	Intestinal brush border
NaCl	100 mM	100	100
NaSCN	100 mM	179	208
Na_2SO_4	50 mM	43	75
KCl	100 mM	—	43
KSCN	100 mM	—	42
K_2SO_4	50 mM	—	41

The medium contained D-[^{3}H]glucose (1 mM), 100 mM mannitol and the salts indicated on the table. Length of incubation was 15 seconds for renal brush border and 10 seconds for intestinal brush border. The values are expressed as percent of the transport observed in the presence of 100 mM NaCl.

inhibited in the presence of a sodium sulphate gradient[39,45]. This indicates an electrogenic transfer of sugars together with sodium across the brush border membrane. It should be mentioned in this context that these differences are not observed[41] under equilibrium conditions for the sodium salts. Therefore the anions can be presumed not to interact directly with the glucose transport system. This is consistent with results obtained earlier with intact cells[46].

Valinomycin is known to increase the electrical conductance of lipid bilayers and biological membranes[47] in the presence of potassium. This compound can also be used to modify the membrane potential. Figure 5.6 presents the results of D-glucose uptake by membrane vesicles preloaded with potassium. The addition of valinomycin produced an overshoot in D-glucose uptake two to three times greater than that at equilibrium. In the absence of K^+, valinomycin has no effect on D-glucose uptake[45]. Owing to the concentration gradient for potassium, an increased inside negative diffusion potential is formed in the presence of the ionophore, since potassium flux via valinomycin is known to be an electrogenic process[47]. The efflux of potassium has to coincide with the flux of another cation because of the requirement of overall electroneutrality. These results strongly suggest that the sodium dependent D-glucose transport proceeds via an electrogenic mode of translocation. In Figure 5.7, a similar experiment is shown for phenylalanine transport in renal brush border membrane vesicles[43].

Figure 5.8 shows experiments which are analogous to those presented in Figures 5.6 and 5.7, except that uncoupler and proton-preloaded vesicles were used. Uncouplers are known to increase the proton conductance of the membranes[47]. Brush border membranes were preloaded by osmotic shock with a pH 5.25 buffer followed by an incubation at pH 7.5 with D-glucose and Na_2SO_4. As seen in Figure 5.8, an accumulation of six times the equilibrium level is observed when the proton ionophore CF–CCP (carbonyl cyanide p-fluoromethoxy-phenylhydrazone) is present[45]. Similar experiments have been

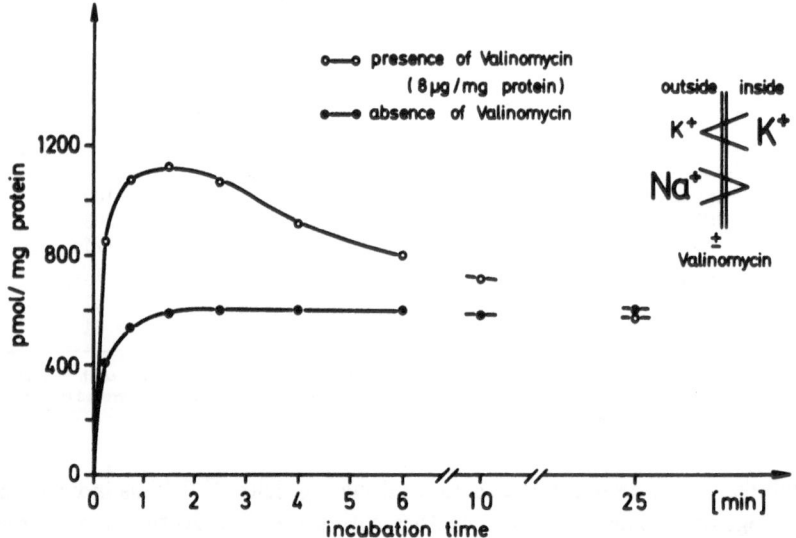

Figure 5.6 Effect of a potassium diffusion potential on D-glucose uptake by isolated brush-border microvilli (intestine). Brush-border membranes were prepared, as described by Hopfer *et al.*[29], in a medium containing 500 mM D-mannitol, 0.1 mM $MgSO_4$, and 1 mM HEPES–Tris (pH 7.5) and preloaded with K_2SO_4 by mixing 1 volume of membrane suspension with 6 volumes of a solution containing 50 mM K_2SO_4, 1 mM HEPES–Tris (pH 7.5), and 0.1 mM $MgSO_4$. The membranes were subsequently collected by centrifugation and resuspended in a solution containing 100 mM D-mannitol, 50 mM K_2SO_4, 0.1 mM $MgSO_4$, and 1 mM HEPES–Tris (pH 7.5). D-glucose uptake was initiated by addition of 1 volume of suspension to 8 volumes of incubation medium with the following final composition: 100 mM D-mannitol, 50 mM Na_2SO_4, 0.1 mM $MgSO_4$, 1.0 mM D-[U^{14}C]glucose, 5.6 mM K_2SO_4, and 1 mM HEPES–Tris (pH 7.5) with or without valinomycin

carried out with amino acids in intestinal and renal brush border membrane preparations[42,43]. The above experiments with such structurally unrelated compounds as SCN^-, valinomycin, and uncouplers all point to the same conclusion: that a positive charge, presumably Na^+, is translocated together with D-glucose or L-phenylalanine by the carrier across the brush border membrane; in other words, that these translocation mechanisms are electrogenic processes. This assumption is also supported by electrophysiological experiments performed in the small intestine[48–53] and the renal proximal tubule[54–56].

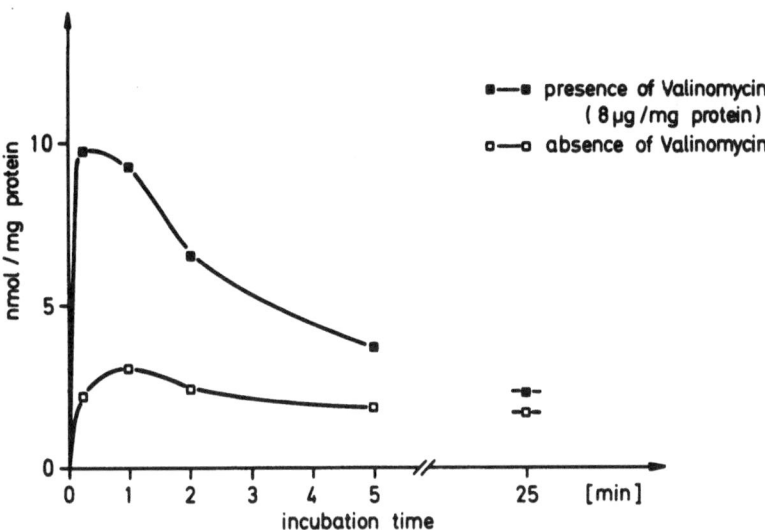

Figure 5.7 Effect of a potassium diffusion potential on L-phenylalanine uptake by isolated brush border microvilli (kidney). Brush border membranes were prepared as described by Heidrich et al.[25], and were preloaded with K_2SO_4 as in Figure 5.6. L-phenylalanine uptake was initiated by addition of 1 volume of membrane suspension to 8 volumes of incubation medium with the final composition: 100 mM D-mannitol, 50 mM Na_2SO_4, 1 mM L-(^3H)-phenylalanine, 5.6 mM K_2SO_4 and 5 mM HEPES–Tris (pH 7.5) with or without valinomycin

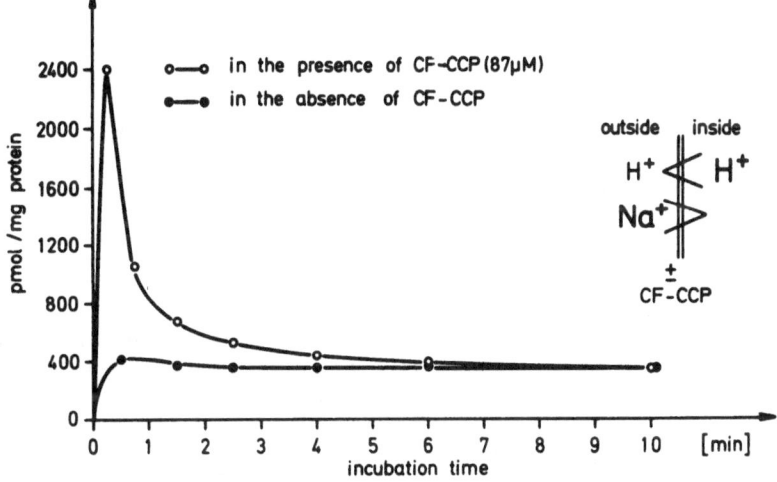

Figure 5.8 Effect of a proton diffusion potential on D-glucose uptake by isolated brush border microvilli (intestine). Brush border membranes were prepared, as described by Hopfer et al.[29], preloaded, and resuspended as in Figure 5.6, but with 50 mM MES–Tris (50 mM MES adjusted with Tris-hydroxide to pH 5.25) instead of K_2SO_4, for the experiments with a pH gradient. D-glucose uptake was initiated by addition of 1 volume of membrane suspension to 8 volumes of incubation medium. The final composition of the medium was 100 mM D-mannitol, 1 mM D-[$U^{14}C$]glucose, 0.1 mM $MgSO_4$, 50 mM Na_2SO_4, 50 mM HEPES–Tris (pH 7.5) and 5.6 mM MES–Tris (final pH 7.5) with or without CF–CCP

SOLUTE TRANSPORT IN BASAL–LATERAL PLASMA MEMBRANES

When basal–lateral plasma membranes were incubated with either labelled D-glucose or L-glucose, different time-courses of uptake were obtained (Figure 5.9). Glucose transport by basal–lateral plasma membrane vesicles was stimulated only slightly by Na^+. Moreover, phlorizin was less effective as an inhibitor in this membrane fraction[30,39]. Stereospecificity, saturability and

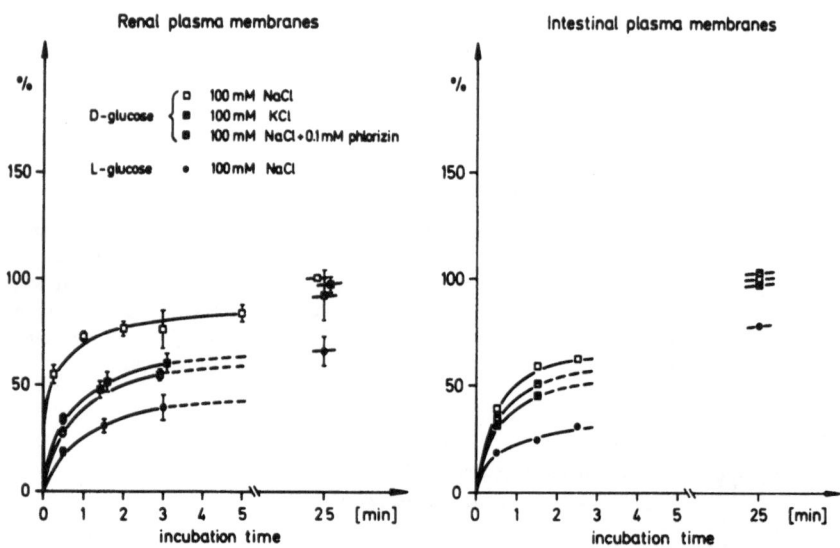

Figure 5.9 Sugar transport by isolated basal–lateral plasma membranes from rat kidney cortex and intestinal epithelial cells. Experimental conditions as in Figure 5.3. The values are expressed as percentages of the amount of D-glucose taken up in the presence of NaCl at equilibrium

counterflow can also be demonstrated for basal–lateral plasma membranes. In Figure 5.10, counterflow experiments with L-valine and D-glucose in brush border membranes and in basal–lateral plasma membranes of small intestinal epithelial cells are presented. L-valine transport was stimulated more than three-fold in the L-valine-preloaded membranes in both the brush border and the basal–lateral fractions compared with the mannitol-preloaded membranes. Similarly, D-glucose uptake was elevated more than five-fold over the control preparation in D-glucose-preloaded brush border vesicles and three-fold in D-glucose-preloaded basal–lateral membranes[40]. In contrast to the glucose or amino acid transport systems in the brush border membranes, different cations or anions or artifically imposed diffusion potentials do not exert a noticeable effect in the basal–lateral plasma membranes[40]. In addition, the D-glucose transport system in the basal–lateral plasma membranes seems to differ from that of the brush border membrane with respect to its different sensitivity towards inhibitors. Phlorizin is more effective than phloretin in inhibiting D-glucose transport in brush border membranes, while phloretin is more potent in the basal–lateral plasma membranes[39,40]. The relative inhibitory potency of phloretin and phlorizin might suggest that the D-glucose transport across the basal–lateral plasma membranes resembles that of the 'facilitated diffusion' system in erythrocytes or other cell types containing a Na^+-independent glucose transport system[57].

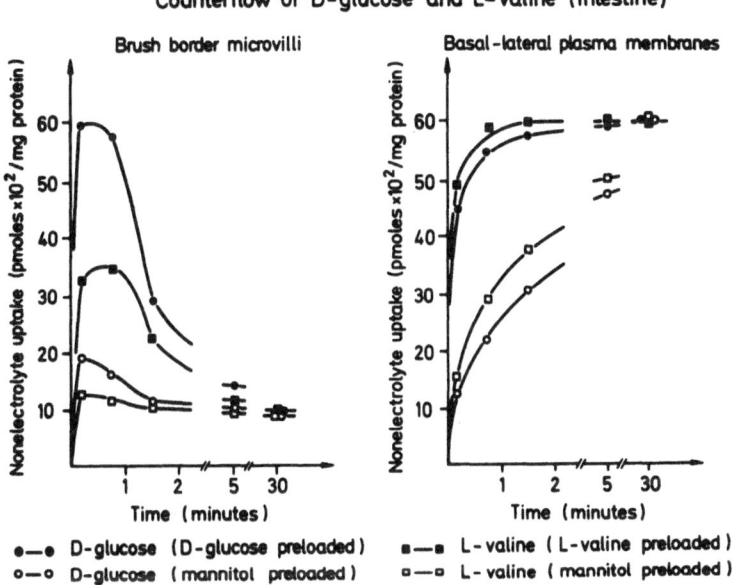

Counterflow of D-glucose and L-valine (intestine)

●—● D-glucose (D-glucose preloaded)   ■—■ L-valine (L-valine preloaded)
○—○ D-glucose (mannitol preloaded)   □—□ L-valine (mannitol preloaded)

Figure 5.10 Effect of preloading with unlabelled non-electrolytes on the uptake of labelled non-electrolytes (counterflow). Intestinal membranes were prepared by density gradient centrifugation[31]. Brush border and basal–lateral plasma membranes were preloaded with a buffer containing 70 mM D-mannitol, 1 mM HEPES–Tris (pH 7.5), and 30 mM L-valine or 30 mM D-glucose. As control, an aliquot of membranes from the same preparation was homogenized in 100 mM D-mannitol, 1 mM HEPES–Tris (pH 7.5) and 0.1 mM $MgSO_4$. The incubation medium contained: NaSCN (100 mM), 100 mM D-mannitol, 0.1 mM $MgSO_4$, and 1 mM HEPES–Tris (pH 7.5). The incubation medium contained in addition (final conc.) either 4 mM D-[³H]glucose or 4 mM L-[³H]valine

SODIUM-DEPENDENT SOLUTE TRANSPORT ACROSS ABSORPTIVE EPITHELIAL CELLS: A MODEL

Transepithelial sodium-dependent sugar and amino acid transport can be reconstructed from the transport events across the isolated plasma membranes

(Figure 5.11). Overall transport can be regarded as the sum of the several transport steps: (a) Sodium-dependent electrogenic uphill movement of solutes across the brush border membrane. This sodium-coupled influx is driven by the downhill flux of the cosubstrate, sodium. (b) Downhill efflux of the accumulated substrates from the cytoplasma through the basal–lateral plasma membrane into the interstitium via transport systems of the 'facilitated diffusion' type. (c) The Na^+-K^+-ATPase in the basal–lateral plasma membranes constitutes the biochemical counterpart to the 'ion pump' which is responsible for maintaining the low intracellular sodium concentration.

Consequences of the electrogenic translocation mechanism in the brush border membrane are coupling of all electrogenic ion and substrate fluxes across the same membrane. Such coupling phenomena have been recently shown to occur between sugar and amino acid uptake by isolated intestinal

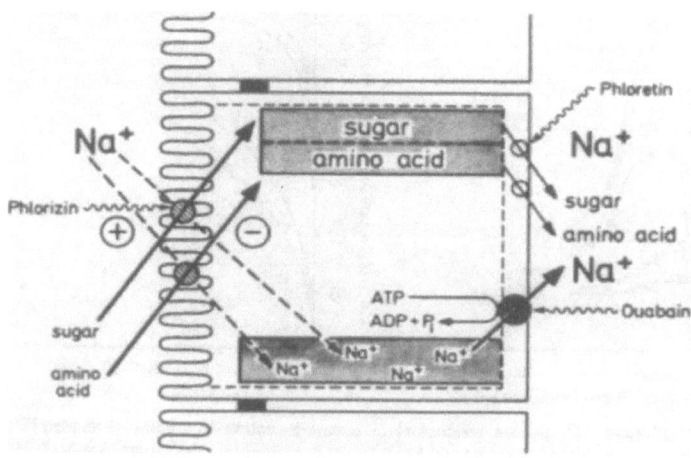

Figure 5.11 Model for glucose and amino acid transport across absorptive epithelial cells

brush border vesicles. Thereby the mutual inhibition could be released by short-circuiting the membrane potential with the ionophores monactin or valinomycin in the presence of potassium[58].

The electrogenic cotransport systems for sugar and neutral amino acids provide an example of the utilisation of the energy of the sodium gradient for transepithelial transport processes. Recently, in studies with isolated renal brush border vesicles, further modes of sodium-coupled transport processes could be demonstrated. Phosphate transport across the brush-border membrane is sodium-dependent but seems not to be electrogenic[59]. There is also evidence for an electroneutral antiport between sodium and protons as indicated by the demonstration of counterflow of both ions under short-circuit conditions[60].

Acknowledgements

We should like to express our gratidue to Professor K. J. Ullrich for valuable discussion during the preparation of the manuscript and to thank Mrs Rentel and Mrs Petzold for the excellent art work of the figures.

References

1. Förster, H. and Hoos, I. (1972). The excretion of sodium during absorption of glucose from the perfused small intestine of rats. *Hoppe-Seylers Z. Physiol. Chem.*, **353**, 88
2. Saltzman, D. A., Rector, F. C. and Fordtran, J. S. (1972). The role of intraluminal sodium in glucose absorption *in vivo*. *J. Clin. Invest.*, **51**, 876
3. Crane, R. K. (1965). Na^+ dependent transport in the intestine and other animal tissues. *Fed. Proc.*, **24**, 1000
4. Crane, R. K. (1968). Absorption of sugars. *Handbook of Physiology*, vol. 3 (Sect. 6), 1323
5. Smyth, D. H. (1971). Sodium–hexose interactions. *Phil. Trans. Roy. Soc. Lond. B*, **262**, 121
6. Bihler, I. and Cybulsky, R. (1973). Sugar transport at the basal and lateral aspect of the small intestinal epithelial cell. *Biochim. Biophys. Acta*, **298**, 429
7. Ullrich, K. J., Rumrich, G. and Klöss, S. (1974). Specificity and sodium dependence of the active sugar transport in the proximal convolution of the rat kidney. *Pflügers Arch.*, **351**, 35
8. Ullrich, K. J., Rumrich, G. and Klöss, S. (1974). Sodium dependence of the amino acid transport in the proximal convolution of the rat kidney, *Pflügers Arch.*, **351**, 49
9. Burg, M. B. and Orloff, J. (1973). Perfusion of isolated renal tubules. *Handbook of Physiology*, Renal physiology, 145
10. Silverman, M., Aganon, M. A. and Chinard, F. P. (1970). D-glucose interactions with renal tubule cell surfaces. *Amer. J. Physiol.*, **218**, 735
11. Foulkes, E. C. and Gieske, T. (1973). Specificity and metal sensitivity of renal amino acid transport. *Biochim. Biophys. Acta*, **318**, 439
12. Silverman, M. (1974). The chemical and steric determinants governing sugar interactions with renal tubular membranes. *Biochim. Biophys. Acta*, **332**, 248
13. Kleinzeller, A. and McAvoy, E. M. (1973). Sugar transport across the peritubular face of renal cells of the flounder. *J. Gen. Physiol.*, **62**, 169
14. Csáky, T. Z. (1963). A possible link between active transport of electrolytes and non-electrolytes. *Fed. Proc.*, **22**, 3
15. Tucker, A. and Kimmich, G. A. (1973). Characteristics of amino acid accumulation by isolated intestinal epithelial cells. *J. Membrane Biol.*, **12**, 1
16. Miller, D. and Crane, R. K. (1961). The digestive function of the epithelium of the small intestine. II. Localization of disaccharide hydrolysis in the isolated brush border portion of intestinal epithelial cells. *Biochim. Biophys. Acta*, **52**, 293
17. Binkley, F., King, N., Milikin, E., Wright, R. K., Neal, C. H. and Wundram, I. J. (1968). Brush border particulates of renal tissue. *Science*, **162**, 1009
18. Kinne, R. and Kinne-Saffran, E. (1969). Isolierung und enzymatische Charakterisierung einer Bürstensaumfraktion der Rattenniere. *Pflügers Arch.*, **308**, 1
19. Berger, S. J. and Sacktor, B. (1970). Isolation and biochemical characterization of brush borders from rabbit kidney. *J. Cell. Biol.*, **47**, 637
20. Wilfong, R. F. and Neville, D. M., Jr. (1970). The isolation of a brush border membrane fraction from rat kidney. *J. Biol. Chem.*, **245**, 6106
21. Stevenson, F. K. (1972). The disaccharidase activity of a membrane fraction obtained from rabbit renal cortex. *Biochim. Biophys. Acta*, **266**, 144

22. Quirk, S. J. and Robinson, G. B. (1972). Isolation and characterization of rabbit kidney brush borders. *Biochem. J.*, **128**, 1319

23. Chertok, R. J. and Lake, S. (1972). A simple method for the preparation of renal brush borders. *J. Cell Biol.*, **54**, 426

24. George, S. G. and Kenny, A. J. (1973). Studies on the enzymology of purified preparations of brush border from rabbit kidney. *Biochem. J.*, **134**, 43

25. Heidrich, H. G., Kinne, R., Kinne-Saffran, E. and Hannig, K. (1972). The polarity of the proximal tubule cell in rat kidney. Different surface charges for the brush-border microvilli and plasma membranes from the basal infoldings. *J. Cell. Biol.* **54**, 232

26. Eichholz, A. (1967). Structural and functional organisation of the brush border of intestinal epithelial cells. III. Enzymatic activities and chemical composition of various fractions of Tris-disrupted brush borders. *Biochim. Biophys. Acta*, **135**, 475

27. Quigley, J. D. and Gotterer, G. S. (1969). Distribution of Na^+-K^+-ATPase activity in rat intestinal mucosa. *Biochim. Biophys. Acta*, **173**, 456

28. Fujita, M., Matsui, H., Nagano, K. and Nakao, M. (1972). Differential isolation of microvillus and basolateral membranes from intestinal mucosa. *Biochim. Biophys. Acta*, **274**, 336

29. Hopfer, U., Nelson, K., Perrotto, J. and Isselbacher, K. J. (1973). Glucose transport in isolated brush border membranes from rat small intestine. |*J. Biol. Chem.*, **248**, 25

30. Murer, H., Hopfer, U., Kinne-Saffran, E. and Kinne, R. (1974). Glucose transport in isolated brush border and lateral–basal plasma membrane vesicles from intestinal epithelial cells. *Biochim. Biophys. Acta*, **345**, 170

31. Murer, H., Ammans, E., Biber, J. and Hopfer, U. (1975). The surface membrane of the small intestinal epithelial cell. I. Localisation of adenylcyclase. (Submitted for publication)

32. Marx, S. J., Fedak, S. A. and Aurbach, G. D. (1972). Preparation and characterization of a hormone responsive renal plasma membrane fraction. *J. Biol. Chem.*, **247**, 6913

33. Manitius, A., Bensch, K. and Epstein, F. H. (1968). ($Na^+ + K^+$)-activated ATPase in kidney cell membranes of normal and methylprednisolone-treated rats. *Biochim. Biophys. Acta*, **150**, 563

34. Ebel, H., Gebhardt, A. and Aulbert, E. (1975). Protein composition of rat kidney basal lateral membranes. *Pflügers Arch.*, **355**, R 51

35. Douglas, A., Kerley, R. and Isselbacher, K. J. (1972). Preparation and characterization of the lateral and basal plasma membranes of the rat intestinal epithelial cell. *Biochem. J.*, **128**, 1329

36. Schmidt, U. and Dubach, U. C. (1971). Na^+–K^+ stimulated adenosine triphosphatase: Intracellular localization within the proximal tubule of the rat nephron. *Pflügers. Arch.*, **330**, 265

37. Stirling, C. E. (1972). Radioautographic localization of sodium pump sites in rabbit intestine. *J. Cell Biol.*, **53**, 704

38. Kinne, R., Schmitz, J. E. and Kinne-Saffran, E. (1971). The localization of the Na^+–K^+-ATPase in the cells of rat kidney cortex. A study on isolated plasma membranes. *Pflügers Arch.*, **329**, 191

39. Kinne, R., Murer, H., Kinne-Saffran, E., Thees, M. and Sachs, G. (1975). Sugar transport by renal plasma membrane vesicles: Characterization of the systems in the brush border microvilli and the basal–lateral plasma membranes. *J. Membrane Biol.*, **21**, 375

40. Sigrist-Nelson, K., Ammans, E., Murer, H. and Hopfer, U. (1975). The surface membrane of the small intestinal epithelial cell. II. Non-electrolyte transport. (Submitted for publication)

41. Sigrist-Nelson, K. (1975). Hexose and amino acid transport in isolated plasma membranes from small intestinal epithelial cells. *Thesis*, ETH-Zürich (Schweiz)

42. Sigrist-Nelson, K., Murer, H. and Hopfer, U. (1975). Active alanine transport in isolated brush border membranes. *J. Biol. Chem.*, **250**, 5674

43. Evers, J., Thees, M. and Kinne, R. (1975). Phenylalanine transport by brush border microvilli vesicles isolated from rat kidney cortex. (Submitted for publication)

44. Segal, S. and Rosenhagen, M. (1974). The effect of extracellular sodium concentration on α-methyl-D-glucoside transport by rat kidney cortex slices. *Biochim. Biophys. Acta*, **332**, 278

45. Murer, H. and Hopfer, U. (1974). Demonstration of electrogenic Na$^+$-dependent D-glucose transport in intestinal brush border membranes. *Proc. Nat. Acad. Sci. (USA)*, **71**, 484

46. Schultz, S. G. and Curran, P. F. (1970). Coupled transport of sodium and organic solutes. *Physiol. Rev.*, **50**, 637

47. Henderson, P. J. F., McGivan, J. D. and Chappell, J. B. (1969). The action of certain antibiotics on mitochondrial, erythrocyte and artificial phospholipid membranes. The role of induced proton permeability. *Biochem. J.*, **111**, 521

48. Rose, R. C. and Schultz, S. G. (1971). Studies on the electrical potential profile across rabbit ileum. *J. Gen. Physiol.*, **57**, 639

49. Rose, R. C. and Schultz, S. G. (1970). Alanine and glucose effects on the intracellular electrical potential of rabbit ileum. *Biochim. Biophys. Acta*, **211**, 376

50. Wright, E. M. (1966). The origin of the glucose dependent increase in the potential difference across the tortoise small intestine. *J. Physiol. Lond.*, **185**, 486

51. White, J. F. and Armstrong, W. McD. (1971). Effect of transported solutes on membrane potentials in bullfrog small intestine. *Amer. J. Physiol.*, **221**, 194

52. Lyon, I. and Sheering, H. E. (1971). Studies on transmural potentials *in vitro* in relation to intestinal absorption. VI. The effect of sugars and amino acids on electrical potential profiles in jejunum and ileum. *Biochim. Biophys. Acta*, **249**, 1

53. Barry, R. J. C. and Eggenton, J. (1972). Membrane potentials of epithelial cells in rat small intestine. *J. Physiol. Lond.*, **227**, 201

54. Kokko, J. P. (1972). Proximal tubule potential difference: dependence on glucose, HCO$_3^-$ and amino acids. *Clin. Res.*, **20**, 598

55. Maruyama, T. and Hoshi, T. (1972). The effect of D-glucose on the electrical potential profile across the proximal tubule of newt kidney. *Biochim. Biophys. Acta*, **282**, 214

56. Frömter, E. and Gessner, K. (1974). Active transport potentials, membrane diffusion potentials and streaming potentials across rat kidney proximal tubule. *Pflügers Arch.*, **351**, 85

57. LeFevre, P. G. (1961). Sugar transport in the red blood cell: structure activity relationship in substrates and antagonists. *Pharmacol. Rev.*, **13**. 39

58. Murer, H., Sigrist-Nelson, K. and Hopfer, U. (1975). On the mechanism of sugar and amino acid interaction in intestinal transport. *J. Biol. Chem.* (In press)

59. Hoffmann, N., Thees, M. and Kinne, R. (1975). Transport of inorganic phosphate by isolated renal plasma membrane vesicles. (In preparation)

60. Murer, H., Hopfer, U. and Kinne, R. (1975). Sodium-proton antiport in brush border membrane vesicles isolated from rat small intestine and rat kidney. (Submitted for publication)

5

Discussion Paper on

Protein Composition of Kidney Cell Membranes

H. Ebel, A. Gebhardt and E. Aulbert

Institut für Klinische Physiologie, Klinikum Steglitz, Freie Universität, Berlin

With respect to the transepithelial transport of sodium, glucose and amino acids, different systems have been demonstrated in the brush borders and the

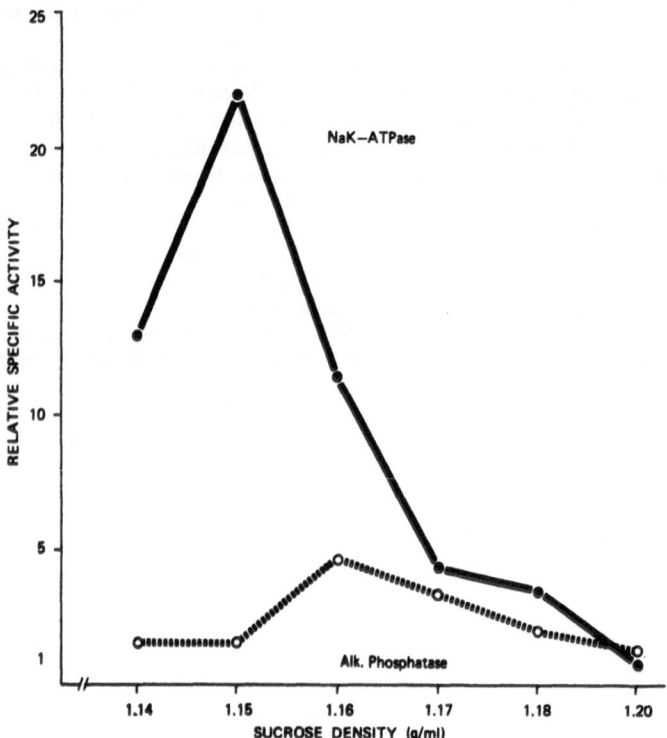

Figure 5.1 Relative specific activities of Na^+-K^+-ATPase and alkaline phosphatase in the membranes collected at different sucrose densities. Basal–lateral membranes accumulated at $d = 1.14$–1.15 g/ml

basal–lateral membranes of renal and intestinal cells. Since transport across membranes is dependent on the membrane structure, it is reasonable to suspect that the brush border and basal–lateral membranes should have different molecular structures. The object of our studies was to investigate the protein composition of renal basal–lateral membranes and to compare it with that of the brush borders.

Basal–lateral membranes were prepared by discontinuous sucrose density gradient centrifugation of crude renal plasma membranes[1]. The membranes were isolated at the sucrose density interface of $d = 1.14/1.15$ g/ml and were characterised by a 22-fold enrichment of Na^+-K^+-ATPase with a Na-K/Mg ATPase ratio of 4.1 (Figure 5.1). The enrichment of the brush-border-bound alkaline phosphatase was only 1.6-fold. The contamination by mitochondria, lysosomes and endoplasmic reticula was negligible. The basal–lateral membranes were extracted first with Triton X100 and the insoluble residue was then treated with sodium dodecylsulphate (SDS). The soluble 100 000 g supernatants were separated by electrophoresis on 5% polyacrylamide gels and stained for proteins and glycoproteins. Both the Triton-soluble and the SDS-soluble protein fraction of the basal–lateral membranes were divided into at least 15 proteins. The protein pattern of the Triton-soluble fraction was quite different from that of the SDS-fraction (Figure 5.2). In the Triton extract, the molecular weights ranged from 23 000 to 400 000. Approximately 60% of the proteins possessed molecular weights within the range of 125 000 to

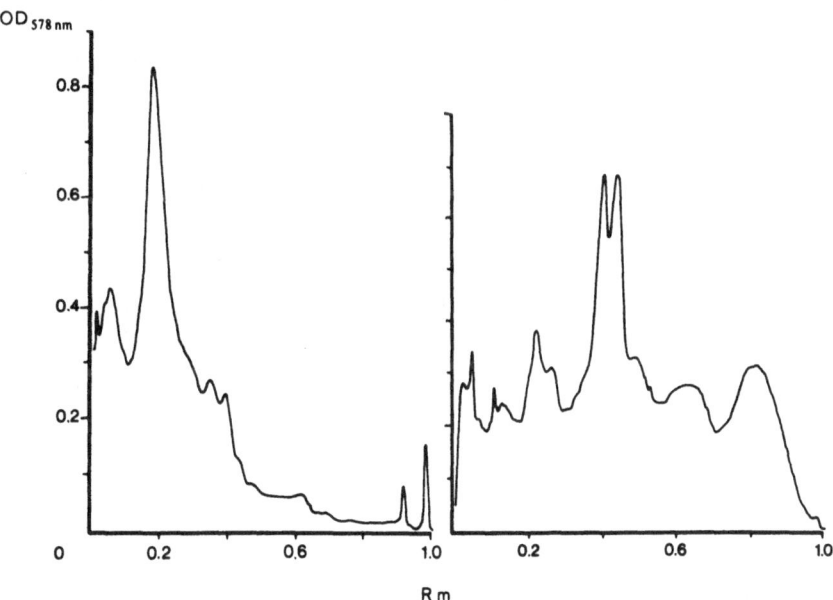

Figure 5.2 Densitometric tracings of solubilized basal–lateral membranes separated on a 5% polyacrylamide gel. (a) Triton fraction; (b) sodium dodecyl sulphate fraction. OD_{578} = optical density at 578 nm; R_m = relative mobility

230 000. The most characteristic sharp peak was found at a molecular weight of 145 000 and included 38% of all proteins. This protein was identified as a glycoprotein that contained ATPase and 5'-nucleotidase activity. The SDS-soluble proteins were distributed over a molecular weight range from 12 000 to more than 1 200 000. In contrast to the Triton fraction, only 17% of the proteins there were found between the weights of 125 000 and 230 000. The SDS fraction was characterised by two distinct peaks at molecular weights of 54 000 and 120 000 that included 22% of the total protein and two further smaller peaks at molecular weights of 14 000 and 22 000 with 23% of the proteins. Only four proteins of the Triton and SDS fraction had the same molecular weights. Whether these are the same proteins or different proteins with identical molecular weights cannot yet be answered and needs further clarification. It therefore seems likely that the renal basal–lateral membranes are composed of 26 if not of 30 different proteins. At least 12 of the proteins were glycoproteins, and six other proteins were identified as enzymes. In contrast to the basal–lateral membranes, a completely different protein subunit composition was found for renal brush border membranes[2]. Only one or two of the 11 brush border glycoproteins were found to have nearly the same molecular weight as the basal–lateral membrane glycoproteins. Thus it is assumed that the two different regions of the renal plasma membrane, that is, the basal–lateral membranes and the brush border membranes have unique and quite different protein compositions. The same has been found in the intestine[3]. This could be interpreted to mean that the different sized protein subunits of the basal–lateral membranes and the brush borders may have different biological functions. However, the subunits with identical molecular weights may serve a function that is common to both regions of the cell.

References

1. Ebel, H., Aulbert, E., and Merker, H. J. (19**). Isolation of the basal and lateral plasma membranes of rat kidney tubule cells. (In preparation)
2. Glossmann, H. and Neville, D. M. (1971). Plasma membrane protein subunit composition. A comparative study by discontinuous electrophoresis in sodium dodecyl sulfate. *J. Biol. Chem.*, **246**, 6339
3. Fujita, M., Kawai, K., Asano, S., and Nakao, M. (1973). Protein components of two different regions of an intestinal epithelial cell membrane. Regional singularities. *Biochim. Biophys. Acta*, **307**, 141

Discussion 5

Alvarado: I agree that sugar transport across the brush border is electrogenic, but it should be emphasised that all evidence in favour of this concept is *indirect*.

Kinne: I agree that all our evidence about the electrogenicity of glucose and neutral amino acid transport across the brush border membrane is indirect in the sense that we did not measure – and are not able to measure, because of the small size of the vesicles – electrical events induced by the sodium-dependent transport systems. However, the three methodological approaches to prove electrogenicity (anion replacement, valinomycin in the presence of potassium gradients, and uncouplers in the presence of a proton gradient) have been shown in model studies with lipid bilayers to provoke changes in membrane potential.

Lauterbach: Could you comment on the concentration gradient for sugars between the medium and your vesicles?

Kinne: The highest vesicle-to-medium ratio reached so far is about 10 in the first 15 seconds of the glucose uptake in the presence of a proton gradient (vesicle > medium) and the uncoupler CF-CCP.

Lauterbach: Are you sure that the transport system in the basolateral membrane is of the facilitated diffusion type? Have you any information about the K_m values there? In our isolated mucosa preparation, we found efflux coefficients for 3-O-methyl-glucose, for example, which were two times higher than the influx coefficients, suggesting a weak exit pump. Furthermore, we found no saturability of influx across the basolateral membrane, suggesting high K_m values in comparison with those referring to brush border influx.

Kinne: At present, we do not have any evidence for an energy input, be it ATP, or a sodium or potassium gradient, at the basolateral plasma membrane during glucose transfer. Concerning the relative affinities of the transport systems, we have to realise that, due to the manipulations to stop transport and to separate the vesicles from the incubation medium, quantitative kinetic analysis is open to severe criticism. Within these experimental limits, the affinities of the two systems are in the range of 1–10 mM for D-glucose.

Caspary: How does the specificity of the hexose transport system in isolated membrane vesicles agree with that of the sodium-dependent hexose transport system in isolated surviving intestine? Did you study the Na^+-dependency of glucose derived from sucrose which seems to be transported Na^+-independently, at least in the hamster small intestine?

Kinne: The specificity of the sodium-dependent sugar transport system in the brush border microvillous vesicles is identical with that found in microperfusion experiments in the proximal tubule of intact rat kidney. The specificity of the sugar transport system in the basolateral membrane vesicles is under study at the moment. Preliminary experiments performed together with Dr Kleinzeller in our laboratory have provided evidence that the facilitated diffusion system found in the vesicle and in cortex slices might also have similar stereospecificities. The sucrose–glucose transport system is not found in the renal brush border.

99

Murer: In small intestinal brush border membrane vesicles, glucose transport is inhibited by galactose but not by mannose or by 2-deoxy-glucose. At the contraluminal pole, mannose and 2-deoxy-glucose are inhibitors. These effects are not dependent on membrane potentials. These results agree with commonly held views on transport specificities. The sucrose–glucose transport system could not be studied owing to the high hydrolytic activity in the brush-border membrane. Glucose is liberated into the medium and then transported via the other system.

Field: Is the sodium leak permeability low enough to make it possible to measure sodium fluxes into, and sodium concentrations in, brush border or basolateral membrane vesicles? If not, are there ways, such as incorporation of Ca^{++}, of decreasing the diffusive permeability of these vesicles sufficiently to enable such measurements to be made?

Murer: Addition of calcium to a final membrane preparation had no effect on ion or solute (glucose) permeability of these membrane vesicles. However, addition of Ca^{++} during earlier steps of the preparation does have such an effect. The membranes become more tight with respect to their sodium permeability. The sodium permeability of brush-border membranes is much lower than that of the basolateral plasma membranes. In the kidney, for technical reasons, the addition of Ca^{++} in early steps of the preparation is not possible. Again, addition of calcium at the end has no effect on permeability changes.

6
Coupled Sodium–Chloride Transport by Small Intestine and Gallbladder

RAYMOND A. FRIZZELL

Department of Physiology,
University of Pittsburgh,
School of Medicine,
Pittsburgh, Pennsylvania

It is now well established that the active transepithelial transport and intracellular accumulation of sugars and amino acids by small intestine requires the presence of Na^+ in the luminal (or mucosal) solution[1,2]. In addition, actively transported sugars and amino acids stimulate Na^+ absorption by the small intestine from a variety of species. Results obtained using intestinal preparations *in vitro* are consistent with the notion that coupled entry mechanisms for Na^+ and sugars or amino acids are localised at the brush border of the transporting cells and that the energy required for cellular accumulation and absorption is derived, at least in part, from the electrochemical potential difference of Na^+ across the mucosal membrane[3].

In recent years, studies[4,5] of electrolyte transport by small intestine *in vitro* have confirmed the results of earlier investigations[6,7] which suggested that mammalian ileum *in vivo* was capable of active Cl^- absorption. These studies have employed preparations of rabbit ileum stripped of serosal musculature which permit better oxygenation of the epithelial cell layer[8]. The results of these studies, and investigations of Na^+ and Cl^- transport by rabbit gallbladder[9], suggest that neutral, coupled NaCl transport plays a major role in the active absorption of these ions. Thus, mechanisms providing for interaction between active Na^+ transport and the absorption of other solutes appear to be ubiquitous phenomena which may provide for the absorption of a variety of substances with minimal energy expenditure.

TRANSEPITHELIAL TRANSPORT OF NaCl

The short-circuit current across stripped rabbit ileum can be accounted for by active Na^+ and Cl^- absorption and HCO_3^- secretion[4,5]. In addition, active Na^+ and Cl^- absorption by isolated rabbit gallbaldder has been recognised for more than a decade[10]. The results of ion replacement studies (Table 6.1) indicate that in both epithelia, the absorptive fluxes of Na^+ and Cl^- are coupled. For ileum, approximately 50% of net Na^+ transport is abolished in the absence of Cl^- in the bathing solutions, whereas active absorption of Cl^- is entirely dependent upon the presence of Na^+. In gallbladder, Na^+ absorption is abolished in the absence of Cl^- and, similarly, net Cl^- transport is abolished in the absence of Na^+. The results obtained from rabbit gallbladder confirm the

Table 6.1 Effects of ion replacement on Na^+ and Cl^- fluxes across rabbit ileum and gallbladder

Ileum	*Na^+ fluxes*		*Cl^- fluxes*	
	Control	Cl^--free	Control	Na^+-free
J_{ms}	12	10	10	8
J_{sm}	8	8	8	8
J_{net}	4	2	2	0
Gallbladder	*Na^+ fluxes*		*Cl^- fluxes*	
	Control	Cl^--free	Control	Na^+-free
J_{ms}	35	22	28	12
J_{sm}	22	21	13	12
J_{net}	13	1	15	0

J_{ms} designates the unidirectional flux from mucosa to serosa; J_{sm}, the unidirectional flux from serosa to mucosa and $J_{net} = J_{ms} - J_{sm}$. All values are in units of $\mu mol/cm^2$ h. Numbers have been rounded off but differences are statistically significant[5,9].

findings of Wheeler[10] that replacement of Na^+ or Cl^- with non-transported ions abolishes net ion absorption without affecting the small, lumen positive, electrical potential difference observed in this tissue. In both tissues, the reductions in net flux of both Na^+ and Cl^- are accounted for by decreases in the mucosa-to-serosa flux of these ions. The serosa-to-mucosa flux is not affected by ion replacement. Similar reductions in the mucosa-to-serosa fluxes of both Na^+ and Cl^- across both ileum[5] and gallbladder[9] are observed in the presence of cyclic AMP or theophylline. These findings suggest that the reduction in absorptive fluxes of Na^+ and Cl^- observed in the presence of agents which elevate intracellular cyclic AMP is due to an inhibition of a neutral, coupled NaCl transport process.

LOCALISATION OF THE COUPLED TRANSPORT PROCESS

Studies of the unidirectional influxes of Na^+ and Cl^- from the mucosal solution into the epithelium have provided direct evidence for a coupled NaCl influx process at the mucosal membranes of both rabbit ileum[11] and gallbladder[9]. The results of these studies are summarised in Table 6.2. In rabbit ileum, approximately 20% of Na^+ influx is inhibited in the absence of mucosal Cl^- and a similar fraction of Cl^- influx is inhibited if the mucosal solution is rendered Na^+-free. In gallbladder, the inhibition of Na^+ influx in the absence of Cl^- from the mucosal solution is equal to the reduction of Cl^- influx observed in the absence of Na^+. These results suggest that a component of the total Na^+ and Cl^- influxes across the mucosal membranes of ileum and gallbladder are mediated by an obligatory one-for-one coupled NaCl influx process, and this stoichiometry was confirmed in rabbit ileum from indepen-

Table 6.2 Effects of ion replacement on Na^+ and Cl^- influxes in rabbit ileum and gallbladder

Ileum	Na+ Influx		Cl- Influx	
	Control	Cl⁻-free	Control	Na⁺-free
	21	17	20	16
		$\Delta = 4$		$\Delta = 4$
Gallbladder	Na+ Influx		Cl- Influx	
	Control	Cl⁻-free	Control	Na⁺-free
	34	22	33	21
		$\Delta = 12$		$\Delta = 12$

All values are in units of $\mu mol/cm^2$ h. Δ is the difference between control and experimental values and designates the coupled NaCl influx.

dent studies[11]. In addition, the inhibitory effects of theophylline and cyclic AMP appear to be restricted to the coupled influx mechanism[5,11]. Although similar data have not been obtained in gallbladder, in rabbit ileum, the inhibitions of Na^+ and Cl^- influx elicited by theophylline are equal. Moreover, the inhibitory effects of this agent on Na^+ or Cl^- influxes are abolished if either Cl^- or Na^+ respectively are removed from the mucosal solution[11]. The observation that theophylline or cyclic AMP reduces the mucosa-to-serosa fluxes of Na^+ and Cl^- in both tissues suggests that their effects on ion transport by rabbit gallbladder are also restricted to inhibition of the coupled NaCl influx process[9].

A KINETIC MODEL OF THE COUPLED TRANSPORT MECHANISM

An analysis of the kinetics of coupled NaCl influx in rabbit ileum suggested the model shown in Figure 6.1 to account for these results[11]. This model is similar to that proposed by Goldner *et al.*[12] for the interaction between sugars and Na^+ at the mucosal membranes of rabbit ileum. The principal features of this model are: (*a*) random combination of Na^+ or Cl^- with a membrane component (X) to form a ternary complex (XNaCl), (*b*) only free carrier and the

INTESTINAL ION TRANSPORT

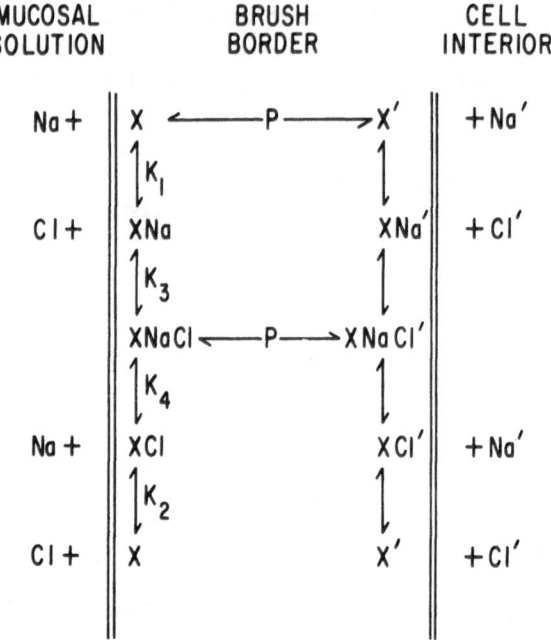

Figure 6.1   Kinetic model for coupled NaCl influx across brush border of rabbit ileum. This model corresponds to a process A of Figure 6.2 and was evaluated[5] using kinetic data for coupled NaCl influx

ternary complex may cross the mucosal membrane, and (c) translocation of X and XNaCl may proceed in either direction and could thus mediate NaCl efflux from cell to mucosal solution. This model was employed to calculate the magnitude of coupled NaCl influx and was found to account for, in a quantitative manner, the experimental data obtained on the kinetics of Na$^+$ and Cl$^-$ influxes[11]. These data indicate that a reduction in either Na$^+$ or Cl$^-$ concentration of the mucosal solution reduces maximal influx via the coupled mechanism and thus simulates the effects of theophylline which acts as a noncompetitive inhibitor of this transport process[13]. Thus, in all respects, theophylline or cyclic AMP mimic the effects of co-ion replacement. Inhibition of NaCl influx across the brush border of rabbit ileum by these agents may result in ion secretion by unmasking an existing coupled NaCl or NaHCO$_3$ efflux process[5]. However, an independent stimulation of *de novo* ion secretion cannot be ruled out from the results of these studies.

ENERGETICS OF Cl$^-$ ABSORPTION

Studies of intracellular ion concentrations[13], the electrical potential profile across the epithelium[14] and the results discussed above, have suggested the

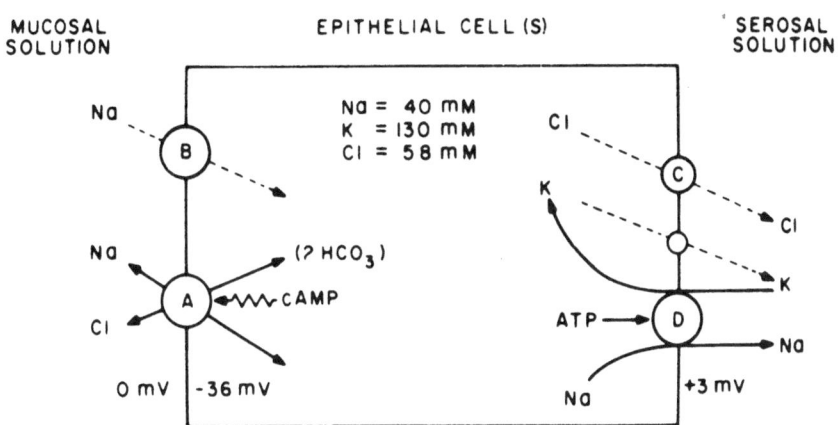

Figure 6.2 Model for Na⁺ and Cl⁻ transport by isolated rabbit ileum. Intracellular concentrations of Na⁺, K⁺ and Cl⁻ and the electrical potential profile under normal conditions are given in this figure. Corresponding values for rabbit gallbladder may be obtained from reference 9

model shown in Figure 6.2 to account for transepithelial Na⁺ and Cl⁻ transport by rabbit ileum[2]. While quantitative differences emerge from studies of rabbit gallbladder[9], the model shown in Figure 6.2 lends itself to a discussion of NaCl transport in this tissue as well. In ileum, approximately 50% of the control rate of Na⁺ absorption persists in the absence of Cl⁻ (Table 6.1) so that Na⁺ appears to cross the mucosal membrane by two routes: one (A) is coupled to the simultaneous uptake of Cl⁻ from the mucosal solution and influx via this process is inhibited by intracellular cyclic AMP. The second (B) is Cl⁻ independent and does not appear to be affected by cyclic AMP. Since net Na⁺ absorption by gallbladder is abolished in the absence of Cl⁻ (Table 6.1), process B does not appear to be present in that tissue. In both tissues, Na⁺ enters the cell down an electrochemical potential difference for this ion and is not affected by inhibitors of energy metabolism[11]. Thus, the coupled NaCl influx process does not appear to require a direct source of metabolic energy.

The entry of Cl⁻ across the mucosal membrane appears to be restricted to process A in both tissues, inasmuch as transepithelial Cl⁻ absorption is abolished in the absence of Na⁺, as shown in Table 6.1. Chloride appears to be accumulated within the cell at a higher electrochemical potential than that of the surrounding media[13]. Thus, Cl⁻ entry across the mucosal membrane, via the coupled influx mechanism, is directed against an apparent electrochemical potential difference for this ion. In rabbit ileum, the Na⁺-dependent entry of Cl⁻ from the mucosal solution into the cell appears to contribute to cellular Cl⁻ accumulation inasmuch as agents which inhibit coupled NaCl influx also result in a decrease in cell Cl⁻ concentration[13]. Thus, the energy required for cellular Cl⁻ accumulation may be derived from the Na⁺ gradient across the mucosal membrane since the transmucosal fluxes of Cl⁻ are linked, in a one-for-one fashion, with those of Na⁺.*

The effects of Na⁺-free incubation media on intracellular Cl⁻ concentrations in rabbit gallbladder, shown in Figure 6.3, support this conclusion. Tissues incubated in Na⁺-free media show a progressive decline in cell Cl⁻ concentration towards the value expected for electrochemical equilibrium

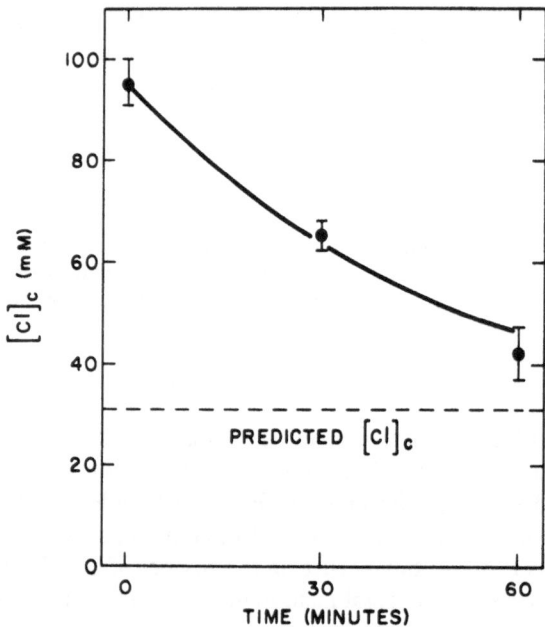

Figure 6.3 Effect of incubation in a Na⁺-free medium on intracellular Cl⁻ concentrations in rabbit gallbladder. Data are presented as a function of incubation time. The value at zero time represents the average of control tissues incubated in media containing a normal Na⁺ concentration for 30 or 60 minutes. These values did not differ significantly. The curve shown is given by the equation

$$[Cl]_c = 64 \exp[-0.023 \, t] + 31$$

where t is the incubation time in hours and $[Cl]_c$ when $t = \infty$ (31 mM) is the cell Cl⁻ concentration expected for electrochemical equilibrium

of this ion. The curve describing these data was calculated to reach an asymptote at a final value of 31 mM which is the cell Cl⁻ concentration expected for passive distribution of Cl⁻ across the cell membrane, calculated from the Nernst equation. These data suggest that the presence of Na⁺ in the bathing

---

* Recently, studies of Na⁺-coupled amino acid and sugar transport by Ehrlich cells[15] and intestinal brush border vesicles[16] have suggested that the electrical potential difference across the cell membrane may directly influence the accumulation of actively transported non-electrolytes within the cell. Sodium-coupled non-electrolyte influx is a rheogenic process[14] and, as such, should be influenced by the electrical potential difference across the mucosal membrane. However, according to the model shown in Figure 6.1, coupled NaCl influx (and efflux) proceeds by movement of neutral carrier species (or components of equal charge) across the mucosal membrane and thus should not be influenced by (nor should it affect) the potential difference across the mucosal membrane.

media is necessary for the accumulation of intracellular Cl⁻ against an apparent electrochemical potential difference[9].

At the basolateral membrane, Na⁺ extrusion from the cell into the serosal solution (process D, Figure 6.2) appears to be an active transport process which has been thought to be coupled with the simultaneous uptake of K⁺ into the cell from the serosal solution via a Na⁺-K⁺ exchange mechanism[2]. However, recent evidence[17] suggests that K⁺ uptake at the serosal membrane of rabbit ileum is not influenced by alterations in Na⁺ absorption, but this complication is not germane to the present discussion.

The movement of Cl⁻ from the cell to the serosal solution (process C) is directed down an electrochemical potential difference for this ion, so that a diffusional transport process might suffice to explain Cl⁻ exit across the basolateral membrane[5,9]. Although information on the Cl⁻ conductance of the basolateral membranes of gallbladder epithelial cells is not available, estimates of total serosal membrane conductance in *Necturus* gallbladder have been made. Frömter[18] and Reuss and Finn[19] estimate serosal membrane resistance to be approximately 2700 Ω cm² serosal surface area, yielding a serosal membrane conductance of 0.4 mmho/cm². If a similar value applies to rabbit gallbladder and *if* the entire conductance of this membrane can be attributed to Cl⁻ diffusion, then the net flux of Cl⁻ can be calculated from

$$\mathcal{J}_{net}^{Cl} = G_{Cl} (E_{Cl} + \psi_{cs})/F$$

where E_{Cl} is the equilibrium potential for Cl⁻ calculated from cell and serosal solution Cl⁻ concentrations and ψ_{cs} is the electrical potential difference across the basolateral membrane (45 mV)[9]. The calculated value for $\mathcal{J}_{net}^{Cl}$ using the conductance value for *Necturus* is 0.3 μmol/cm² h, which is approximately 40 times less than the observed net Cl⁻ flux in rabbit gallbladder under normal conditions. However, rabbit gallbladder, unlike that of *Necturus*, is a villous structure, and although the extent to which the villi increase the area of the epithelial cell layer per unit serosal area in rabbit gallbladder is not known, for small intestine Wilson[20] has estimated this factor to be 30–40-fold. This would raise the calculated value of $\mathcal{J}_{net}^{Cl}$ to 12 to 16 μmol/cm² h which does not differ from the net Cl⁻ flux given in Table 6.1. Thus, current evidence may be compatible with a diffusional exit of Cl⁻ from the cell across the basolateral membranes of rabbit gallbladder, but further speculation on this issue is clearly unwarranted.

Sodium-coupled transport: conservation of metabolic energy

Several aspects of active Cl⁻ transport by rabbit ileum and gallbladder resemble the active transport of sugars and amino acids by small intestine[3]: (*a*) active Cl⁻ absorption is abolished when the mucosal solution is rendered Na⁺-free; (*b*) Na⁺ and Cl⁻ enter the cell across the mucosal membrane via a coupled carrier-mediated mechanism; (*c*) the electrochemical potential of intracellular Cl⁻ exceeds that in the surrounding media so that net Cl⁻ entry into the cell from the mucosal solution is directed against an electrochemical potential difference (chemical potential difference for the case of non-electrolytes); (d) in the absence of Na^+, the intracellular Cl^- concentration (in rabbit gallbladder) declines toward the value expected for electrochemical equilibrium (chemical equilibrium for sugars and amino acids). All of these findings suggest that the energy necessary for Cl^- entry into the cell against an electrochemical potential difference, for intracellular Cl^- accumulation, and for subsequent transepithelial Cl^- transport, may be derived, at least in part, from the electrochemical potential difference for Na^+ across the mucosal membrane. For rabbit gallbladder, the calculated electrochemical gradient for Na^+ across the mucosal membrane is 1.5 kcal/mol, which is likely to be an underestimate since direct determinations of cell Na^+ activity are approximately one half the intracellular concentration. The energy required for the apparent uphill movement of Cl^- is 0.7 kcal/mol. These calculations suggest that the energy inherent in the Na^+-gradient is more than sufficient to provide for cellular Cl^- accumulation and that the efficiency of energy conversion need be only 50%.

According to the model shown in Figure 6.2, metabolic energy is linked only to the active Na^+ extrusion mechanism at the basolateral membranes. As discussed above, and elsewhere[3], a similar model has been proposed for the absorption of sugars and amino acids by small intestinal epithelium. Thus, transepithelial transport of solutes whose entry into the cell from the mucosal solution is coupled to that of Na^+ may be energised by the Na^+ gradient across the mucosal membrane. Recent studies by Rubino and Field[21] suggest that dipeptides may also fall into this category in the small intestine. In addition, there is now abundant evidence that water absorption is dependent upon and directly related to net solute absorption[22]. Thus, active solute transport mechanisms appear to establish gradients of osmotic pressure which ultimately provide the driving force for passive water absorption. For small intestine, and in the majority of mammalian epithelia, the absorption of solutes and water proceeds against minimal transepithelial concentration gradients and thus may be characterised as operating at 'level flow'[23]. The inefficiency which would be involved in directly coupling energy conversion to the transport of individual solutes between compartments of essentially equal concentration is obvious. On the other hand, coupling between the absorptive fluxes of Na^+ and a variety of solutes would allow the absorption of large quantities of nutrients, Cl^- and H_2O but the energy required would be no greater than that invested in the active absorption of Na^+ alone.

Acknowledgements

The author wishes to thank Dr Stanley G. Schultz for stimulating discussions and a critical reading of the manuscript. Work from these laboratories was supported by research grants from the USPHS (NIAMDD) (AM16275) and the American Heart Association (73-620).

References

1. Schultz, S. G. and Frizzell, R. A. (1975). Amino acid transport by small intestine. In T. Z. Csáky (ed.) *Intestinal Absorption and Malabsorption*, pp. 77–93, (New York: Raven Press)
2. Schultz, S. G., Frizzell, R. A. and Nellans, H. N. (1974). Ion transport by mammalian small intestine. *Ann. Rev. Physiol.*, **36**, 51
3. Schultz, S. G. and Curran, P. F. (1970). Coupled transport of sodium and organic solutes. *Physiol Rev.* **50**, 637
4. Field, M., Fromm, D. and McColl, I. (1971). Ion transport in rabbit ileal mucosa. I. Na and Cl fluxes and short-circuit current. *Amer. J. Physiol.*, **220**, 1388
5. Nellans, H. N., Frizzell, R. A. and Schultz, S. G. (1974). Brush-border processes and transepithelial Na and Cl transport by rabbit ileum. *Amer. J. Physiol.*, **226**, 1131
6. Curran, P. F. and Solomon, A. K. (1957). Ion and water fluxes in the ileum of rats. *J. Gen. Physiol.*, **41**, 143
7. Kinney, V. R. and Code, C. F. (1964). Canine ileal chloride absorption: Effect of carbonic anhydrase inhibition on transport. *Amer. J. Physiol.*, **207**, 998
8. Frizzell, R. A., Markscheid-Kaspi, L. and Schultz, S. G. (1974). Oxidative metabolism by rabbit ileal mucosa. *Amer. J. Physiol.*, **226**, 1142
9. Frizzell, R. A., Dugas, M. C. and Schultz, S. G. (1975). Sodium chloride transport by rabbit gallbladder: Direct evidence for a coupled NaCl influx process. *J. Gen. Physiol.*, **65**, 769
10. Wheeler, H. O. (1963). Transport of electrolytes and water across wall of rabbit gallbladder. *Amer. J. Physiol.*, **205**, 427
11. Nellans, H. N., Frizzell, R. A. and Schultz, S. G. (1973). Coupled sodium-chloride influx across the brush border of rabbit ileum. *Amer. J. Physiol.*, **225**, 467
12. Goldner, A. M., Schultz, S. G. and Curran, P. F. (1969). Sodium and sugar fluxes across the mucosal border of rabbit ileum. *J. Gen. Physiol.*, **53**, 362
13. Frizzell, R. A., Nellans, H. N., Rose, R. C., Markscheid-Kaspi, L. and Schultz, S. G. (1973). Intracellular Cl concentrations and influxes across the brush border of rabbit ileum. *Amer. J. Physiol.*, **224**, 328
14. Rose, R. C. and Schultz, S. G. (1971). Studies on the electrical potential profile across rabbit ileum: Effects of sugars and amino acids on transmural and transmucosal electrical potential differences. *J. Gen. Physiol.*, **57**, 639
15. Gibb, L. E. and Eddy, A. A. (1972). An electrogenic sodium pump as a possible factor leading to concentration of amino acids by mouse ascites tumor cells with reversed sodium ion concentration gradients. *Biochem. J.*, **129**, 979
16. Murer, H. and Hopfer, U. (1974). Demonstration of an electrogenic Na^+-dependent D-glucose transport in intestinal brush border membranes. *Proc. Nat. Acad. Sci. (USA)*, **71**, 484
17. Nellans, H. N. and Schultz, S. G. (1975). Potassium influx across the basolateral membranes of rabbit ileum. *Fed. Proc.*, **34**, 285
18. Frömter, E. (1972). The route of passive ion movement through the epithelium of Necturus gallbladder. *J. Memb. Biol.*, **8**, 259
19. Reuss, L. and Finn, A. L. (1975). Circuit analysis in Necturus gallbladder epithelium. *Fed. Proc.*, **34**, 327
20. Wilson, T. H. (1962). *Intestinal Absorption*. (Philadelphia: W. B. Saunders Co.)
21. Rubino, A., Field, M. and Shwachman, H. (1971). Intestinal transport of amino acid residues of dipeptides. I. Influx of the glycine residue of glycyl-L-proline across mucosal border. *J. Biol. Chem.*, **246**, 3542
22. Schultz, S. G. and Curran, P. F. (1968). Intestinal absorption of sodium chloride and water. In C. F. Code (ed.). *Handbook of Physiology, Sect. 6, Alimentary Canal*, pp. 1245–1275. (Washington, DC: Amer. Physiol. Soc.)
23. Kedem, O. and Caplan, S. R. (1965). Degree of coupling and its relation to efficiency of energy conversion. *Trans. Faraday Soc.*, **61**, 1897

6

Discussion Paper on
Model for Ileal Transport in Congenital Chloridorrhoea

J. Rask-Madsen

Medical Department F, Glostrup Hospital,
Copenhagen

The kinetic model for ileal transport proposed by Dr Frizzell implies that brush border transport processes are the major determinants of transepithelial Na^+ and Cl^- movements. Although the model satisfies most of the data obtained in human studies, it may seem hazardous to relate brush-border transport by animal ileum *in vitro* to net transepithelial transport by human ileum *in vivo* — and in any case unfruitful. However, the surprising results obtained in perfusion studies in an 8-month-old child with congenital chloridorrhoea has offered an opportunity to test the adequacy of the proposed model and the apparent need to invoke electrogenic Na^+ absorption in the human ileum.

In this rare condition — which is the only apparently specific disturbance of ion transport in human ileum — fluid diarrhoea was present from birth, and the stool Cl^- concentration was characteristically greater than the sum of the Na^+ and K^+ concentrations (see Table 6.1). This results in persistent hypochloraemic, hypokalaemic alkalosis and episodes of severe Na^+ and K^+ dehydration.

In collaboration with J. Kamper and E. Krag of Copenhagen, three steady-state perfusions of the ileum, and one of jejunum have been performed on two occasions. We used a five-luminal perfusion tube with a proximal occlusive balloon, one of the lumina being a KCl electrode for measuring the electrical

Figure *6.1a and b* Technique for perfusion of the human small intestine. A five-lumen polyvinyl tube with a proximal occlusive balloon features one lumen for aspiration of proximal intestinal secretions, another for inflation of the balloon, a third for infusion of perfusates, and a fourth (with aspiration holes 15 cm distal to the perfusion site) for sampling. The fifth lumen is a flowing KCl electrode for measuring the electrical potential of intestinal lumen relative to blood. An intravenous electrode of saline was used as reference

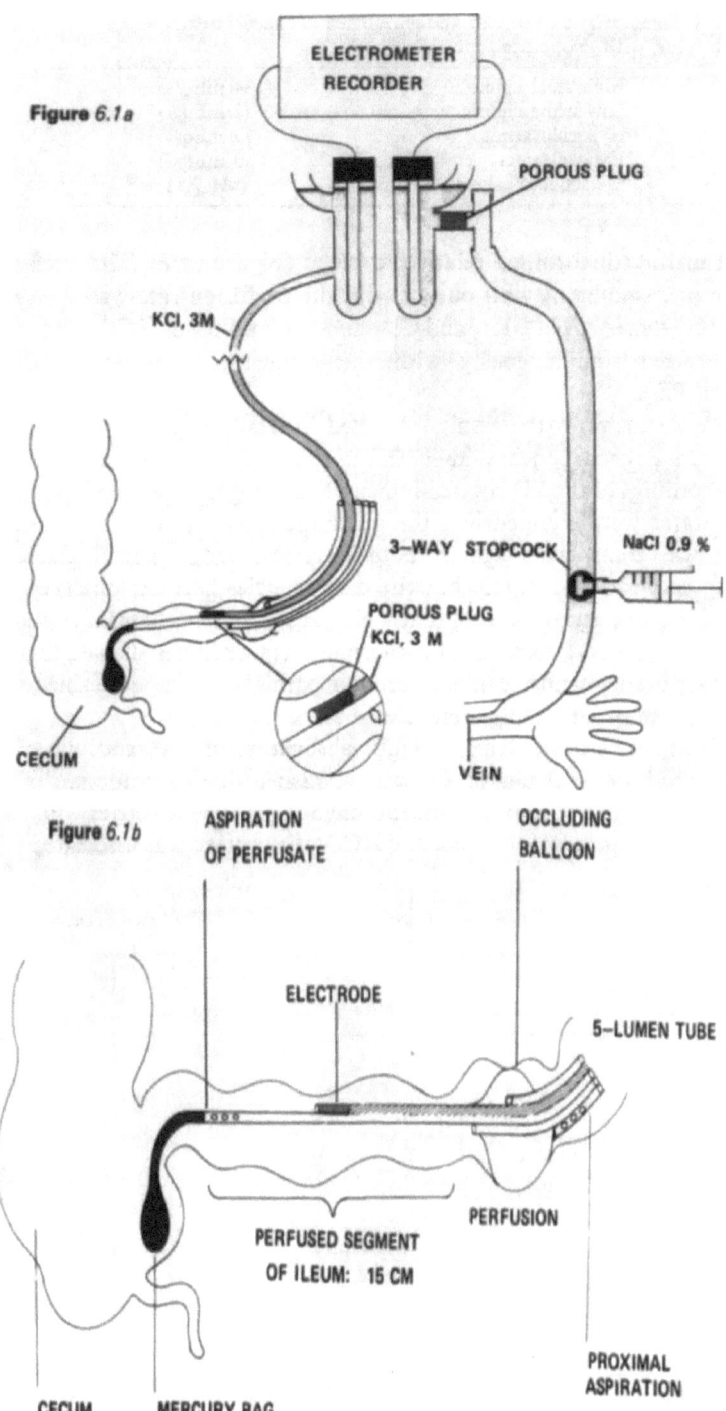

Figure 6.1a

ELECTROMETER RECORDER

POROUS PLUG

KCl, 3M

3-WAY STOPCOCK

NaCl 0.9 %

POROUS PLUG
KCl, 3 M

CECUM

VEIN

Figure 6.1b

ASPIRATION OF PERFUSATE

OCCLUDING BALLOON

ELECTRODE

5-LUMEN TUBE

PERFUSION

PERFUSED SEGMENT OF ILEUM: 15 CM

PROXIMAL ASPIRATION

CECUM   MERCURY BAG

Table 6.1 **Characteristic chemical abnormalities of faeces, urine, and serum in an 8-month-old male with congenital chloridorrhoea**

High stool chloride	(134 mEq/1)
Low urine chloride	(1 mEq/1)
Hypochloraemia	(77 mEq/1)
Hypokalaemia	(2.0 mEq/1)
Metabolic alkalosis	(pH 7.51)

potential of intestinal lumen relative to blood (Figure 6.1a). The perfusates were isotonic, simulating ileal output, and the perfusion rate was 5 ml/min. Bidirectional fluxes of Na^+, K^+, and Cl^-, and net transfer of HCO_3^- and water were measured simultaneously with the transmural electrical potential difference (PD).

Figure 6.2 illustrates the results obtained in ileal perfusions without and with 2.5 mM glycochenodeoxycholic acid in the luminal fluids. In the control period, recordings of the PD showed lumen 95 mV negative to blood. Na^+, K^+, Cl^-, and water were secreted into the gut lumen, and HCO_3^- net absorbed. Only Cl^- was transported against both electrical and chemical gradients, suggesting active Cl^- secretion, but the discrepancies between observed and predicted Na^+ flux ratios indicate that a Na^+ absorbing mechanism is also active in spite of net Na^+ secretion. Furthermore, tracer fluxes showed that the mucosal membrane, inclusive of extracellular pathways, is impermeable to diffusional passage of Cl^-, but permeable to Na^+.

In the presence of bile acids, a slight absorption of Na^+ and water was observed, while net transfer of Cl^- was abolished due to reduction of the plasma-to-lumen fluxes. No significant changes in the electrical PD and luminal pH could be demonstrated, and HCO_3^- absorption was associated with

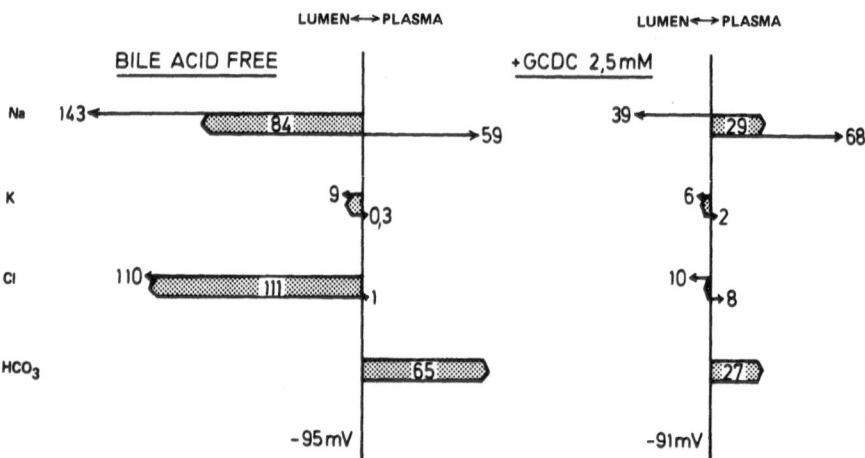

Figure 6.2 Bidirectional fluxes of Na^+, K^+, and Cl^-, and net transport rates of HCO_3^- in ileum of an 8-month-old male with congenital chloridorrhoea (μEq/min/15 cm ileum)

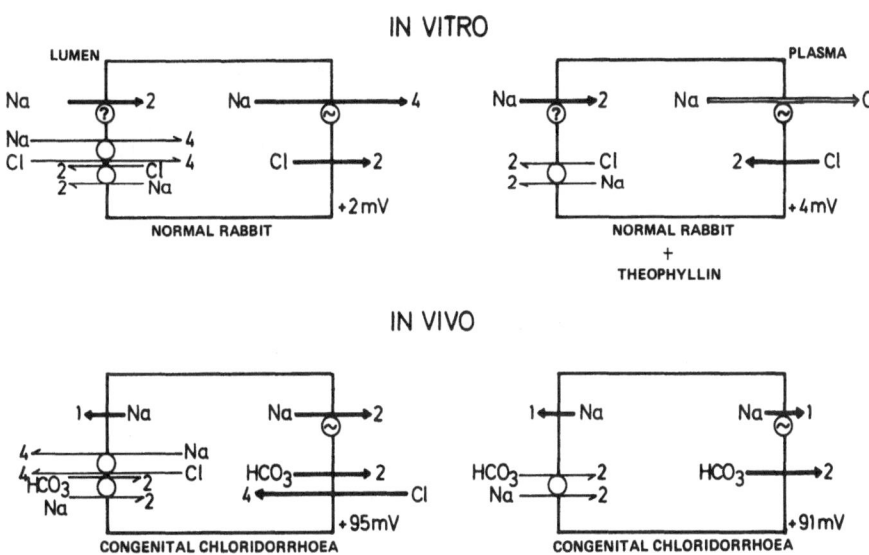

Figure 6.3 Turnberg's[2] model representing ileal electrolyte transport in normal subjects and in a patient with congenital chloridorrhoea

an insignificant fall in the CO_2 of the lumen fluid. In contrast, water and electrolyte absorption in jejunum was normal, and the transmural PD was -3 mV.

The present results obtained in ileum appear incompatible with the double

Figure 6.4 Models relating transport across rabbit brush border to transepithelial transport by rabbit ileum *in vitro* (from reference 3) and human ileum in an 8-month-old male with congenital chloridorrhoea *in vivo* (present study)

ion exchange mechanism previously proposed by Turnberg and colleagues[1] for normal ileal transport, *viz.* absorption of Na^+ in exchange for H^+, and Cl^- in exchange for HCO_3^-. The fact that luminal fluids were acidified in Turnberg's[2] patient with chloridorrhoea and not in ours suggests the existence of different defects within this clinical syndrome. However, the presence of a large electrical PD in the ileum of our patient speaks against a model featuring a defect in one of two independent electroneutral exchange mechanisms.

In contrast, our observations in congenital chloridorrhoea can be explained by the model of Frizzell and colleagues[3] (Figure 6.4), by only proposing an inversion of the coupled NaCl–influx–Na–anion efflux mechanism, which normally mediates net entry of NaCl and is inhibited by theophylline. Na^+ transport via the Cl^--independent and theophylline-insensitive mechanism need not be affected, but our data fit exactly if reversal of this movement is also postulated.

Consequently, a clinical trial with theophylline was performed. The diarrhoea stopped, but since the compound provoked vomiting — probably due to jejunal hypersecretion — we are now in the process of preparing coated theophylline to be released in the ileum only.

References

1. Turnberg, L. A., Bieberdorf, F. A., Morawski, S. G. and Fordtran, J. S. (1970). Interrelationships of chloride, bicarbonate, sodium, and hydrogen transport in the human ileum. *J. Clin. Invest.*, **49**, 557
2. Turnberg, L. A. (1971). Abnormalities in intestinal electrolyte transport in congenital chloridorrhoea. *Gut*, **12**, 544
3. Nellans, H. N., Frizzell, R. A. and Schultz, S. G. (1974). Brush-border processes and transepithelial Na and Cl transport by rabbit ileum. *Amer. J. Physiol.*, **226**, 1131

Discussion 6

Armstrong:	How would your estimates of the Cl^- electrochemical potential gradient be influenced if there is a significant difference between intracellular Cl^- activity and apparent intracellular Cl^- concentration? Specifically, what fraction of the intracellular Cl^- would have to be 'bound' or sequestered in order to reverse the direction of the Cl^- electrochemical potential gradient across the serosal cell membrane?
Frizzell:	We are aware of the problems in determining intracellular ion concentrations by these techniques; however, I should point out that these determinations employed ^{36}Cl, so that the exchangeable fraction of intracellular Cl^- was measured. Nevertheless, our data suggested that two-thirds of the intracellular Cl^- would have to be compartmentalised in order for Cl^- to be distributed at electrochemical equilibrium. At the serosal or basolateral membrane, we have suggested that Cl^- exits from the cell by diffusion because the apparent electrochemical potential within the cell exceeds that of the bathing media. As pointed out in the accompanying paper, current estimates of serosal membrane chloride conductance in Necturus gall bladder are compatible with this view, provided that this conductance is entirely due to Cl^- diffusion.
Binder:	To what extent is the apparent effect of theophylline on NaCl influx influenced by the changes in conductance produced by cyclic AMP?
Frizzell:	The decrease in conductance of rabbit ileum exposed to theophylline or cyclic AMP averaged 15% in our studies. Thus, this effect could account for only a small decline in the influxes of Na^+ and Cl^- observed in tissues preincubated with these agents. In other studies, such as those of Powell,[*] a larger conductance change is observed, but Dr Field and ourselves find only a small change. The most telling information in this regard is that the decrease in Cl^- influx observed in tissues incubated with theophylline is more than twice as great as the entire movement of Cl^- via passive conductance pathways across this tissue.
Murer:	It is not possible that coupled NaCl absorption is the sum of two electroneutral exchange processes, for instance Na^+ exchanged for H^+ and Cl^- for HCO_3^-?
Frizzell:	Yes, the model shown on p. 105 makes provision for $NaHCO_3$ efflux to explain the observations *in vivo* that ileum secretes HCO_3^-, apparently in exchange for luminal Cl^-. I should emphasize that our estimates of cell-to-mocosal solution efflux are based upon steady-state assumptions (in other words, that the net flux of each ion across the apical and basolateral membranes is the same as that across the tissue). They are not based on direct measurements, as are the influx data. Thus, they are derived values. The exact identities of the efflux species require further elucidation. However, our data do suggest that at least a fraction of this ion efflux is composed of NaCl.
Munck:	The very low passive permeability and extremely high transmural PD necessitates that, in the patient reported by Dr Rask-Madsen, the PD profile shown for the frog skin by Dr Armstrong must apply.

---

[*] *Amer. J. Physiol.*, **227**, 1436, 1974

Armstrong: Our observations indicate that the intrinsic e.m.f., as well as the measured membrane potential across the mucosal membrane of bullfrog small intestinal epithelia is orientated so that the cell interior is negative with respect to the mucosal medium.

Levin: I reckon that the PD mentioned by Dr Rask-Madsen must qualify for inclusion in the Guinness Book of Records!

7
Sodium-Driven Transport
A Re-evaluation of the
Sodium-Gradient Hypothesis

FRANCISCO ALVARADO*

Department of Physiology and Biophysics,
School of Medicine, University of Puerto Rico,
San Juan, Puerto Rico

INTRODUCTION

The sodium-gradient hypothesis (SGH) was originally proposed to explain the uphill transport of certain organic solutes,† particularly sugars and amino acids, in the small intestine as well as in several other cells and tissues[1,2,3,4]. The molecular basis of this transport is assumed to consist of a typical *mobile carrier* mechanism[5] that is made asymmetrical by virtue of its being coupled to the opposite transmembrane gradients of the alkali metal ions, Na^+ and K^+. The fundamental concept underlying the hypothesis is that of *cotransport*[6]. Organic solute and Na^+ would interact at the level of a carrier with distinct but (allosterically) related binding sites for each of these two species. The concept of cotransport includes the twin concepts of *reciprocal activation* and *coupled flows*: binding and the ensuing influx of one species activates the binding and influx of its partner. As a corollary, reciprocal *inhibitory effects* and *countertransport* may also be explained through, and be a part of, the same mechanism[6]. In fact, such opposite activating and inhibitory roles were assigned by Crane to Na^+ and K^+ respectively[2]. The prevailing extracellular

---

* On special leave from the University of Puerto Rico. Present address: Laboratorie de Physiologie Comparée, Université de Paris-Sud, Centre d'Orsay, 91405-Orsay, France.
† Since essentially identical mechanisms are involved in the Na^+-dependent transport of sugars and amino acids[6], the term *organic solute* or, simply, *solute* or *substrate* will be used throughout to refer collectively to either or both of these chemical species.

cation, Na^+, would stimulate solute influx by cotransport, while the prevailing intracellular cation, K^+, would inhibit the efflux and perhaps move out of the cell by countertransport. The concerted effect of the two cations would be the net accumulation of the organic solute within the enterocyte.

According to the SGH, therefore, the energy for organic solute accumulation comes entirely from the electrochemical potential energy stored in the Na^+/K^+ gradient. In this concept resides precisely the most far-reaching theoretical implication of the SGH; it clearly allows for the distinction between two types of *active transport* mechanisms, depending on the exact origin of the energy directly implicated in the substrate accumulation: *primary* and *secondary* active transport processes[7,8].

Although all energy for active transport must ultimately come from some exergonic metabolic reaction, the question remains as to the exact manner in which the coupling is accomplished. The sodium pump, for instance, would be a clear example of a primary active transport process, since a direct link between Na^+ transport and ATP hydrolysis has been demonstrated in all cells studied[9]. On the contrary, the question of whether organic solute transport constitutes a true case of secondary active transport, as claimed by the proponents of the SGH, is today a matter of heated controversy. Some workers, particularly Kimmich[10,11], claim that organic solute transport in the small intestine is linked directly to ATP hydrolysis, and in fact may share the same Na^+-K^+-ATPase that has been implicated in the transport of Na^+ and K^+. The possibility is also entertained by others that solute transport in the intestine and other cells (for example the ascites tumour cell) may have both primary and secondary components. Some workers deny that the energy stored in the Na^+/K^+ gradient is sufficient to account fully for all organic solute uphill transport[12,13].

In the present paper, I intend to analyse some of the experimental evidence supporting the SGH, particularly with reference to the small intestine. Although some of the experimental evidence appears to be incompatible with the SGH, particularly if the hypothesis is understood in a rigid or 'static' manner, other results to be discussed here suggest the possibility of modifying the SGH in such a way that no source of energy other than that stored in the electrochemical potential gradient for Na^+ and K^+ need be invoked to explain organic solute uphill transport in the small intestine. According to the dynamic reformulation of the SGH, the factor determining the unidirectional influx and accumulation of an organic solute is not the Na^+/K^+ gradient *per se*. Solute influx is driven by a coupled flow of Na^+ that is made essentially irreversible by virtue of a coupling between the influx across the brush border and extrusion by the pump at the basolateral membrane. Intracellular K^+ is postulated to play a key role in making the coupled Na^+ and organic solute fluxes across the brush border essentially irreversible. This role of K^+ takes place through a specific *capacity effect* of this ion acting at a site other than the Na^+-binding site involved in solute activation.

118

LACK OF A DIRECT ROLE OF ATP IN ORGANIC SOLUTE TRANSPORT IN SMALL INTESTINE

The strongest arguments in favour of a direct role of ATP in solute transport in the intestine have been marshalled by Kimmich[10,11]. In this work, technically first-rate, Kimmich used isolated epithelial cells from chicken small intestine. The use of isolated cells constitutes an innovation that in theory would simplify things, making interpretation of the results easier. On the contrary, in practice, the analysis of the results is severely complicated by the fact that the enterocyte is a polar cell; it is limited by two functionally very distinct boundaries, the *brush-border* and the *basolateral* membranes. In whole-tissue experiments, where the two-dimensional structure of the intestinal epithelium is preserved, it is possible to interpret results in terms of fluxes across only the luminal (brush border) face of the enterocyte. This is no longer possible when the individual cells are in free suspension and both membranes are equally accessible to substrate, ions, and any other effector that may have been added to the incubation medium. Both in the analysis of his own data, and in the ensuing generalizations to the results found by others using the intact epithelium, Kimmich has largely ignored these facts, treating the enterocyte as if, in his experiments, only a single membrane, the brush border, were operative. The untenability of such an approach has been amply exposed by other work also involving the use of isolated cells[14,15].

The hypothesis that solute transport in the intestine may share a common transport ATPase with Na^+ has been refuted by work from several laboratories, which indicates a different localization of the sugar and amino acid carriers (located in the brush border) with respect to the Na^+-K^+-ATPase (located in the basolateral membrane). Particularly worth mentioning in this regard is the work of Hopfer, Murer and colleagues demonstrating Na^+-dependent solute transport in brush-border membrane vesicles that have no ATPase activity[16,17].

One of Kimmich's experiments may be mentioned here for its high relevance to arguments to be made later in this paper. Using isolated chicken cells, Kimmich found that ouabain inhibits sugar transport almost instantaneously (Figure 3 in reference 10). He considered this as strong evidence that the Na^+-K^+-ATPase (known to be ouabain sensitive) is directly involved in active sugar transport. However, if ouabain is added to free cells, it may have ready access to the outer face of the basolateral membrane, its locus of action, a situation that would not hold in the case of the intact epithelium. It is known that, in whole-tissue experiments, ouabain added to the mucosal solution is inactive, while if added to the serosal solution it may become active only after a lag period, which is presumably required for the inhibitor to diffuse across several layers of tissue until it can reach its target at the basolateral membrane level[18]. An alternate interpretation of the early effect of ouabain in

Kimmich's experiments is that, as suggested later in this paper, active solute transport requires a fully active sodium pump, together with a functional coupling between Na^+ influx across the brush border and its active extrusion at the basolateral membrane. Any interference with the functioning of the pump would be accompanied immediately by a decrease in solute influx. If a medium-to-cell Na^+ concentration gradient is not *per se* the determining factor underlying active solute transport, there is no need to expect any delay in the action of ouabain; in other words, this inhibitor need not act, as is widely believed, simply by abolishing the Na^+/K^+ gradient.

Finally, and further supporting the argument of a lack of direct participation of ATP in solute transport, it may be mentioned that no one has ever been able to show any correlation between ATP hydrolysis and solute uphill transport[19]. More recently, Heinz again analysed this question in very careful experiments with ascites tumour cells, once more with negative results[13].

EXPERIMENTAL BASIS OF THE SODIUM-GRADIENT HYPOTHESIS: KINETIC EVIDENCE

Two main lines of evidence support the SGH. On the one hand, we have the kinetic evidence for the *activation* of solute transport by Na^+, and for its converse. On the other hand, we have the question of the *reversal* of a substrate flux when the sodium gradient (the transmembrane concentration gradient of sodium) is inversed. The question of activation will be dealt with first, since it was also the first to be observed. There is little doubt that reciprocal activations occur in organic solute and Na^+ transport, so that the experimental basis for the concept of cotransport is solid. However, whether this activation plays a central role in uphill solute transport is a different question that may only be elucidated from experiments on flux reversal. We shall see that, even though evidence for such a reversal has been around for more than ten years, interesting questions in this respect remain unanswered.

Crane, Forstner and Eichholz[3] were the first to provide direct kinetic evidence that the apparent affinity of the carrier for sugars (in hamster intestine) is a direct function of $(Na^+)_o$, the external (bulk) concentration of Na^+. The experiments involved a demonstration that apparently simple Michaelis kinetics were followed, even at $(Na^+)_o = 0$, using the tissue-accumulation method[20] and incubation times of 10 minutes. Since Lineweaver-Burk plots at various concentrations of Na^+ all gave the same intercept, the conclusion seemed warranted that V_{max} was constant and independent of $(Na^+)_o$, that is, Na^+-activation in hamster intestine represented a pure case of *affinity* or *K-kinetics* (for an explanation of the terminology, see reference 6).

Similar kinetic studies of solute activation by Na^+ have been performed with other substrates and other animal species with similar results. Particularly worth mentioning is the work of Schultz and Zalusky demonstrating the reverse side of the coin, namely, the activation of Na^+ transport by organic solutes (for review, see reference 18).

A general model for cotransport

It is known that the active transport of many solutes, both organic (for example sugars, amino acids, bile salts, uracil, ascorbic acid) and inorganic (such as sulphate, chloride) is activated by the sodium ion[18]. The possibility became apparent that this general dependence on Na^+ may not be coincidental, but rather could reflect the existence of a common mechanism of great physiological significance. Two schools of thought relative to this question developed in the last ten years. Since sugars and amino acids (particularly the neutral, but also the basic) were the most studied among the above solutes, the controversy centred around them, although a possible extrapolation to the case of other solutes was always implied. As one school has it, sugars and amino acids are transported by entirely different, 'parallel' mechanisms, the common trait of a dependency on sodium being a mere coincidence[18]. According to the other school, the common Na^+-dependency has a profound meaning, and identical mechanisms are postulated to be involved in all these transport processes. The possibility has also been suggested that the carriers for sugars and amino acids may be associated functionally, and they may even share common Na^+-binding sites[21-24]. Following this last possibility, a general model for the activation of solute transport in the small intestine has been proposed[6] and is schematised in Figure 7.1. Some of the salient features of this model will be summarised here, using for illustration purposes some still unpublished results on sugar transport in guinea-pig jejunum[25].

The carrier, C, is bifunctional and has two separate but allosterically interrelated sites for both the substrate, S, and the allosteric modifier (activator), A. Although in the experiments to be shown here A is Na^+, the model is entirely symmetrical and allows for an analysis of the activation of Na^+ transport by the organic solutes. Formation of the ternary complex S–C–Na^+ occurs in a stepwise manner by either of two possible routes, namely with either S or A binding first. By definition, the model is *non-compulsory*. The overall dissociation constant (K_{sa}) of the ternary complex S–C–A is the product of the two (partial) dissociation constants involved in each reaction sequence:

$$K_{sa} = K_s \cdot K_a' = K_a \cdot K_s' \qquad (1)$$

which can be rearranged in this manner:

$$K_s/K_s' = K_a/K_a' = R \qquad (2)$$

For the case we are dealing with at present, namely that of activation, R is always greater than 1.

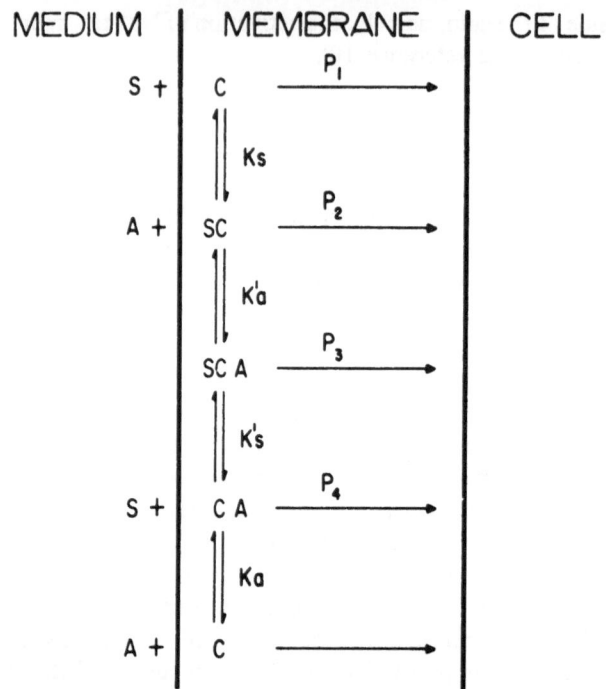

MEDIUM | MEMBRANE | CELL

Figure 7.1 The general model for cotransport. The two reaction sequences for the stepwise formation of the ternary complex S–C–A at the external face of the membrane are schematized, together with the respective dissociation constants. The horizontal arrows and permeability constants, P, illustrate the translocation step that is considered essentially irreversible. Taken from reference 6

The *translocation, permeability* or *rate constants, P_1* to P_4 (Figure 7.1) need not be equal, thus allowing for possible effects on V_{max} (*capacity* or *V-effects*). However, since all Na^+-activations of solute transport to be discussed in this paper constitute pure cases of *affinity* or *K-kinetics*, the simplification may be made that all P constants are equal. If we further assume that, under appropriate experimental conditions (see later), the influx reaction is irreversible, the general equation may be obtained:

$$v = V_{max}/\ 1 + (K_s/(S))(K_a + (A)/K_a + (A)\,R) \qquad (3)$$

At each concentration of A, this equation simplifies to that of Michaelis and Menten, where K_T is equivalent to the Michaelis constant, K_m:

$$K_T = K_s(K_a + (A)/K_a + (A)\,R) \qquad (4)$$

Using guinea-pig jejunum, saturation curves were obtained using the two methylglucosides as substrates, in the presence of fixed Na^+ concentrations in the range 0–134 mM. The results of a preliminary survey (Table 7.1) demonstrate quite convincingly that: (a) Methylglucoside transport follows Michaelis–Menten kinetics at any value of $(Na^+)_o$ and (b) increasing $(Na^+)_o$

Table 7.1 Kinetics of the activation of methylglucoside transport by the sodium ion

(n)	(Na^+) (mM)	V_{max} (μmoles/min)	K_T (mM)
Substrate: β-methylglucoside			
(5)	—	1.32	10.0
(5)	57.9	1.25	2.53
(4)	101.3	1.15	1.50
(6)	133.9	1.33	1.62
		(mean: 1.26)	
Substrate: α-methylglucoside			
(6)	—	1.53	31.60
(4)	57.9	1.51	6.35
(5)	101.3	1.85	5.54
(6)	133.9	1.30	4.03
		(mean: 1.55)	

Rings from everted guinea-pig jejunum were incubated for 5 minutes in 5 ml phosphate buffer containing 8.5 mM K$^+$ and Na$^+$ concentrations as indicated: Li$^+$ was used to replace the Na$^+$. Experimental procedure and handling of the data was as described[6]. (n) is the number of experiments (animals).

causes K_T to decrease, leaving V_{max} essentially unaffected. The conclusion seemed inescapable that, as in the case of the amino acids[6], sugar transport in the guinea-pig intestine constitutes a pure case of affinity kinetics that may in principle be described by equations (3) and (4).

To demonstrate the fitting of the data to the general model, the results in Table 7.1 were subjected to the kinetic analysis developed previously[6] for this purpose: detailed calculations will be published elsewhere[25]. For the moment, it is enough to show (Figure 7.2) that theoretical curves (solid lines) calculated on the basis of equation (4) fit quite well the experimental results obtained with either glucoside. Furthermore, the similarity of these curves with that previously published for the case of an amino acid in the same animal (cycloleucine, Figure 4 in reference 6) seems obvious. Further evidence indicating a similar mechanism for the activation of organic solute transport by Na$^+$ is shown in Table 7.2, where data currently available on the kinetics of transport of two sugars and two amino acids in guinea-pig jejunum are directly compared. The most striking fact emerging from these data is the essentially identical value for K_a obtained in all cases. If allowance is made for a certain variability of the results (the data at this stage may be considered as only preliminary), the value of K_a (the dissociation constant for Na$^+$) is approximately equal to 180 mM in all cases. An identical value for K_a is precisely the result to be expected if the hypothesis is correct that sugars and amino acids conform to identical mechanisms for sodium activation and may even share common Na$^+$-binding sites.

Another interesting fact emerging from the data in Table 7.2 is that the ratios K_a/K_s range in value from 5 to 20. As argued previously, this means that organic solutes 'are about ten times better as activators of Na$^+$ than Na$^+$

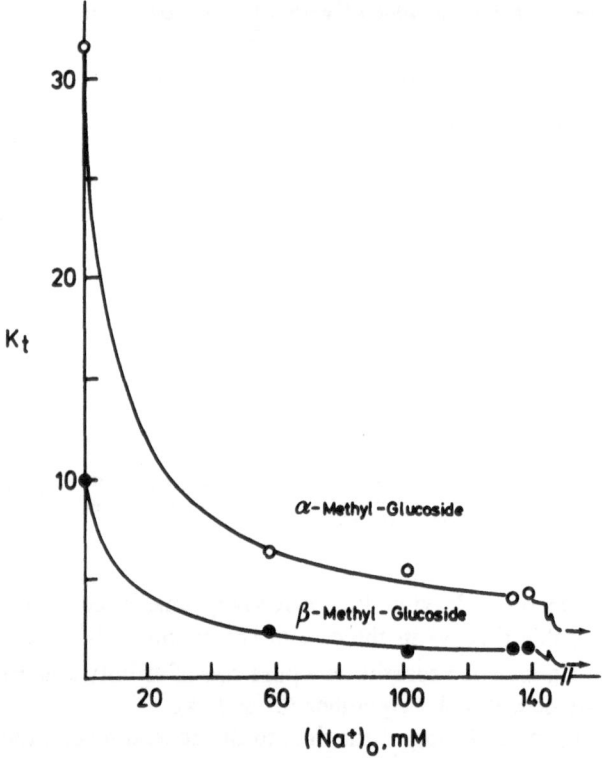

Figure 7.2 The effect of $(Na^+)_o$ on the K_T for the transport of the methylglucosides in guinea-pig jejunum. Data from Table 7.1: The solid lines show the theoretical fit of the data according to equation (4) and using the constants shown in Table 7.2. The arrows indicate the limiting value of K_T (K'_s) at infinite $(Na^+)_o$

is' of organic solute transport[6]. The significance of this observation will become evident later in this paper when the concept of sodium-driven transport is formulated. In effect, it can be calculated from the equations of the general model for cotransport that, under conditions of similar *relative* concentration of solute and Na^+ (identical values for the ratios $(S)/K_s$ or $(A)/K_a$),

Table 7.2 Cotransport of organic solutes and sodium ion in guinea-pig jejunum

Substrate	K_s (mM)	K_a (mM)	K_{sa} (mM)	R	K_a/K_s
Cycloleucine	28.2	247	0.64	10.9	8.8
L-alanine	22.7	132	0.50	6.0	5.9
α-Methylglucoside	31.6	163	0.34	15.1	5.2
β-Methylglucoside	9.9	184	0.12	15.0	18.5

Summary of preliminary data concerning dissociation constants for the solute (K_s), the sodium ion (K_a), the overall ternary complex (K_{sa}), and appropriate ratios between constants. Taken from reference 45.

all solute-activated fluxes of Na^+ are greater than any corresponding Na^+-activated flux of solute.*

EVIDENCE THAT A MOBILE CARRIER IS INVOLVED IN ORGANIC SOLUTE TRANSPORT IN THE SMALL INTESTINE. SOLUTE-FLUX REVERSAL EXPERIMENTS

The kinetic evidence summarized above constitutes a solid theoretical basis for the concept of cotransport of Na^+ and solutes, the cornerstone of the SGH. In the following, evidence will be discussed that this cotransport involves a mobile carrier mechanism. Emphasis will be placed on the operational nature of the carrier concept, which will involve evidence of reversibility, competition between analogues, and countertransport[5].

The first demonstration that a gradient of Na^+ can drive the uphill transport of an organic solute was probably that of Vidaver[26], using pigeon red blood cells and glycine as substrate. Shortly thereafter, a similar demonstration of Na^+-linked flux reversal was achieved using the sugar transport system in hamster small intestine. Of these experiments, carried out independently and almost simultaneously by Crane[27] in Chicago and by Alvarado[4] in Madrid, only the former are widely recognized, in spite of the fact that the second represented an equivalent but considerably more thorough demonstration that a mobile carrier is involved in this system. In the following, a summary of the Madrid work will be given because it constitutes an approach with possibilities that have not been fully exploited and also because it can be used as the point of departure for discussing facts of high relevance to the argument being developed in this paper.

The two key experiments are reproduced in Figure 7.3. Accumulation of a glucose analogue, arbutin, requires both Na^+ and oxygen. If, after a short period of incubation in which the substrate is allowed to accumulate against the gradient, the uncoupler 2,4-dinitrophenol (DNP) is added to the medium, the substrate is seen to leave the tissue downhill, to approach a tissue/medium (T/M) concentration ratio of 1, that is, *equilibration*. It is as if, upon withdrawing the supply of energy that supports uphill transport (by uncoupling ATP synthesis with the DNP), the asymmetrical (uphill) carrier system had become symmetrical (downhill). That the energy directly involved in sugar uphill transport comes from the sodium gradient is shown by the fact that, if $(Na^+)_o$ is reduced to zero, the accumulated substrate rapidly leaves the tissue and in fact accumulates in the medium against its own concentration gradient (the lower curve in Figure 7.3A falls below the T/M ratio of 1). Furthermore, the energy for this uphill transport in the reverse (tissue-to-medium) direction only comes from the inverted sodium gradient since it may be equally well demonstrated in tissue poisoned with DNP (Figure 7 in reference 4).

---

* Of course, this statement applies only to conditions of lack of saturation with substrate. If the system is saturated with regard to both S and A, the two fluxes become equal: by definition, the *coupling coefficient* is unity.

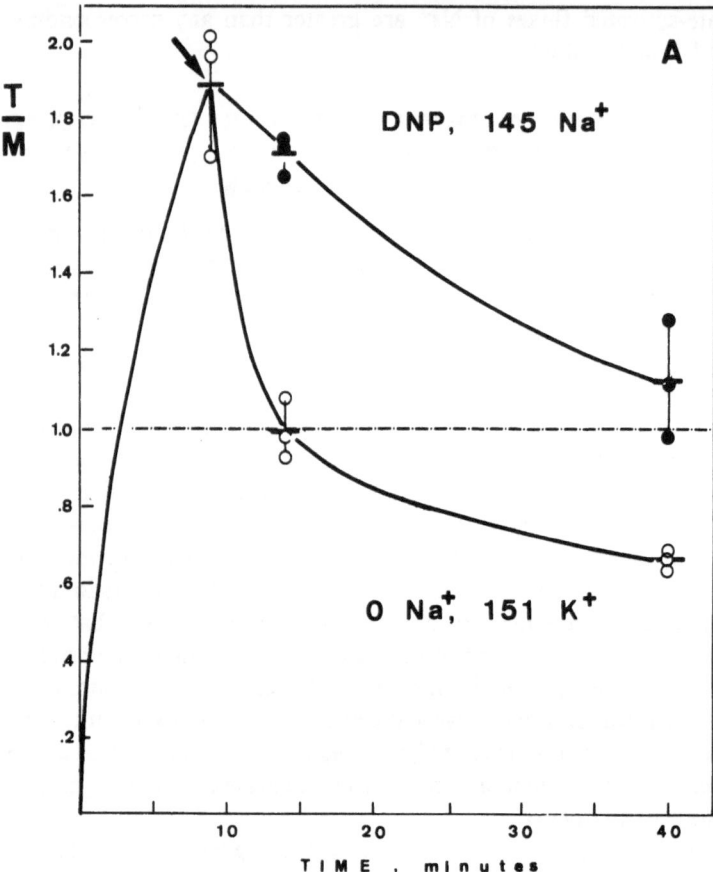

Figure 7.3 Flux reversal experiments. Rings of everted intestine from hamsters were loaded with substrate, S, by a *first incubation* in presence of 5 mM S in oxygenated bicarbonate buffer[48] containing 6 mM K[+] (sodium buffer). At the arrow, the tissues were transferred for a *second incubation* as indicated. *Part A. Upper curve:* Sodium buffer with 5 mM S and 0.5 mM DNP. *Lower curve:* Na[+]-free, K[+]-substituted buffer with 5 mM S. *Part B.* Sodium buffer, 4.5 mM S, 0.23 mM DNP and 27.3 mM *elicitor*, that is, D-mannitol (*upper curve*) or D-glucose (*lower curve*). The results are expressed as the substrate concentration ratios, tissue/medium (T/M), where a ratio of 1 indicates equilibration. Redrawn from reference 4, figures 2 and 4 respectively

The experiment in Figure 7.3B demonstrates the phenomenon of *countertransport*, which can be considered as a proof that a mobile carrier is involved[5]. In the highly asymmetrical system of the intestine, substrate influx in the first few minutes is practically irreversible, as we shall discuss in detail later and demonstration of countertransport is not as easy as it usually is in the case of symmetrical carrier systems. Nevertheless, two experimental devices have been used to demonstrate countertransport in the intestine. First, the system may be allowed to run for some time and approach the steady state, a condition in which inward and outward substrate fluxes become approx-

126

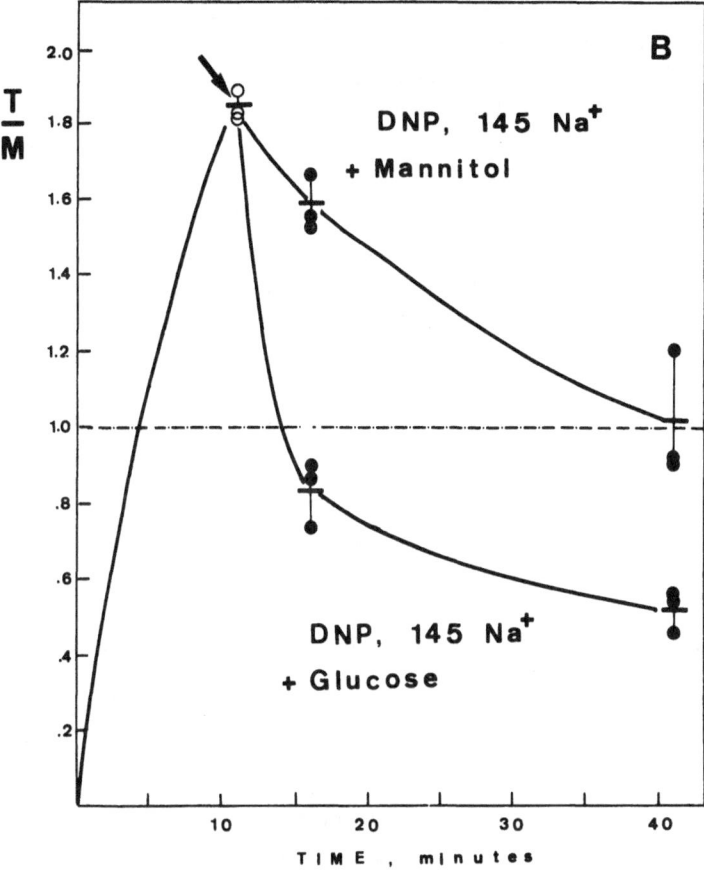

Figure 7.3B

imately equal. Under these conditions, addition to the incubation medium of an analogue (the *elicitor*) that competes for the same carrier would cause a net efflux of the substrate, or countertransport[24,28]. Second (this was the approach first used by Alvarado[4]), after a short incubation period in which the substrate is allowed to enter the tissue essentially unidirectionally, DNP is added to make the system reversible as in the experiment described above (upper curve in Figure 7.3A). Under these conditions, the substrate flows downhill into the medium, and addition to this medium of some inert analogue such as mannitol would have no effect on the rate of substrate efflux (compare the two upper curves in Figure 7.3A and B respectively). But substitution of the mannitol by an analogue capable of competing with the substrate for the carrier will elicit a very significant increase in the rate of substrate efflux, that is, countertransport. In fact, the net efflux may be such that the substrate accumulates in the external medium against its own concentration gradient, as demonstrated by the fact that the lower curve in Figure 7.3B falls below the equilibration value of T/M = 1. Using this technique, Alvarado was able to demonstrate that Na^+ is required for countertransport to occur in hamster intestine, indicating that the affinity of the carrier for the sugars is a function of $(Na^+)_o$. Cations such as $Tris^+$ behave essentially in an inert manner in this regard, but K^+ has a specific inhibitory effect since countertransport could not be demonstrated when this cation was used to substitute for all the Na^+ ions[4]. The experiments just described permitted the following conclusions:

(1) Sugar transport in the intestine involves a typical mobile carrier.

(2) This carrier system, however, is made asymmetrical by coupling to some energy source, as evidenced by its dependence on an adequate oxygen supply.

(3) Withdrawal of the energy source, for instance, by poisoning with DNP, renders the carrier symmetrical or downhill.

(4) The affinity of the substrate for the carrier is a function of $(Na^+)_o$.

(5) Na^+ acts as an allosteric activator of the sugar–carrier interaction.

(6) K^+ has an opposite effect to that of Na^+, probably through the same site.

(7) The relative medium-to-tissue concentration ratio of Na^+ (the sodium gradient) determines the direction of net sugar transport.

(8) The reversal of sugar flux caused by an inversion of the Na^+ gradient is independent of metabolic energy since it can be readily demonstrated in tissues poisoned with DNP.

(9) Therefore, Na^+-dependent sugar transport may be fully explained in terms of the classical *affinity–gradient hypothesis*.

THE SODIUM-GRADIENT HYPOTHESIS AS A SPECIAL CASE OF THE AFFINITY-GRADIENT HYPOTHESIS. DIFFICULTY IN RECONCILING THE EXPERIMENTAL FACTS WITH THE THEORY

Mobile carriers are, by definition, freely reversible[5]. The classical equation shown below defines v_{net} (the net substrate flow) as the difference between an inward and an outward flux $(v_{in} - v_{out})$, each given by a Michaelis relationship:

$$V_{net} = \frac{V_{max1}\,(S_1)}{(S_1) + K_{T1}} - \frac{V_{max2}\,(S_2)}{(S_2) + K_{T2}} \tag{5}$$

where suffixes 1 and 2 indicate the extra- and the intracellular fluids respectively. In the absence of an external energy supply, both the capacity (V_{max}) and the affinity (K_T) factors at either side of the membrane are equal $(V_{max1} = V_{max2}$ and $K_{T1} = K_{T2})$ the system being entirely symmetrical. Obviously, under these conditions and at steady state, it should hold that $(S_1)/(S_2) = 1$: the carrier necessarily leads simply towards substrate equilibration.

A giant theoretical advance in the transport field took place when it was shown that any carrier system may achieve uphill transport provided an asymmetry is introduced at some point of the cycle. This showed for the first time that there is no essential difference between uphill and downhill transport systems, except for the coupling in the former case to some metabolic energy source[5]. The *affinity–gradient* hypothesis assumes that, while the capacity factor remains unchanged, coupling to some energy source at a given point in the cycle may render the two affinity factors unequal, thereby causing a net accumulation of substrate at that side of the membrane where K_T is greater, that is, the affinity lower. The well-known assumptions just described are summarised in Figure 7.4. It seems obvious that, according to this hypothesis, Michaelis kinetics may be expected only when true initial velocities are measured, so that (S_2) is essentially equal to zero. As soon as (S_2) begins to build up, the kinetics will deviate from the expectations of the Michaelis theory, unless the value of K_{T2} is exceedingly large. The relevance of these considerations to the argument being developed in this paper will become obvious in what follows.

UPHILL TRANSPORT:

THE AFFINITY-GRADIENT HYPOTHESIS

$$V_{\max_1} = V_{\max_2}$$
$$K_{T1} < K_{T2}$$

And, at the steady-state:

$$\frac{(S_2)}{(S_1)} = \frac{K_{T2}}{K_{T1}} > 1$$

Figure 7.4 The postulates of the affinity-gradient hypothesis

From the facts summarised earlier, it seems clear that the SGH constitutes a special case of the affinity-gradient hypothesis. For the last ten years, many workers, including myself, have accepted at face value the idea that the uphill transport of organic solutes in the intestine may be explained simply by the gradient of affinity across the brush border, caused by the transmembrane concentration gradient of Na^+ and K^+. However, a close scrutiny of the experimental data would have shown very early that the situation is not so simple. For instance, we have mentioned that the affinity-gradient hypothesis may explain *net* substrate accumulation, but Michaelis kinetics may be expected to hold only under rather restricted experimental conditions. The fact that sugar transport in hamster intestine apparently follows simple Michaelis kinetics for considerable periods of time (up to at least 10 minutes), even when the medium Na^+ concentration is zero[3], appears to be incompatible with observations also summarised above (Figure 7.3) that the flux of sugar is inversed when $(Na^+)_o$ is made equal to zero. Specifically, the gradient of affinity (given by the ratio K_{T2}/K_{T1}) would be at a very low value and may even be reversed; for example, it may be smaller than 1 at $(Na^+)_o = 0$, in contrast with a value greater than 1 required by the affinity-gradient hypothesis (Figure 7.4). This situation would be particularly true when K^+ is used as the Na^+-substituting cation, as in some of the experiments of Crane and colleagues[3]. Since both the kinetic experiments under discussion and those on flux reversal discussed earlier were performed using the same experimental animal, hamster, and even the same substrate, 6-deoxyglucose[4,27], there seems to be no way of reconciling the two sets of experimental observations.

Possible differences between animal species

In view of the preceding comments, it would appear that the question of the reversal of organic solute fluxes by inversion of the Na^+ gradient deserves further investigation, and work along these lines has been reinitiated in our laboratory. In relation to this, it seems appropriate at this moment to re-emphasise the importance of taking into consideration possible differences between species. This is a facet of physiology that is all too frequently overlooked. Particularly in the intestinal transport field, we seem to suffer from a chronic malaise according to which results are freely extrapolated from species to species, leading to constant controversy and confusion.

I would like to start from the proposition that essentially identical mechanisms underlie the Na^+-dependent transport of organic solutes in mammals, birds, and perhaps most vertebrates. A few years ago, for instance, Alvarado and Monreal marshalled the evidence that, in these animals, the sugar carriers may have a common phylogenetic origin[29]. A similar argument may be made, perhaps, for the case of other solutes. At the same time, it does not necessarily follow that all species must exhibit identical transport characteristics macroscopically. Rather, it can be conceived that, even though in a given instance the same basic mechanism might be involved, relatively minor differences between two species may lead to operationally quite different behaviour, in terms of a given physiological parameter or test. In the following, some examples will be mentioned suggesting the existence of meaningful differences between some of the species commonly used in intestinal transport studies.

Using chicken intestine, Alvarado and Monreal[29] demonstrated a mechanism for the Na^+-dependent transport of phenylglucosides, essentially identical to that previously shown in the hamster[4]. In both species, the direction of net glucoside flux was shown to be dictated by the medium-to-tissue Na^+-concentration gradient. However, and in contrast with the results found using the hamster, a net efflux of arbutin from tissue to medium at zero values of $(Na^+)_o$ was not achieved using the chicken (see reference 29, Figure 3). At the time, we ignored this apparent quantitative difference between species, considering it as unimportant. The more recent work of Kimmich with isolated chicken enterocytes, however, made us reconsider the possibility that there may indeed be some meaningful difference in the behaviour of hamster and chicken intestine with regard to the precise role of the sodium gradient in organic solute transport. Kimmich was unable to obtain a reversal of the flux of galactose when he inversed the gradient for Na^+, although it must be emphasised that Kimmich never used values of $(Na^+)_o$ below the 20 mM level in his experiments[10].

More recently, experiments similar to those shown in Figure 7.3 were carried out in our laboratory, using guinea-pig intestine. To our surprise, the results so reproducibly obtained using the hamster could not be repeated; namely no net efflux of substrate from tissue to medium at $(Na^+)_o = 0$ could be achieved using the guinea-pig jejunum. Lack of time has prevented us from further investigating the possible meaning of these observations. Nevertheless, the data available clearly suggest that the differences mentioned above are meaningful. In the last part of this paper, attention is focused mainly on the recent results obtained in our laboratory using the guinea-pig jejunum. More work will be required to ascertain to what extent the conclusions drawn from these observations apply to other animal species.

Before proceeding, however, mention must be made of a hitherto neglected property of solute transport in the intestine: its high asymmetry, manifested operationally by the essential irreversibility of the carrier-mediated substrate influx across the brush-border membrane.

UNIDIRECTIONALITY OF ORGANIC SOLUTE TRANSPORT IN THE SMALL INTESTINE

Although, as we have seen, a mobile carrier mechanism seems to be involved in solute transport in the intestine, there exists, nevertheless, an obvious implication that the transport includes at some point an irreversible step. There is no other way of explaining the good agreement of the experimental results with the predictions of simple Michaelis–Menten kinetics, even when rather long incubations are used. Finch[30] was probably the first to point out that amino acid transport in the small intestine is 'non-reversible'. This concept of irreversibility, of course, is merely operational and specifically refers to the initial period of uptake, before much substrate accumulation has taken place. In long-term experiments involving steady-state conditions. It is possible experimentally to demonstrate that the process is reversible, as would be expected[31], and has been mentioned above in relation to the experimental demonstration of countertransport[24,28].

The situation as I see it is schematised in Figure 7.5. In the upper part, the reactions involved in the carrier cycle are shown according to common usage. The external substrate, S, combines with the carrier, C, to give the Michaelis complex, S–C: this is translocated to the inner side, releasing S′ to the intracellular fluid and regenerating C, which *returns empty*. In this last assumption, the model differs from classical carrier theory, the cornerstone of which

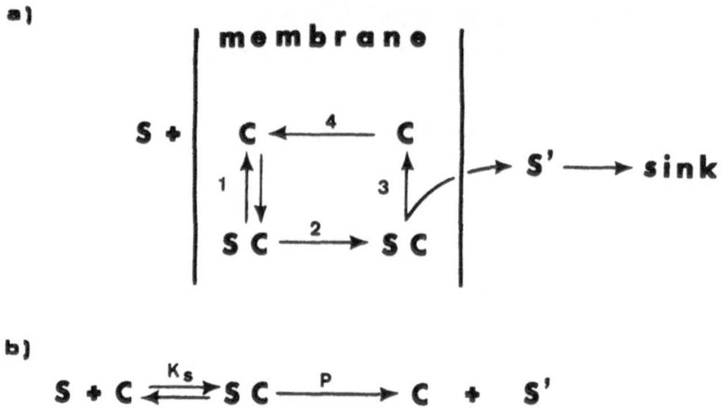

Figure 7.5 Schematic representation of an asymmetric mobile carrier system that may give Michaelis–Menten kinetics for long time periods

is the concept of a reversible mechanism[5]. Any unorthodoxy, however, is milder than it may appear at first sight. While the existence of reversibility is granted, the asymmetry of the system may be such that, in operational terms, and under appropriate conditions, reaction 3 may be considered as *practically* irreversible, as drawn. The passive movement of substrate to other layers of tissue across the basolateral membrane (represented in the scheme by the 'sink'), would further contribute to the irreversibility of the system.

If all the above assumptions are correct (and there is much evidence to support them, as we shall see in the following), the carrier cycle might be simplified drastically, as shown in Figure 7.5b. Here, the reversible interaction between S and C at the external face of the membrane, defined by a dissociation constant, K_s, is shown to be followed by an irreversible translocation step that is rate-limiting, governed by the permeability constant, P. Of course, this unidirectional arrow encompasses reactions 2–4 in Figure 7.5a. It means that, for all practical purposes, the presence of C at the inner side of the membrane, either bound or free, may be ignored: this is the assumption made in developing the general model discussed above (Figure 7.1). Needless to say, the sequence proposed in Figure 7.5b is coincident with the basic assumption in Michaelis kinetics.

A direct demonstration that substrate efflux from tissue to medium across the mucosal border is negligible under the conditions of our kinetic experiments would appear to be essential for the argument that the influx of substrate across this membrane is to all intents and purposes irreversible. Without entailing a detailed discussion of unidirectional fluxes across the intestinal epithelium, the following simple experiment will serve to provide such a demonstration. Sacs of hamster intestine were prepared according to Crane and Wilson[36]. This technique permits the measurement of the mucosal-to-serosal flux $(\mathcal{J}_{m \to s})$ by taking samples periodically from the serosal compartment (SC) of a well-oxygenated sac of everted intestine, with labelled substrate initially added only to the mucosal compartment (MC). Results obtained using

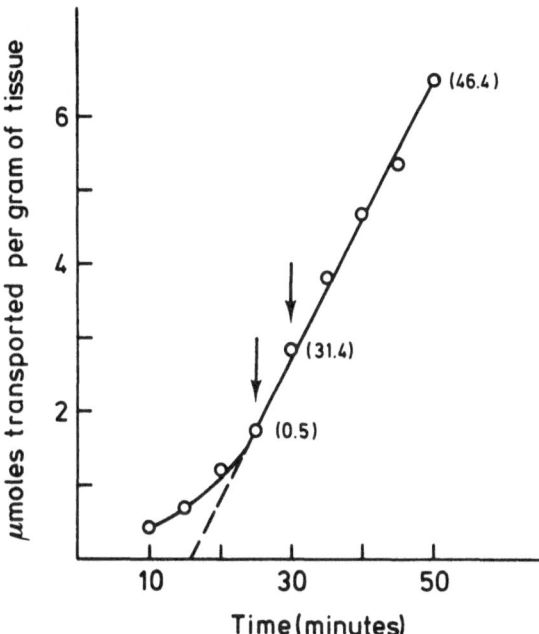

Figure 7.6 Asymmetry of substrate influx across the intestinal brush-border membrane. One sac from the everted intestine of one hamster was mounted on the apparatus described by Crane and Wilson[36]. The serosal compartment was filled with 1.2 ml phosphate buffer[48] without substrate (serosal fluid, SF), and the entire preparation was immersed in 15 ml of the same buffer (mucosal fluid, MF). After a 10-minute equilibration period at 37 °C, the experiment was initiated by transferring the sac preparation to fresh MF containing 1.12 mM [³H]cycloleucine. Aliquots (20 μl) were withdrawn at intervals from the SF for radioactivity measurement. At 25 and 30 minutes (arrows), two consecutive transfers of the sac were made to fresh MF without substrate, while the sample collection from the SF was continued. The appearance of substrate in the SF is plotted in μmol/g of fresh tissue as a function of time. Figures in parenthesis indicate substrate concentration ratios, serosal/mucosal

cycloleucine are shown in Figure 7.6: similar results were also found using sugars such as D-galactose. As has been repeatedly observed using this or similar techniques, the appearance of substrate in the SC occurs only after a lag period of 5–10 minutes. This lag clearly represents the time required for any substrate entering through the brush border to diffuse across the various layers of tissue until the serosal membrane is reached. Substrate trapped in the tissue during this lag period constitutes the 'sink' in Figure 7.5.

The experiment in Figure 7.6, however, also illustrates a very simple but revealing procedure that, to the best of my knowledge, has not been used or published before. At minutes 25 and 30, the sacs were transferred to fresh buffer without substrate in the mucosal compartment: two transfers were used to remove effectively most of the substrate possibly carried over into the extracellular spaces. It is seen that, even under these conditions, where the gradient of substrate across the brush border is very large (since (S_1) is zero), the unidirectional flux from the tissue to the SC continues linearly for no less than 20 minutes. This result could not be obtained unless there is a very effective barrier to the efflux of substrate from the cells and back into the mucosal compartment.

A COMMENT ON METHODOLOGY: THE TISSUE-ACCUMULATION METHOD

Kinetics is a powerful tool for the study of mechanisms and has been widely used in the transport field for the last 20 years. However, for the kinetic approach to be really effective, one must be certain that the methods used serve the intended purpose, for example, in the present case, to measure the rate of substrate flux across the brush border. Only a flux taking place at this level may be interpreted as involving the carrier.

A large part of the kinetic work quoted here has been performed using the *tissue-accumulation method* (TAM), because of its simplicity and suitability for use with small animals such as the hamster and guinea-pig. The method[20] consists of measuring the uptake of a given substrate by pieces (usually *rings*) of everted intestine. By allowing for the randomisation of the intestinal rings, the use of short incubation periods, and a number of possible duplicates and internal controls, the TAM permitted for the first time the application of simple kinetic concepts to the study of intestinal transport. Because of this, the TAM was at the root of the enormous conceptual revolution that took place in the transport field in the early sixties. Granted, the system is deceptively simple, and I myself was rather sceptical when I was first introduced to the TAM. For instance, I wished to demonstrate that phlorizin was a fully competitive inhibitor of sugar transport, but it took me many months before I decided that a direct kinetic demonstration of that fact, using the TAM, could, after all, be attempted. The results[32] were surprisingly successful. They demonstrated quite convincingly that the TAM works and that kinetics can indeed by used to study intestinal transport. The fact that somewhat more sophisticated methods have since been developed does not necessarily mean, as claimed by some, that all the results obtained with the TAM must be discarded. Indeed, the variability encountered with the TAM is remarkably small and probably lower than that of any other method. We have also demonstrated recently that the results obtained with the TAM may be directly compared with those found by others using supposedly 'unequivocal' techniques (see reference 6).

The main objection often raised against the TAM is that it does not distinguish whether a given flux occurs through the brush border or other boundaries also exposed to the incubation medium: the serosal membrane or the cut ends. This objection would be unbeatable if the TAM were used without reference to supporting data. It is very easy to demonstrate, however, that among a number of possible fluxes, in and out of the rings, only the unidirectional influx across the brush border is quantitatively important when the method is used judiciously, for example, when adequate oxygenation and relatively short incubation periods are employed. In terms of area, for instance, mucosal and serosal borders can in no way be compared. It is known and may be calculated[33] that, because of the multiplying effect of the intestinal villi and microvilli lining the epithelium, the mucosal-to-serosal surface ratio is of the order of 200/1. But the question is not merely one of area. Crane and colleagues[34] went to considerable trouble to localize the active step in sugar transport right at the tip of the enterocytes, that is, the brush border. Frozen-section autoradiography confirmed these results, both for sugars and for amino acids[35]. Finally, experiments with sacs (that eliminate possible uncertainties by preventing fluxes other than those across the mucosal border) have, in our laboratory, consistently confirmed our assumption that, in correctly performed kinetic experiments, only fluxes across the brush border may be measured (examples illustrating this fact are given later in this paper).

THE POSSIBLE PHYSIOLOGICAL ROLE AND KINETIC CONSEQUENCES OF THE EXISTENCE OF A SODIUM-RICH MICROENVIRONMENT EXTERNAL AND IMMEDIATELY ADJACENT TO THE BRUSH BORDER MEMBRANE

Using guinea-pig intestine, we have been performing in our laboratory for the last couple of years a kinetic analysis of the activation of solute transport by Na^+. Although some of our results, described above, appear to be consistent with the proposed general model for cotransport, a detailed quantitative description of the situation is not yet available for two main reasons. One reason is the considerable variation between animals that we have encountered and which has slowed our progress. The other reason, to be dealt with in detail in this paper, has to do with the uncertainty involved in the determination of K_T in kinetic experiments, particularly when buffers without Na^+ are used. According to the allosteric model, the value of K_T at $(Na^+)_o = 0$ is, in theory, identical with K_s, the true dissociation constant of the S–C complex. However, the possible presence of a significant concentration of Na^+ in a region external and immediately adjacent to the brush border membrane, even when the tissues have been washed and are incubated in buffers without Na^+, would drastically alter the results, and in particular may yield false K_s values that may be orders of magnitude different from the authentic ones. Since a precise knowledge of the value of K_s is essential for the application of the equations developed for the calculation of all the other constants involved[6], it seems clear that all quantitative data available, either from our laboratory or from those of others, will have to be revised. Until a series of questions are answered, all cotransport data, therefore, will have to be regarded only as semiquantitative*.

All the above considerations apply particularly well to the case of the guinea-pig. The values of K_s for sugars and amino acids calculated in our laboratory for this animal (Table 7.2) appear to be rather small and, in particular, a value of $K_s = 10$ mM for the β-methylglucoside seems suspiciously low. Earlier mention was made of the reasons why the determination of the apparent value of K_T at $(Na^+) = 0$ may be difficult and even impossible. Therefore, before attempting to ascertain why in the guinea-pig the values calculated for K_s are so low, it would appear essential to clarify first the reliability of the measurement itself. Because the data on β-methylglucoside are the most complete, our attention will be focused on the kinetic behaviour of this sugar. However, it must be emphasised that similar data have been ob-

Table 7.3 β-Methylglucoside transport in guinea-pig jejunum: kinetics in sodium-free buffers

(n)	Prep.	Prewashing		Transport assay		V_{max} (μmol/m)	K_T (mM)
		Time (26 °C)	Buffer	Time (37 °C, min)	Buffer		
(3)	ES	40 s	PL	5	PL	0.45	10.2
(5)	ES	40 s	TL	2	TL	1.21	10.9
(5)	R	40 s	PL	5	PL	1.32	10.0
(3)	R	40 s	PL	5	PL	0.86	9.0
(4)	R	40 s	TL	5	TL	0.96	8.8
(4)	R	30 m	TCH	2	TL	1.01	10.7
					(Means):	(0.97)	(9.9)

Transport was assayed as in Table 7.1, but always in the absence of Na⁺. PREP refers to the tissue preparation used (tissue-accumulation method): R = rings and ES = empty sacs, that is, sacs containing neither buffer nor air (see reference 24). Prewashing means a period of preincubation in Na⁺-free buffer at room temperature, prior to the assay for transport. Buffers used were modifications of the Krebs–Henseleit phosphate[46] in which the Na⁺ had been fully substituted by either Li⁺ or choline⁺ (134 mM). PL is a potassium phosphate–Li⁺ buffer containing 8.5 mM K⁺. TL and TCH indicate Li⁺ and choline⁺ buffers respectively, containing zero K⁺ since all the potassium phosphate had been replaced by Tris chloride (pH 7.2).

tained in our laboratory using other sugars and amino acids, in agreement with the notion that identical mechanisms operate in the cotransport of Na⁺ and these two classes of organic solute.

The results of a series of experiments on the kinetics of β-methylglucoside transport in Na⁺-free buffers, under various experimental conditions, are

* It should be emphasised that such changes in the numerical value of the K_s constant will result in a modification of the value of the remaining dissociation constants, but will in no way affect the overall validity of the allosteric model. For instance, we have calculated theoretical curves of $K_T = f(A)$, using K_T data such as those shown in Table 7.1, but assigning increasing numerical values to the reference constant, K_r. As this constant is increased, K_s falls but rapidly reaches a plateau, so that the value of K_s remains essentially constant even when K_r is increased by several orders of magnitude. As K_r increases, however, the value of R also increases linearly.

collected in Table 7.3. First, the results reveal the existence of considerable variability in the value of V_{max} from one series to another. However, this variability is inconsistent: because of its lack of relevance to the present discussion, it will not be considered further. Second, the results demonstrate a great constancy in the value of K_T under all conditions used, indicating that we are not dealing with an artefact. Let us examine in some detail the evidence contained in Table 7.3 (1) Results obtained with the tissue accumulation method may be ascribed to events taking place only at the level of the mucosal border of the enterocyte and therefore to the carrier. In effect, identical K_T values are obtained using either open *rings* (preparation R) or *sacs* (preparation ES). (2) At an 8.5 mM concentration, K^+ is unable to modify the apparent affinity of the carrier for the sugar since identical values for K_T are found using lithium buffers with (buffer PL) or without (buffer TL) potassium. This finding may have two explanations. First, the affinity of K^+ for the carrier may be exceedingly low. Second, at this concentration, K^+ may have no access to the Na^+-binding site at which level, according to the SGH, it would have an inhibitory effect opposite to that of Na^+. At higher concentrations (see later) K^+ can be shown to compete for the Na^+-binding site, in agreement with the postulates of the SGH. (3) Washing of the tissues in Na^+-free buffers prior to the assay for transport does not affect the result. This is true both for short (40 seconds) or long (30 minutes) incubations using either Li^+ or choline$^+$ as the substituting cation. The significance of the apparent inertness of these two cations, in contrast with K^+, will be discussed in detail later. (4) Significantly, the results in Table 7.3 demonstrate that sugar transport in the absence of Na^+ follows simple Michaelis kinetics since identical K_T values are obtained using incubation periods of either 2 or 5 minutes. As mentioned before, these results show that, for all practical purposes, sugar influx under the conditions of these experiments is irreversible, a result that is in principle incompatible with the postulates of the SGH (see page 128). Earlier in this paper I have marshalled the evidence in favour of the unidirectionality of sugar and amino acid influx across the brush border in the small intestine. However, that the system continues to behave as if it were irreversible, even in the absence of external (bulk) Na^+, is amazing. In the conditions of these experiments, the Na^+ gradient clearly has been reversed, since $(Na^+)_o$ is zero: according to our experience with the hamster (Figure 7.3A), the net flow of sugar must take place in an outward direction. Since the results, on the contrary, indicate that the substrate is, in fact, flowing into the cell in a practically irreversible fashion for periods up to at least 5 minutes, it seems clear that a simple Na^+-dependent transmembrane gradient of affinity, as postulated by the SGH, cannot explain the situation. Therefore, it appears necessary to invoke the existence of some additional source of asymmetry that would render the influx across the brush border, in effect, irreversible. This hypothesis will be discussed in detail later (page 142). It must be emphasised, however, that the above conclusion refers in particular to the case of the guinea-pig: it seems conceivable, as we have seen earlier, that the situation in the hamster may be slightly different. Unfortunately, at this moment, no detailed study has been made of the kinetics of organic solute transport in Na^+-free buffers, using hamster intestine.

Once established that the value of $K_T = 10$ mM for β-methylglucoside transport by guinea-pig intestine, in Na^+-free buffers, probably represents a correct measurement, the question may be made: what is the explanation for the very low values for the K_s of sugars and amino acids found in our experiments? It seems obvious that an explanation of this fact might be found in the presence of significant concentrations of Na^+ in a region external and immediately adjacent to the brush border. Under this condition, the carriers would be partially activated and the K_T values at $(Na^+)_o = 0$ would not be true K_s values. Accordingly, the question now becomes: where exactly is this Na^+? *Unstirred water layers* (UWL) have lately attracted considerable attention, and for good reason. The evidence is clear that such layers of water may severely complicate the study of transport kinetics since they represent an additional barrier to the diffusion of substrate from the bulk of the incubation solution to the membrane[37,38]. It seems quite possible that Na^+ could be retained in one such UWL, particularly if we take into consideration the existence of a negatively charged region immediately external to the brush-border membrane[39,40].

At the beginning of these studies, we generally used 40-second washings in Na^+-free buffer prior to the determination of transport. Our reasoning was that such washings in a large volume of buffer (buffer/tissue ratios on the order of 100/1 were habitually used) should be sufficient to remove any previous buffer sticking to the tissues. A second incubation (for transport assay) with a similar excess of Na^+-free buffer should further dilute to negligible levels any Na^+ still present in the UWL. However, in recent correspondence with J. W. L. Robinson, our 'ritual' washings were criticised as insufficient. In his experiments, Robinson washes for at least 5 minutes (generally with potassium buffer), while Curran, Schultz and colleagues habitually wash their preparations for 30 minutes in choline buffer prior to the determination of influx[18].

This question of the apparent difficulty of washing away traces of Na^+ from a necessarily small volume of water, such as the one involved in the UWL, seemed puzzling. In my naïveté, I felt that a (passive) layer of water that needs 5 or more minutes to equilibrate with the (stirred) bulk solution, is a very sticky layer indeed. In Table 7.3, for instance, we see that, even after washing the tissues in choline buffer (TCH) for 30 minutes, the K_T for the glucoside at $(Na^+)_o = 0$ is identical to that found after 'ritual' washings for only 40 seconds. It seems possible that, perhaps, one may not be dealing with a problem of simple diffusion across a thin layer of water, but rather with a question of chemical specificity. Would it not be possible that the glycocalix, a substance known to be rich in negative charges, may act as an ion-exchange resin, with a preference for Na^+?

THE ION-EXCHANGE REGION

Therefore, rather than a simple unstirred water layer, it seems necessary to postulate the existence of an *ion-exchange region* (IER) specific for Na$^+$ and directly external and adjacent to the carriers in the brush border membrane. The glycocalix would logically appear to be the best candidate for the physical substratum of this IER, both because of its chemical composition (mucoproteins rich in negatively-charged groups) and because it is an integral part of the membrane, endowed with considerable stability[39].

Suggestions that Na$^+$ may be concentrated in the *fuzzy coat* or *outer membrane region, in vivo,* have already been made[40]. Particularly worth mentioning in this regard are the studies of Saltzman, Rector and Fordtran[41], who probably were the first to suggest that the 'fuzzy coat is electrically charged in such a way as to trap sodium ions on the luminal surface'. As far as I know, however, this and similar suggestions always implied a rather passive role for the glycocalix, which in general was regarded simply as a physical barrier to the free diffusion of Na$^+$ as well as other ions or molecules, such as the sugars. For instance, in order to explain the lack of agreement between experiments on Na$^+$-activation of organic solute transport either *in vivo* or *in vitro*, it has been suggested that, *in vivo,* Na$^+$ may diffuse from the blood across the intercellular spaces and the leaky 'tight' junctions into the glycocalix region, where the mucopolysaccharides and adjacent layers of mucus would somehow retard the diffusion of Na$^+$ into the bulk mucosal solution.

In contrast, what I should like to propose here is the concept of a very active participation of the glycocalix or IER in retaining Na$^+$ by a specific ion-exchange mechanism, *in vitro* as well as *in vivo*. Negative charges, present in this region, would certainly be responsible for the attraction of the sodium ions. However, an element of specificity must be invoked to explain the preferential concentration of Na$^+$ instead of other alkali metal ions (see later). The postulate is deliberately made, therefore, that the IER consists of a specific ion exchanger with considerable specificity for Na$^+$, rather than a simple sink for positively charged ions.

The difference mentioned earlier in the behaviour of chicken, hamster and guinea-pig intestine with regard to the role of Na$^+$ on the net directionality of organic solute transport, *in vitro,* may in principle be explained in terms of the different size and/or chemical specificity of the IER in each of these species. Results to be shown later indicate that the IER in the guinea-pig is very stable and specific for Na$^+$: it is little affected by the presence of a large excess of either choline$^+$ or Li$^+$ in the bulk mucosal solution, suggesting a rather negligible affinity of these two ions for the Na$^+$ receptors. Only K$^+$ has been found to exhibit noticeable affinity and to be able to exchange — although rather inefficiently — with the Na$^+$ in the IER. In the following section, the functional implications of these findings will become apparent.

THE SODIUM ION CYCLE

A logical consequence of the concept of a very stable Na^+ microenvironment at the external face of the brush-border membrane is the formulation of the existence of a *sodium ion cycle*, as schematised in Figure 7.7. The IER may be considered as a Na^+ reservoir separating the membrane from the bulk mucosal solution: although the IER may have considerable affinity for Na^+, the cation would be freely exchangeable, and therefore readily available for transport. I represent this free Na^+ as the black dot in the IER compartment. *Step 1* in the cycle is then the reversible association of this Na^+ with the Na^+-binding site of the organic solute carrier, represented by the rectangle with two circles inside. According to the general model for cotransport, binding of Na^+ to this site and its subsequent translocation into the cell, *step 2*, is stimulated by binding of the external solute to its own site (for didactic purposes the organic solute is not represented in the figure and therefore the corresponding binding site is empty: compare with Figure 7.10). According to the views marshalled in this paper, step 2 is depicted as irreversible. However, the only truly irreversible reaction in the cycle is *step 4*, the extrusion of Na^+ into the intercellular spaces by the action of the sodium pump. Accordingly, it is only at this level that a

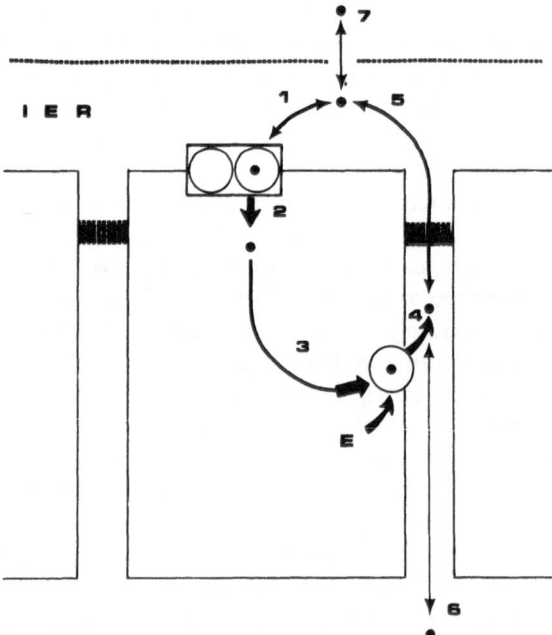

Figure 7.7 The sodium ion cycle. The rectangle in the centre represents an enterocyte separated from its neighbours by the intercellular spaces and connected to them through the tight junctions. Above the junction is the brush border, and below it the basolateral membrane. For further details, see the text

provision is made for the direct participation of an exergonic chemical reaction, represented by E in the figure. It can be argued (see later) that the sodium pump 'pulls' step 2 by means of the coupling reaction depicted by the unidirectional arrow, *step 3*. Once in the lateral spaces, Na^+ may move back into the IER by diffusion across the 'tight' junction (represented by the vertical bars), which is known to be very 'leaky' to both Na^+ and water, in the small intestine[40]. This is *step 5* that closes the cycle. Of course, the cycle is also in communication with the blood or tissue Na^+ pools, *step 6*, and with the external or mucosal medium through *step 7*.

As described, the Na^+ cycle would appear to be on solid ground, with the possible exception (some would say) of the unidirectional sense given to arrows 2 and 3 in Figure 7.7. Although, in order to defend this position, it will be necessary to engage for a moment in speculation, I feel justified in doing this. The proposals to be made in what follows constitute, in my opinion, the best working hypothesis that may be construed with the available data. An analogy between the enterocyte and an idealised epithelial cell from the frog skin may be useful at this point. We may regard both epithelia as formed by similar polar cells: slight variations in a central theme may explain the differences as well as the parallelisms in the function of the two epithelia. Both cells have a *mucosal membrane* facing either the intestinal lumen or the pond, that is, the outside world; and a *basolateral membrane* facing the internal milieu. The two membranes are clearly separated by the *tight junction*. In the frog skin, the mucosal membrane is believed to be poorly permeable to Na^+. This means that, rather than by simple diffusion, Na^+ influx across this membrane is thought to be mediated by a specific, saturable *carrier*. Also, the frog skin is known to exhibit *rectification*: the mucosal membrane has the properties of a *diode*[42]. In our terminology, Na^+ influx across this membrane may be considered *irreversible*. Although the exact manner in which Na^+ crosses the intestinal brush border membrane is not known with precision[40], there are some indications (see below) that it may behave in a similar manner. One difference between the intestine and the frog skin with regard to the mucosal membrane is that, in the former, the Na^+-binding site in the carrier(s) is associated with another specific site, capable of carrying into the cell another substrate by *cotransport*. Although this paper deals only with sugars and amino acids, we know that there are many other solutes, both organic and inorganic, that in principle may be thought as possible cotransport partners for Na^+. The question to investigate, therefore, is twofold: (a) Whether most, if not all, Na^+ entry across the intestinal brush border is carrier-mediated; and (b) Whether this Na^+ influx is essentially irreversible. Strong support for the above two points comes from the work of Hopfer and Murer[17]. Using vesicles prepared from intestinal brush borders, these workers have demonstrated quite convincingly that substrate-activated Na^+ influx across this membrane is electrogenic. No such electrogenicity could be expected if these membranes were permeable to Na^+, nor if the carrier-mediated influx of Na^+ were readily reversible. In relation to mechanism, the same conditions causing the irreversibility of organic solute influx (to be discussed in detail later) may explain in principle the postulated irreversibility of Na^+ influx in the intestine. In relation to the experiments with vesicles, however, it may be worth emphasising at this time that any results obtained with this technique can be extrapolated only with considerable caution to the whole-cell situation. According to the concept of the sodium ion cycle, any charge being carried into the cell by the influx of Na^+ across the brush border may be compensated immediately by the movement of an equivalent charge across the basolateral membrane and back into the IER across the tight junction. In other words, although Na^+ transport across the brush border is in theory electrogenic, and may be so in practice in the vesicle experiments, it need not necessarily always be so in the case of the whole cell. Small differences between species in this regard may in principle explain the conflicting results quoted by Hopfer and Murer[17].

With regard to the coupling (*step* 3) between influx across the brush border and extrusion at the basolateral membrane, this is a logical assumption to make. The existence of such coupling in the frog skin has been propounded by Candia[43]: a similar approach may be used to demonstrate the phenomenon in the intestine.

An interesting difference between the intestine and the frog skin concerns the leakiness of the tight junction. The frog skin is an epithelium whose main function is sodium transport. The irreversibility of *step* 2 and the tightness of the junction (*step* 5 in Figure 7.7 does not occur in the frog skin) are both conditions conducive to the unidirectional transport of Na^+ in the inward (pond to blood) direction. On the contrary, in the small intestine, the leakiness of the junction permits the establishment of the sodium ion cycle, as described. Both *in vivo* and *in vitro*, the ion exchange region would be loaded at all times with Na^+, a situation conducive to the optimal absorption from lumen to blood of a host of solutes, all known to be Na^+-dependent, and including the organic and inorganic solutes already mentioned. The sodium ion cycle, therefore, makes the intestine an organ optimally adapted for its main function, *absorption*. Although outside of the scope of this paper, similar arguments may be applied to the case of another important function of the intestine, *digestion*. It has been known since the pioneer studies of Crane and Miller[44] that some digestive enzymes are localised in the brush border and are also activated by Na^+. It has been demonstrated recently that the activation by Na^+ of a digestive enzyme such as sucrase conforms to an allosteric mechanism essentially identical to that described earlier for organic solute and Na^+ cotransport[45].

CAPACITY EFFECT OF POTASSIUM: A POSSIBLE NEW SOURCE OF ASYMMETRY IN ORGANIC SOLUTE TRANSPORT

Even if we argue that the glycocalix acts as a trap for sodium ions, creating a Na^+-rich microenvironment at the external face of the brush border, the results discussed in the Section on page 135 would still be hard to reconcile with a simple version of the SGH. In effect, we have seen that substrate influx in Na^+-free buffers follows simple Michaelis kinetics, at least in the case of the guinea-pig intestine. If the affinity of the carrier for organic solutes under these conditions is as high as that suggested by the low K_s values shown in Table 7.2, it should be expected from equation (5) that significant rates of substrate efflux would be established after a period of only seconds, even if the intracellular Na^+ *activity* is as low as 14 mEq/l[46]. But the results, on the contrary, show that the rate of efflux is negligible, even after 5 minutes. As mentioned, the conclusion seems inescapable that an additional source of asymmetry needs to be postulated to explain completely the apparent irreversibility of substrate influx. The question is whether this asymmetry has a chemical origin or whether the potential energy inherent in the Na^+/K^+ gradient could be sufficient to explain it. Experimental observations to be discussed presently suggest that a hitherto unrecognised *capacity effect of K^+*, probably acting at a locus other than the Na^+-binding site of the carrier, might constitute the molecular basis of this new source of asymmetry.

The evidence that the effect of Na^+ on organic solute transport in guinea-pig intestine constitutes a simple case of K-kinetics may appear at first sight to conflict with previous observations indicating that, in this animal, activation of sugar transport by alkali metal ions may exhibit *mixed effects*[23]. In this work, an analysis was made of the effect of a change in the ratios $(Na^+)_o/(K^+)_o$ at constant $(Na^+)_o + (K^+)_o$ on the kinetics of transport of the two methylglucosides. The α-glucoside presented an apparently pure case of K-kinetics, but the β-isomer gave a mixed effect. Since, according to the results in this paper, Na^+ is a pure K-activator, the inference is quite clear that the V-effect observed using β-glucoside must have been caused by K^+. Experiments were carried out to verify this hypothesis, as follows.

Old and new saturation experiments with β-methylglucoside as the substrate are shown in Figure 7.8. The plot of Eadie-Hoffstee was used to illustrate better the fall in V_{max} as $(K^+)_o$ increases (this plot gives V_{max} directly as the y intercept). It seems quite clear that both series of experiments, carried out some three years apart, fully agree with each other. Small differences between the two sets of curves reflect the considerable variability between animals already mentioned. Without entering into a discussion of this variability, the results in Figure 7.8 demonstrate that there is a very consistent fall in V_{max} as $(K^+)_o$ increases, the average inhibition being on the order of 40%. In the case of the α-glucoside, a similar study (not illustrated) revealed that the effect of K^+ was inconsistent, in agreement with the earlier observations[23]. However, the apparently different behaviour of the two glucosides in this regard is only quantitative. In other experiments using even smaller $(Na^+)_o/(K^+)_o$ ratios (not shown), a clear V-effect of K^+ on α-methylglucoside transport also became evident.

A new series of experiments was carried out in which Li^+ and K^+, each at

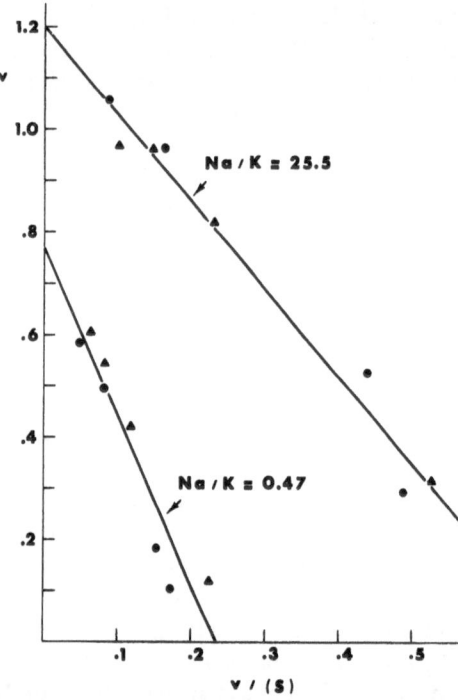

Figure 7.8 The capacity effect of potassium. The kinetics of β-methylglucoside transport was assayed according to standard procedures[6], using guinea-pig jejunum and 5-minute incubations. For one series (upper curve, $V_{max} = 1.2$ μmol/min), a regular Krebs–Henseleit phosphate buffer[48] was used with 138.5 mM Na^+ and 5.4 mM K^+ (ratio $(Na^+)/(K^+) = 25.5$). For the other series ($V_{max} = 0.77$); a low-Na^+, high K^+ buffer was used (ratio $(Na^+)/(K^+) = 46.4/97.7 = 0.47$). The results are the pooled data from two separate series of experiments. One group ($\blacktriangle$, four animals) is the same as in reference 23, using an (S) range from 0.6 to 9.6 mM. The other series ($\bullet$, three animals) involved a (S) range from 0.6 to 12 mM. Because the two groups could not be averaged, regression lines were calculated using eight points per curve, as shown. Regression coefficients were 0.988 and 0.944 for upper and lower curves respectively

Table 7.4 Time-dependent capacity effect of potassium on β-methylglucoside transport

(n)	Time (min)	Lithium buffer		Potassium buffer	
		V_{max} (μmol/min)	K_T (mM)	V_{max} (μmol/min)	K_T [mM]
(4)	5	0.96	8.8	0.37	14.3
(5)	2	1.31	10.9	1.12	35.6

Transport was assayed as in Table 7.1, using guinea-pig jejunum and Na^+-free buffers as indicated. The lithium buffer is identical with TL in Table 7.3 (it contains neither Na^+ nor K^+). The potassium buffer is equivalent to TL, but with all Li^+ replaced with K^+. Before assay, the tissues were washed for 40 seconds at room temperature in buffer TL.

134 mM, were directly compared in the absence of Na$^+$. From the results (Table 7.4), an interesting fact seems to emerge. When transport was assayed for 5 minutes, as was the case in the experiments in Figure 7.8, K$^+$ produced a very significant effect on V_{max} (62% inhibition). But when transport was assayed for only 2 minutes, the inhibition was negligible (14%). This apparent time-dependence of the K$^+$ action, furthermore, refers only to the capacity effect. A time-dependent, non-competitive effect such as the one just described may be interpreted in one of two ways: (1) It could involve an interaction of K$^+$ with the Na$^+$-binding site, resulting in the formation of the ternary complex S–C–K$^+$. If the permeability constant of this complex were smaller than that of complexes S–C or S–C–Na$^+$, an *allosteric V-effect* would be obtained. But there is no reason to expect that K$^+$ would behave in such a peculiar manner, nor that the interaction of K$^+$ with the Na$^+$-binding site would be time-dependent. One would rather expect a very fast, freely reversible interaction, similar to that postulated for Na$^+$. Therefore, the possibility seems more likely that: (2) In addition to a competition of K$^+$ for the Na$^+$-binding site (the

Table 7.5 Long-lasting capacity effect of potassium on β-methylglucoside transport

Preincubation (26 °C, 30 min)	Choline buffer	Potassium buffer
Na$^+$ released to medium (mM)	0.91	1.31
Transport-assay (37 °C, 2 min)	Lithium buffer	Lithium buffer
Na$^+$ released to the medium (mM)	0.14	0.13
V_{max} (μmol/min)	1.0	0.6
K_T (mM)	10.7	9.9

Using guinea-pig jejunum, transport was assayed in Li$^+$ buffer (TL), as in Table 7.4. Before assay, the tissue rings had been washed at room temperature in 10 ml of Na$^+$-free buffers similar to the TL, except that the Li$^+$ had been totally replaced by either choline$^+$ or K$^+$. The content of Na$^+$ in the incubation media was determined both after the preincubation and after the assay periods. The results indicate the mean of four experiments.

data reveal this type of *affinity-effect*, which is in agreement with the premises of the SGH), K$^+$ may also have an action at some point other than this site, resulting in the inactivation of the carrier. Such K$^+$-dependent inactivation of the carrier would be in agreement with, and in principle may explain, some of Robinson's earlier results. In these experiments, transport activity was apparently lost when guinea-pig intestinal rings were preincubated for 30 minutes in Na$^+$-free, K$^+$-substituted buffers[47].

A *non-competitive inhibition* of the *IIa type* is therefore suggested here for K$^+$. Additional evidence for this interpretation comes from the experiment shown in Table 7.5. Intestinal rings were incubated for 30 minutes at room temperature in either choline$^+$ or K$^+$ buffers: transport was determined immediately afterwards for 2 minutes in Li$^+$ buffer. The pretreatment with K$^+$ resulted in a very clear effect on V_{max} (40% inhibition). On the contrary, and very significantly, there was no effect on K_T, demonstrating that: (*a*) withdrawal of K$^+$ from the bulk of the incubation solution by transfer to the Li$^+$ buffer removed all the K$^+$ that might have been available to compete for the Na$^+$-site; and (*b*) sufficient K$^+$ remained bound to the hypothetical additional sites to cause a very significant effect on the V_{max}. Clearly, the *affinity* and the *capacity* effects of K^+ have different loci of action in the guinea-pig. It must be emphasised that an interpretation of the above experiment in terms of an intracellular action of K^+ seems unwarranted. An increase in $(K^+)_i$ would favour rather than inhibit sugar influx, according to the Na^+-gradient hypothesis. Also, an increase in $(K^+)_i$ would not interfere with metabolism nor the functioning of the sodium pump. It seems reasonable to conclude on the contrary, that the capacity effect of K^+ has its site of action at the external face of the brush border, that is, at the carrier level: the implications of this suggestion will now be discussed.

To say that K^+ acts on solute transport as a *non-competitive* inhibitor gives, unfortunately, no clue as to the possible mechanism. However, and in view of the fact that K^+ is the main intracellular cation, it is tempting to speculate that the effect observed may have physiological significance. Perhaps we have come upon the additional source of asymmetry that, as we have seen, seems necessary to explain fully the unidirectionality of solute influx across the brush border. A detailed study of the role of K^+ on solute transport therefore seems warranted, although it is severely complicated by the existence of the ion-exchange region separating the external face of the brush-border membrane, and therefore the carrier, from the bulk of the incubation medium. In the following, a brief summary is given of some of the work initiated in our laboratory to characterise the IER, particularly with regard to the way it handles the two main alkali–metal ions, Na^+ and K^+.

In order to obtain Michaelis kinetics for periods of 5 minutes or more, we have seen that the second term in equation (5) must be kept essentially equal to zero (page 129). If the affinity effects of Na^+ and K^+ are not sufficient to meet this condition, an additional capacity effect of K^+ would be able to achieve this goal, as postulated above, only if V_{max} in the presence of K^+ were very strongly depressed. In the experiments just shown, however, inhibitions caused by K^+ were never greater than 60%. This apparent inability of K^+ fully to inactivate the carrier from the outer face of the membrane could be explained, however, if the IER were very selective for Na^+ in such a way that, even after a prolonged incubation (for example 30 minutes, Table 7.5) in the absence of Na^+ and in the presence of 140 mM K^+, the IER would still contain sufficient Na^+ to partially counteract the effects of K^+. In support of this idea is the observation made earlier (Table 7.3) that low (8.5 mM) K^+ concentrations do not affect the values of K_T observed in Na^+-free buffers. As already suggested, this fact could be explained if K^+ at this concentration could not displace Na^+ from the IER. Only considerably greater values of $(K^+)_0$, such as 100 mM or more, are able to increase significantly the K_T values, as compared with those observed, for instance, in the presence of a comparable concentration of Li^+, as in the experiment in Table 7.4.

The type of Na^+-selective exchange mechanism under consideration would also explain other results, shown in Table 7.5. After a 30 minute incubation period in Na^+-free buffers, sacs from guinea-pig intestine appear to release a rather small amount of Na^+ to the medium. This amount, however, is always consistently greater in K^+ (1.3 mM Na^+) than in choline (0.9 mM Na^+) buffers, indicating that both ions would compete poorly with the Na^+ in the IER, but that K^+ would have a greater affinity for this region than choline$^+$. One can think in terms of a *batch exchange mechanism* of an ion in the external medium, X_0^+, with Na^+ in the IER, which may be represented in a very simplified manner as follows:

$$R\text{--}Na + X_0^+ \rightleftharpoons R\text{--}X + Na_0^+ \qquad (6)$$

where R represents the ion-exchange 'resin' that is highly specific for Na^+. If this type of situation were present in the intestine, changing the external Na^+-free medium a series of consecutive times would result in a greater withdrawal of Na^+ from the IER than that achieved by a single exposure to the same buffer, for an equivalent total length of time. The results of one such experiment are shown in Figure 7.9.

Here, sacs of everted guinea-pig jejunum were incubated in various Na^+-free buffers, using either choline$^+$, Li^+ or K^+ as the substituting cations. The

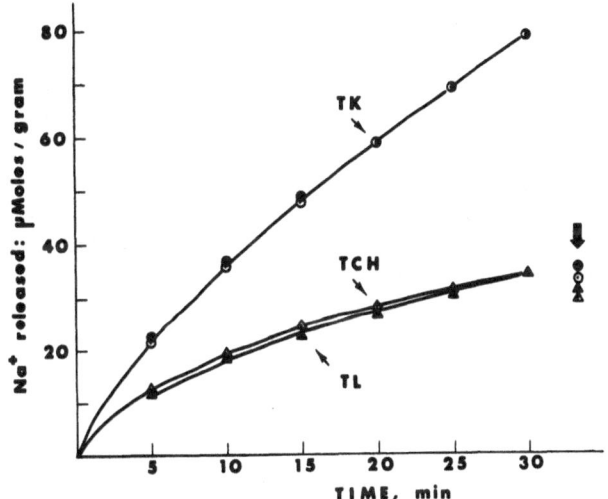

Figure 7.9 The exchange of sodium ions with extracellular cations. Sacs from everted guinea-pig jejunum were prepared in Krebs–Henseleit phosphate[48] and subjected to exchange in Na^+-free buffers at room temperature, as described in the text. Buffers (and symbols) used were: TL (▲, a Tris–Li^+ buffer, described in Table 7.3); TCH (△) and TK (○, ●). The latter two buffers were similar to TL, but with the Li^+ fully substituted with either choline$^+$ or K^+. Before the exchange, all sacs were washed for 20 seconds in buffer TCH. Two different animals were used, represented by the empty and filled symbols respectively. Each point is the average of two sacs. The results are shown as Na^+ (measured with a Corning flame photometer) released to the medium in μmoles per gram of fresh tissue. Individual points under the arrow show the result of a single 30-minute incubation. The curves illustrate the cumulative Na^+ release using the repetitive exchange procedure

appearance of Na^+ in the medium was measured either after a single incubation at room temperature for 30 minutes (points under the arrow) or after six consecutive changes to fresh media for the same total length of time. As predicted, the Na^+-exchanging effect of K^+ was considerably greater (by a factor larger than 2) when the repetitive exchange procedure was used. On the contrary, both choline$^+$ and Li^+ were very inefficient in exchanging for Na^+, confirming the assumption that their affinity for the IER is negligible.

When the repetitive exchange procedure was used, a total of about 80 μmoles of Na^+ per gram of wet tissue was released to the medium (Figure 7.9). However, it seems highly relevant that, when the parameters for β-methylglucoside transport were determined after such a treatment, the results (not shown here) were essentially the same as if a single incubation for the same total length of time had been performed, as in the experiment of Table 7.5. This result speaks strongly in favour of the concept of a very stable Na^+-rich microenvironment in the IER. In effect, as each new exchange with K^+ is performed, it can be conceived that a constant fraction of the Na^+ removed from the IER is probably immediately replaced by Na^+ moving from the tissue pool and into the IER through steps 5 and 6 of the sodium–ion cycle (Figure 7.7). In this way, the concentration ratios $(Na^+)/(K^+)$ in the IER are kept very constant, as evinced by the constancy of the kinetic parameters of β-methylglucoside transport, mentioned above.

A logical consequence of this argument is that, after repeated exchanges of K^+ for Na^+, all available tissue Na^+ would eventually be lost. Once this stage is reached, the IER would also begin to deplete of Na^+ and become loaded with K^+. It can be predicted, therefore, that if such a situation could be attained experimentally, K^+ might be demonstrated to be able to exert fully its capacity effect on solute transport from the external face of the membrane, thereby inhibiting very strongly the influx of substrate across the brush border. Experiments to test this hypothesis have been initiated in our laboratory. The results seem to support the prediction, but they can be considered only as preliminary and no details may be given at this time.

CONCLUSION: THE CONCEPT OF SODIUM-DRIVEN TRANSPORT

Summarising the above ideas, the 'static' concept of the sodium-gradient hypothesis may be changed into a 'dynamic' model in which the emphasis is placed on the *coupling of fluxes* of the organic solutes and Na^+ at the level of the brush border, by *cotransport* (Figure 7.10). These fluxes are not necessarily driven by the sodium gradient: within certain limits, the intracellular concentration of Na^+ may have little effect on the unidirectionality of the influx. More fundamental to the existence of an irreversibility of influx is the idea of two functionally opposite ionic microenvironments at each side of the

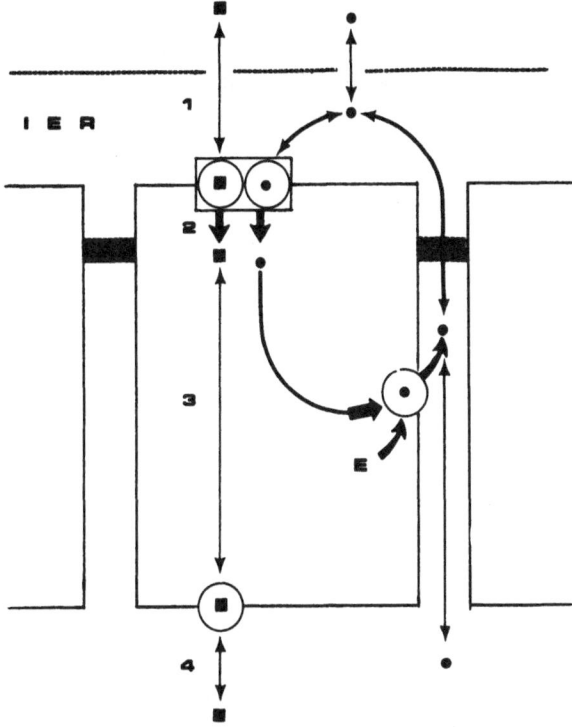

Figure 7.10 Sodium-driven transport. The sodium ion cycle is represented as in Figure 7.7. In addition, this figure illustrates the coupled flow of solute (■) that enters the cell by cotransport with Na⁺ (●). *Step 1* is the interaction of external substrate, S, with the carrier (diffusion across the IER is assumed); *step 2* is the irreversible carrier-mediated influx; *step 3* is the physical diffusion of S across the intracellular fluid; *step 4* is the carrier-mediated efflux at the basolateral membrane. Note that this last carrier is not coupled to Na⁺ and is freely reversible

membrane. Because of the existence of a Na⁺-specific exchanger at the outer face of the brush border, the ion-exchange region, the carrier at this point is in a state of activation due to the Na⁺. On the contrary, the inner face of the membrane has no such exchange region and may be conceived instead as covered by an unstirred water layer loaded with K⁺, the prevailing intracellular cation*. This K⁺ would cause an inactivation of the carrier due to a *capacity effect* specific for this ion, which in turn will cause the selective inhibition of substrate efflux. The carrier may be conceived, therefore, as being switched 'on' and 'off' depending on the side of the membrane with which it is in contact.

* The inner face of the brush-border membrane faces the 'core' of the microvilli formed of fibrillar material directly connected with the terminal web. As argued by Crane[44], this region constitutes an organelle physically, as well as functionally, distinct from the rest of the cell. Any model of transport in the enterocyte would depend ultimately on a knowledge of the exact ionic composition of the fluid filling this region.

Central to the concept of sodium-driven transport, therefore, is the idea of the ionic asymmetry across the brush-border membrane. This asymmetry is maintained on the one hand by the characteristic ionic selectivity of the IER, and on the other hand by the sodium pump that keeps $(K^+)_i$ high. The model is therefore one of *secondary active transport*, as in the original sodium-gradient hypothesis. No provision is made for the coupling to some exergonic chemical reaction at the level of the carrier (the brush border): the chemical energy input remains exclusively at the level of the sodium pump located at the basolateral membrane.

The premises of the model are summarised in Figure 7.11. Two distinct factors are believed to act synergistically. On the one hand, the opposite *affinity effects of Na$^+$ and K$^+$* may contribute quite definitely to the net asymmetric distribution of the substrate at the steady state, in agreement with the premises of the affinity-gradient hypothesis (compare with Figure 7.4). On the other

---

SODIUM-DRIVEN TRANSPORT

(1) The *affinity* effect of the Na^+/K^+ concentration gradient:

$$K_{T1} < K_{T2}$$

(2) The *capacity* effect of (intracellular) potassium:

$$V_{max_1} \gg V_{max_2}$$

Figure 7.11 Factors underlying the concept of sodium-driven transport

hand, a new *capacity effect of K$^+$* is postulated to contribute quite decisively in rendering the second term in equation (5) negligible for considerable periods of incubation, thus explaining the apparent irreversibility of substrate influx, before the steady state is reached.

Acknowledgements

It is a pleasure to acknowledge my indebtedness to J. W. L. Robinson who, with characteristic forcefulness, attracted by attention to the very peculiar behaviour of the potassium ion. A. Mahmood participated in some of the most recent experiments quoted in this paper. The excellent technical assistance of Mrs B. Robillard and, in the early work here quoted, Miss L. Argomaniz, is also greatly appreciated. The most recent work was supported by NIH Grant AM17750: the consistent support provided by the National Institutes of Health, USPHS, from the beginning of our studies in this field is also gratefully acknowledged.

References

1. Crane, R. K., Miller, D. and Bihler, I. (1961). Restrictions on the possible mechanisms of intestinal active transport of sugars. In A. Kleinzeller and A. Kotyk (eds.). *Membrane Transport and Metabolism*, p. 439 (New York: Academic Press)
2. Crane, R. K. (1965). Na⁺-dependent transport in the intestine and other animal tissues. *Fed. Proc.*, **24**, 1000
3. Crane, R. K., Forstner, G. and Eichholz, A. (1965). Studies on the mechanism of intestinal absorption of sugars. X. An effect of Na⁺ concentration on the apparent Michaelis constants for intestinal sugar transport, *in vitro*. *Biochim. Biophys. Acta*, **109**, 467
4. Alvarado, F. (1965). The relationship between Na⁺ and the active transport of arbutin in the small intestine. *Biochim. Biophys. Acta*, **109**, 478
5. Wilbrandt, W. and Rosenberg, T. (1961). The concept of carrier transport and its corollaries in pharmacology. *Pharmacol. Revs.*, **13**, 109
6. Alvarado, F. and Mahmood, A. (1974). Cotransport of organic solutes and sodium ions in the small intestine: A general model. Amino acid transport. *Biochemistry*, **13**, 2882
7. Alvarado, F. (1970). La membrana celular como mosaico de funciones. *Bol. R. Soc. Esp. Hist. Nat., Biol.*, **68**, 33
8. Curran, P. F. and Schultz, S. G. (1968). Transport across membranes: general principles. In C. F. Code (ed.). *Handbook of Physiology. Alimentary Canal.* Sect. 6, vol. III, p. 1217 (Washington, D.C.: Amer. Physiological Soc.)
9. Glynn, I. M. and Karlish, S. J. D. (1975). The sodium pump. *Ann. Rev. Physiol.*, **37**, 13
10. Kimmich, G. A. (1970). Active sugar accumulation by isolated intestinal epithelial cells. A new model for sodium-dependent metabolite transport. *Biochemistry*, **9**, 3669
11. Kimmich, G. A. (1973). Coupling between Na⁺ and sugar transport in small intestine. *Biochim. Biophys. Acta*, **300**, 31
12. Heinz, E. (1972). *Na-linked Transport of Organic Solutes*. (Berlin: Springer-Verlag)
13. Heinz, E. (1974). Coupling and energy transfer in active amino acid transport. In F. Bronner and A. Kleinzeller (eds.). *Current Topics in Membranes and Transport*, Vol. 5, p. 137 (New York: Academic Press)
14. Bihler, I. and Cybulsky, R. (1973). Sugar transport at the basal and lateral aspect of the small intestinal cell. *Biochim. Biophys. Acta*, **298**, 429
15. Gall, D. G., Butler, D. G., Tepperman, F. and Hamilton, J. R. (1974). Sodium ion transport in isolated intestinal epithelial cells. The effect of actively transported sugars on sodium ion efflux. *Biochim. Biophys. Acta*, **339**, 291
16. Hopfer, U., Nelson, K., Perrotto, J. and Isselbacher, K. J. (1973). Glucose transport in isolated brush-border membrane from rat small intestine. *J. Biol. Chem.*, **248**, 25
17. Murer, H. and Hopfer, U. (1974). Demonstration of electrogenic Na⁺-dependent D-glucose transport in intestinal brush-border membranes. *Proc. Nat. Acad. Sci. USA*, **71**, 484
18. Schultz, S. G. and Curran, P. F. (1970). Coupled transport of sodium and organic solutes. *Physiol. Revs.*, **50**, 637
19. Saunders, S. J. and Isselbacher, K. J. (1965). Inhibition of intestinal amino acid transport by hexoses. *Biochim. Biophys. Acta*, **102**, 397
20. Crane, R. K., and Mandelstam, P. (1960). The active transport of sugars by various preparations of hamster intestine. *Biochim. Biophys. Acta*, **45**, 460
21. Alvarado, F. (1966). Transport of sugars and amino acids in the intestine: evidence for a common carrier. *Science*, **151**, 1010
22. Alvarado, F. (1971). Interrelation of transport systems for sugars and amino acids in small intestine. In W. McD. Armstrong and A. S. Nunn (eds.). *Intestinal Transport of Electrolytes, Amino Acids and Sugars*, p. 281 (Springfield: Ch. C. Thomas)
23. Alvarado, F. (1972). Sodium activation of intestinal sugar and amino acid transport: A general or an individual effect? In E. Heinz (ed.). *Na-linked Transport of Organic Solutes*, p. 147. (Berlin: Springer-Verlag)

24. Robinson, J. W. L. and Alvarado, F. (1971). Interaction between the sugar and amino acid transport systems at the small intestinal brush borders: a comparative study. *Pflügers Arch.-Europ. J. Physiol.*, **326**, 48

25. Alvarado, F. and Mahmood, A. (19**). Cotransport of organic solutes and sodium ions in the small intestine: A general model. II. Sugar transport. (In preparation)

26. Vidaver, G. A., (1964). Some tests of the hypothesis that the sodium ion gradient furnishes the energy for glycine active transport by pigeon red cells. *Biochemistry*, **3**, 803

27. Crane, R. K. (1964). Uphill outflow of sugar from intestinal epithelial cells induced by reversal of the Na$^+$ gradient: Its significance for the mechanism of Na$^+$-dependent active transport. *Biochem. Biophys. Res. Commun.*, **17**, 481

28. Robinson, J. W. L. (1974). The question of countertransport in the intestine. *Biochim. Biophys. Acta*, **367**, 88

29. Alvarado, F. and Monreal, J. (1967). Na$^+$-dependent transport of phenylglucosides in the chicken small intestine. *Comp. Biochem. Physiol.*, **20**, 471

30. Finch, L. R. (1962). Non-reversibility in the uptake of amino acids by isolated segments of rat intestine. *Biochim. Biophys. Acta*, **64**, 556

31. Christensen, H. N., Feldman, B. H. and Hastings, A. B. (1963). Concentrative and reversible character of intestinal amino acid transport. *Amer. J. Physiol.*, **205**, 255

32. Alvarado, F. and Crane, R. K. (1962). Phlorizin as a competitive inhibitor of the active transport of sugars by hamster small intestine *in vitro*. *Biochim. Biophys. Acta*, **56**, 170

33. Wilson, T. H. (1962). *Intestinal absorption*, p. 2 (Philadelphia: W. B. Saunders).

34. McDougal, D. B., Little, K. S. and Crane, R. K. (1960). Studies on the mechanism of intestinal absorption of sugars. IV. Localization of galactose concentrations within the intestinal wall during active transport. *Biochim. Biophys. Acta*, **45**, 483

35. Kinter, W. B. and Wilson, T. H. (1965). Autoradiographic study of sugar and amino acid absorption by everted sacs of hamster intestine. *J. Cell. Biol.*, **25**, 19

36. Crane, R. K. and Wilson, T. H. (1958). *In vitro* method for the study of the rate of intestinal absorption of sugars. *J. Appl. Physiol.*, **12**, 145

37. Winne, D. (1973). Unstirred layer, source of biased Michaelis constant in membrane transport. *Biochim. Biophys. Acta*, **298**, 27

38. Dugas, M. C., Ramaswamy, K. and Crane, R. K. (1975). Analysis of the D-glucose influx kinetics of *in vitro* hamster jejunum, based on considerations of the mass-transfer coefficient. *Biochim. Biophys. Acta*, **382**, 576

39. Ito, S. (1956). The enteric surface coat on cat intestinal microvilli. *J. Cell Biol.*, **27**, 475

40. Schultz, S. G., Frizzell, R. A. and Nellans, H. N. (1974). Ion transport by mammalian small intestine. *Ann. Rev. Physiol.*, **36**, 51

41. Saltzman, D. A., Rector, F. C. and Fordtran, J. S. (1972). The role of intraluminal sodium in glucose absorption *in vivo*. *J. Clin. Invest.*, **51**, 876

42. Candia, O. A. and Chiarandini, D. J. (1973). Transport of lithium and rectification by frog skin. *Biochim. Biophys. Acta*, **307**, 578

43. Candia, O. A. and Reinach, P. (1975). The Na pool and Na fluxes across inner and outer barriers of frog skin epithelium. *Biophys. J.*, **15**, 228a

44. Crane, R. K. (1966). Structural and functional organization of an epithelial cell brush border. In K. B. Warren (ed.). *Intracellular Transport*, p. 71. (New York: Academic Press)

45. Mahmood, A. and Alvarado, F. (1975). The activation of intestinal brush-border sucrase by alkali metal ions: An allosteric mechanism similar to that for the Na$^+$-activation of non-electrolyte transport systems in intestines. *Arch. Biochem. Biophys.*, **168**, 585

46. Lee, C. O. and Armstrong, W. McD. (1972). Activities of sodium and potassium ions in epithelial cells of small intestine. *Science*, **175**, 1261

47. Robinson, J. W. L. (1970). Comparative aspects of the response of the intestine to its ionic environment. *Comp. Biochem. Physiol.*, **34**, 641

48. Krebs, H. A. and Henseleit, K. (1932). Untersuchungen über die Harnstoffbildung im Tierkörper. *Z. Physiol. chem.* **210**, 33

7

Discussion Paper on

Ionic Dependence of Glucose Transport from Disaccharides

W. F. Caspary

*Division of Gastroenterology and Metabolism,
Department of Medicine, University of Göttingen*

Despite some negative comments on Dr Crane's work, it has been pointed out by Dr Alvarado that the Na^+-gradient hypothesis for Na^+-coupled hexose transport, originated by Dr Crane is still alive and seems to be less disputed than ever in view of the experimental results of Hopfer, Murer and Kinne.

We have been working in Dr Crane's laboratory since 1969 on the transport mechanism of glucose derived from disaccharides[1,2]. It had been pointed out earlier that a close functional and structural relationship exists in the brush-border membrane between disaccharidases and the carrier-mediated hexose transport system. In order to explain the very efficient uptake of glucose from disaccharides we examined the relationship between the transport of glucose from disaccharides and from free glucose in the medium. It could be shown that glucose derived from disaccharides (maltose, sucrose, trehalose, lactose) was at least partially transported in hamster small intestine by a translocation process other than the Na^+-dependent active hexose pathway. This evidence emerged from experiments showing that under conditions of nearly complete saturation of the hexose transport system additional tissue uptake of glucose from disaccharides could be achieved[1]. Interaction of substrates of the hexose pathway (β-methyl-D-glucoside, D-galactose) with transport of glucose from disaccharides was of a non-competitive nature[1]. More recent data demonstrated that the transport of glucose from disaccharides was—in contrast to free glucose uptake—virtually Na^+-independent[2]. This observation was further substantiated by transmural potential measurements showing that addition of sucrose did not lead to a further increase of D-glucose induced PD[3].

Parsons and Prichard[4] had studied the relationship of hydrolysis of disaccharides to the transport of the resulting glucose with a perfused preparation of amphibian small intestine *in vitro*. They concluded that the process of disaccharide hydrolysis and transfer of related glucose are sequential and independent processes. Glucose from disaccharides and free glucose would contribute to a common pool of hexose and would compete for a common transport site. By measuring uptake rates of glucose from disaccharides and free glucose at short incubation intervals, we could demonstrate that addition of free glucose (30 mM) did not affect the specific activity of the tissue [^{14}C]glucose derived from the labelled sucrose under Na$^+$-free incubation conditions[2]. Uptake of glucose from sucrose in a Na$^+$-free medium exhibited saturation kinetics[2]. Since sucrose is activated in the presence of Na$^+$, the minor degree of inhibition of glucose absorption from sucrose has to be explained by a decrease in sucrose hydrolysis in the absence of Na$^+$ [2].

Trehalase, unlike other disaccharidases, is insensitive to Na$^+$. Hence glucose uptake from trehalose was not inhibited in the absence of Na$^+$. Under Na$^+$-free incubation conditions other disaccharides did not affect glucose absorption from trehalose and *vice versa* trehalose did not affect glucose uptake from other disaccharides (maltose, sucrose)[2].

In the absence of Na$^+$, uptake of glucose from disaccharides was clearly additive, whereas in the presence of Na$^+$ and various disaccharides interaction took place. The same phenomenon was observed for the interaction of β-methylglucoside with the transport of glucose from disaccharides: in the presence of Na$^+$, β-methylglucoside exhibited a non-competitive type of inhibition of glucose uptake from disaccharides; in the absence of Na$^+$ β-methylglucoside had no effect on glucose transport from disaccharides.

In conclusion: transport of glucose from disaccharides across the brush-border membrane occurs through a transport system which differs from the active Na$^+$-dependent hexose pathway. Glucose transport from disaccharides is Na$^+$-independent, but in the presence of Na$^+$ interaction between transport of glucose from disaccharides and free hexoses occurs by some unknown mechanism.

References

1. Malathi, P., Ramaswamy, K., Caspary, W. F. and Crane, R. K. (1973). Studies on the transport of glucose from disaccharides by hamster small intestine *in vitro*. I. Evidence for a disaccharidase-related transport system. *Biochim. Biophys. Acta*, **307**, 613
2. Ramaswamy, K., Malathi, P., Caspary, W. F. and Crane, R. K. (1964). Studies on the transport of glucose from disaccharides by hamster small intestine *in vitro*. II. Characteristics of the disaccharidase-related transport system. *Biochim. Biophys. Acta*, **345**, 39
3. Caspary, W. F. (1972). Evidence for a sodium-independent transport system to glucose derived from disaccharides. In E. Heinz (ed.). *Na-linked Transport of Organic Solutes*. p. 99 (Berlin, Heidelberg, New York: Springer-Verlag)
4. Parsons, D. S. and Prichard, J. S. (1971). Relationships between disaccharide hydrolysis and sugar transport in amphibian small intestines. *J. Physiol. Lond.*, **212**, 299.

Discussion 7

Smith: If you believe that the glycocalyx has specific ion-binding properties, why do you not strip it from the membrane and measure it?

Alvarado: We are indeed doing work along these lines. We have found evidence of Na^+-binding to brush-border membrane particles low in nucleic acid but enriched in mucopolysaccharide. The data are only preliminary and cannot be presented here. Nevertheless, it is obvious that this type of work has high preference in the near future in our laboratory.

Dowling: May I ride an old hobby-horse, which follows on from Dr Caspary's presentation? He suggested that *in vivo*, most of our sugars are absorbed from disaccharides and most of our proteins from oligopeptides. But Olsen and Ingelfinger's (*J. Clin. Invest.*, **47**, 1133, 1968) results have clearly shown that, in man *in vivo*, the luminal concentrations of glucose after a meal often reach 20 mM and occasionally 40 mM, but that Na^+-dependent glucose transport ceased at 2–5 mM (about 50 mg%). If that is the case, what is the relevance of all these *in vitro* models of Na^+-dependent transport mechanisms?

Caspary: I agree that active Na^+-dependent hexose or amino acid transport as defined in the small intestine *in vitro* may not be the only mechanism operating *in vivo* after heavy glucose loads. Perfusion experiments *in vivo* in the presence of high concentrations of phlorizin reveal the existence of a diffusional component, which increases with increasing substrate concentration (Förster and Menzel, *Z. Ernährungswiss.* **11**, 24, 1972). Whether this is a passive diffusional process or a carrier-mediated transport process with very low affinity is open for discussion. Recently it has been shown by Cook (*Clin. Sci.*, **44**, 425, 1973) with intestinal perfusions in man, that glucose is absorbed more efficiently from maltose than from equimolar free glucose; this observation could be taken as evidence for the efficiency of the disaccharidase-related glucose transport system.

Field: Differences in the sodium-dependence of sugar absorption *in vivo* and *in vitro* are unlikely to result from any fundamental difference in the transport mechanisms involved. In slow perfusions *in vivo*, there is probably a large poorly stirred layer over the brush border with a high effective sodium concentration, this sodium arising in part from the blood. This effective sodium concentration may be close to that of the blood, despite the low sodium concentration in the bulk perfusate. *In vitro*, under better mixing conditions and with a low sodium concentration present on both sides of the epithelium, the Na^+-dependence of glucose absorption can be more readily demonstrated.

Dowling: I still tend to believe that our whole discussion this morning relates only to a tiny part of sugar transport at the very end of the absorption process, whereas the vast bulk of absorption *in vivo* occurs by mechanisms that we have not discussed.

Caspary: A recent paper has shown that amino acids are absorbed from a mixture of various amino acids at the same rate as when given alone. How can this be explained in terms of the competitive effect of different amino acids for the same carrier site?

Smith: We can explain that by the fact that the concentration of each individual amino acid used was considerably below its apparent K_m-value. In these circumstances, uptake is proportional to V_{max}/K_m. The work referred to, however, was not performed by me!

Alvarado: May I conclude by emphasizing to Dr Caspary that my work does not disprove Crane's hypothesis. On the contrary, my work supports the early concept suggested by Crane, namely that sugar and amino acid transport is driven by the *transport* of sodium. My work slightly modifies and extends the Crane hypothesis in the sense of taking away emphasis from the sodium *gradient* and emphasising instead the coupling to the *flux* of sodium. I am sure Dr Crane would fully agree with me since he suggested a similar thing a couple of years ago.

8
The Influence of Harmaline on Sodium and Sodium-Dependent Transport Mechanisms

F. V. SEPÚLVEDA and J. W. L. ROBINSON

Département de Chirurgie Expérimentale,
Hôpital Cantonal Universitaire,
Lausanne

Harmaline is a psychotomimetic alkaloid extracted from *Banisteriopsis caapi*, a Colombian liana. A recent study[1] has disclosed its action as an inhibitor of various transport systems in epithelial tissues, where its mode of action differs from that of other known transport inhibitors. Thus the drug reduces both sugar and amino acid uptake by the guinea-pig intestine *in vitro*; furthermore[1] this inhibition can be extrapolated to zero time, revealing that the effect of the drug, at least in short incubations, is on the first step of the transport process, namely the translocation of the substrate across the brush-border membrane of the enterocyte.

Harmaline also inhibits other sodium-dependent transport mechanisms in other epithelia, such as sugar and amino acid uptake *in vitro* by renal cortex slices and dog colonic mucosa.

In the guinea-pig intestine, the fraction of phenylalanine influx which is independent of the presence of sodium ions in the incubation medium is not affected by the drug[1], although it can be inhibited by another neutral amino acid[2]. These facts, as well as the finding that the sodium influx is also inhibited by harmaline, led us to suggest that the drug may interact with a sodium transport site in the brush border membrane of the enterocyte.

In the present paper, we present some data on the interaction of harmaline with the influx of sodium in the guinea-pig intestine, as well as some further aspects of the effect of the drug on the transport of phenylalanine in this tissue.

METHODS

Experiments were performed on the small intestine of guinea-pigs. Under ether anaesthesia, an appropriate length of the ileum was rinsed free of its contents with Krebs bicarbonate buffer and then cut into rings for studies of uptake into the tissue, or opened longitudinally and cut into flat sheets for studies on transmural fluxes.

Tissue uptake experiments

The influx of ^{14}C-L-phenylalanine (1 mM in Krebs bicarbonate buffer) into intestinal rings was determined using methods described in detail elsewhere[3]. The tissues were preincubated at 37 °C in a substrate-free buffer for about 10 minutes and then transferred to a solution containing the radioactive amino acid for incubations of either 2 or 5 minutes. Following the incubation, the tissues were briefly rinsed in icecold buffer, gently blotted, weighed and dissolved in 30% KOH, prior to counting in a liquid scintillation spectrometer as described[3]. Exactly analogous methods were employed for the determination of sodium influx. The incubation medium was labelled with tracer doses of ^{22}Na, and the tissues were counted after weighing in a well-type γ-counter.

Transmural flux measurements

Transmural fluxes of sodium across sheets of guinea-pig ileum were determined essentially as reported previously[4]. The tissue was mounted between two lucite chambers. The area of the window between them was 0.64 cm^2 and the temperature of the system was maintained at 37 °C by means of a water-jacket. The volume of each compartment was 3.5 ml of Krebs bicarbonate buffer containing 0.2% glucose. The solutions were circulated with the help of a gas-lift system, using 95%/5% O_2/CO_2. The two unidirectional transmural fluxes of Na$^+$ were measured simultaneously by using ^{22}Na and ^{24}Na added on opposite sides of the tissue; 50 μl samples were taken from each chamber every 10 minutes for a period of one hour, and from the appearance of each isotope in the opposite compartment the two unidirectional transmural fluxes were determined. Details concerning the counting procedures for the separation of the isotopes have been described elsewhere[5].

Solutions

Two different buffers were employed. The Krebs bicarbonate buffer was used in some of the experiments on the kinetics of sodium influx and in all the measurements of amino acid uptake. Its composition (mM) was: NaCl 119, KCl 4.8, $CaCl_2$ 2.5, KH_2PO_4 1.2, $MgSO_4$ 1.2, $NaHCO_3$ 24.6.

In some of the kinetic experiments on sodium influx, a K^+-free buffer was used; its composition, in mM, was: NaCl 120, $NaHCO_3$ 15.1, NaH_2PO_4 0.6, Na_2HPO_4 2.4, $MgSO_4$ 1.2, Na_2SO_4 0.6, $CaCl_2$ 1.0. Choline was employed in every case as the Na^+-substituting cation. In sodium uptake experiments, L-phenylalanine was present at 20 mM concentration.

Materials

(U)-^{14}C-L-phenylalanine was obtained from New England Nuclear, Boston; [22]NaCl originated from the Radiochemical Centre, Amersham; [24]Na was purchased from the Eidgenössisches Institut für Reaktorforschung, Würenlingen. Harmaline hydrochloride was purchased from Fluka, Buchs.

RESULTS

Effect of harmaline on transepithelial fluxes

It was previously suggested on the basis of tissue uptake experiments that harmaline affects processes located in the brush-border membrane of the enterocyte[1]. To investigate this point further, we examined the effect of 4 mM

Table 8.1 Influence of harmaline on unidirectional Na^+ fluxes across guinea-pig ileum

	Flux ($\mu Eq/cm^2 \cdot h$)		
	m → s	s → m	net
Control	10.3 ± 0.68	10.1 ± 0.63	0.2 ± 0.63
Harmaline-m	6.3 ± 0.49*	6.6 ± 0.45*	0.3 ± 0.36
Harmaline-s	10.0 ± 0.64	8.4 ± 0.55	1.6 ± 0.53

Each flux is quoted as means ± SEM of nine experiments, in each of which two determinations of the unidirectional fluxes of sodium were made. Both sides of the tissue were bathed with Krebs bicarbonate buffer containing 11 mM glucose under open-circuit conditions. Harmaline was added to the mucosal (m) or to the serosal (s) face of the tissue at a concentration of 4 mM. *indicates a significant difference with the control series at the 1% level (according to a two-way analysis of variance with replicates[5]).

harmaline on the unidirectional fluxes of Na^+ across sheets of guinea-pig ileum (Table 8.1). When the drug was added to the mucosal solution, both unidirectional fluxes of sodium were significantly decreased, whereas no effect could be detected when harmaline was present in the serosal medium.

Na^+ influx at different Na^+ concentrations

Curran et al.[6] have suggested that the influx of Na^+ across the brush-border membrane of the rabbit ileum in the absence of amino acid is a linear function of the Na⁺ concentration, at least up to 140 mM. In an attempt to detect any mediated component of this process in the guinea-pig ileum, we have measured the uptake of Na⁺ from solutions of different sodium concentrations in the presence of 20 mM phenylalanine. Sodium influx, assessed after 2-minute incubations, is shown in Figure 8.1, as a function of the Na⁺ concentration. The relationship is clearly non-linear, and the fact that the points at the five highest concentrations fall on a straight line suggests that the curve

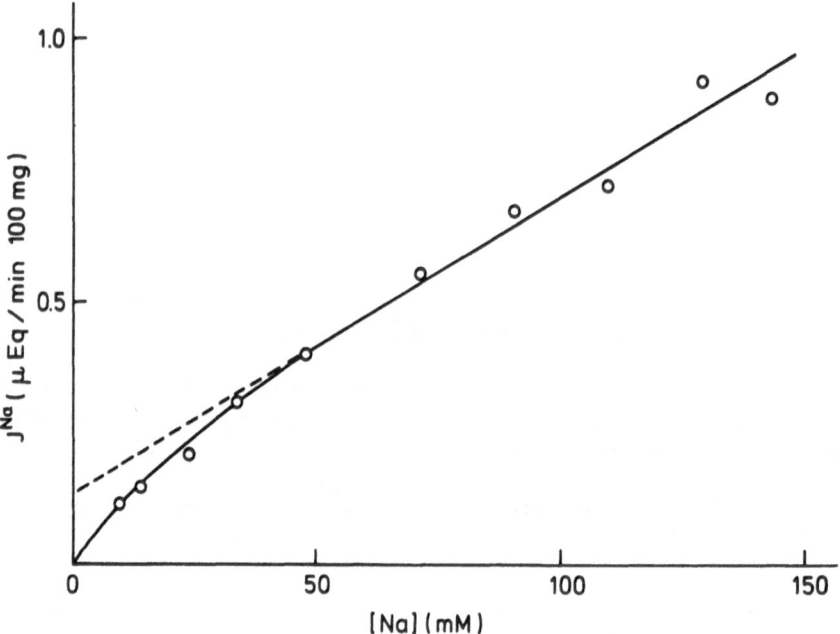

Figure 8.1 Dependence of sodium uptake on the sodium concentration of the incubation medium. The amount of ^{22}Na⁺ taken up by intestinal rings was measured after exposure of the tissue to the isotope for 2 minutes. The tissues were preincubated in a Krebs bicarbonate buffer containing 143 mM Na⁺. The incubation media were modifications of this buffer replacing sodium by choline to obtain the desired sodium concentration; each incubation medium contained 20 mM phenylalanine. The values are means of six experiments using the tissue from different animals. The straight line, constructed by least squares analysis of the last five points, was used to compute the linear component of uptake ($K_D = 0.0053$)

may be a combination of a saturable and a linear component. Thus the uptake into the tissue would be expressed by:

$$J^{Na} = \frac{J^m \cdot (Na^+)}{K_{Na} + (Na^+)} + K_D \cdot (Na^+) \tag{1}$$

where J^m is the maximal influx of Na⁺ across the brush-border membrane via a saturable system, K_{Na} is the apparent Michaelis constant for this process,

(Na^+) is the sodium concentration in the incubation medium, and K_D is a constant describing the passive penetration of sodium into the tissue. When the values in Figure 8.1 are plotted in the form $(Na^+)/J^{Na}$ vs. (Na^+), the Woolf plot[7], a straight line is not obtained. But if the non-saturable component, computed from the slope of the straight line in Figure 8.1, is subtracted from each point, the data can be replotted to give a straight line as shown in Figure 8.2. From this graph a value of $K_{Na} = 37$ mM is obtained.

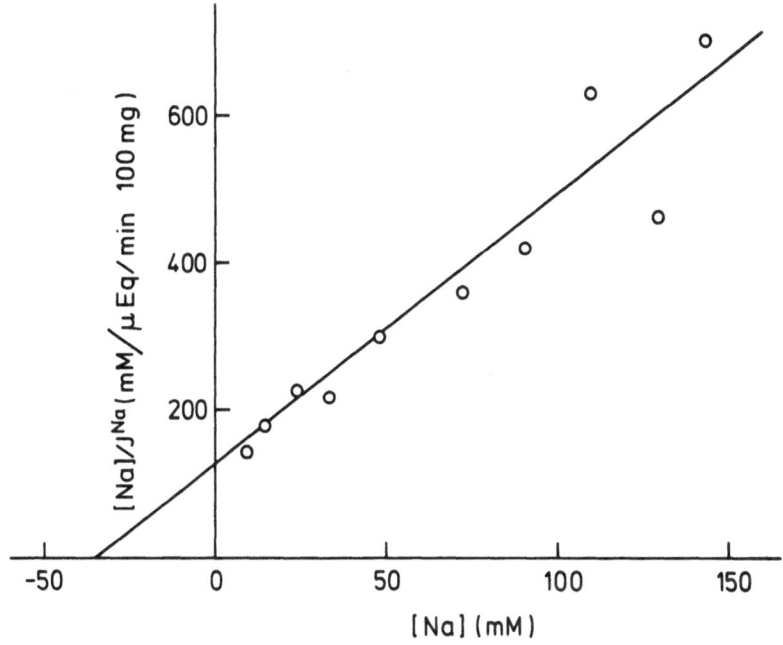

Figure 8.2 Woolf plot of the data from Figure 8.1 after subtraction of the linear component of uptake, calculated on the basis of K_D of 0.0053 (determined from Figure 8.1). The extrapolated constants were $K_{Na} = 36$ mM and $J^m = 0.28$ μEq/min 100 mg fresh tissue. The line was drawn from least squares analysis

Inhibition of the sodium influx by harmaline

Influx measurements were made at five different sodium concentrations in tissues from the same animal in the presence and absence of 4 mM harmaline (Table 8.2). Sodium uptake was always decreased in the presence of harmaline, but the inhibition was relatively smaller at higher Na^+ concentrations. This behaviour is suggestive of a competition between the alkaloid and the sodium ion and should therefore only involve the saturable component of influx. To test this possibility, the linear component of influx was calculated using $K_D = 0.0053$ and subtracted from the total uptake. The reciprocal of the corrected uptake was then plotted against the reciprocal of the Na^+ concentration

Table 8.2 Inhibition on Na⁺ uptake by harmaline

Na⁺ concentration (mM)	$J^{Na}(\mu Eq/min\ g\ fresh\ tissue)$	
	Without harmaline	*4 mM harmaline*
10	1.38	0.93
14.3	1.87	1.36
28	2.80	2.34
50	5.04	4.05
143	11.70	10.09

Values are the means of six experiments performed with different animals. The tissues were preincubated for 10 minutes in a Krebs bicarbonate buffer and then transferred to a modified buffer containing harmaline 4 mM, 20 mM phenylalanine and the desired concentration of ²²Na⁺, choline being used to maintain osmolality.

(Figure 8.3): The results indicate that harmaline behaves as a competitive inhibitor of the saturable component of sodium influx.

The above calculations involve the implicit assumption that the passive penetration of the tissue by sodium is not altered by the presence of harmaline in the incubation medium. To decide whether this assumption was justified, the uptake of Na⁺ was measured at nine different sodium concentrations in the presence and absence of 4 mM harmaline in order to permit the evaluation

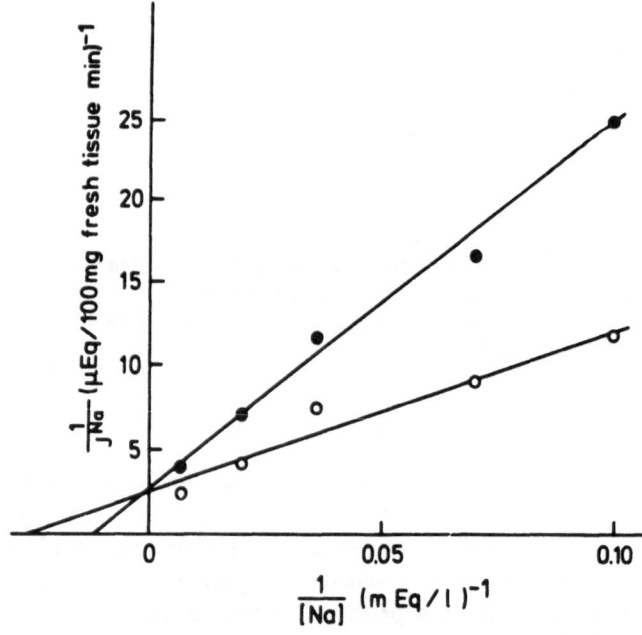

Figure 8.3 Double reciprocal plot of the saturable component of sodium influx at different sodium concentrations. Open circles represent control values and closed circles the values measured in the presence of 4 mM harmaline in the incubation medium. Experimental conditions identical to those described in Figure 8.1

of the linear component of the uptake under both conditions. The experimental points were then fitted to Equation (1) by iterative simulation to obtain the most likely values of the constants. The best fits were obtained with the following equations:

$$\mathcal{J}_c = \frac{0.375 \cdot (Na^+)}{(Na^+) + 33} + 0.0050 \cdot (Na^+)$$

$$\mathcal{J}_i = \frac{0.375 \cdot (Na^+)}{(Na^+) + 115} + 0.0045 \cdot (Na^+)$$

It is evident that harmaline induces no change in $\mathcal{J}^m$ and only a slight modification of K_D. Its major effect is on K_{Na} which increases from 33 to 115 mM. Hence a value of K_i of 1.6 mM can be calculated. In Figure 8.5 the same values are presented on a Woolf plot[7] after subtracting the linear component from each point.

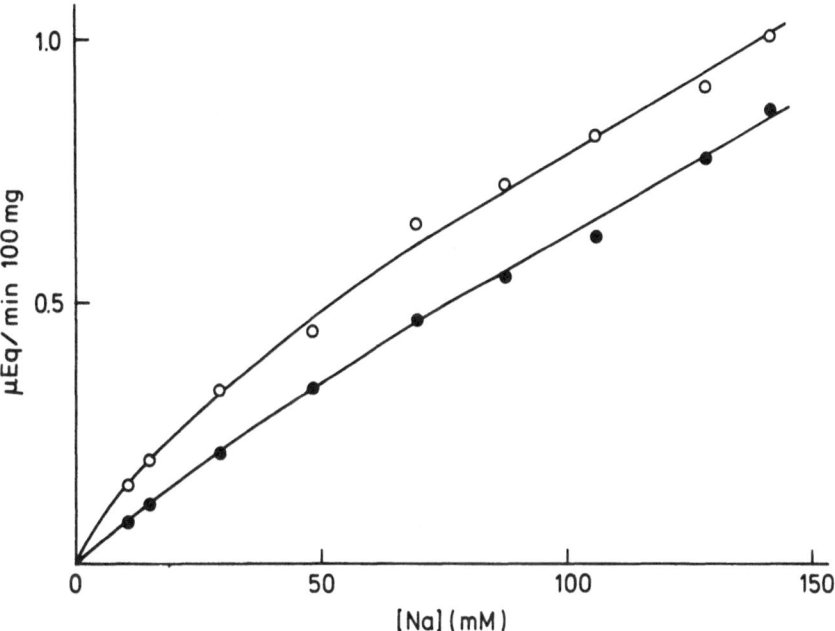

Figure 8.4 The effect of harmaline on sodium influx measured at different external concentrations of sodium. The tissues were preincubated in a K⁺-free buffer containing 142 mM Na⁺. The incubation media were modifications of this buffer, containing 20 mM phenylalanine, and where sodium was replaced by the appropriate quantities of choline. The uptakes were measured 2 minutes after exposure of the intestine to radioactive solution. Open circles represent control uptakes (means of six animals), filled circles are uptakes in the presence of 4 mM harmaline (means of eight guinea-pigs) The lines represent the best fits to the experimental data obtained by iterative simulation. χ^2 for the fits was 3.12 for the control points and 1.34 for the harmaline points

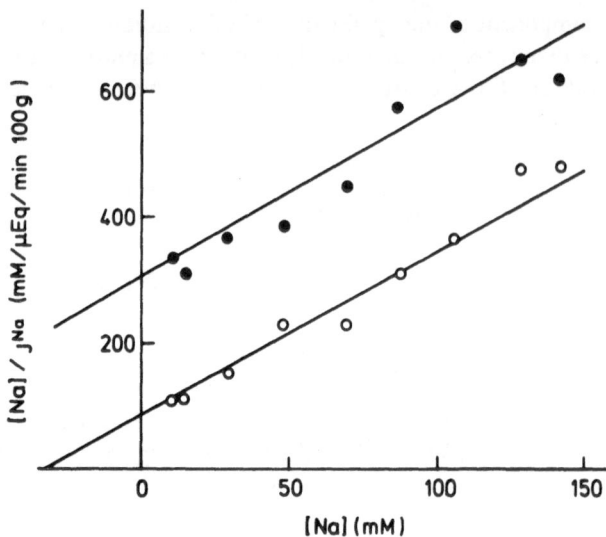

INTESTINAL ION TRANSPORT

Figure 8.5 Experimental points in Figure 8.4 represented as a Woolf plot after subtraction of linear component of uptake. The lines were drawn using the constants obtained from the simulation described in Figure 8.4

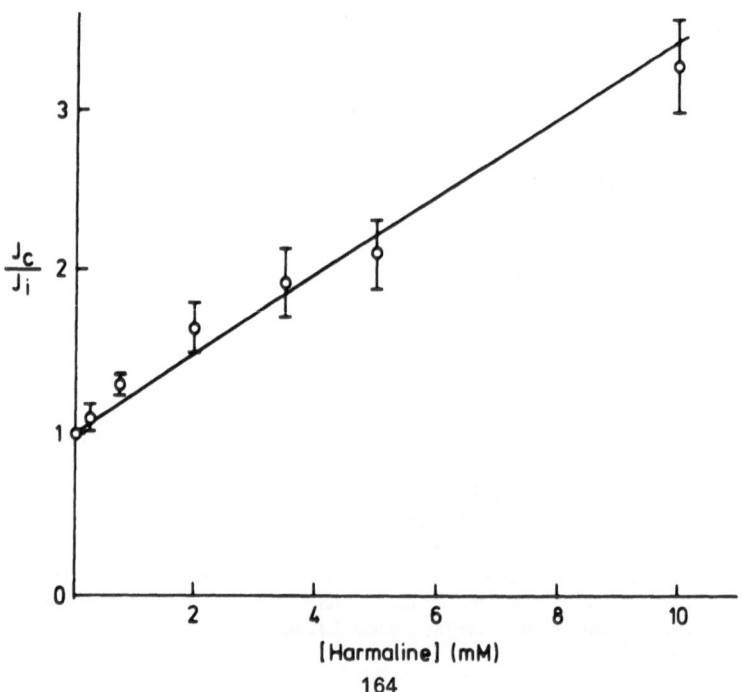

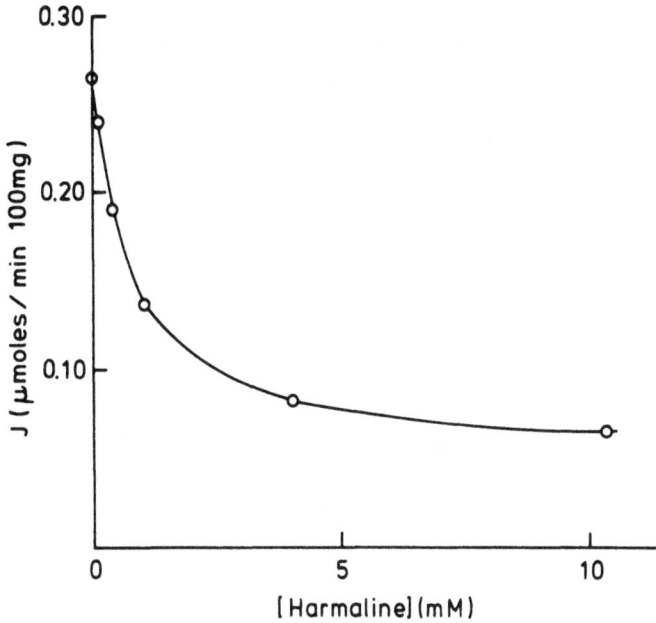

Figure 8.7 Dose-response curve of the inhibition by harmaline of phenylalanine uptake by guinea-pig intestinal rings. Incubations for 5 minutes performed in 1 mM phenylalanine in Krebs bicarbonate buffer in the presence of different concentrations of harmaline. Results are the means of six experiments

For a strictly competitive inhibitor[7], the ratio of control influx $\mathcal{J}_c$ to the influx in the presence of the inhibitor $\mathcal{J}_i$, will be given by:

$$\frac{\mathcal{J}_c}{\mathcal{J}_i} = 1 + \frac{(I)}{\left(1 + \dfrac{(Na^+)}{K_{Na}}\right) \cdot K_i} \qquad (2)$$

in which (I) is the concentration of the inhibitor in the incubation medium and K_i is the inhibitor constant. According to equation (2), $\mathcal{J}_c/\mathcal{J}_i$ should be a linear function of (I) with an intercept on the ordinate of 1.0. The slope depends on K_{Na}, K_i and the Na$^+$ concentration employed. An experiment to test whether

---

Figure 8.6 Kinetics of harmaline inhibition of sodium influx. Ratio of inhibited to un-inhibited Na$^+$ influx, corrected for the linear component of uptake, is plotted against the harmaline concentration in the incubation medium. Sodium concentration was 50 mM. The line was drawn assuming strictly competitive inhibition of the mediated component of Na$^+$ influx and using the constants calculated from the experiment illustrated in Figure 8.4. $K_i = 1.61$ mM, $K_{Na} = 33$ mM. The difference between experimental values and calculated points is not significant, $\chi^2 = 4.64$. Points are the means ($\pm$ SEM) of six experiments performed with different animals

harmaline inhibition of sodium influx conforms to such a relationship is shown in Figure 8.6. The line is calculated using the values of K_{Na} and K_i obtained from the experiment in Figure 8.4. The experimental values were corrected for the linear component of uptake using $K_D = 0.00475$, the average constant in the experiment described in Figure 8.4. The close agreement between the experimental values and the predicted line confirms that harmaline acts as a competitive inhibitor of the sodium site for mediated entry into the enterocyte across the brush border membrane.

The effect of harmaline on phenylalanine uptake

The more complex nature of the interaction between harmaline and L-phenylalanine influx is illustrated in Figure 8.7. A significant inhibitory effect is already present at a harmaline concentration of 0.1 mM. If the experiment is presented as a Dixon plot[7], a linear relationship between the reciprocal of the influx and the inhibitor concentration is not obtained (Figure 8.8), suggesting that the inhibition of phenylalanine influx by harmaline is not strictly competitive.

Comparison of the effects of ouabain and harmaline on the uptake of phenylalanine

Canessa et al.[8] have described harmaline as being an inhibitor of the Na^+-K^+-activated ATPase extracted from brain cortex and from the squid giant axon membranes. In our previous publication[1] we did not consider this effect to be a

Table 8.3 Influence of ouabain and harmaline on phenylalanine transport by the intestine

Preincubation	Phenylalanine uptake (μmol/min g fresh tissue)
Krebs	0.156
Krebs + harmaline	0.089
Krebs + ouabain	0.097
Na^+-free Krebs	0.199
Na^+-free Krebs + harmaline	0.085
Na^+-free Krebs + ouabain	0.124
$D_{0.05}$	0.030
$D_{0.01}$	0.040

Tissues were preincubated for 10 minutes either in a Krebs bicarbonate buffer, or in an equivalent buffer in which all sodium ions had been replaced by choline; 4 mM harmaline or 0.5 mM ouabain were also added to the appropriate flasks; the uptake was then measured from a Krebs bicarbonate buffer (143 mM Na^+) containing 1 mM L-phenylalanine in incubations of 2 minutes.
  Statistical evaluation by two-way analysis of variance[16] from which is extracted the value of the least significant difference at a given probability level ($D_{0.05}$, $D_{0.01}$). The results are the means of six experiments.

very likely explanation for the action of the alkaloid in the intestinal preparation in view of the rapid onset of the inhibition. An experiment was therefore designed to underline the different characteristics of the inhibitory actions of harmaline and ouabain in the intestine (Table 8.3). Preincubation of the tissue in the presence of either inhibitor in a 143 mM Na$^+$ buffer produces a strong inhibitory effect of the subsequent phenylalanine uptake. The action of ouabain in this type of experiment has been interpreted previously[9] as indicating that during the preincubation the cells take up sodium and thus abolish the sodium gradient across the brush-border membrane which is mandatory for normal phenylalanine influx. If the preincubation is carried out in a sodium-free buffer, the effect of ouabain is partially reversed since sodium can no longer flood the cells during the preincubation. On the other hand, harmaline causes its inhibition both in the presence and absence of sodium in the pre-incubation medium, suggesting that indeed it does not act by inhibiting a sodium-pumping mechanism.

DISCUSSION

It has been recently shown that the uptake of Na$^+$ across the mucosal border of intestinal preparations consists of two components[10,11]: one involves movement across the apical membrane of the enterocytes into its intracellular space, whereas the other embraces penetration of the tissue through relatively high conductance extracellular pathways according to the laws of strict ionic diffusion.

Our results on the kinetics of Na$^+$ uptake by intestinal rings were interpreted on this basis. The total radioactive sodium recovered from the tissue in fact consists of three components, namely that which has invaded the extracellular space via the cut edges or via the muscular layers (or is trapped in unstirred layers), that which has penetrated the epithelium through the paracellular pathways and finally that which has entered the enterocyte across its apical membrane. The first two components are nonsaturable and together are represented by the linear part of the function plotted in Figure 8.1. Subtraction of this linear component provides a saturable compartment as shown in Figure 8.2. It has previously been suggested that in the absence of the amino acids, the influx of Na$^+$ is a linear function of the sodium concentration[6]. The fact that in the presence of 20 mM phenylalanine a saturable function can be obtained suggests that the kinetics we are investigating involve a Na$^+$-phenylalanine coupled transport. These arguments, together with the goodness of fit revealed in Figure 8.4, represent a powerful validation of our methodology, which incidentally does not appear to have been used previously for a kinetic study of intestinal sodium influx.

Our results showing that harmaline inhibits transmural Na$^+$ flux only when added to the mucosal face of the intestinal tissue (Table 8.1), together with the rapid onset of its inhibition of Na⁺ uptake by the tissue[1], constitute strong evidence that this substance inhibits transport of sodium through the brush-border membrane of the enterocyte. Furthermore, the finding that the major effect of harmaline is on the mediated component of Na⁺ penetration into the cell, and more specifically on the affinity of a hypothetical carrier for coupled amino acid-Na⁺ transport, suggests that harmaline may interact with a sodium transport site in the brush-border membrane. The inhibitory effect on other Na⁺-dependent transport systems could be due to the similar nature of these sites[12], or to the existence of common binding sites for the cation shared by the different transport systems[13].

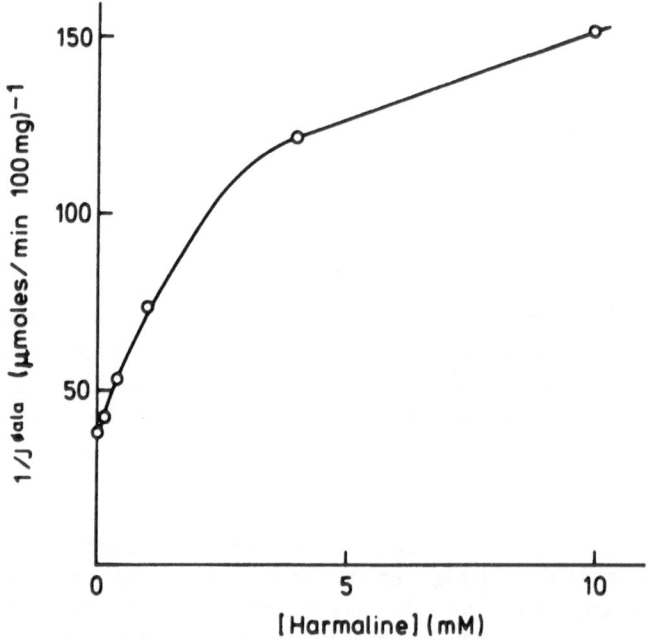

Figure 8.8 Dixon plot of the inhibition of phenylalanine transport by harmaline. The points were taken from the experiment in Figure 8.7. The deviation from the linearity, calculated from the regression of grouped points, is very significant: $F_{4,30} = 19.8$

An alternative explanation may be considered for the action of harmaline which could conceivably give rise to kinetics of the competitive type: The alkaloid could act as a lipophilic cation sticking to the membrane and adding positive charges to the microenvironment of the membrane carriers and thus preventing sodium interaction with its sites. This explanation would account for both the lack of inhibition of the drug on the Na⁺-independent phenylalanine influx and the relatively smaller inhibition of Na⁺ influx at high sodium concentrations. However, the fact that harmine, a very similar compound but more liposoluble, has almost identical effects in the intestine (unpublished results) suggests that the mechanism of action is not related to the liposolubility of the drugs.

As illustrated in Figures 8.7 and 8.8, the characteristics of the effect of harmaline on phenylalanine uptake are different and do not represent strict competition. This is not inconsistent with the hypothesis that harmaline interacts with sodium site in the carrier, since the binding sites for sodium and nonelectrolytes are evidently distinct.

The results presented in Table 8.3 show that the inhibition of phenylalanine transport by ouabain can be reversed, at least partially, when the tissues were preincubated in the absence of sodium. A similar result has been obtained by Chez et al.[14] for alanine influx, by Goldner et al.[15] for 3-O-methylglucose uptake in rabbit ileum, and by ourselves[9] with kidney slices. This procedure does not affect the inhibition provoked by harmaline, indicating that the mechanism of action of the two drugs must be different.

SUMMARY

Previous studies have suggested that the alkaloid harmaline may interact with the Na^+ transport processes in the brush-border of guinea-pig intestine. This hypothesis was strengthened by the results in the present report.

The kinetics of sodium influx were studied in order to separate the carrier-mediated and the linear components of this process. K_{Na} for the saturable process was increased by harmaline from 33 to 115 mM. A Dixon plot of the inhibition revealed that the action of the drug was that of a strictly competitive inhibitor. The alkaloid reduces sodium transmural fluxes only when added to the mucosal side of the tissue. The inhibitory effect of ouabain on the influx of phenylalanine was prevented by maintaining low intracellular sodium levels. This manipulation had no effect on the harmaline inhibition. Thus harmaline does not appear to act a a sodium-pump inhibitor.

Acknowledgements

This work was supported by Zyma S.A., Nyon, and the Fonds National Suisse. We are indebted to Dr J.-A. Antonioli (Nestlé, Orbe) for help with the computer programmation. We are grateful to Mmes H. Capt and P. Ganguillet and Mlle D. Mettraux for their skilful technical assistance.

References

1. Sepúlveda, F. V. and Robinson, J. W. L. (1974). Harmaline, a potent inhibitor of sodium-dependent transport. *Biochim. Biophys. Acta*, 373, 527
2. Robinson, J. W. L. (1974). The question of countertransport in the intestine. *Biochim. Biophys. Acta*, 367, 88

3. Robinson, J. W. L. (1970). Comparative aspects of the response of the intestine to its ionic environment. *Comp. Biochem. Physiol.*, **34**, 641

4. Robinson, J. W. L., Rausis, C., Basset, P. and Mirkovitch, V. (1972). Functional and morphological response of the dog colon to ischaemia. *Gut*, **13**, 775

5. Robinson, J. W. L. (1975). Inhibition of transport processes in the dog colon. This Proceedings, p. 287

6. Curran, P. F., Schultz, S. G., Chez, R. A. and Fuisz, R. E. (1967). Kinetic relations of the Na-amino acid interaction at the mucosal border of intestine. *J. Gen. Physiol.*, **50**, 1261

7. Dixon, M. and Webb, E. C. (1964). *Enzymes*, 2nd Ed., p. 316 (London: Longmans)

8. Canessa, M., Jaimovich, E. and de la Fuente, M. (1973). Harmaline: a competitive inhibitor of Na ion in the $(Na^+ + K^+)$-ATPase system. *J. Memb. Biol.*, **13**, 263

9. Robinson, J. W. L. and Luisier, A.-L. (1973). Inhibition of renal sugar and amino-acid transport by n-butyl-biguanide. *Naunyn-Schmiedeberg's Arch. Pharmacol.*, **278**, 23

10. Frizzell, R. A. and Schultz, S. G. (1972). Ionic conductances of extracellular shunt pathway in rabbit ileum: Influence of shunt on transmural sodium transport and electrical potential differences. *J. Gen. Physiol.*, **59**, 318

11. Munck, B. G. and Schultz, S. G. (1974). Properties of the passive conductance pathway across *in vitro* rat jejunum. *J. Memb. Biol.*, **16**, 163

12. Frizzell, R. A. and Schultz, S. G. (1970). Effects of monovalent cations on the sodium–alanine interaction in rabbit ileum: Implication of anionic groups in sodium binding. *J. Gen. Physiol.*, **56**, 462

13. Alvarado, F. and Mahmood, A. (1974). Cotransport of organic solutes and sodium ions in the small intestine, a general model. Amino acid transport. *Biochemistry*, **13**, 2882

14. Chez, R. A., Palmer, R. R., Schultz, S. G. and Curran, P. F. (1967). Effect of inhibitors on alanine transport in isolated rabbit ileum. *J. Gen. Physiol.*, **50**, 2357

15. Goldner, A. M., Hajjar, J. J. and Curran, P. F. (1972). Effect of inhibitors on 3-O-methylglucose transport in rabbit ileum. *J. Memb. Biol.*, **10**, 267

16. Pearce, S. C. (1965). *Biological statistics. An introduction.* p. 34. (New York: McGraw-Hill).

Discussion 8

Love: Can I confess complete ignorance? What is harmaline and why did you choose it to alter transport processes?

Sepúlveda: It is related structurally to tryptamine. It is a hallucinogenic drug, first shown to inhibit Na^+-K^+-ATPase in neural tissue by Canessa *et al.* (reference 8 on p. 170). We expected it to have an effect on sodium pumps in our tissues, but even though it does inhibit Na^+-K^+-ATPase at high concentrations, it is much more powerful as an inhibitor of sodium influx.

Whittembury: What concentrations of harmaline are required?

Sepúlveda: We use 4 mM harmaline for routine work. The first significant effects in the guinea-pig ileum are encountered at a concentration of 0.1 mM.

Case: Does harmaline have actions on transport processes which are not normally linked with amino acid or sugar transport, for example in the transport processes of the gall bladder?

Sepúlveda: We have studied the effect of harmaline on amino acid transport by mucosal slices of dog gall bladder and in this tissue it has a similar effect to that in the intestine. But dog gall bladder mucosa absorbs amino acids by a sodium-dependent process (Mirkovitch *et al.*, *Pflügers Arch.*, **355**, 319, 1975). We have not studied sodium fluxes in tissues where sodium movement is not linked to non-electrolyte transport.

Sharp: On seeing your slide of the structure of harmaline, I was reminded of the structure of other agents which block sodium entry processes, agents such as tetrodotoxin which acts on nerve, and amiloride and triamterene which act on the distal portion of the nephron and on the large intestine. The ability to block Na^+ entry appears to reside in the guanidinium moiety or a guanidinium-like portion of the molecule, and it may be that tissue specificity is conferred by the remaining part of the molecule. Have you compared the action of harmaline with that of these other agents, and have you studied, for example, the effects of the guanidinium ion on sodium entry and Na^+-dependent transport processes?

Sepúlveda: No, we have not performed experiments with guanidinium ions, but one indication in that sense is the fact that under conditions similar to those we have employed to demonstrate an effect of harmaline on Na^+ transport in the intestine, there is no effect of amiloride.

Love: Is it reasonable to suggest carrier-binding as an action of harmaline, since the drug seems to affect influx and efflux equally. As a carrier-binder, one might expect more action on influx and only a small effect on efflux.

Sepúlveda: The experiments suggesting an action of harmaline on efflux were carried out by measuring transmural fluxes across the epithelium under steady state conditions. To do this, we have to make measurements over a one-hour period, and probably after such a long contact between the drug and the tissue, side effects may be present.

171

Kinne: In the proximal tubule of the rat kidney, harmaline has the following effects: Given intratubularly at a concentration of 5 mM, harmaline does not influence isotonic volume reabsorption nor sugar transport; given peritubularly, it strongly inhibits the volume flow and depolarizes the cell (Baumann, Frömter and Samarzija, personal communication). In isolated brush-border membranes, harmaline inhibits D-glucose and L-phenylalanine uptake mainly by decreasing the overshoot observed in the presence of sodium. However, its action is not competitively inhibited by sodium nor by the substrate concentration. Moreover, harmaline inhibits phlorizin binding to the glucose-sensitive high affinity receptor in the brush-border membrane. Again, the inhibition is independent of the sodium and phlorizin concentrations (Evers, Bode and Kinne, unpublished observations). Thus, in the proximal tubule, harmaline does not seem specifically to inhibit the sodium-dependent transport systems. Its action probably involves other mechanisms such as unspecific alterations of membrane properties by an interaction with the lipid phase of the membrane, for example.

Robinson: I should like to comment on these remarks. We have studied the effect of harmaline on 2-deoxyglucose transport in the dog kidney cortex slice, and we found that it inhibited the uptake of this sugar both in the presence and absence of sodium. This indicates that the situation in the kidney is not the same as in the intestine. Your results would indicate that harmaline acts as a sodium-pump inhibitor, though we have preliminary evidence that it does not alter intracellular ion contents of dog kidney cortex slices to any great extent. As remarked earlier, harmaline may act both as a Na^+-K^+-ATPase inhibitor and as an inhibitor of Na^+ influx, but it appears that in the guinea-pig ileum, the latter inhibition is predominant. Measurements of transmural fluxes of sodium or non-electrolytes across both ileum and dog colon have revealed that harmaline *only* acts when present in the mucosal medium, which makes it less likely that it inhibits via an effect on the sodium pump. Furthermore the results in Table 8.3 underline the differences in mode of action of ouabain and harmaline at least in the intestine.

9
Effect of Vasopressin on Water Transport in the Kidney: Possible Role of Microtubules and Microfilaments

M. ABRAMOW

Laboratoire de Médecine Expérimentale,
Fondation Médicale Reine Elisabeth, Brussels

Antidiuretic hormone (ADH) plays an important role in water conservation[1]. In the mammal, ADH may have some effects on urinary sodium[2] and phosphate[3] excretion but this is of minor physiological importance as compared with the regulation of water metabolism. The control of water excretion depends on a unique characteristic of the permeability to water of the renal collecting tubule epithelium. This permeability increases under the influence of ADH.

Some of the mechanisms of action of vasopressin are well known and are based on the model of Orloff and Handler[4] which ascribes a central role to cyclic AMP as a second messenger.

The initial step of hormone action is the binding of vasopressin to its receptor in the peritubular membrane. The binding is coupled to the activation of adenylate cyclase. These early steps have recently been well studied in plasma membranes derived from renal medulla[5,6]. The resulting accumulation of cAMP is responsible for the permeability changes that occur in the apical membrane of the cells. The level of cyclic AMP—a balance between production by adenylate cyclase and degradation by phosphodiesterase—modulates the permeability to water.

We have investigated some aspects of the model using as a physiological approach the collecting tubule isolated from the rabbit kidney[7].

After isolation, the tubule is sucked at both ends in holding pipettes and cannulated at one end with an inner pipette connected to the perfusion system. The bath is an oxygenated, well-stirred bicarbonate buffer. The perfusion fluid is hypotonic and contains iodothalamate-^{125}I as a volume marker[8,9]. Ten to twenty minutes' collections are made at the distal end. Thus water absorption and hydraulic conductivity (*Lp*) can be measured accurately.

In Figure 9.1, the osmotic water permeability is plotted as a function of time after starting the perfusion. Initially it is high, presumably reflecting the influence of endogenous ADH at the time of sacrifice. The permeability spontaneously drops and reaches a steady state low level after about three hours of perfusion.

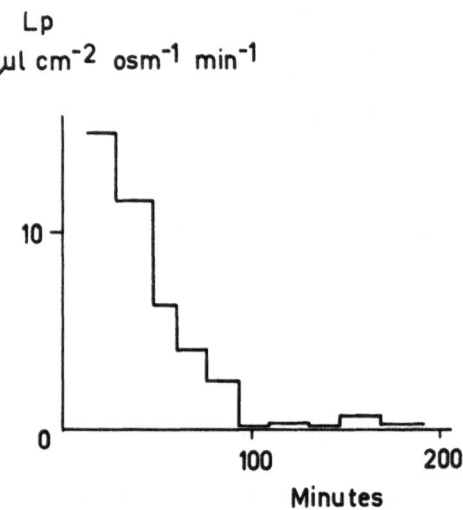

Figure 9.1 Hydraulic conductivity of a collecting tubule as a function of time; the perfusion starts at time 0

The hydro-osmotic effect of vasopressin is depicted in Figure 9.2. The addition of small amounts of ADH to the bath produces a rapid and considerable increase in permeability. This high level is sustained for hours, as long as the hormone is present.

We have conducted similar studies with dibutyryl-cyclic AMP which mimics vasopressin in our system[8]. Another compound with ADH-like action is theophylline[8]. It is supposed to increase the hydraulic conductivity by inhibiting phosphodiesterase. These results are consistent with the Orloff and Handler's model[4] as applied to the collecting tubule. However, neither the model nor its experimental confirmation can directly shed any light on the mechanisms by which the metabolic events in the cells are translated into permeability changes. In other words, the nature of the coupling between the stimulus and the permeability change remains unknown. Some physical alterations in the membrane must occur. Grantham[10] has shown that the deformability of the apical membrane of collecting duct cells is increased and that the viscosity of the cytoplasm underneath is probably decreased under the influence of vasopressin or cyclic AMP.

We found it interesting to investigate whether contractile proteins of the microfilamentous system play any role in the stimulus-permeability coupling, since this system has been implicated in some of the actions of cAMP on several processes in other cells[11,12]. Similarly the microtubular system has been thought to be involved in water transfer in toad bladder[11].

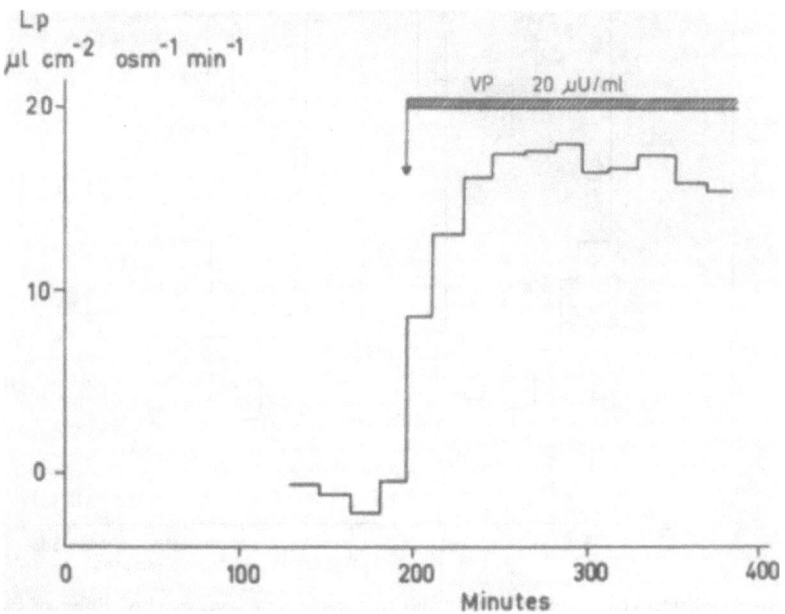

Figure 9.2 Hydro-osmotic effect of vasopressin; hormone is added to the bathing medium when osmotic water permeability has reached steady-state low values

Experiments with cytochalasin B

The drug cytochalasin B, a mold metabolite, is known to interfere with a number of cellular events while it disrupts microfilaments[12]. It blunts[11,13] or even completely blocks[14] the hydro-osmotic effect of vasopressin in toad bladder. We studied how this drug affects water transfer in our system. A typical study with cytochalasin B is represented in Figure 9.3. When osmotic water flow has reached low values, cytochalasin B does not seem to affect it. Moreover, the subsequent vasopressin response is not prevented, as in toad bladder, but is rather dramatic. This does not reflect a deterioration of the preparation since the permeability drops again when both agents are removed. A second response can be obtained following a new challenge with the hormone. This indicates a good reversibility of the system.

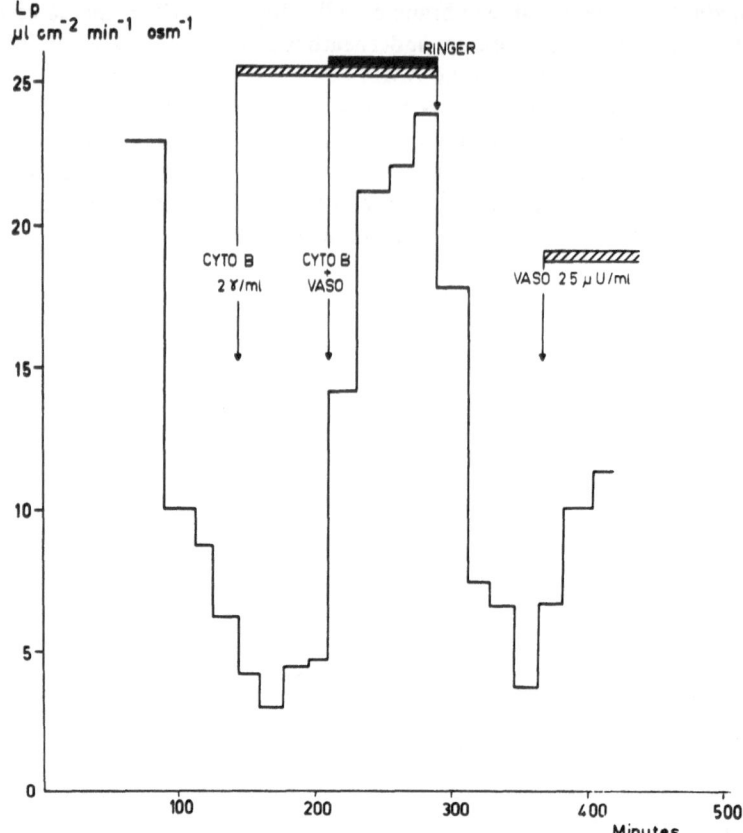

Figure 9.3 Effect of cytochalasin B (2 γ/ml) on osmotic water permeability. Effect of vasopressin (2.5 μU/ml) in the presence of cytochalasin B and effect of the removal of these agents. Effect of a new challenge with vasopressin in the absence of cytochalasin B

The sequence of adding the agents has been reversed and cytochalasin B was also included in the perfusate in the study represented in Figure 9.4. The hormonal response is very good. When cytochalasin B is added to the external medium, the permeability continues to rise and reaches the highest level we observed so far with vasopressin alone at this low concentration[8].

In other experiments, cytochalasin B was added only on the peritubular side, as summarized in Figure 9.5. On the left-hand side of the panel are studies without ADH. Each point is the average hydraulic conductivity of one tubule both with and without cytochalasin B. The drug does not alter the low basal water flow. On the right, in other experiments, under steady-state vasopressin-mediated high water flows, cytochalasin B, in combination with vasopressin, produces a significant increase in hydraulic conductivity. The magnitude of the effect is 20% of the vasopressin response.

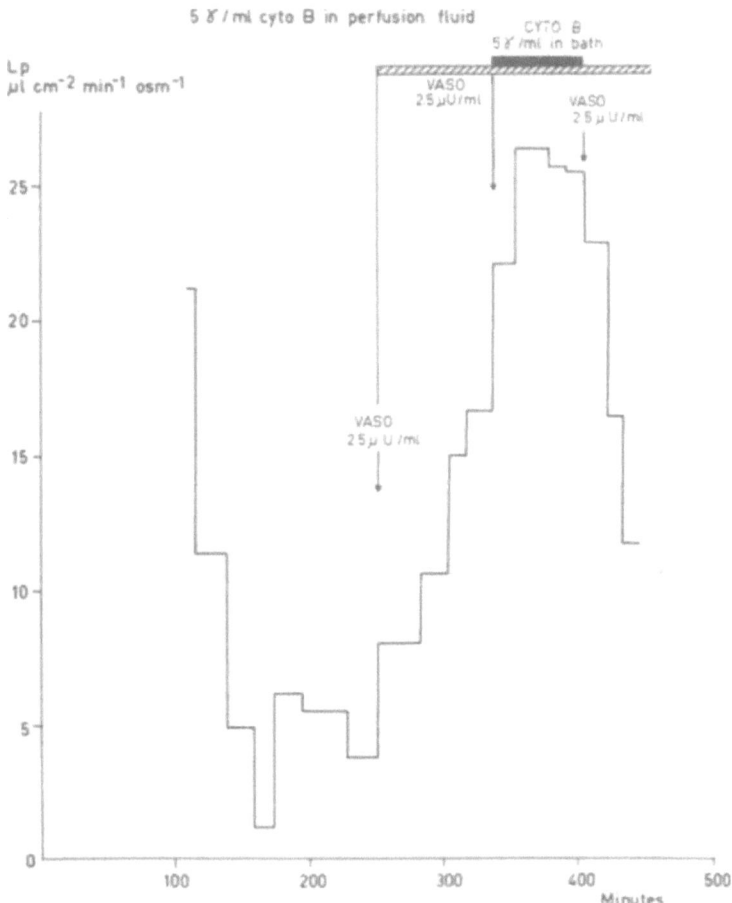

Figure 9.4 Effect of cytochalasin B (5 γ/ml) added to the bathing medium on the permeability response to vasopressin (2.5 μU/ml). Cytochalasin B in the perfusate throughout the experiment

An independent line of evidence suggesting an action of cytochalasin B on the response of the tubules to vasopressin is provided by the morphological changes we observed during the measurement of permeability. In the collecting tubule during the steady-state period of low water permeability, the cells are flat and the intercellular spaces are nearly invisible. In contrast, the cells swell and the intercellular spaces are dilated under the effect of vasopressin[15]. We have confirmed these observations. Moreover, we discovered that a few minutes after addition of cytochalasin B, numerous vacuoles are formed, some becoming very large.

Figure 9.6 provides a summary of the morphological changes under various conditions. Transverse sections of tubules are depicted. In the upper row, the

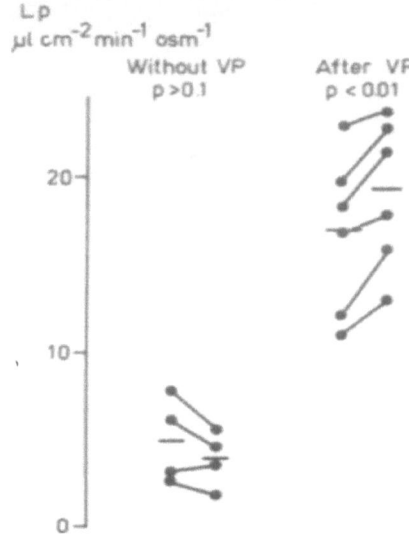

Lp
$\mu l\ cm^{-2}\ min^{-1}\ osm^{-1}$

Without VP
p >0.1

After VP
p < 0.01

Figure 9.5 Effects of cytochalasin B (2–5 y/ml) on hydraulic conductivity in the absence (left) or presence (right) of vasopressin. Each point is the mean of two to three collection periods in the steady state; the points connected by lines belong to the same tubule. Statistical analysis by Student's t-test for paired values

perfusate is hypotonic relative to the bath. With vasopressin, the cells swell, with enlargement of the intercellular spaces, the arrows showing the proposed pathways for net water flow[15]. When such a tubule is incubated with

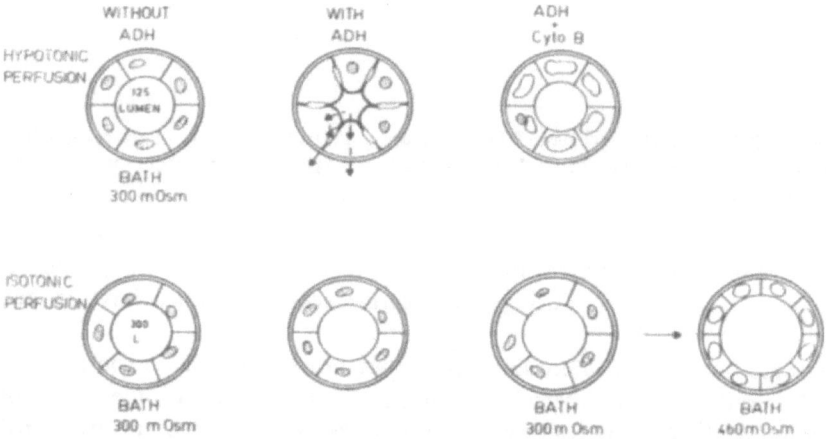

Figure 9.6 Diagram of the morphological changes under vasopressin and cytochalasin B. *Upper row:* luminal fluid hypotonic. *Lower row:* luminal fluid (L) isotonic. In the experimental condition on the right of the figure, the bathing medium is suddenly rendered hypertonic (300 to 460 mols/kg)

178

cytochalasin B, the large vacuoles appear. In contrast, when water flow is small, in the absence of vasopressin, cytochalasin B alone has no visible effect.

With an isotonic perfusate, net water flow is zero and the cells have the same appearance as in the upper left of the figure, even when ADH and cytochalasin B are present. However if in the latter condition, the bath is made hypertonic, the cells shrink, as expected, and the vacuoles appear immediately.

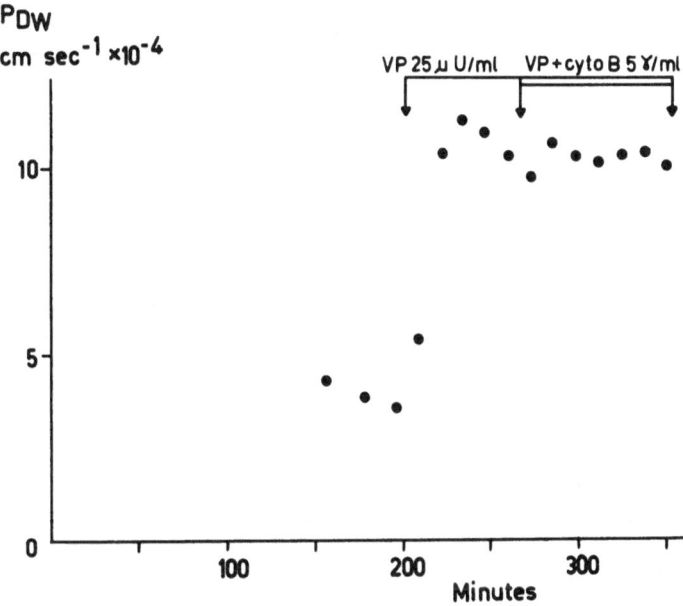

Figure 9.7 Effect of vasopressin (25 μU/ml) followed by the combination of vasopressin plus cytochalasin B (5γ/ml) on diffusional water permeability (P_{Dw})

This demonstrates that simple osmotic swelling of the cells cannot be responsible for the vacuolar changes. The vacuoles are produced when a transtubular osmotic gradient favouring large net water flows from lumen to bath under vasopressin is present.

We also investigated the functional effects of vasopressin and cytochalasin B in the absence of an osmotic gradient. This required the measurement of diffusional water permeability using tritiated water in the perfusion fluid. A representative experiment is shown in Figure 9.7. The diffusional water permeability coefficient (P_{Dw}) has a dependence on time and vasopressin which is quite similar to that of the hydraulic conductivity[16]. Cytochalasin B, however, does not increase the permeability further, even after more than 90 minutes incubation.

In eight experiments of this kind, the steady-state diffusional water permeability in the absence of vasopressin was 46 ± 3.98 cm s$^{-1} \times 10^{-5}$. Vasopressin 25–250 μU/ml produced a significant increase in permeability ($p < 0.02$ as evaluated by paired t-test analysis). The mean value of P_{D_w} in the steady state under vasopressin was 138.8 ± 34.7 cm s$^{-1} \times 10^{-5}$. After cytochalasin B, there was no further change. P_{D_w} during cytochalasin B + vasopressin was 143.7 ± 37.7 cm s$^{-1} \times 10^{-5}$ ($p > 0.1$). An increase in P_{D_w} of a magnitude comparable to that produced by cytochalasin B on the hydro-osmotic response to vasopressin would have been detected in our studies. We have shown for example that, after maximal stimulation by vasopressin, theophylline significantly increases P_{D_w}. Moreover, under vasopressin, P_{D_w} and Lp increase *pari passu* with the dosage level of the hormone from 2.5 to 250 μU/ml (unpublished).

Thus, cytochalasin B by itself has no effect on hydraulic conductivity. It potentiates the hydro-osmotic response to vasopressin, but does not alter the vasopressin effect on diffusional water permeability. The morphological and functional effects of cytochalasin B can be detected only in the presence of both the vasopressin and a transtubular osmotic gradient. This has been observed independently in toad bladder[13]. Taken together, the results suggest that the action of cytochalasin B is not at a single step such as the hormone receptor, adenylate cyclase or phosphodiesterase.

The effects of colchicine on water flows

We have also studied in preliminary experiments the effects of colchicine on water flows. Colchicine has been shown to inhibit the hydro-osmotic effect of vasopressin in toad bladder[11] and the antidiuretic effect of exogenous vasopressin in the rat[17].

Colchicine does not interfere with an established effect of vasopressin in the isolated collecting tubule. In contrast, as shown in Figure 9.8, when a tubule was preincubated with colchicine, the full response to vasopressin was prevented. When colchicine was subsequently removed from the bathing medium, the response to vasopressin became apparent after a considerable delay. In tubules not preincubated with inhibitors, the vasopressin response is half-maximal after only 12 minutes (unpublished, see also Figure 9.2).

Our study confirms that microtubules may be involved in the action of vasopressin on water transport in the kidney. The hormone may promote polymerization of microtubular protein[17]. The results with cytochalasin B suggest that microfilaments may also play a role in the stimulus–permeability coupling. However, in contrast to the conclusions derived from experiments using toad bladder[11,12,13], disruption of microfilaments would facilitate rather than depress bulk water transfer in the isolated collecting tubule. In our view, cytochalasin B presumably opens additional channels for transtubular flow of bulk water without altering the diffusional water permeability of the rate-limiting barrier in the apical membrane.

It is possible that ADH, in addition to its effect on the apical barrier, also decreases the viscosity of the underlying cytoplasm by interacting with the microfilaments. The exact mechanisms involved require further study.

However, the results do not indicate with certainty whether the microtubular and microfilamentous system is involved in the effects of the drugs, since colchicine[18] and cytochalasin B[19] are also known to interact with cell membranes.

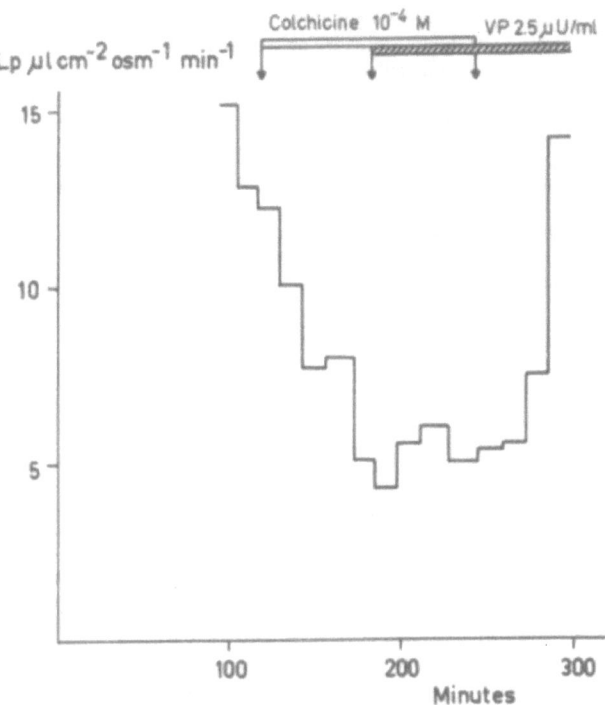

Figure 9.8 Effect of colchicine (10^{-4} M) and vasopressin on the hydraulic conductivity of a collecting tubule; the response to the hormone becomes apparent more than 30 minutes after removal of colchicine and more than 100 minutes after exposure to vasopressin

We have undertaken ultrastructural studies in an attempt to answer this question and correlations between structure and function will be sought in order to progress further in this field.

Acknowledgements

The collaboration of Dr M. Dratwa in some of these experiments and the technical assistance of Mrs S. Foulon is acknowledged.

References

1. Handler, J. S. and Orloff, J. (1973). The mechanism of action of antidiuretic hormone. In: *Handbook of Physiology*, p. 791, Section 8, Orloff J. and Berliner, R. W. (eds.). *Renal Physiology* (Washington: Amer. Physiol. Soc.).

2. Antoniou, L. D., Burke, T. J., Robinson, R. R. and Clapp, J. R. (1973). Vasopressin-related alterations of sodium reabsorption in the loop of Henle. *Kidney Int.*, **3**, 6

3. Wen, S. F. (1974). The effect of vasopressin on phosphate transport in the proximal tubule in the dog. *J. Clin. Invest.*, **53**, 660

4. Orloff, J. and Handler, J. S. (1962). The similarity of effects of vasopressin, adenosine 3'5'-monophosphate (cyclic AMP) and theophylline on the toad bladder. *J. Clin. Invest.*, **41**, 702

5. Bockaert, J., Roy, C., Rajerison, R. and Jard, S. (1973). Specific binding of ^{3}H lysine-vasopressin to pig kidney plasma membranes. Relationship of receptor occupancy to adenylate cyclase activation. *J. Biol. Chem.*, **248**, 5922

6. Rajerison, R., Marchetti, J., Roy, C., Bockaert, J. and Jard, S. (1974). The vasopressin-sensitive adenylate cyclase of the rat kidney. Effect of adrenalectomy and corticosteroids on hormonal receptor–enzyme coupling. *J. Biol. Chem.*, **249**, 6390

7. Burg, M. B., Grantham, J., Abramow, M. and Orloff, J. (1966). Preparation and study of fragments of single rabbit nephrons. *Amer. J. Physiol.*, **210**, 1293

8. Abramow, M. (1974). Effects of ethacrynic acid on the isolated collecting tubule. *J. Clin. Invest.*, **53**, 796

9. Abramow, M. and Dratwa, M. (1974). Effect of vasopressin on the human collecting duct. *Nature (London)*, **250**, 492

10. Grantham, J. J. (1970). Vasopressin: effect on deformability of urinary surface of collecting duct cells. *Science*, **168**, 1093

11. Taylor, A., Mamelak, M., Reaven, E. and Maffly, R. (1973). Vasopressin: possible role of microtubules and microfilaments in its action. *Science*, **181**, 347

12. Wessels, N. K., Spooner, B. S., Ash, J. F., Bradley, M. O., Ludvena, M. A., Taylor, E. L., Wrenn, J. T. and Yamala, K. M. (1971). Microfilaments in cellular and developmental processes. *Science*, **171**, 135

13. Davis, W. L., Goodman, D. B. P., Schuster, R. J., Rasmussen, H. and Martin, J. H. (1974). Effects of cytochalasin B on the response of toad urinary bladder to vasopressin. *J. Cell. Biol.*, **63**, 986

14. De Sousa, R. C., Grosso, A. and Rufener, C. (1974). Blockade of the hydro-osmotic effect of vasopressin by cytochalasin B. *Experientia*, **30**, 175

15. Grantham, J. J., Ganote, C. E., Burg, M. B. and Orloff, J. (1969). Paths of transtubular water flow in isolated renal collecting tubules. *J. Cell. Biol.*, **41**, 562

16. Grantham, J. J. and Burg, M. B. (1966). Effect of vasopressin and cyclic AMP on permeability of isolated collecting tubules. *Amer. J. Physiol.*, **211**, 255

17. Dousa, T. P. and Barnes, L. D. (1974). Effects of colchicine and vinblastine on the cellular action of vasopressin in mammalian kidney. A possible role of microtubules. *J. Clin. Invest.*, **54**, 252

18. Wunderlich, F., Muller, R. and Speth, V. (1973). Direct evidence for a colchicine-induced impairment in the mobility of membrane components. *Science*, **182**, 1136

19. Kletzien, R. F. and Perdue, J. F. (1973). The inhibition of sugar transport in chick embryo fibroblasts by cytochalasin B. Evidence for a membrane-specific effect. *J. Biol. Chem.*, **248**, 711

9

Discussion Paper on

Effect of ADH on Intestinal Electrolyte and Water Absorption

R. Dennhardt

Intitut für Angewandte Physiologie der Philipps-Universität, Marburg/Lahn

Vasopressin enhances the permeability to electrolytes and water of epithelial structures in a number of organs. One such organ is the intestine.

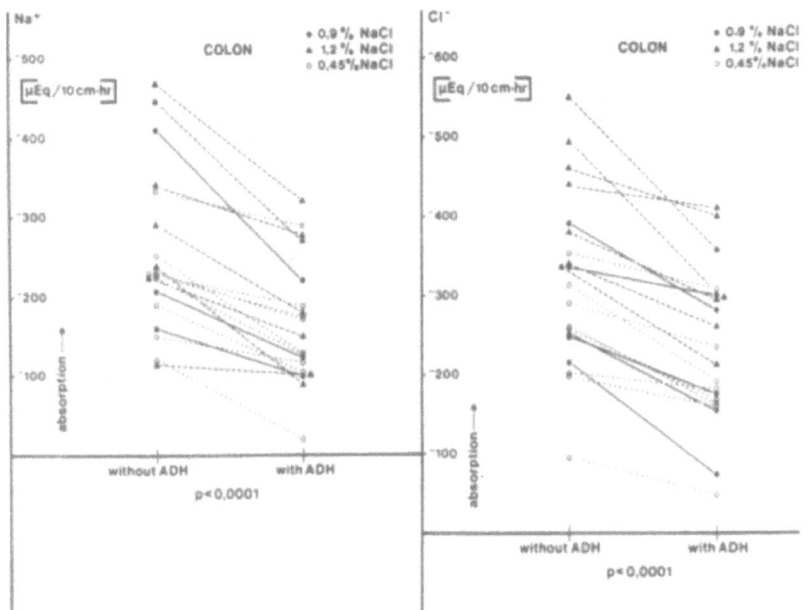

Figure 9.1 Net Na+ and Cl- fluxes in the colon without and with intravenous ADH-infusion (189 μU/min). The perfusion medium contains 0.9% NaCl, 1.2% NaCl or 0.45% NaCl

We have tested the effect of arginine–vasopressin in physiological doses on electrolyte and water absorption in the jejunum, ileum and colon of rats. For this purpose, it is necessary to carry out the experiments on unanaesthetised rats which are operated at least three days in advance. The chosen intestinal segment can be temporarily isolated and subsequently perfused in a closed system under recirculation conditions.

The following data are obtained:

(1) Continuous intravenous infusions of ADH (between 40 and 200 μU/min) diminish the absorption of sodium, chloride and water over the whole in-

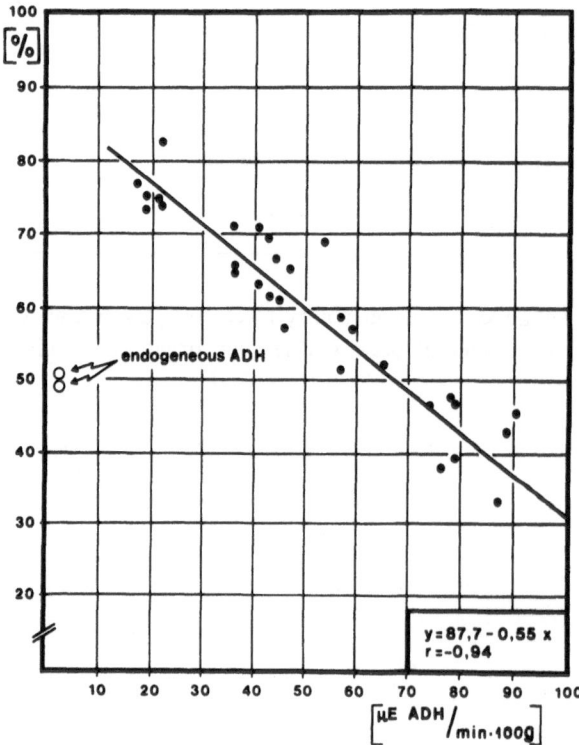

Figure 9.2   Effect of different ADH doses on volume transport in the small intestine. *Abscissa:* intravenous doses of ADH, *ordinate:* percentage reduction of net volume absorption related to control values

testinal tract (Figure 9.1). The effect of ADH shows an oral–aboral gradient (jejunum > ileum > colon).

(2) The effect is also observed when significant osmotic gradients are induced by a hypotonic or hypertonic perfusion medium. Vasopressin is effective only when applied to the serosal (blood) side.

(3) Within the physiological dosage range, we find a linear dose-response curve (Figure 9.2).

(4) The relationship between transported sodium and transported volume (Na^+-H_2O equivalent) remains unchanged under ADH (Figure 9.3).

(5) The change in net sodium transport is basically due to a decrease in Na^+ efflux, whereas the behaviour of the influx is not homogeneous. The unidirectional volume fluxes show the same behaviour as the sodium fluxes (Figure 9.4).

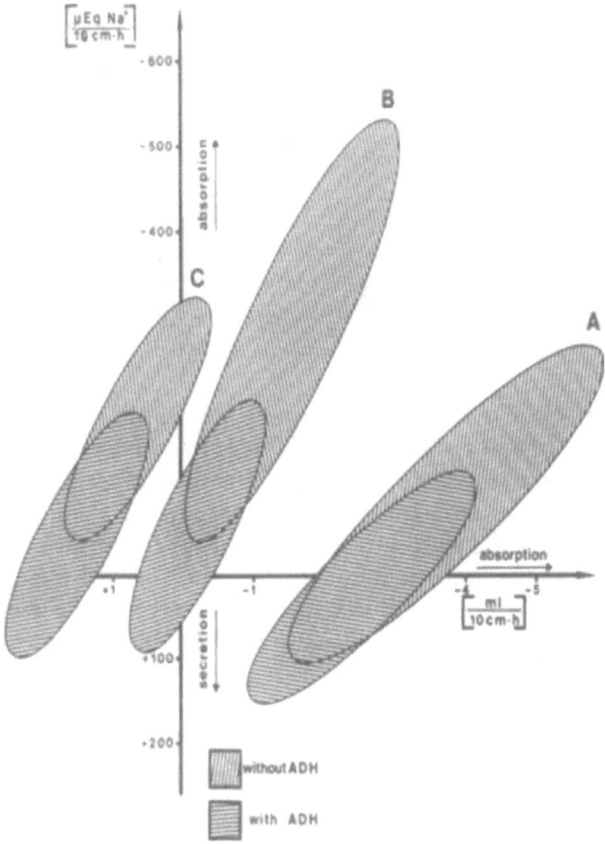

Figure 9.3 Sodium–water equivalent without and with ADH. *Abscissa:* Net volume transport, *ordinate:* Net sodium transport, A: perfusion with hypotonic (0.45% NaCl) solution; B: perfusion with isotonic (0.9% NaCl) solution; C: perfusion with hypertonic (1.8% NaCl) solution

(6) If 30 mM glucose is added to the perfusion solution, no significant influence of ADH on the net sodium and water transfer rates are observed (Table 9.1).

(7) ADH does not affect the transfer of actively transported sugars, but it influences that of passively transported substances, for example sorbose or urea.

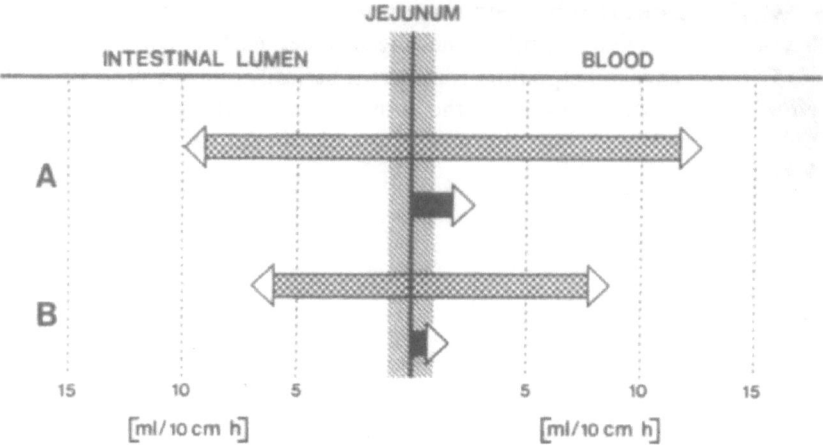

Figure *9.4* Unidirectional water fluxes in rat jejunal loops; experiments with and without ADH. The chequered arrows represent the mean values of the two unidirectional fluxes; the heavy arrows indicate the net water transport

According to these results, the following mechanism, based on a two-membrane model, can be postulated: ADH leads to a decreased permeability of the luminal membrane system. The passive transport processes are reduced while the absorption of actively transported substrates (for example glucose, amino acids, 3-O-methyl-glucose) remains practically unchanged. Similarly the passive sodium permeability is changed by ADH but not its active transport. Since passive movements of electrolytes take place to a different degree in the upper and lower intestinal tract, the above mentioned oral–aboral gradient can be explained in these terms.

Table *9.1* Effect of ADH of volume and sodium absorption in the presence of glucose

	Net volume absorption (N = 11) (ml/10 cm h)	Net Na$^+$ absorption (N = 10) (μEq/10 cm h)
Without ADH	2.8 ± 0.75	359.0 ± 79.3
	n.s.	n.s.
With ADH	2.7 ± 0.68	370.1 ± 59.3

Perfusion solution: 30 mM glucose + NaCl (osmolality: 291 ± 2 m osmol/kg)

Discussion 9

Maetz: Am I right in thinking that the contact time in your experiments with colchicine was rather short? Four hours, rather than two hours, were required in the studies published by Taylor *et al.* (reference 11, p. 182) and Carasso *et al.* (*J. Microsc. Paris*, **18**, 383, 1973).

Abramow: It is certain that the time of incubation with colchicine after vasopressin response has been obtained was rather short. However, periods of incubation of three hours were also employed before adding vasopressin, with a consequent blunting of the vasopressin response. Whether the optimal duration of incubation may be, the results are in agreement with those of Taylor. I am not aware of toad bladder experiments showing an inhibition of an established hydro-osmotic effect of vasopressin. Dousa and Barnes (reference 17 on p. 182) could prevent the antidiuretic effect of exogenous vasopressin with colchicine in the rat, but they were unable to counteract the established effect of endogenous vasopressin. Our results, although preliminary, are consistent with their findings.

Kinne: Do you have any information about the specificity of the colchicine action in the collecting duct? What other cellular functions are altered?

Abramow: It would be difficult to test directly other cellular functions in one single isolated collecting tubule. From very preliminary experiments, we have the impression that even the effect of vasopressin on diffusional water permeability is not changed by colchicine, just as it is unaffected by cytochalasin B. From experiments on toad bladders, it is apparent that colchicine does not block the natriferic action of vasopressin.

Kinne: Do you have any information about the state of the microtubules in the collecting duct epithelial cell after colchicine treatment?

Abramow: The effect of colchicine on the state of the microtubules in the collecting duct epithelial cell is presently under investigation. Even if we see a disruption of microtubules, we will not be certain that the relevant interaction does not take place at the surface of the membrane itself. This is where the problems of specificity appear to be the most critical.

Caspary: Dr Abramow, if you give a patient with an acute attack of gouty arthritis one tablet of colchicine every hour, he usually gets severe diarrhoea after the sixth or seventh hour. This effect is usually explained in terms of the inhibitory effect of colchicine on mitotic activity. Could it not be possible that colchicine acts by affecting the microfilamentous system? This would seem to be more likely, since inhibitors of mitotic activity such as methotrexate induce diarrhoea much later.

Abramow: This is an interesting question. I was going to ask it to the intestinologists. In my view, diarrhoea could well be due to the disruptive effect of colchicine on microtubules in the intestinal cells. How this effect could be dissociated from the antimitotic effect is not clear to me.

Smith: Would you care to speculate on the anatomical origin of vacuoles formed in the presence of vasopressin by the action of cytochalasin?

Abramow: At this time, only speculations are possible. I believe that the vacuoles contain water that accumulates in some intracellular compartment, where hydrostatic pressure builds up for some unknown reason. Recent electron microscopic studies of Davis *et al.* (reference 13 on p. 182) in the toad bladder exposed to cytochalasin B, plus an osmotic gradient plus vasopressin, also show large intracellular vacuoles, which seem to be membrane-bound. We are at present studying the morphological findings in the isolated collecting tubule by different ultrastructural methods.

Wingate Dr Dennhardt, to what extent are the changes described by you perhaps due to modifications in splanchnic blood flow?

Dennhardt: We did not measure the splanchnic blood flow directly, but the pressures in the portal vein and the superior mesenteric artery revealed no changes in the presence of physiological doses of vasopressin. We cannot exclude, however, modifications in the microcirculation of the intestinal mucosa.

Skadhauge: It is well known that dehydration reduces the water content of faeces. May I ask: (*a*) Whether you saw any effect on the colon, and (*b*) whether similar effects as those caused by ADH could be seen when hydrated and dehydrated animals were compared?

Dennhardt: The effect of ADH on colonic water and electrolyte absorption is also evident, but the response is significantly lower than that encountered in the jejunum or ileum. Similar effects can be seen with dehydrated rats. After 24 hours without drinking, the volume absorption drops to 50% of the control values; this is the same response as obtained with an ADH dose of 70 μU/min 100 g body weight.

Robinson: Do you think that vasopressin might exert its effect by acting on the adenyl cyclase system to increase secretion?

Dennhardt: Yes. We could show that during ADH administration, cAMP appears in the perfusion medium in higher concentrations than in control experiments. This would appear to indicate that ADH stimulates cAMP release.

10
Pathway of Sodium Moving from Blood to Intestinal Lumen under Influence of Oxyphenisatin and Deoxycholate

G. NELL, W. FORTH, W. RUMMEL and R. WANITSCHKE

Institut für Pharmakologie und Toxikologie der Universität
des Saarlandes, Homburg

Laxatives of the diphenolic type and dihydroxy bile acids do not only inhibit the absorption of water and sodium from the intestine but cause a net transfer of fluid and electrolytes into the intestinal lumen. This was shown by Forth *et al.*[1,2] for the rat colon and by Mekhjian *et al.*[3] for the human colon using bile acids. Ewe and Hölker[4] confirmed these results with respect to bisacodyl, a diphenolic laxative, in the human colon. The transferred fluid contains sodium and chloride at the same concentrations as blood plasma[3,5,6].

The question concerning the reversal of the direction of net transfer of water and sodium arises as to whether the flux from lumen to blood is decreased or the flux from blood to lumen is increased. In order to answer this question, the unidirectional sodium fluxes were measured.

Table 10.1 shows that the main effect of oxyphenisatin, as well as deoxycholate, is a massive increase in the sodium flux from blood to lumen, whereas the flux in the opposite direction is almost unaffected. The increase in the flux from blood to lumen is nearly entirely responsible for the complete reversal of the net transfer of sodium.

During the last few years, the existence of two pathways across epithelia has been confirmed (for literature, see Schultz *et al.*[5]). One is a low and the other a high conductance pathway. From electrophysiological and morphological investigations, it was concluded that the shunt pathway is an extracellular route

Table 10.1 Unidirectional sodium fluxes in rat colon *in vivo* under the influence of oxyphenisatin and deoxycholate[7,8]

	$L \to B$ (μEq cm^{-1} min^{-1})	$B \to L$ (μEq cm^{-1} min^{-1})	Net transfer (μEq cm^{-1} min^{-1})
Control ($n = 13$)	0.44 ± 0.03	0.17 ± 0.01	$+0.27 \pm 0.2$
Oxyphenisatin 6.5×10^{-5}M ($n = 5$)	0.39 ± 0.04	$0.88^* \pm 0.05$	$-0.38^* \pm 0.08$
Deoxycholate 3×10^{-3} M ($n = 5$)	0.45 ± 0.04	$0.73^* \pm 0.07$	$-0.26^* \pm 0.04$

Tied-off loops filled with 2 ml Tyrode solution; ^{22}NaCl and ^{24}NaCl were administered simultaneously intraluminally and intravenously. Oxyphenisatin and deoxycholate were administered intraluminally (see Nell *et al.*[7] for further experimental details). Mean values $\pm$ SEM; L = lumen, B = blood; *signifies $p < 0.05$ as compared with the controls; + signifies net transfer from lumen to blood; − signifies net transfer from blood to lumen.

through the mucosal epithelium across the intercellular spaces and the tight junctions. The shunt pathway is of particular importance in a low resistance epithelium like the intestinal mucosa.

What is the pathway of sodium moving across the colonic mucosa from blood to lumen under the influence of oxyphenisatin and deoxycholate, the transcellular or the intercellular pathway? With respect to the driving forces for the net transfer of sodium into the lumen, preference for the transcellular pathway would support the assumption that oxyphenisatin and deoxycholate activate a secretory process in the epithelial cells, whereas predominance of the intercellular pathway would speak in favour of a driving force from behind the intestinal epithelium.

In order to discriminate between these two pathways, the transfer through the colonic mucosa of well established markers of the extracellular space was measured with and without oxyphenisatin and deoxycholate respectively. Oxyphenisatin raises the transfer of [^{51}Cr]EDTA and [^{14}C]inulin from blood to

Table 10.2 Influence of oxyphenisatin on the transfer of [^{51}Cr]EDTA and [^{14}C]inulin through rat colonic mucosa *in vivo*[10]

	Blood $\to$ Lumen	
	[^{51}Cr]EDTA (Imp. cm^{-1}. h^{-1})	[^{14}C]inulin
Control ($n = 6$)	116 ± 6	52 ± 7
Oxyphenisatin 3.5×10^{-5} M	$392^* \pm 6$	$123^* \pm 8$

	Lumen $\to$ Blood			
	[^{51}Cr]EDTA		[^{14}C]inulin	
	conc. in intestinal fluid (imp. ml^{-1}. 10^{-3})	conc. in plasma (imp. ml^{-1})	conc. in intestinal fluid (imp. ml^{-1}.(10^{-3})	conc. in plasma (imp. ml^{-1})
Control ($n = 6$)	500 ± 7.7	84 ± 17.5	2200 ± 136	281 ± 37
Oxyphenisatin 3.5×10^{-5} M ($n = 5$)	380 ± 6.3	$207^* \pm 17$	2000 ± 92	$765^* \pm 76$

Tied-off loops filled with 2 ml isotonic choline chloride solution; [^{51}Cr]EDTA and [^{14}C]inulin were added intravenously (blood to lumen), or intraluminally (lumen to blood); duration of the experiment: 1 hour. The transfer rates in the direction from blood to lumen are normalised on the basis of 100 000 counts per ml and minute. Mean values $\pm$ SEM; *signifies $p < 0.05$ as compared to controls.

lumen by a factor of two to three (Table 10.2, upper part). When [^{51}Cr]EDTA and [^{14}C]inulin are administered in the colonic lumen, the disappearance rate out of the lumen is too small to be measured exactly. Therefore we measured the plasma level of these substances after intraluminal administration with and without oxyphenisatin (Table 10.2, lower part) The plasma levels are also increased by a factor of two to three.

In the presence of deoxycholate, there is a tremendous increase in the transfer of [^{51}Cr]EDTA from blood to lumen by a factor of 130 (Table 10.3, upper part). The lower part of Table 10.3 shows the influence of the bile acid on the transfer of [^{14}C]sucrose from lumen to blood. In the control case, the disappearance rate of [^{14}C]sucrose lies below the limits of experimental error but under the influence of deoxycholate, the disappearance rate is readily measurable and rises to about 10% of the amount administered. Deoxycholate increases the permeability of the colonic mucosa *in vivo* to a greater extent

Table 10.3 Influence of deoxycholate on the transfer of [^{51}Cr]EDTA and [^{14}C]sucrose across rat colonic mucosa *in vivo*[10,11]

	Blood → Lumen ([^{51}Cr]EDTA) Imp. cm^{-1} h^{-1}
Control ($n = 6$)	116 ± 6
Deoxycholate 3×10^{-3} M ($n = 5$)	$15\,300^* \pm 1200$
	Lumen → Blood ([^{14}C]sucrose) Imp. cm^{-1} h^{-1}
Control ($n = 6$)	360 ± 342
Deoxycholate 3×10^{-3} M ($n = 6$)	$6240^* \pm 840$

Tied-off loops filled with 2 ml Tyrode solution, duration of the experiment: 1 hour. In order to measure the transfer of [^{51}Cr]EDTA from blood to lumen, [^{51}Cr]EDTA was administered intravenously; to measure the transfer of [^{14}C]sucrose from lumen to blood, the disappearance rate of [^{14}C]sucrose from the lumen was determined. The transfer rates are normalised on the basis of 100 000 counts per ml and minute either in plasma ([^{51}Cr]EDTA) or in luminal fluid ([^{14}C]sucrose). Mean values ±SEM. *signifies $p < 0.05$ as compared to controls.

than does oxyphenisatin. This agrees well with the observation that deoxycholate renders the colonic mucosa permeable to choline whereas oxyphenisatin does not[12].

Therefore it can be stated that both oxyphenisatin and especially deoxycholate raise the permeability of the colonic mucosa for substances which do not enter living cells. This speaks in favour of the intercellular pathway for sodium moving from blood to lumen.

The homeostasis of the sodium and potassium distribution between the extra- and the intra-cellular space is a function of the activity of the pumping system and the passive permeability of cell membranes. If oxyphenisatin and deoxycholate induce a net transfer of sodium from blood to lumen along a transcellular pathway, an alteration in the tissue content of sodium and potassium would be expected. A net transcellular sodium movement from blood to lumen would necessarily involve changes in the activity of the pumping system.

Table 10.4 Influence of oxyphenisatin on the tissue content and the intracellular concentrations of sodium and potassium in rat colon *in vivo*[10]

	Control (n = 5)	Oxyphenisatin 3.5 × 10⁻⁵ M (n = 5)
Na μEq/g d.w.	137 ± 7	157 ± 7
K μEq/g d.w.	374 ± 26	361 ± 6
Extracellular fluid		
[⁵¹Cr]EDTA % of w.w.	14.3 ± 0.1	14.6 ± 1.7
Na μEq/g cell water	11.2 ± 1	15.5 ± 2
K μEq/g cell water	112 ± 9	113 ± 4

Tied-off loops filled with 2 ml isotonic choline chloride solution; [⁵¹Cr]EDTA was administered intravenously; duration of the experiment: 30 minutes; mean values ± SEM; w.w. = wet weight, d.w. = dry weight.

Table 10.4 shows the influence of oxyphenisatin on the content of sodium and potassium in the mucosal tissue. Based on the [⁵¹Cr]EDTA space, the intracellular concentrations of sodium and potassium were calculated. The mucosal part of the gut wall was scraped off after lyophilisation. Therefore all data refer to mucosa only. There is no significant change either in the tissue contents or in the intracellular concentrations, under the influence of oxyphenisatin.

In principle the same results were obtained with deoxycholate. Again the tissue content of electrolytes in the presence of the bile acid remains unchanged (Table 10.5). The control values differ from the data given in Table 10.4 since the tied-off loops were filled with Tyrode solution in these experiments.

From these measurements, the conclusion can be drawn that the pump and leak ratio of the epithelial cells of the colonic mucosa is not changed appreciably by oxyphenisatin and deoxycholate in spite of the fact that the amount of sodium transferred into the lumen during 30 minutes under the influence of oxyphenisation is thirty times greater than the intracellular sodium pool[6]. Therefore the most plausible explanation for these results is that sodium crossing the mucosa from blood to lumen follows the intercellular pathway.

Table 10.5 Influence of deoxycholate on the tissue content and the intracellular concentrations of sodium and potassium in rat colon *in vivo*[10]

	Control (n = 5)	Deoxycholate 3 × 10⁻³ M (n = 5)
Na μEq/g d.w.	280 ± 7	250 ± 19
K μEq/g d.w.	445 ± 15	441 ± 8
Extracellular fluid		
[⁵¹Cr]EDTA % of w.w.	14.7 ± 0.7	15 ± 1.9
Na μEq/g cell water	31 ± 2	26 ± 7
K μEq/g cell water	119 ± 5	112 ± 5

Tied-off loops, with ml Tyrode solution (for further details see Table 10.4).

If the transcellular path was preferred, not only an exchange of the extracellular sodium with ^{22}Na but also a rapid mixing of intracellular sodium with the tracer would be expected. A more rapid uptake of ^{22}Na, when administered from the blood side, into the mucosal tissue due to the influence of oxyphenisatin or deoxycholate would occur. If the ^{22}Na appearing in the lumen comes mainly from the sodium pool inside the mucosal cells, then an increase in the appearance of ^{22}Na in the lumen should correspond with a simultaneous increase of the ^{22}Na content in the mucosal cells.

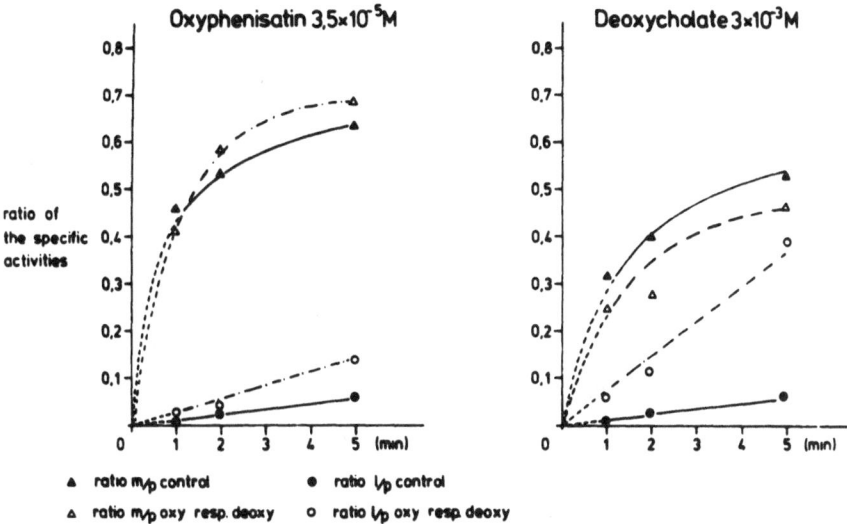

Figure 10.1 Time-course of the ratio of the specific ^{22}Na activities m/p and l/p after intravenous administration of ^{22}Na under the influence of oxyphenisatin and deoxycholate[10]. Rat colon *in vivo*. Tied-off segments filled with 2 ml Tyrode solution; ^{22}Na was given i.v. at zero time. Mean values $\pm$ SEM; $n = 5$–10.

$$\text{ratio m/p} = \frac{^{22}\text{Na specific activity in mucosal tissue}}{^{22}\text{Na specific activity in plasma}}$$

$$\text{ratio l/p} = \frac{^{22}\text{Na specific activity in lumen}}{^{22}\text{Na specific activity in plasma}}$$

Figure 10.1 shows the time course of the sodium specific activity in the mucosal tissue in relation to the plasma specific activity (ratio m/p, upper curves) and the time course of the sodium specific activity in the lumen in relation to the plasma specific activity (ratio l/p, lower curves).

Under the influence of both substances, the values of the ratio l/p (lower curves) are statistically significantly higher than the controls, particularly in the case of deoxycholate. This reflects the significant increase of the unidirectional sodium flux from blood to lumen which was shown in Table 10.1.

In spite of this tremendous increase in the specific activity in the luminal fluid, there is no difference in the time course of labelled sodium uptake into the mucosal tissue (upper curves, ratio m/p) in the presence of either substance within the limits of experimental error.

In order to elucidate the meaning of these values the distribution volumes of ^{22}Na were calculated (Table 10.6). A comparison of the distribution volumes of ^{22}Na in the mucosal tissue after an exposure time of 5 minutes shows that values for the respective controls and the two groups with oxyphenisatin and deoxycholate are not statistically different. They are also not greater than the values of the [^{51}Cr]EDTA space.

Therefore it can be concluded: firstly, the exchange of ^{22}Na with tissue sodium is not altered by either drug in spite of the massive increase in the unidirectional sodium flux from blood to lumen; secondly, within the exposure time of 5 minutes, ^{22}Na is mainly mixed with the extracellular sodium pool under all experimental conditions, whereas the intracellular sodium pool is obviously not involved to a measurable degree during this short period. This is a further argument against the significance of the transcellular pathway.

Table 10.6   Distribution volume of [^{51}Cr]EDTA and ^{22}Na in the colonic mucosa[10]

	Distribution volume (ml/g d w)
^{22}Na control (5 min)	1.04 ± 0.04 ($n = 10$)
^{22}Na oxyphenisatin 3.5×10^{-5} M (5 min)	1.16 ± 0.05 ($n = 10$)
^{22}Na control (5 min)	0.84 ± 0.04 ($n = 7$)
^{22}Na deoxycholate 3×10^{-3} M (5 min)	0.70 ± 0.02 ($n = 6$)
[^{51}Cr]EDTA control (30 min)	1.01 ± 0.04 ($n = 5$)

The distribution volumes were calculated on the base of the plasma concentrations. Mean values ±SEM (see Table 10.4 and Figure 10.1 for experimental details).

Our evidence in favour of the intercellular way is based mainly on three arguments. Firstly, the transfer of extracellular markers is increased. This corresponds to the increase in tissue conductance in the presence of bile acids *in vitro* described by Binder and Rawlins[13].

Secondly, the measured tissue sodium and potassium content and calculated intracellular concentrations remain unchanged. This speaks against a significant alteration of the pump mechanisms or the permeabilities of the cell membranes, but of course this argument alone cannot exclude the possibility that changes in the transport mechanisms and the leaks occur which just balance each other.

Thirdly, there is an increased sodium flux from blood to lumen under the influence of oxyphenisatin and deoxycholate, whereas the uptake of labelled sodium administered from the blood side into the mucosal tissue did not increase.

Taking these three points together, we think that at present the most plausible hypothesis is the assumption that sodium moving into the colonic lumen in the presence of oxyphenisatin and deoxycholate takes an intercellular pathway through the intercellular spaces and the so-called tight junctions. There are some other arguments which support this hypothesis. Preliminary results show that *in vitro* ionic lanthanum permeates the tight junctions of rat colon more readily under the influence of oxyphenisatin[14] and the electrical conductance of the rat colon increases under the influence of oxyphenisatin and deoxycholate[15].

It cannot be definitely excluded that the sodium transfer from blood to lumen induced by oxyphenisatin and deoxycholate is at least partially transcellular and involves only a small intracellular sodium compartment or a particular type of epithelial cell which represents only a small part of the total cell population. However, this explanation seems rather improbable in view of the fact that the permeability of the shunt pathway is increased.

Finally, the results obtained *in vitro* do not favour the assumption of a stimulation of the cellular secretion by oxyphenisatin and deoxycholate as the *primum movens* for the net transfer of sodium and fluid from blood to lumen. *In vitro*, a net transfer from the serosal to the mucosal side in the presence of these substances was only obtained after imposing a hydrostatic pressure on the serosal side. Therefore, we prefer the hypothesis that under *in vivo* conditions the hydrostatic pressure in the extracellular space is the main driving force (see reference 16).

Acknowledgement

These investigations were supported by a grant of the SFB 38 'membrane research' at the Universität des Saarlandes, BRD

References

1. Forth, W., Rummel, W. and Baldauf, J. (1966). Wasser- und Elektrolytbewegung am Dünn- und Dickdarm unter dem Einfluss von Laxantien, ein Beitrag zur Klärung ihres Wirkungsmechanismus. *Nauny-Schmiedebergs Arch. Pharmak. Exp. Path.*, **254**, 18
2. Forth, W., Rummel, W. and Glasner, H. (1966). Zur resorptionshemmenden Wirkung von Gallensäuren. *Naunyn-Schmiedebergs Arch. Pharmak. Exp. Path.*, **254**, 363
3. Mekhjian, H. S., Phillips, S. F. and Hoffmann, A. F. (1971). Colonic secretion of water and electrolytes induced by bile acids: perfusion studies in man. *J. Clin. Invest.*, **50**, 1569
4. Ewe, K. and Hölker, B. (1974). Einfluss eines diphenolischen Laxans (Bisacodyl) auf den Wasser- und Elektrolyttransport im menschlichen Colon. *Klin. Wschr.*, **52**, 827
5. Overhoff, H., Forth, W., Nell, G., Pfleger, K. and Rummel, W. (1970). Zur Klärung der Ursachen des durch Oxyphenisatin bedingten Nettotransfers von Wasser und Na⁺ am Colon der Ratte. *Naunyn-Schmiedebergs Arch. Pharmak.*, **266**, 419

6. Nell, G., Overhoff, H., Forth, W. and Rummel, W. (1973). The influence of water gradients and oxyphenisatin on the net transfer of sodium and water in the rat colon. *Naunyn-Schmiedebergs Arch. Pharmak.*, 277, 363

7. Nell, G., Overhoff, H., Forth, W., Kulenkampff, H., Specht, W. and Rummel, W. (1973). Influx and efflux of sodium in jejunal and colonic segments of rats under the influence of oxyphenisatin. *Naunyn-Schmiedebergs Arch. Pharmak.*, 277, 53

8. Wanitschke, R., Nell, G. and Rummel, W. (1975). Influence of deoxycholate and oxyphenisatin on the movement of water and sodium in rat colon. (In preparation)

9. Schultz, S. G., Frizzell, R. A. and Nellans, H. N. (1974). Ion transport by mammalian small intestine. *Ann. Rev. Physiol.*, 36, 51

10. Nell, G., Forth, W., Rummel, W. and Wanitschke, R. (1975). Pathway of sodium moving from blood to intestinal lumen under the influence of oxyphenisatin and deoxycholate. (In preparation)

11. Freiberger, T. (1975). Der Einfluss von Desoxycholsäure auf die Permeabilität des Colons der Ratte *in vivo*. *Thesis*, Medizinische Fakultät der Universität des Saarlandes. (In preparation)

12. Nell, G., Forth, W., Rummel, W. and Wanitschke, R. (1972). Abolition of the apparent Na^+ impermeability of the colon mucosa by deoxycholate. In: *Bile acids in human diseases. Second Bile Acid Meeting*, p. 263 (Stuttgart, New York: F. K. Schattauer Verlag)

13. Binder, H. J. and Rawlins, C. L. (1973). Effect of conjugated dihydroxy bile salts on electrolyte transport in rat colon. *J. Clin. Invest.*, 52, 1460

14. Specht, W., Nell, G., Rummel, W. and Wanitschke, R. (Unpublished results)

15. Soergel, K. H., Nell, G., Rummel, W. and Wanitschke, R. (Unpublished results)

16. Rummel, W., Nell, G. and Wanitschke, R. (1975). Action mechanism of antiabsorptive and hydragogue drugs. In: T. Z. Csáky (ed.). *Intestinal Absorption and Malabsorption*, p. 209 (New York: Raven Press)

10

Second Main Paper
Bile Acids and Bulk Flow

David L. Wingate

Gastroenterology Unit and Department of Physiology,
London Hospital Medical College

In common usage, the terms 'intestinal absorption' and 'intestinal secretion' are still used to refer to the direction of net fluid flow, unless we qualify them with the name of an individual solute species such as 'glucose' for 'glucose absorption'. Perhaps this is in deference to the pioneers of absorption physiology, such as Cohnheim and Waymouth Reid, Goldschmidt and Dayton, who thought in terms of solutions rather than solute or solvent. Physiologically, bulk flow is important; even if we drink nothing for 24 hours, we must still absorb several litres of secretion, and failure to do this has serious consequences[1]. The cholera victim does not see his problem as one of cation or anion secretion, but would probably understand the term 'bulk flow'. This is by way of introducing the suggestion that physiologists and membrane biologists are not always appraising similar aspects of identical phenomena, or even the same phenomena at all, and the assumption that they are speaking a common language may generate confusion. Until the work of Visscher and his colleagues[2], no serious attempt was made to separate the net transport of solute and solvent across the intestinal mucosa: when the Minneapolis group, using isotopes, made such an attempt, they found the net fluxes invariably coupled to form an approximately isotonic stream.

The growth of studies *in vitro* in England led by Fisher and Parsons[3] from Oxford, and Smyth[4] and his group from Sheffield was at first directed at the study of solute absorption. It was Curran[5] who gave us the concept of local osmosis which linked the transport of solute and solvent; refined by Diamond[6] into the standing gradient model, we have an accepted working hypothesis linking ion and water transport which has resolved the problem of earlier studies which apparently demonstrated the existence of active water transport[7]. But, during recent years, we have seen an explosive growth in the number of ion flux studies across sheets of intestinal mucosa isolated in Ussing chambers, an explosion to which this symposium bears witness. The reasons for this growth are debatable; statistically, there is a significant association with the rise of colour television and the decline in the value of sterling. More seriously, such studies are simple, elegant, and provide decisive answers; moreover, they can be done in profusion by an average PhD student. Scientifically, in relation to the problems of absorption, many such studies are open to the criticism that bulk flow, or net solvent changes are not measured in conjunction with unidirectional flux studies. The answer that net volume changes in such situations are probably small and introduced only trivial errors into the calculation of unidirectional ion fluxes is not enough; the question is, are such studies made on tissue which is mediating bulk flow during the period of study?

Historically, an important ancestor of the Ussing chamber was the Waymouth Reid chamber[8]; we have to thank Dennis Parsons[9] for drawing our attention to the neglected but important work of this early enthusiast. The important differences between the Reid chamber and the Ussing chamber is that Reid was measuring volume change; in other words, bulk flow. Reviewing his demonstrations of secretion, one may feel that his enthusiasm exceeded his objectivity. Lee[10], many years later, reported an elegant series of experiments in which he showed the failure of isolated mucosa, removed from an experimental animal secreting due to cholera toxin, to continue secretion *in vitro*. Net fluid secretion cannot be convincingly shown *in vitro*. This we should all remember, but I shall shortly forget, in the interests of science.

And so to the bile acids. Conjugated bile acids have a unique effect on intestinal absorption, and as such, are valuable tools for the scientific study of absorption. The phenomenon of net intestinal secretion due to bile acids was first reported by Forth and his colleagues[11] from Homburg-Saar. Because of the possibility that this might be important in pathophysiological terms, an extensive programme of investigating this phenomena in man was carried out at the Mayo Clinic by Sidney Phillips, Alan Hofmann, and a long succession of collaborators among whom I was privileged to be included.

For present purposes, one may summarise the findings in man very briefly. In the human jejunum, ileum, and colon, glycine-conjugated dihydroxy bile acids provoke fluid secretion when present in low concentrations — 5–10 mM — in physiological solutions perfused through the intestinal lumen. The unusual characteristics of this secretory effect are that (a) it is rapidly reversible when the bile acid is removed, (b) it is associated with no more than a modest decline in glucose absorption, and (b) the molecular configuration of the bile acid is important in that while dihydroxy conjugates provoke secretion, trihydroxy conjugates do not. The unique value of the conjugated bile acids as experimental substances is that these effects are achieved with very low concentrations which only alter the osmotic and ionic differences between lumen and plasma by insignificant amounts; we know that the difference is insignificant because the trihydroxy conjugates act as controls in this respect.

My contribution[12] to this massive perfusion programme was the study of the jejunal effects, working with Sidney Phillips. When we came to sort out our data, we tested various regressions of net ion transport against net water transport; like so many absorption physiologists before and since, we found these regressions to be statistically significant, but, at first, conceptually insignificant.

On further reflection, we realised that we had net ion transport data over a very wide range of net water transport, ranging from absorption at 2 ml/min^{-1} to secretion at 2 ml/min^{-1}. Because the luminal conditions in all these studies differed little, we plotted data from all of our studies together, and calculated the regression $y = bx + a$ for net water movement on the x axis against net solute movement on the y axis. The correlation coefficients (r) were satisfyingly high (Table 10.1). Much more strikingly, the regression coefficients (b) were virtually identical to the luminal ion concentrations (c). In other words the ratio of net solute to net solvent was isotonic with the lumen, apparently irrespective of the magnitude or direction of net flow. By contrast with the regressions for sodium and potassium, which passed close to the

Table 10.1 Calculated regression of net ion movement against net water movement in the human jejunum

Ion	c	b	a	r
Na$^+$	139	137	−10	0.99
K$^+$	5	6	—1	0.92
Cl$^-$	100	95	−92	0.98
HCO$_3^-$	40	48	80	0.89

a and b are the values for the equation $y = a + bx$ calculated for the linear regression of net ion movement (y axis) against net water movement (x axis) in 44 human jejunal perfusion studies, and r are the values of the correlation coefficients; c are the concentrations of the ions in the luminal perfusate. Data from Wingate et al.[14]

origin, there were large and highly significant intercepts (a) for chloride and bicarbonate. These would correspond to the chloride–bicarbonate exchange in the jejunum, which Turnberg and his colleagues[13] had previously shown. The hypothesis which I wish to make here is this; if (and this must remain hypothetical) the linear regression equation corresponds to our data, the implication is that the bulk flow of fluid across the intestinal mucosa is an isotonic stream, while the ion-exchange — in this case chloride and bicarbonate — is a constant, unaffected by solvent drag, or the rate and direction of bulk flow. From this, two further suggestions arise. First, bulk flow and ion-exchange may be carried out through different pathways across the mucosa; and secondly, they are unrelated processes.

Subsequently[14], we calculated the data from the ileal and colonic data in the same way, and, essentially, the findings were similar. In particular, the regression statistics from the colonic data (Table 10.2) are interesting by comparison with the jejunal statistics, for they show, once more, a close correspondence between the regression coefficients (b) and the luminal ion concentrations (c).

Table 10.2 Calculated regression of net ion movement against net water movement in the human colon

Ion	c	b	a	r
Na^+	130	122	26	0.98
K^+	20	28	—14	0.85
Cl^-	95	116	127	0.96
HCO_3^-	48	35	—125	0.73

a and *b* are the value for the equation $y = a + bx$ calculated for the linear regression of net ion movement (*y* axis) against net water movement (*x* axis) in 35 human colonic perfusions studies, and *r* are the values of the correlation coefficients; *c* are the concentrations of the ions in the luminal perfusate. Data from Wingate *et al.*[14]

In this case, the intercepts (*a*) for chloride and bicarbonate are again very large, but the signs are reversed, suggesting a fixed excretion of bicarbonate in exchange for chloride. As might be imagined, the regression statistics for the ileum suggest a situation midway between that found at the proximal and distal ends of the intestine[14].

I have suggested one interpretation for our data; others are possible. Clearly, *in vitro* study was required. And so again recurs the problem of studying bulk flow problems *in vitro* without measuring bulk flow. While acknowledging that the perfused intestine *in vivo* tends to reveal phenomena without offering explanations, I attempted a compromise in extending the study of the bile acid phenomenon by choosing an *in vitro* model which allows bulk flow measurement — but not precise unidirectional ion flux studies. The model I chose was the isolated rat intestine with oxygenated mucosal recirculation, the Fisher and Parsons preparation[3], modified by using an accurate gravimetric method of measuring volume change[7]. In these experiments, both the mucosal and serosal fluids were identical Krebs–Ringer bicarbonate solutions, either glucose-free, or both containing 28 mM glucose. In the experiments where glucose was present, the mucosal fluid either contained no bile acid or a 5 mM concentration of one of the three glycine conjugates, glycocholate (GC), glycochenate (glycochenodeoxycholate, GCDC), or glycodeoxycholate (GDC). By contrast with the perfused intestine *in vivo*, the experimental design did not allow testing for the reversibility of the bile acid effect; in isolated tissue, which is not in a steady state, this can be complicated.

Using the *in vitro* system, glucose-stimulated net fluid transport was demonstrated in both jejunum and ileum, and the *in vivo* effects of bile acids were, to a considerable extent, reproduced[15]. At this, you may consider that the views that I expressed above on the difficulty or impossibility of reproducing net fluid secretion *in vitro* are inconsistent with the attempt to investigate the secretogenic properties of bile acids on isolated tissue. This question was anticipated in the experimental design. In the human studies, a 5 mM concentration of dihydroxy conjugate arrested net fluid transport rather than induced net secretion; by selecting the same concentration in the isolated model, its validity would not depend upon the production of frank fluid secretion,

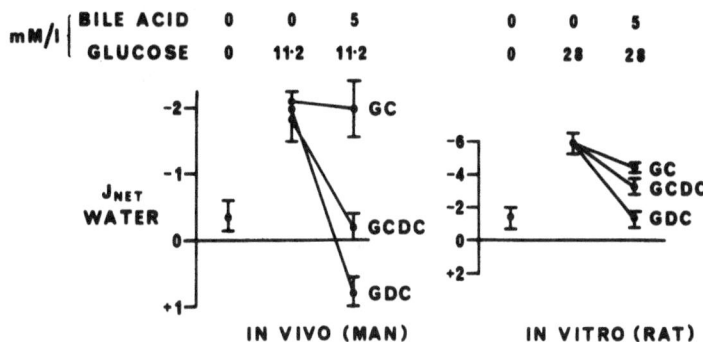

Figure 10.1 The effect of bile acids and glucose on net water movement in the perfused and isolated jejunum. The effects of glycocholate (GC), glycochenate (GCDC), and glycodeoxycholic (GDC) on net water movement in the perfused human jejunum and the isolated human ileum. Rates of net water movement (J_{net}) are expressed as $ml^{-1} min^{-1}$. 25 cm segment in man and $ml^{-1} h^{-1} g^{-1}$ dry tissue in the rat. Values for studies *in vivo* are the mean ±SEM of four studies, and for studies *in vitro* are the mean ±SEM of six studies. Data from Wingate *et al*.[12], and Wingate[15]

which I did not expect to demonstrate. Using this possibly devious stratagem, the results were reasonably gratifying. In the jejunum (Figure 10.1), the dihydroxy conjugates diminished or abolished glucose-stimulated net fluid transport; the slight fall with glycocholate was not significant. As in man, GDC appeared to be most potent in the jejunum. In the ileal experiments (Figure 10.2) I have compared the rat data with the human data published by Krag and Phillips[16]. In the rat ileum, the trihydroxy conjugate was as inhibitory as the dihydroxy conjugate; perhaps this is because taurocholate rather than glycocholate is normally secreted in rat bile.

The replication in isolated tissue of inhibited transport is none too convincing; it is only too easy to inhibit vital activity in a tissue which has a precarious and diminishing hold on life. Much more interesting was the fact

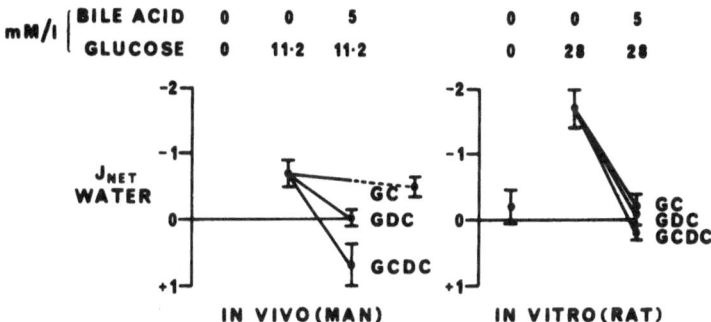

Figure 10.2 The effect of bile acids and glucose on net water movement on the perfused and isolated ileum. For explanation of symbols and abbreviations, see Figure 10.1. Note that no value is given for the effect of 5 mM GC in human ileum; the interpolated value is for 10 mM GC. Data from Krag and Phillips[16], and Wingate[15]

that in the isolated jejunum, the effect on glucose uptake was much less marked than on fluid transport (Figure 10.3). *In vivo*, glucose absorption was diminished by about 25% by 5 mM GDC; *in vitro* the inhibition was about 40%, but the inhibitory effect was on glucose translocation[3] to the serosal surface and not on glucose catabolism which was only slightly reduced. This effect on glucose transport *in vitro* is more significant, because the luminal glucose concentration *in vivo* initially exceeded plasma glucose, favouring absorption; *in vitro*, on the other hand the concentrations on either side of the tissue were initially identical.

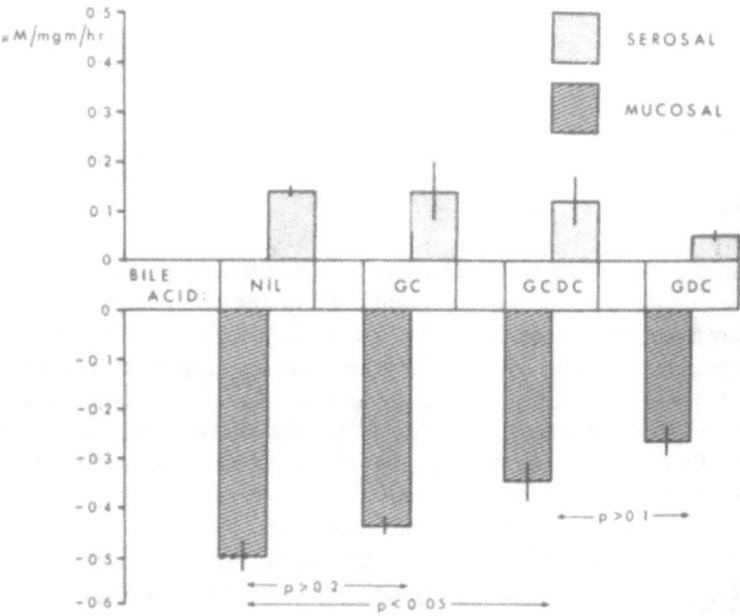

Figure 10.3 The effect of glycine-conjugated bile acids on net glucose transport across the isolated rat jejunum. Each column represents the mean ±SEM of six experiments. Positive values show glucose appearance in the serosal fluid; negative values show glucose uptake from the mucosal fluid. Data from Wingate[15]

The transmural potential difference was followed during the experiments *in vitro*. Although I have no comparable *in vivo* data, the observations are of some interest. In the jejunum (Figure 10.4), GC did not affect the glucose-stimulated potential difference, whereas both the dihydroxy conjugates depressed the glucose-stimulated PD without altogether abolishing it. In the ileum, the changes were rather different (Figure 10.5). Both the dihydroxy conjugates consistently abolished the glucose-stimulated PD, but whereas glycocholate initially appeared to do the same, but more slowly, the ileal segments with glycocholate showed a complete recovery of the glucose-stimulated PD by the end of the experiment. Whether relevant or not, the only significant absorption of bile acid in the series *in vitro* was of glycocholate by the ileal segments where the luminal concentration of GC fell by 7% during the experiments.

The results described so far do not increase our understanding of the bile acid effect. But illumination came from the distribution of lactate. The isolated intestinal mucosa takes up glucose from the mucosal fluid, of which a moiety may be translocated to the serosal fluid; of the rest, about 80% is

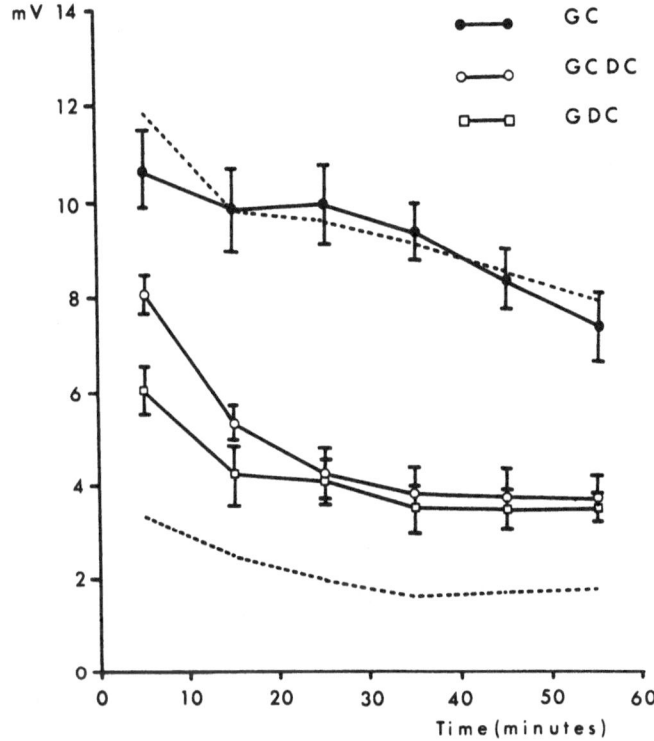

Figure 10.4 The effect of glycine-conjugated bile acids on transmural potential differences in the isolated rat jejunum. Potential difference (serosa electropositive) in millivolts on the vertical axis. Time in minutes from the start of each experiment on the horizontal axis. Each point shows the mean ±SEM of six experiments. The lower broken line shows the time course of PD change in the absence of both glucose and bile acid. The upper broken line shows the time-course of PD change in the presence of glucose but the absence of bile acid. Data from Wingate[15]

recovered as lactate[17]. Invariably, the concentration of lactate in the serosal fluid is three to four times that on the mucosal side. This distribution of lactate is not altered even when net fluid transport across the tissue is altered osmotically[7]. The effect of bile acids on the distribution in the jejunal segments was dramatic (Figure 10.6, Glycocholate, which did not reduce water transport or alter PD, did not affect the lactate distribution whereas the dihydroxy conjugates abolished the expected concentration difference.

Although lactate concentrations are illustrated in Figure 10.6, the heights of the columns are proportional to lactate production; comparison of the results with the glucose-free experiments shows that most of the lactate is derived from the added glucose. In the ileum (Figure 10.7), the situation was similar except that, as might be expected, all three bile acids abolished the concentration difference.

Since the lactate is produced in the enterocyte, and since its distribution between mucosal and serosal fluids is not normally changed by altered bulk

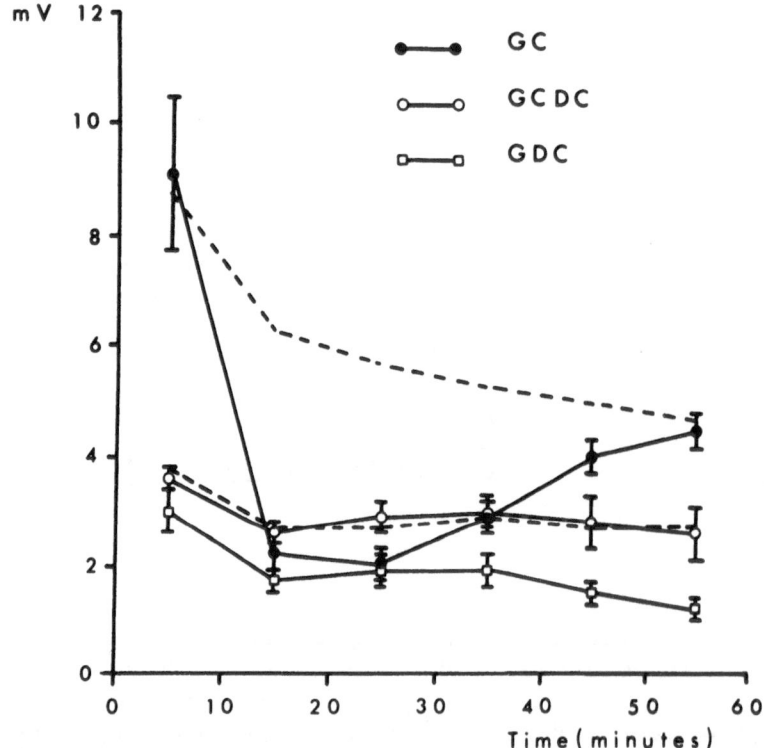

Figure 10.5 The effect of glycine-conjugated bile acids on transmural potential difference in the isolated rat ileum. For explanation of symbols, see Figure 10.3. Data from Wingate[15]

flow, the rate at which lactate diffuses out of the enterocyte must depend upon the relative permeabilities of the two faces. If this is so, then the bile acids have increased the permeability of the mucosal pole of the enterocyte. We know that the permeability of the mucosa as a whole is not increased, since increased leakiness of the tissue *in vitro* would have given increased apparent water absorption because of the effect of hydrostatic pressure.

The tentative hypothesis which results from all this runs as follows. *In vivo*, the majority of bulk flow is an isotonic stream which is independent of ion exchange, and presumably, predominantly intercellular through the gap junctions[18]. The experiments *in vitro* suggest that the effect of the bile acids is a physical effect on the mucosal face of the enterocyte, rendering them leaky, and allowing the enterocyte, or part of the enterocyte to act as a short circuit both in terms of bulk flow and electrical activity. If this is true, a cation which becomes entrained in the normal bulk flow might, under the influence of bile acids, be diverted back to the lumen when it was only halfway through the mucosal layer. Conventional isotopic unidirectional flux studies would not be able to distinguish between this particular ion, and an ion which had never become involved in a transmucosal flux, but had simply stayed in the mucosal fluid.

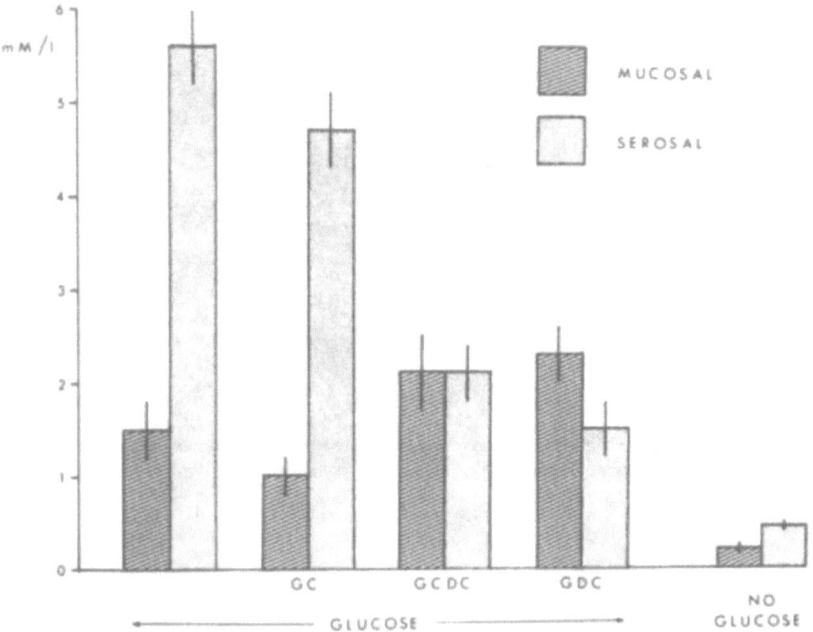

Figure 10.6 The effect of glucose and glycine-conjugated bile acids on lactate concentrations in fluids bathing isolated rat jejunum. Each column represents the mean ±SEM of six experiments and shows the lactate concentration after one hour in the mucosal or serosal fluid. Data from Wingate[15]

This interpretation is as leaky as some of the phenomena that I have described. It seems to me an open question whether my *in vitro* model is truly a valid model of the situation *in vivo* or merely happens to resemble the perfused human intestine in certain kinetic respects. I can at least claim that both show bulk flow changes in the same direction, but I cannot prove the causes for the bulk flow changes to be identical, and I suspect that they may not be so. Symposia are gatherings for the discussion of problems, and I make no apology for concluding with more questions that I posed at the beginning. Having devoted a measurable quantum of my research career to the effects of bile acids on the transport of fluid across the intestinal mucosa, I would like to know exactly how they work. I conclude leaving this problem open, and adding to it the problem of how valid experiments on bulk flow change can be carried out in model systems where these changes may be non-existent, or artefactual. It was said many years ago by the American humorist, Dorothy Parker, that 'If all the girls at the Yale prom were laid end to end, I wouldn't be surprised'. Perhaps I am saying the same thing about studies of bidirectional movements in acrylic chambers.

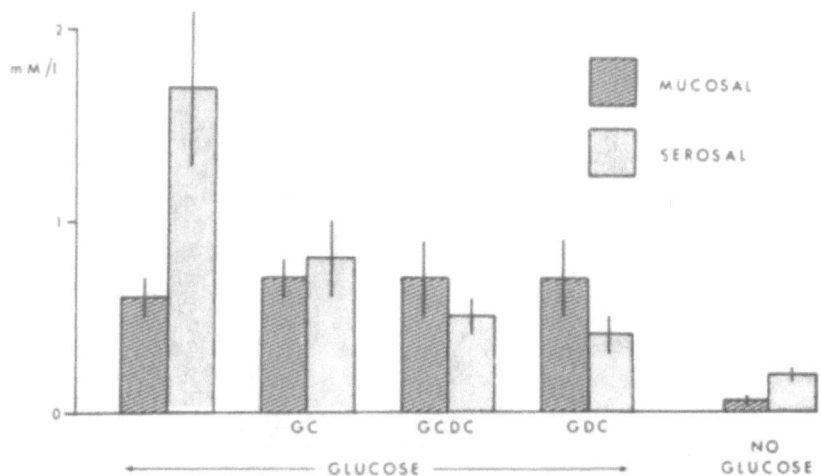

Figure 10.7 The effect of glucose and glycine-conjugated bile acids on lactate concentrations in fluids bathing isolated rat ileum. For explanation of symbols, see Figure 10.6. Data from Wingate[15]

Acknowledgements

I wish to take this opportunity of thanking Sidney Phillips and Alan Hofmann for introducing me to the bile acid problem and for their subsequent help and encouragement. It is a pleasure to be able to acknowledge the skilled assistance of Anne Dand with the animal experiments and also her expertise in the preparation of illustrations. I am indebted to the Mayo Foundation and to the Wellcome Trust for financial support at various stages of this work.

References

1. Phillips, S. F. (1972). Diarrhea: a current view of the pathophysiology. *Gastroenterology*, **63**, 495
2. Visscher, M. B., Fetcher, E. S., Carr, C. W., Gregor, H. P., Bushey, M. S. and Barker, D. E. (1944). Isotopic trace studies on the movement of water and ions between intestinal lumen and blood. *Amer. J. Physiol.*, **144**, 457

3. Fisher, R. B. and Parsons, D. S. (1949). Glucose absorption from surviving rat small intestine. *J. Physiol. Lond.*, **110**, 281.

4. Newey, H., Smyth, D. H. and Whalen, B. C. (1955). The absorption of glucose by the *in vitro* intestinal preparation. *J. Physiol. Lond.*, **129**, 1

5. Curran, P. F. (1960). Na, Cl, and water transport by rat ileum *in vitro*. *J. Gen. Physiol.*, **42**, 1137

6. Diamond, J. M. (1971). Standing gradient model of fluid transport in epithelia. *Fed. Proc.*, **30**, 6

7. Parsons, D. S. and Wingate, D. L. (1961). The effect of osmotic gradients of fluid transfer across rat intestine *in vitro*. *Biochim. Biophys. Acta*, **46**, 170

8. Reid, E. W. (1892). Preliminary report on experiments upon intestinal absorption without osmosis. *Brit. Med. J.*, **i**, 1133

9. Parsons, D. S. (1968). Methods for investigation of intestinal absorption. In: *Handbook of Physiology*, sect. 6, Alimentary Canal, C. F. Code (ed.), vol. III: Intestinal Absorption, chap. 64. p. 1177 (Washington DC: American Physiol. Society)

10. Lee, J. S. and Silverberg, J. W. (1972). Effect of cholera toxin on fluid absorption and villus lymph pressure in dog jejunal mucosa. *Gastroenterology*, **62**, 993

11. Forth, W., Rummel, W. and Glasner, H. (1966). Zur resorptionshemmenden Wirkung von Gallensauren. *Naunyn-Schmiedebergs Arch. Exp. Path. Pharmak.*, **254**, 364

12. Wingate, D. L., Phillips, S. F. and Hofmann, A. F. (1973). Effect of glycine-conjugated bile acids with and without lecithin on water and glucose absorption in perfused human jejunum. *J. Clin. Invest.*, **52**, 1230

13. Turnberg, L. A., Fordtran, J. S., Carter, N. W. and Rector, F. C. (1970). Mechanism of bicarbonate absorption and its relationship to sodium transport in the human jejunum. *J. Clin. Invest.*, **49**, 548

14. Wingate, D. L., Krag, E., Mekhjian, H. S. and Phillips, S. F., (1973). Relationships between ion and water movement in the human jejunum, ileum, and colon during perfusion with bile acids. *Clin. Sci. Mol. Med.*, **45**, 593

15. Wingate, D. L. (1974). The effect of glycine-conjugated bile acids on net transport and potential difference across isolated rat jejunum and ileum. *J. Physiol., Lond.*, **242**, 189

16. Krag, E., and Phillips, S. F. (1973). Bile acids in human ileum: effect on water, electrolyte, glucose, and bile acid absorption. (Abstract) *Gastroenterology*, **64**, 756

17. Wilson, T. H. (1954). Concentration gradients of lactate, hydrogen, and some other ions across the intestine *in vitro*. *Biochem. J.*, **56**, 512

18. Diamond, J. M. (1974). Tight and leaky junctions of epithelia; a perspective on kisses in the dark. *Fed. Proc.*, **33**, 2220

10

Discussion Paper on

Effect of Bile Salts on Electrolyte Transport in the Rat Colon

H. J. Binder

Department of Internal Medicine, Yale University

Bile salts alter fluid and electrolyte transport in all parts of the gastro-intestinal tract[1,2]. We have performed a series of experiments designed to evaluate the mechanism by which bile salts affect colonic ion transport. The following observations have been obtained in the study of taurochenodeoxy-cholic acid (TCDC) in the rat colon:

(1) 2 mM TCDC, but not 2 mM taurocholic acid, increases I_{sc}, decreases J_{net}^{Na}, reduces J_{net}^{Cl} to zero and increases the residual ion flux, which probably represents HCO_3^- secretion.

(2) The increase in I_{sc} requires the presence of both HCO_3^- and Cl^-.

(3) These changes are qualitatively similar to those produced by theophylline and dibutyryl-cAMP in the rat colon and by cholera enterotoxin in the rabbit ileum.

(4) TCDC increases mucosal cyclic AMP levels.

Although bile salts increase mucosal permeability *in vivo* and increase tissue conductance *in vitro*, we propose that bile salt-induced changes in fluid and electrolyte movement in the colon is secondary to active anion secretion, which is most likely controlled by mucosal cyclic AMP concentrations.

References

1. Binder, H. J. and Rawlins, C. L. (1973). Effect of conjugated dihydroxy bile salts on electrolyte transport in rat colon. *J. Clin. Invest.*, 52, 1460
2. Binder, H. J., Filburn, C. and Volpe, B. T. (1975). Bile salt alteration of colonic electrolyte transport: Role of cyclic adenosine monophosphate. *Gastroenterology*, 68, 503

Discussion 10

Love: Dr Nell, I am surprised at the movement of [^{51}Cr]EDTA that you described across the mucosa. We have used this substance in whole bowel perfusions and have found it to be the best non-absorbable marker — 100 $\pm$ 1% recovery! Can you comment?

Nell: The permeation of [^{51}Cr]EDTA is very low in the control case. The luminal level after intravenous administration lies below 1% after one hour.

Levin: Did you measure the PD *in vivo*? This would enable you to get a better estimate of how ions would move into the lumen of the intestine from the plasma.

Nell: We did not measure PD *in vivo*, but we did measure it *in vitro* in the presence of glucose, and we found a decrease.

Parsons: I should like to suggest to Dr Wingate that his results *in vitro* confirm the view of Dr Nell that certain bile acids increase the leakiness of the zonula occludens. *In vitro*, with no capillary blood flow in the mucosa, the fluid and solutes dumped into the intercellular space may have difficulty in passing forward across the muscle and serosal layers. If bile acids increase the conductance of the zonula occludens, Dr Wingate's findings with respect to fluid, lactate and glucose can be explained without recourse to invoking additional actions on the brush border membranes.

Wingate: I agree that intercellular permeability may be increased by dihydroxy bile acids, but this does not, *per se*, explain the altered *direction* of bulk flow. Altered permeability is non-vectorial!

Robinson: Do you think there is any change in the permeability of the tight junctions to glucose under the influence of bile acids?

Wingate: This cannot be excluded, but I have no evidence of a permeability increase in the tight junctions.

Munck: The role of the paracellular pathway in passage across the epithelium of the small intestine is indicated by data on the serosa–to–mucosa fluxes of the short-circuited rat mid small intestine mounted according to the technique described by Ussing and Zerahn (Munck, *J. Physiol. Lond.*, **223**, 699, 1972; Munck and Schultz, *J. Memb. Biol.*, **16**, 174, 1974). Measured in the presence of 28 mM D-glucose using [^{14}C]PEG-4000, [^{3}H]mannitol, [^{14}C]L-lysine, and ^{22}Na, the relative permeabilities of these substances were: 1 : 3 : 5 : 15, that of [^{14}C]PEG-4000 being 6.4 $\pm$ 1.2 $\cdot$ 10^{-3} cm/h. In this connection, it should be pointed out that the presence of glucose enhances the apparent permeability of PEG-4000 by a factor of approximately 10 whereas the fluxes of the other substances are increased only by a factor of about 2.

May I also point out to Dr Wingate that the distribution between the mucosal and serosal bathing media of endogenous lactic acid is very much dependent on the experimental conditions? This can be illustrated by the following observations (Munck and Schultz, unpublished observations). Using rat mid small intestine mounted in Ussing chambers bathed on each side with 5 ml Krebs phosphate buffer containing 28 mM D-glucose, the time-course and distribution of lactate was measured. The ratio of distribution (m/s) between mucosa (m) and serosa (s) bathing media was, with bilateral oxygenation, 1.5 ± 0.2 ($n = 8$) in the open-circuit state and 2.0 ± 0.2 ($n = 9$) in the short-circuit state. With mucosal side oxygenation maintained but with gassing with 100% N_2 on the serosal side, the ratio of distribution was 0.8 ± 0.1 ($n = 4$) both in the open and in the short-circuit state.

Wright: I wish to clarify the importance of the paracellular pathway in transport across epithelia. The most important case is for small monovalent ions where in 'leaky' epithelia the tight junctions are the major pathway, the reason being that the permeability of the cellular pathway is so low. Similar considerations apply to molecules such as sucrose and inulin. However, with molecules, like water, which permeate across cellular membranes very readily, the paracellular pathway is of minor importance. We have estimated that the flow of water across the tight junction is insignificant mainly because: (a) the area of the junctional complex is small in relation to the total membrane area; (b) the solute reflection coefficients (σ's) for the paracellular pathway are likely to be close to zero; and (c) the water permeability of the cell membranes is very high. Furthermore, it is clear that hydrostatic pressures in the physiological range produce insignificant volume flows across epithelia compared to those produced by osmotic gradients. Thus I feel that hydrostatic gradients are not the driving force for water flow across the intestine and also that the tight junctions are not the major route for water flow. However, the lateral intercellular spaces do provide a common pathway for all molecules crossing the epithelium, and diffusion along these spaces may provide the rate-limiting step in transport across the epithelium (Smulders *et al.*, *J. Memb. Biol.*, **5**, 297, 1972; Wright *et al.*, *J. Memb. Biol.*, **7**, 198, 1972; Bindslev *et al.*, *J. Memb. Biol.*, **19**, 357, 1974; and Wiedner and Wright, *Pflügers Arch.*, **358**, 27, 1975).

Caspary: Dr Binder reported an increase in short-circuit current and PD induced by bile acids, but Dr Wingate, taking measurements after 5 minutes, reported a decrease in glucose-induced PD. We observed that taurocholate did not induce a PD increase in the rat jejunum, but in the ileum a transient increase in PD lasting for up to 2 minutes was observed; thereafter, the D-glucose-induced PD declined to below baseline-levels. I would therefore like to know whether Dr Wingate ever did observe an initial PD increase and whether Dr Binder observed a persistent rise in PD and short-circuit current.

Wingate: I have no complete data on the effects of bile acids on PD *in vitro* earlier than 5 minutes after exposure to bile acids, but occasionally the decrease was observed after about 3 minutes. No evidence of an initial rise was seen.

Binder: We observed the increase in PD for approximately 40 minutes. It is important to recognise that, although bile salts increase PD *in vitro*, they also increase conductance. Therefore, I do not think that there is any significant discrepancy between the different results.

Alvarado: I should like to ask the bile-salt gentlemen what kind of controls they have to show that the effects observed are not simply due to the detergent action of the compound. Bile salts are used to solubilise membranes. Have any measurements been made of the possible appearance of brush-border enzymes in the soluble fraction at the end of the experiments?

Dowling: I think the best evidence comes from the demonstration that the inhibitory or stimulatory effects of bile acids on net fluxes are rapidly reversible when they are removed from the perfusion medium. This would suggest that the bile acids have not had a detergent effect on the intestinal epithelial membranes.

Wingate: It seems unlikely that bile acids are disrupting cell membranes. During bile acid perfusion, there is no evidence of the appearance of phospholipid in the perfusate. Moreover, morphology appears to be intact. The best evidence for intact cells is the rapid reversibility of bile-acid-induced secretion *in vivo* which occurs within 30 minutes.

Dowling: Dr Nell and Dr Wingate's results clearly show that bile acids may *inhibit* water and electrolyte absorption from the colon. But under certain circumstances, it seems that dihydroxy bile acids can have the opposite effect and may actually *enhance* absorption. To illustrate this, I should like to show some results obtained by my colleague, Dr Chadwick, which he presented almost one year ago at the Third International Bile Acid Meeting in Freiburg (Chadwick, Elias, Bell and Dowling, in *Bile Acids in Human Diseases*, edited by Back, Hackenschmidt and Matern, 1975, in press). When rat colon was perfused *in vivo* using a recirculation perfusion system with a Krebs–Ringer phosphate buffer containing glucose (21 mM), a non-absorbable marker polyethylene glycol (mol.wt. 4000) and ^{14}C-labelled oxalate, there was net absorption of both water and oxalate. In keeping with Dr Wingate and Dr Nell's findings, when glycodeoxycholate was added to the perfusion medium (10 mM), net water movement changed from absorption to secretion but paradoxically, the addition of bile acids to the perfusion *enhanced* oxalate absorption/unit length of colon. Since these results in a closed colonic circuit perfused with a watery bile acid solution may be quite different from the physiological effects of bile acids in the large bowel containing normal colonic contents, we turned to another experimental model, that of the restrained Rhesus monkey with normal intestinal contents. A 1 mM solution of ^{14}C-labelled oxalate was infused continuously into the colon through a caecal catheter for 12–14 days. During a baseline period of 3–5 days, steady-state conditions were reached when 5–10% of the infused oxalate was absorbed and excreted in the urine. But when chenodeoxycholate was added to the colonic infusate, in quantities (100 mg/day) calculated to simulate the amount of bile acids which would 'spill' into the colon in the absence of a normal active transport system in the ileum, oxalate absorption increased by 200 and in some cases 400% promptly returning to baseline values when the bile acid infusion stopped.

These results in both rats and monkeys are consistent with Dr Nell's hypothesis that the effect of bile acids on net ion movement in the intestine depends on the molecular size of the substrate and that while dihydroxy bile acids inhibit water and electrolyte absorption, they increase the absorption of small molecular size substances such as oxalate. This stimulatory effect of bile acids on intestinal oxalate absorption has recently been confirmed by Dr Binder and his colleagues (Dobbins and Binder, *Gastroenterology*, **68** A27, 1975 (Abstract)).

Caspary: We have measured oxalate absorption in the colon and ileum in the presence of bile acids and cholestyramine; 10 mM taurocholate markedly increased oxalate absorption and extracellular space (PEG 4000 and [^{14}C]inulin). Cholestyramine normalised the increased oxalate absorption induced by bile acids, but had no effect itself on oxalate absorption. It therefore seems to me that the beneficial effect of cholestyramine when reducing hyperoxaluria following ileal resection may be mediated by the bile acid-binding property of cholestyramine. The latter would thus reduce the stimulation of oxalate absorption by bile acids, rather than bind to the oxalate itself. Administration of cholestryamine *in vivo* did not reduce oxalate absorption following administration of [^{14}C]oxalate.

Dowling: I am interested to hear that you too have found increased oxalate absorption when bile acids are added to the perfusate. It would seem therefore, that several groups have confirmed Dr Chadwick's original observation. As regards the question of cholestyramine, it binds oxalate almost as well as bile acids so whether the reduction in oxalate absorption and resultant hyperoxaluria is due to binding of bile acids or of oxalate itself to cholestyramine is, as yet, an open question.

Forth: Dr Binder, you mentioned the similarity between the effect of taurochenodeoxycholate and that of cholera toxin on the rat colon. Could you please comment on the time-courses of the effects?

Binder: The effect of bile acids on the electrical parameters can be seen within 5 minutes. As you know, the effect of cholera enterotoxin is delayed for 60–120 minutes. However, this different time response does not constitute evidence that the action of bile salts is different from that of cholera enterotoxin. *E. coli* enterotoxin is generally believed to stimulate adenyl cyclase and resembles cholera enterotoxin in many ways. However, the time of onset of *E. coli* enterotoxin is also significantly shorter than that of the toxin of cholera.

Nell: I have a number of comments on Dr Binder's presentation. Although he did not measure the movement of different anions, he concludes that there was a bicarbonate secretion from his values of the residual current. Measurement of residual currents is subject to considerable methodological error. Furthermore, Dr Binder noted a striking resemblance between the effects of cholera toxin and those of bile acids. In fact, with respect to the cholera toxin, anion secretion was evidently shown, though in the case of bile acids, this secretion was not clear-cut. Finally, cholera toxin increased the electrical resistance of the epithelium, whereas bile acids reduced it. We observed in everted sacs of rat colon mucosa no net transfer of water and sodium from the serosal to the mucosal side in the presence of deoxycholate, unless a hydrostatic pressure was imposed on the serosal side.

Binder: Thank you. Additional studies are required to determine the relative contributions of active secretion and altered permeability in the overall production of fluid under the influence of bile salts.

Simmonds: Can the speakers reconcile the apparent molecular specificity of the bile acid action — that is to say, that dihydroxy but not trihydroxy conjugates are effective — with the increasing effects at concentrations above the critical micellar concentration? This suggests a solubilisation phenomenon with elution of a surface component. But why should this be specific for the dihydroxy acid micelles?

Binder: Trihydroxy bile acids are less effective than dihydroxy bile acids. If the concentration of taurocholic acid is increased, then this may become as effective a secretogogue as taurochenodeoxycholic acid. I am not certain that the critical micellar concentration (CMC) is the determining factor, since Dr Wingate has shown that the addition of lecithin to form mixed micelles (and which also lowers the CMC) results in a marked decrease in the secretory effect of the bile acids.

Love: As a concluding remark, may I be permitted to muse whether bile acids are relevant to real life bowel function? The secretory effect seems to be abolished by the presence of phospholipid and micelles which are normally also present in the normal intestine. Pure free bile acids are not!

11
Sodium Transport by the Newborn Pig Intestine: Functional Changes During the First Few Days of Postnatal Life

M. W. SMITH

A.R.C. Institute of Animal Physiology, Babraham, Cambridge

INTRODUCTION

The small intestine of the newborn pig shares with some other mammals the ability to absorb different immune proteins from ingested colostrum. Much of the ingested protein subsequently appears in the blood in a degraded form, but sufficient is transported intact to provide the pig with an initial passive immunity to disease. The piglet is entirely dependent upon intestinal transport in this respect, placental transfer of immunoglobulins being virtually nonexistent.

Intestinal absorption of proteins, which takes place along the whole length of the small intestine, is accompanied by pronounced changes in mucosal morphology. Much effort has been invested recently in deciding how these changes might relate to the way proteins are absorbed by and degraded within the mucosal cell. Three unusual types of vesicle exist in the intestinal mucosa of the newborn pig. First there are the tubular vesicles in the apical cytoplasm of the cell. These make occasional contact with the intestinal lumen through the formation of apical pits across the terminal web. Present at birth, they increase in size and number during the process of protein absorption. They are thought to be responsible both for the initial selective binding of immunoglobulins and for their subsequent entry into the mucosa. The second type of vesicle, the coated vesicle, is thought to be formed from the tubular vesicle. They can apparently fuse with the lateral membranes of the mucosal cell, expelling their contents into the intercellular space by a process of reverse pinocytosis[1]. The third type of vesicle is smooth-walled and far larger than the two previous types. It probably exists as an extension to the tubular vesicle. Expanding considerably during periods of protein absorption, these vesicles can come to measure up to 30 μm in length. The presence of a vesicle approaching these dimensions in a cell roughly the same size inevitably leads to physical distortion. There is a lengthening of the cell itself and often a displacement of the nucleus towards the brush-border membrane. The function of this type of vesicle remains unclear; it could be involved in the transport of protein across the cell, but it also probably acts as a site for the lysosomal degradation of exogenous protein.

One might imagine that the gross morphological changes seen to take place within the mucosal epithelium might have a generally adverse effect on normal intestinal function. The present work describes how the intestine copes with the absorption of other substances at a time when its main preoccupation is with the transport of proteins. During the course of this work it soon became apparent that colonic function was also being modified during the immediate postnatal period. These findings were investigated further to assess the efficiency of the colon in compensating for an impaired absorptive function in the small intestine. The measurement of sodium transport was the chosen parameter for study in these experiments. Part of the work also involved examination of the changing ability of the brush-border membrane to increase its permeability to sodium in the presence of various activity transported non-electrolytes.

TRANSPORT OF SODIUM ACROSS THE SMALL INTESTINE OF THE NEWBORN PIG

The transport of sodium across the ileum of piglets taken at birth or after a short period of suckling is shown in Table 11.1. Bidirectional fluxes were measured under short-circuit conditions using a conventional Ussing-type chamber. Both the short-circuit current and open-circuit voltage remained stable in these preparations for up to 2 hours making them particularly suitable for this type of *in vitro* work[2]. The net mucosal-to-serosal flux of sodium across the ileum of the newborn pig corresponded to that calculated from the

Table 11.1 Bidirectional sodium fluxes determined across short-circuited preparations of pig ileum maintained at 37 °C in Krebs–Henseleit bicarbonate medium gassed with 95% O_2 + 5% CO_2

Treatment	Sodium flux (μEq cm^{-2} h^{-1})			scc	Conductance (mmho cm^2)
	Φ_{ms}	Φ_{sm}	Φ_{Net}		
Newborn unsuckled (31)	13.5 ± 1.5	9.4 ± 1.0	4.1 ± 1.2	3.7 ± 1.0	16.7 ± 1.6
Newborn suckled 5 h (15)	9.1 ± 0.9	7.5 ± 0.6	1.6 ± 0.4	2.0 ± 0.8	12.0 ± 1.2

Values give means $\pm$ SEM (number of observations in parentheses)

short-circuit current, assuming that current to be carried by a monovalent cation. Both the mucosal-to-serosal and serosal-to-mucosal flux of sodium was reduced by suckling. The conductance also fell significantly. The net flux of sodium to the serosa was reduced by approximately the same amount as the short-circuit current. This equivalence between short-circuit current and net sodium flux is not, however, maintained under all experimental conditions. Situations where divergences occur are dealt with in a later section.

These initial experiments establish the fact that the mucosa is unable to transport sodium with the same efficiency following a period of protein absorption. Separate experiments showed this inhibition to take place without any significant change in ATP/AMP ratios (2.35 $\pm$ 0.41 and 2.11 $\pm$ 0.17 for mucosa taken from newborn and suckled piglets respectively[1]). There is no evidence to suggest that suckling changes either the total amount of adenine nucleotides present or the quantity of ATP available within the cell. Further experiments were undertaken to see whether the fall in net sodium transport could be related to changes occurring within the microvillar membrane following a period of endocytosis. Endocytosis is used here to describe the mechanism whereby tubular vesicles undergo temporary fusion with the microvillar membrane. It does not necessarily imply that any part of the microvillar membrane is actually lost to the interior of the cell. The experiments to be described fall into three categories, experiments on sodium uptake, experiments to measure the effects of non-electrolytes on microvillar membrane function and protection experiments using purified brush-border membranes.

Measurements of sodium uptake

The technique for measung sodium uptake into intestinal mucosal tissue, used *in vitro* over short periods of time, was similar to that described originally[3]. The total isotopic uptake of sodium was measured and corrected for extracellular contamination using a second, non-penetrating, radioactively labelled substance in the incubation fluid. Inulin normally serves this purpose[3,4], but in the pig ileum, where endocytosis may be taking place, one has to use a much larger space marker to avoid anomalous results. Mildly sonicated liposomes, of average diameter 1 to 2 μm, labelled with radioactive cholesterol, were found to be satisfactory markers of extracellular space in this tissue. The rapid uptake of sodium by pig ileum taken at birth or after suckling, corrected for liposome space, is shown in Figure 11.1. Uptake was linear with time for at least 1 minute for the newborn and up to 3 minutes for ileum taken from suckled animals. Extrapolation of these lines to zero time gave an apparent sodium uptake of 0.1 μEq cm^{-2} in both cases. This is probably an artefact due to the presence of a few very large liposomes in the incubation medium. The corrected uptake by ileum from newborn pigs was

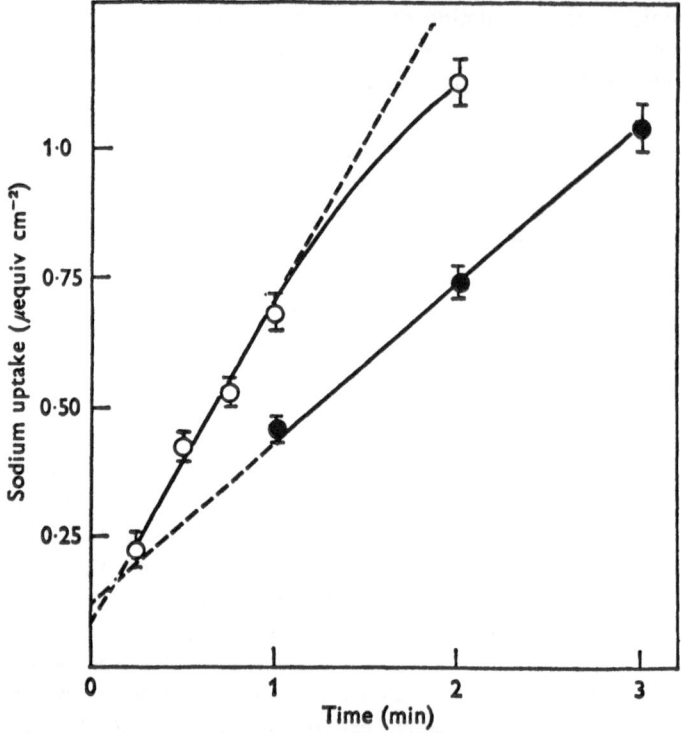

Figure 11.1 Sodium uptake by pig ileum. [³H]cholesterol-labelled liposomes were used to correct total radioactive sodium recovered, for extracellular space. (O), uptake of sodium by newborn pig ileum; (●), sodium uptake by pig ileum taken after a 24-hour period of suckling. Values given means ±SE of from eight to sixteen determinations.

about twice that measured in the suckled animal (0.63 as opposed to 0.33 μEq cm^{-2} min^{-1}). This provided the first piece of evidence that the permeability of the microvillar membrane to sodium, measured in the absence of glucose, was being inhibited by the previous transport of protein.

Sodium-glucose interactions in the newborn pig ileum

The presence of an actively transported non-electrolyte such as glucose in contact with the mucosa stimulates sodium transport, in part at least, by increasing the ease with which sodium enters the cell[5]. Measuring the kinetics of glucose-dependent increases in short-circuit current gives a useful, though indirect, measure of the efficiency with which the sodium—glucose interaction takes place within the microvillar membrane. The results of some of these experiments, carried out on ileum taken from newborn and suckled animals, is shown in Figure 11.2a. The interaction of glucose with the microvillar membrane appeared to follow Michaelis—Menten kinetics in both cases. The

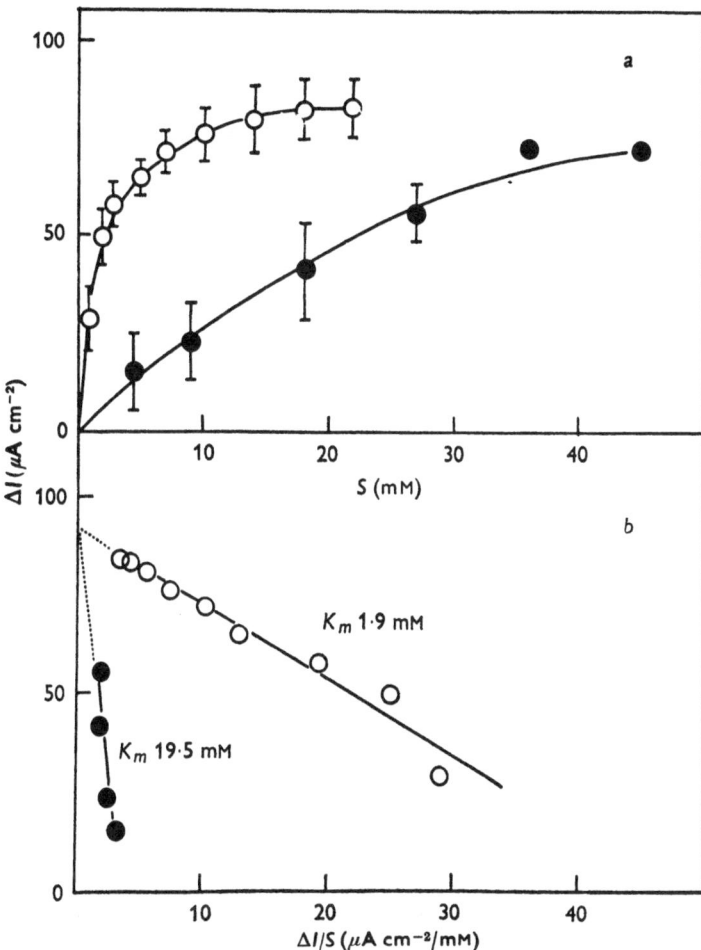

Figure 11.2 Glucose dependence of short-circuit current in the newborn and suckled pig intestine. (a) ΔI gives the increase in short-circuit current when different concentrations of glucose (S) are presented to the mucosal surface. Intestines were from newborn unsuckled (—O—) or suckled (—●—) pigs. Increases in current were measured not later than 60 seconds following the addition of glucose. Values give means $\pm$SE of estimates carried out in three to six pigs; (b), Hofstee plot of values shown in (a). The maximal glucose effect is given by the intercept on the ordinate and the apparent K_m by the negative slope. Signs and symbols as for (a)

data have been redrawn in the form of a Hofstee plot in Figure 11.2b. The apparent affinity constant of glucose for its ternary carrier is 1.9 mM for the newborn and 19.5 mM for ileum taken from suckled pigs. The maximal response elicited by glucose was the same in both cases (about 85 μA cm^{-2}). This provides the first piece of evidence that specific (that is, a glucose interaction with a membrane component) as well as non-specific (glucose-independent sodium uptake) changes take place in the microvillar membrane as a result of suckling.

Glucose and phlorizin protected sulphydryl groups in microvillar membrane proteins

p-Chloromercuriphenyl sulphonic acid has recently been shown to inhibit the ability of galactose to interact with the intestinal mucosa of rabbits[6]. This effect is also seen when measuring the influx of phenylalanine in rabbit intestine. Kinetic analysis would suggest that the main effect of this compound

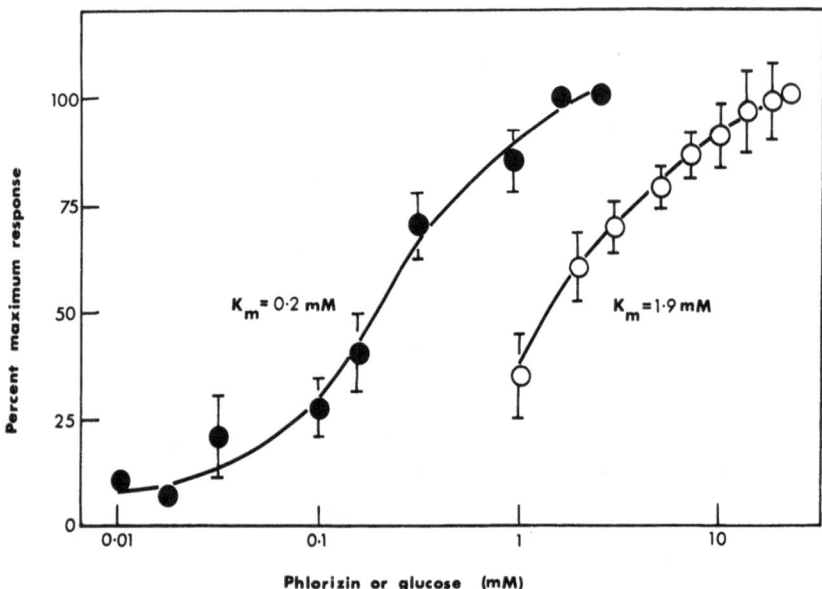

Figure 11.3 Effect of glucose and phlorizin on the short-circuit current of newborn pig intestine. The intestine was mounted in an Ussing chamber in Krebs bicarbonate saline, gassed with 95% O_2 + 5% CO_2, containing 5 mM glucose, at a temperature of 37 °C. This medium was replaced with one containing no glucose and the short-circuit current allowed to decay to a constant level. Different amounts of glucose were then added in small volume to the mucosal side of the preparation; increments in short-circuit current were measured and represented as a percentage of the maximal response to glucose (—O—). In a second series of experiments different concentrations of phlorizin and 5 mM glucose were added simultaneously to the intestine bathed in glucose-free solution. The increment in short-circuit current was then compared with that found using 5 mM glucose. Results are expressed as percent inhbition of a mean response to 5 mM glucose (—●—). Each point gives the mean ±SE of nine to twelve observations

is to inhibit the binding of sodium to the ternary carrier within the microvillar membrane. *p*-Chloromercuriphenyl sulphonic acid also modifies the ability of glucose to increase the short-circuit current in the newborn pig ileum[7]. Experiments were therefore undertaken to investigate the long-term binding of radioactively labelled *p*-chloromercuriphenyl sulphonic acid to microvillar membranes prepared from the ileum of newborn and suckled pigs to see, first, whether glucose or phlorizin could inhibit this binding and, second, if this did occur, what effect suckling would have on this protection.

Initial experiments to determine the concentrations of glucose and phlorizin to be used on the binding experiments are shown in Figure 11.3. The concentration of glucose to produce half-maximal response, that is half the maxi-

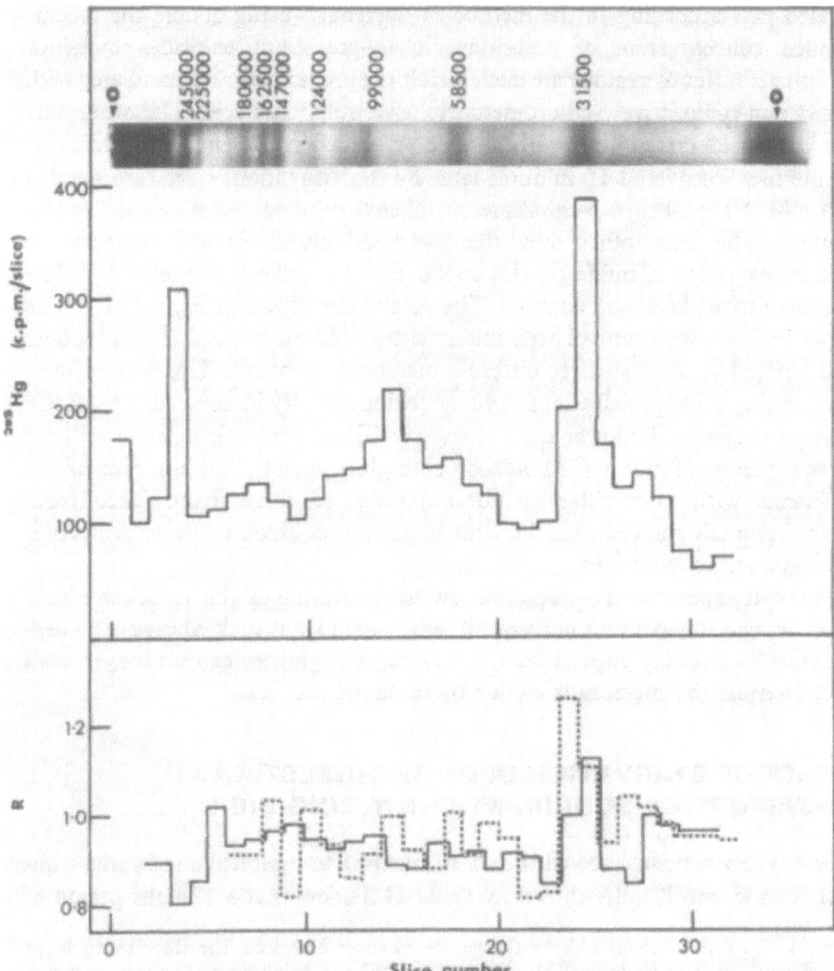

Figure 11.4 Polyacrylamide-gel electrophoresis of pig intestinal brush-border membranes. Purified brush borders, previously incubated in ^{203}Hg-labelled p-chloromercuriphenyl sulphonic acid, were dissolved in 3% w/v sodium lauryl sulphate for electrophoresis. Bands are numbered according to their estimated mass in daltons calculated from their respective R_f values in relation to cytochrome c (C). The origin (O) is marked to the left of the gel. The upper trace shows the distribution of ^{203}Hg in a control experiment. The lower trace shows the ratio of counts for glucose or phlorizin-treated membranes to control membranes. Values of R represent, in each case, the mean of three experiments using either 2.5 mM glucose (————) or 0.2 mM phlorizin (- -) to protect proteins against the initial binding of non-radioactive p-chloromercuriphenyl sulphonic acid

mal increase in short-circuit current, was 1.9 mM; the concentration of phlorizin to cause a 56% inhibition of a response to 5 mM glucose was 0.2 mM. It was decided, on the basis of these results, to use 2.5 mM glucose or 0.2 mM phlorizin for the subsequent binding experiments.

Microvillar membranes were prepared from the ileum of newborn and suckled pigs according to the method of Porteous[8], using double the recommended concentration of potassium citrate–potassium chloride–potassium phosphate buffer to agglutinate nuclei. Half the preparation was incubated with 5 mM non-radioactive p-chloromercuriphenyl sulphonic acid. The other half was treated identically but with glucose or phlorizin present. The microvilli membranes, recovered 15 minutes later by centrifugation, were resuspended in 5 mM ^{203}Hg-labelled p-chloromercuriphenyl sulphonic acid and left for 60 minutes. The membranes were then washed, solubilized and subjected to preparative polyacrilamide-gel electrophoresis as described previously[9,10]. The gels were then sliced and counted. The results are shown in Figure 11.4. The upper trace shows a control experiment with p-chloromercuriphenyl sulphonic acid binding to at least three different membrane proteins. This is in spite of the fact that these preparations were incubated initially in non-radioactive sulphydryl reagent. The lower trace shows significant protection of one of these three proteins, of mol. wt. 31 500, by both glucose and phlorizin. Similar experiments with microvillar membranes prepared from ileum taken from suckled animals showed a similar control pattern of binding but no protection with glucose or phlorizin.

Previous experiments showed this low concentration of glucose to have little effect on the short-circuit current of ileum taken from suckled pigs. The present results strongly suggest that this is because glucose can no longer bind effectively to the membrane under these circumstances.

EFFECT OF STARVATION UPON THE INTESTINAL TRANSPORT OF SODIUM BY THE YOUNG PIG

Previous experiments showed the act of suckling to inhibit the intestinal transport of sodium. Results shown in Table 11.2 show that a 12-hour period of

Table 11.2 Bidirectional sodium fluxes across short-circuited intestines taken from pigs during the first 10 days of life. Piglets were taken straight from the sow (suckled) or after a 12-hour period of starvation (suckled–starved).

| Age of pig | Sodium flux (μEq cm^{-2} h^{-1}) | | | | | |
| | Suckled | | | Suckled–starved | | |
	Φ_{ms}	Φ_{sm}	Φ_{net}	Φ_{ms}	Φ_{sm}	Φ_{net}
5–24 hours	8.0 ± 0.8	5.8 ± 0.8	2.2 ± 0.9	16.5 ± 0.8	10.7 ± 0.6	5.8 ± 0.5
5 days	4.0 ± 0.3	2.9 ± 0.2	1.1 ± 0.2	14.8 ± 0.7	7.4 ± 0.5	7.4 ± 0.5
10 days	9.0 ± 0.3	4.3 ± 0.2	4.7 ± 0.2	21.7 ± 0.8	10.5 ± 0.7	11.2 ± 0.7

Values give means ± SE of from 23–60 determinations of four to twelve piglets.

starvation, following suckling, will restore the capacity of the intestine to transport sodium to levels approaching, or even exceeding, those measured in the newborn. Both the mucosal-to-serosal and the serosal-to-mucosal flux of sodium is doubled following overnight starvation, the net transport of sodium to the serosal side being increased by a factor of three. This applies to all pigs tested from 1 to 10 days of age.

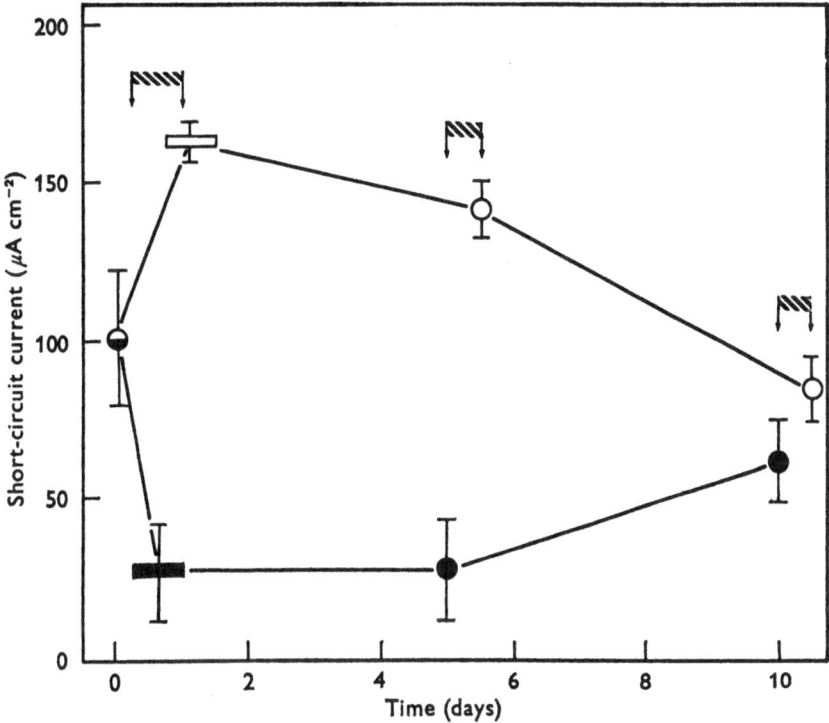

Figure 11.5 Short-circuit current of pig ileum taken from pigs during the first 10 days of postnatal life. Piglets were either taken straight from the sow (filled symbols) or kept apart from the sow for 12 hours before use (open symbols). The cross-hatched areas show the times during which piglets were denied access to the sow. Values give means ±SE of from 23–60 determinations on four to twelve piglets

The short-circuit current of these intestinal preparations also responds to starvation. Figure 10.5 shows the current to be consistently lower in the suckled animals. Starvation for 12 hours causes the current to increase significantly using the 1 and 5-day-old, but not the 10-day old pigs. The failure of the current to increase in 10-day old animals at a time when the net flux of sodium is increasing by a factor of two (Table 11.2), shows the first major discrepancy between measured short-circuit current and net sodium transport.

The response of the short-circuit current to stimulation by glucose also returns to normal following a period of starvation. The kinetics of the glucose response, determined on the ileum of a 1-day old suckled pig following a 12-hour period of starvation, is compared with that of the newborn pig in Figure

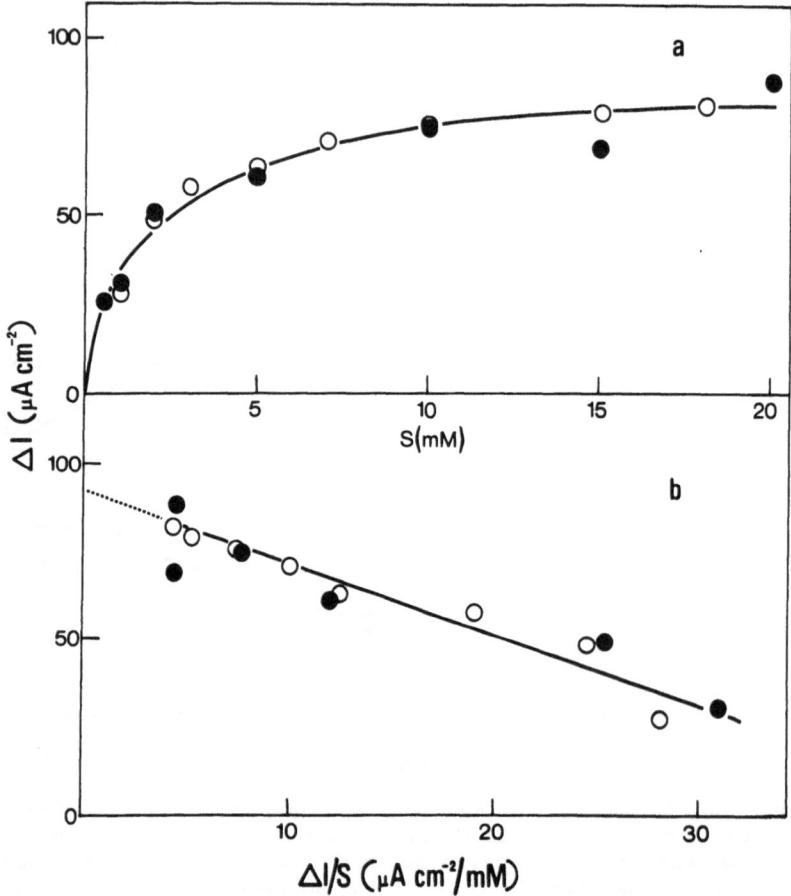

Figure 11.6 Glucose dependence of short-circuit current in newborn pig intestines and in intestines taken from 1-day old suckled pigs following a 12-hour period of starvation. (a), ΔI gives the increase in short-circuit current when different concentrations of glucose (S) are presented to the mucosal surface. Intestines were from newborn unsuckled (—O—) or 1-day old suckled pigs following a 12-hour period of starvation (—●—). Values give means of estimates carried out on six pigs; (b), Hofstee plot of values shown in (a)

11.6a. The substrate dependency of the effect follows Michaelis–Menten kinetics in both cases with one line fitting both sets of values. A Hofstee plot of these values (Figure 11.6b) shows identical K_m and V_{max} values for newborn and suckled–starved intestines.

Endocytosis in other cells is said to involve a loss of plasma membrane to the interior without loss of membrane carriers[11]. It is as if the carriers were anchored in an otherwise mobile membrane. The maintenance of a constant maximal effect for glucose on ileum taken from newborn, from suckled and from suckled–starved intestines would agree with such a concept. The lowered affinity for glucose in the suckled intestine could reflect some condensation of membrane components following a period of endocytosis. The subsequent recovery on starvation may be due to a replenishment of membrane surface or to replacement of specific components within that membrane.

The quick recovery of intestinal function following food deprivation might also have some importance to the overall metabolism of the animal, though the minimal time of starvation needed to produce these effects has yet to be determined. The colon plays a more obvious role in compensating for a reduced sodium absorption in the small intestine. This is dealt with in the following section.

Sodium transport in the helicoidal colon of the newborn pig

The helicoidal colon of the pig consists of a proximal part folded into four complete turns followed by a further 3.5 turns formed within the circumference of the more proximal loops. The average length at birth is 75 cm (cf. small intestine with an initial length of about 400 cm). Both the colon and the small intestine increase in length during the first few days of postnatal life, the colon of the 1-day pig measuring 100 cm and the small intestine growing at a rate of about 0.8 cm/hour over the first 10 days of postnatal life.

Pieces of colon were taken at the end of the first outer loop (proximal colon), and at the end of the last complete inner loop (distal colon). The ability of these tissues to transfer sodium in the presence of 5.5 mM glucose is shown in Table 11.3. The net flux of sodium in newborn proximal and distal colon is similar (about 4 μEq cm^{-2} h^{-1}) and equal to that found in the newborn pig ileum (4.1 μEq cm^{-2} h^{-1}). The conductance of the colon is, however, only about one-third that of the newborn pig small intestine (5 vs. 16.7 mmho cm^{-2}). This is reflected in the smaller backflux of sodium in the colon (3 vs. 9.5 μEq cm^{-2} h^{-1} for the ileum).

Table 11.3 Unidirectional Na$^+$ fluxes across short-circuited preparations of pig colon taken at birth or after a 24-hour period of suckling

| | Na$^+$ transport (μEq cm^{-2} h^{-1}) | | |
	influx	efflux	net flux
Newborn proximal	7.06 ± 0.60	3.24 ± 0.37	3.82
1-day old proximal	12.0 ± 0.75	4.14 ± 3.36	7.86
Newborn distal	7.20 ± 1.09	3.10 ± 0.35	4.10
1-day old distal	11.9 ± 0.97	3.50 ± 1.26	8.40

The effect of suckling is to *double* the net absorption of sodium by the colon, the exact opposite to that found in the ileum, where the flux is halved. This increase in sodium transport following a period of suckling, which is seen with both proximal and distal colon, is accompanied by a modest increase in tissue conductance, from about 5 to 8 mmho cm^2. The short-circuit current, which remains stable for both proximal and distal colon throughout these measurements, only accounts for about half the net transport of sodium[12]. The non-equivalence between current and sodium transport is discussed more fully in a later section.

Sections of pig colon were next examined at birth and after a 1-day period of suckling to see whether the increased sodium transport could be associated with any change in mucosal structure. The cellular structure of the proxin.al colon taken at birth appeared normal, while that taken 24 hours later showed numerous large vesicles present in the apical cytoplasm of cells situated at the tips of the mucosal folds. These vesicles were shown histochemically to contain fat. Tests for the presence of protein proved negative. The distal colon showed none of these changes in mucosal morphology.

Glucose and methionine induced increases in short-circuit current measured across newborn pig colon

Pieces of newborn proximal and distal colon were incubated in Ussing chambers in the presence of 5.5 mM glucose. The fluid bathing the mucosa was then replaced by an identical one, but containing no glucose. The short-circuit current fell for both the proximal and distal colon. Adding 5 mM glucose to the mucosal side of these preparations caused a rapid increase in current for both the proximal and the distal colon. Similar results were obtained using 5 mM methionine. The results of further experiments with the proximal colon, showing the substrate dependency of this effect, are shown in Figure 11.7. Both glucose and methionine cause substantial increases in measured short-circuit current. The apparent K_m and V_{max} values are identical for these two substrates (K_m 0.17 mM; V_{max} 24 μA cm^{-2}). Suckling has no effect on either of these two parameters.

It is natural to equate these effects with those seen to take place in the small intestine. There are, however, important differences showing that the proximal colon does more than act as a temporary extension of the small intestine during the early postnatal period. The apparent affinity of glucose for the system is, for instance, ten times greater in the colon and the same is probably also true for methionine. The V_{max} for the glucose effect in the proximal colon is only one-third of that in the ileum. Methionine produces hardly any rise in current in the ileum, higher concentrations inhibit, and yet it is as effective as glucose in the proximal colon. Finally the effect of non-electrolytes persists unchanged in the colon but not in the small intestine.

224

This persistence of effect with time is shown in greater detail, for the proximal colon, in Figure 11.8. In this case, 3 mM glucose or methionine has been
used as a standard challenging concentration, this having been shown
previously (Figure 11.7) to produce a near maximal response. The ability of
glucose or methionine to increase the short-circuit current persisted for 1 day

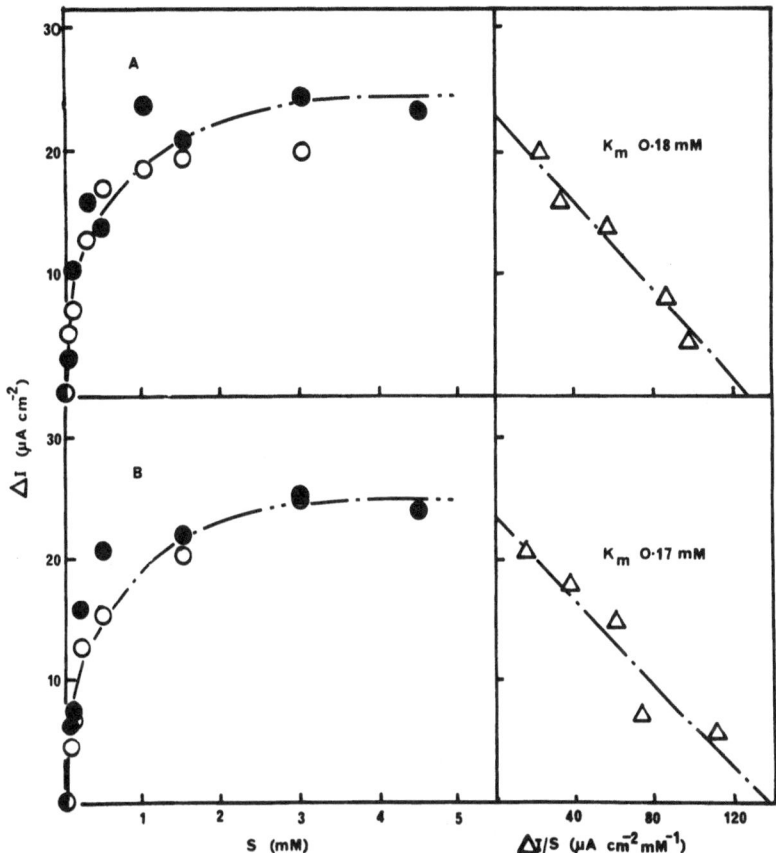

Figure 11.7 Glucose and methionine dependence of short-circuit current in proximal colons
taken from newborn and 1-day old suckled pigs. S gives the concentration of glucose (A) or
methionine (B) in the mucosal solution. ΔI gives the increase in short-circuit produced by the
addition of non-electrolyte to the mucosal side of the preparation. Colons were from newborn
(—●—) or 1-day old suckled (—○—) pigs. Each value gives the mean of multiple estimations
carried out on four to seven pigs

and then declined, disappearing altogether sometime between 2 and 4 days
after birth. Starving a one day suckled pig for a period of 24 hours did not
change this pattern. The subsequent glucose response of the now 2-day-old
proximal colon might appear greater, but the scatter was such as to make this
difference insignificant.

Sodium transport in the proximal colon operates most efficiently during the early postnatal period and if non-electrolytes are present in the colon at this time, they will be able to stimulate this transport still further. Sodium transport in the distal colon is also increased at a time when the intestinal transport of sodium is likely to be low. This increase is not connected with the presence or absence of non-electrolytes. These effects will all tend to act in the same way, aiding the reabsorption of sodium and possibly of non-electrolytes which have escaped into the colon due to a temporary inhibition of transport in the more proximal regions of the intestinal tract.

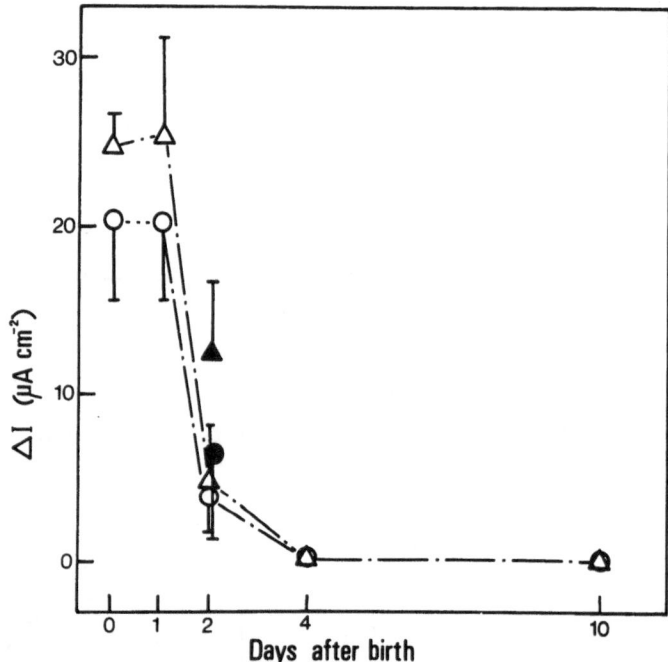

Figure 11.8 Glucose and methionine dependence of short-circuit current on pig proximal colon measured during the first 10 days of postnatal life. Glucose or methionine were used in the mucosal solution at a final concentration of 3 mM. △▲, glucose; ○●, methionine; ▲●, piglets starved 24 hours before the experiment. Values give means ±SE of from five to ten determinations

NON-EQUIVALENCE OF SODIUM TRANSPORT WITH SHORT-CIRCUIT CURRENT

Mention has already been made of occasions when the net transport of sodium does not equal that calculated from the measured short-circuit current. These discrepancies always occur in the same direction, that is with the net transport of sodium being greater than that calculated from the short-circuit current. The most likely explanation for this finding is that some anion accompanies sodium, either as a neutral transport of salt, or as a parallel electrogenic transfer mechanism. Sometimes it is possible to introduce a discrepancy between short-circuit current and sodium transport as a dynamic event during the course of a single experiment. One such case is shown, for the newborn pig

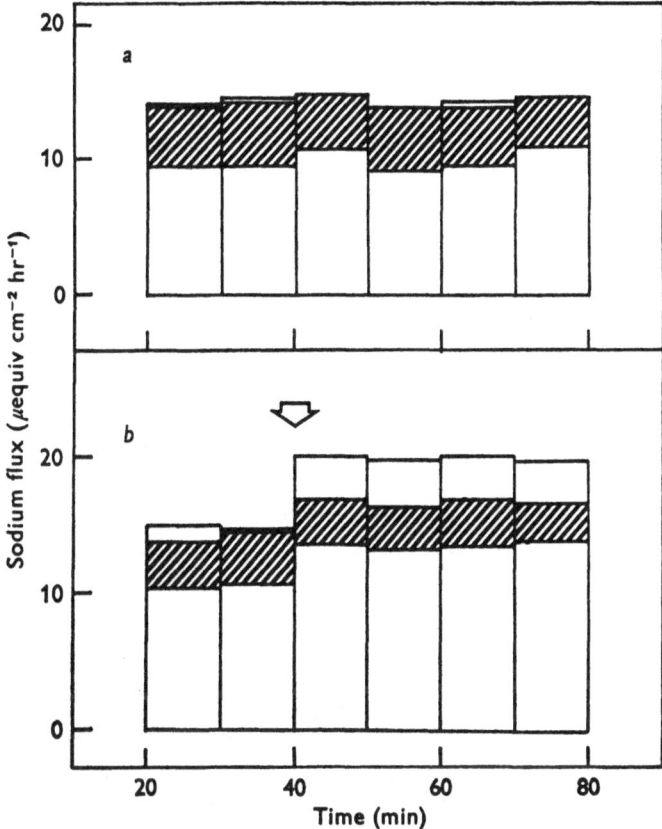

Figure 11.9 Time-dependent stability of bidirectional sodium fluxes measured across newborn pig intestine. Effect of bovine γ-globulin on the agreement between net sodium transport and short-circuit current. Cross-hatched areas give the short-circuit current represented as μEq Na cm^{-2} h^{-1}. Lower open histograms give the serosal-to-mucosal and upper open histograms the mucosal-to-serosal flux of sodium. Time of incubation is measured from the moment radioisotopes are added to the two bathing solutions; (a), control experiment showing the stability of sodium flux with time in the absence of protein; (b), similar to (a), but bovine γ-globulin was added to the mucosal solution at the point shown by the arrow, to give a final concentration of 1% w/v

ileum, in Figure 11.9. The top half of the figure shows the normal agreement between current and net flux, the cross-hatched area (short-circuit current calculated as net flux of cation) matching the difference between influx and efflux over a period of 60 minutes. The lower half of the figure shows what happens when 1% bovine immunoglobulin is added to the mucosal solution halfway through an experiment. The current remains constant but the net absorption of sodium doubles. This change, which is not seen in ileum taken from fed pigs[7], is accompanied by a significant increase in tissue conductance. This is shown in Figure 11.10. The conductance of the newborn unsuckled pig

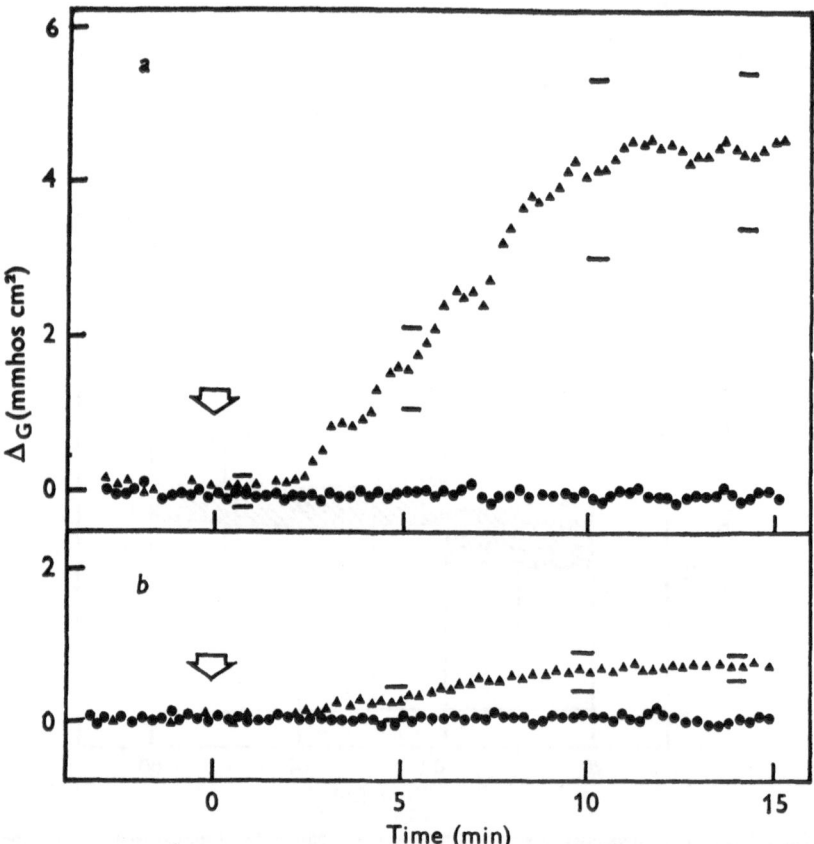

Figure 11.10 Conductance changes in the newborn pig ileum induced by the presence of bovine γ-globulin. —▲—, test conditions, the mucosal solution being changed for one containing 1% bovine γ-globulin at time 0, shown by the arrow; —●—, control conditions, no protein present; Δ_G, time-dependent changes in conductance. The solid bars give the range of results in both cases; (*a*), newborn unsuckled pig ileum giving mean results from five pigs. The initial tissue conductance varied from 14 to 18 mmho cm²; (*b*), newborn pig ileum used after a 24-hr period of suckling giving the mean of results obtained from two pigs. Starting tissue conductance 11 and 12 mmhos cm².

ileum begins to increase soon after the addition of globulin to the mucosal solution. The maximal increase, about 4 mmho cm², represents a 25% increase over the conductance measured at the start of the experiment. The slight increase in conductance seen in ileum taken from suckled pigs is probably not significant.

Separate experiments showed the unidirectional influx of chloride to increase from 8.3 to 11.4 μEq cm^{-2} h^{-1} in the presence of immunoglobulin. This increase is in fairly good agreement with the globulin-dependent increase in sodium influx (3.8 μEq cm^{-2} h^{-1}).

Conclusions

Figure 11.11 summarises the changes thought to take place in the newborn pig ileum as immunoglobulin reacts with the microvillar membrane. The

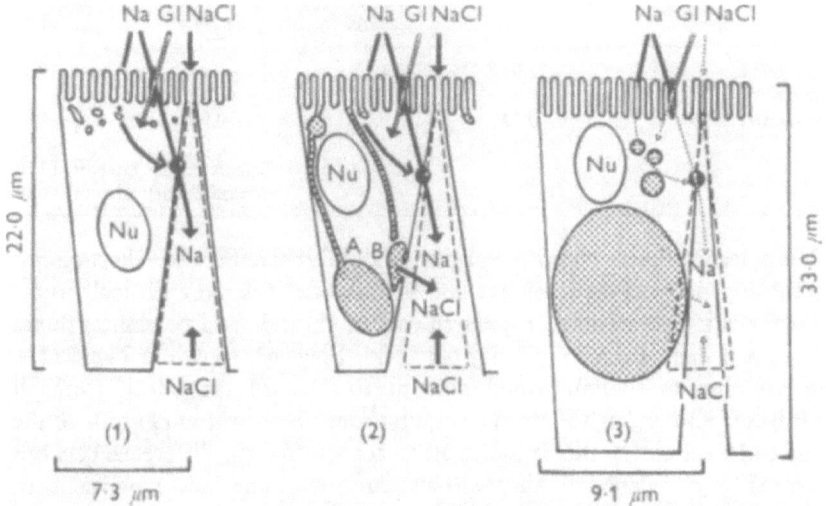

Figure 11.11 Schematic representation of how sodium transport changes during the first 24 hr of postnatal life. (1) Newborn unsuckled pig ileum, no globulin present. The dashed triangle represents the intercellular space, reproduced in (2) and (3) for comparison. Nu, nucleus; Gl, glucose. The measurements of cell height and width give mean values obtained from three pigs. (2) Newborn unsuckled pig ileum incubated *in vitro* in the presence of 1% (w/v) bovine globulin. The dotted areas represent vacuoles filled with protein. (3) Newborn pig ileum incubated *in vitro* following a 24-hour period of suckling. The presence of globulin in medium bathing the mucosa will not change sodium transport. The dashed lines indicate that both the active and passive movement of sodium is reduced

apical vesicles, present at birth, appear not to affect the normal pattern of sodium transport in the absence of protein. The short-circuit current is fully accounted for by the net transfer of sodium. The initial effect of immunoglobulin is to increase the net absorption of sodium by a non-electrogenic pathway (Figure 11.11 (2) giving a diagrammatic representation for results shown in Figures 11.9 and 11.10). Larger vesicles are formed but the short-circuit current remains unchanged at this stage. Independent electron microscopic evidence shows these vesicles to form *in vitro* in the presence of protein[13]. Tissue conductance increases, either because the endocytotic pathway has a high conductance, or because the tight junctions spread due to a widening of the intercellular spaces. A new stable state is reached within a few hours and the vesicle-filled cells are then considerably larger. Both passive and glucose-mediated entry of sodium is reduced at this time and the tissue conductance is low. All these parameters can be reversed, up to 4 days after birth, by a 12-hour period of starvation.

Table 11.4 Unidirectional fluxes of ions measured across short-circuited preparations of pig proximal colon taken after a 24-hour period of suckling

| | Transport (μEq cm^{-2} h^{-1}) | | | Equivalent current μA cm^{-2} |
	influx	efflux	net flux	
Sodium	12.0	4.1	+7.9	+212
Chloride	4.7	3.4	+1.3	−35
Potassium	0.12	0.17	−0.05	−1

Calculated net current +176
Measured net current +80

The colon of the newborn pig also shows differences between short-circuit current and net sodium transport and in this case it is more difficult to account for the discrepancies. Measurements of chloride and potassium fluxes across the proximal colons of 1-day old suckled pigs are shown in Table 11.4. The net flux of sodium would amount to 212 μA cm^{-2} if it were all electrogenic and, though there is a simultaneous movement of chloride to the serosa (−35 μA cm^{-2}), this is too small to account for the difference between measured and calculated short-circuit currents. The net movement of potassium is negligible in this tissue. The passive movement of sodium with another anion such as bicarbonate may take place, but this is unlikely to be through an endocytotic route, for the discrepancy is seen both in newborn proximal colon, where the presence of vesicles is not obvious, and in distal colons at birth and after suckling. Obviously more work needs to be carried out to investigate this difference further and to test for the presence of mechanisms capable of actively transporting different non-electrolytes.

Acknowledgements

I should like to acknowledge the help provided by different people in taking this work to its present state: To Dr de Jesus who used the pig ileum recently to obtain a Cambridge PhD; to Professor Bentley who convinced me that time spent with the pig colon would not be wasted; to Dr Ferguson for providing his expertise on protein separation; to Mr Burton for preparing microvillar membranes in a surprisingly pure form and to Mr James for his dedicated attachment to the measurement of things electrical.

References

1. Rodewald, R. (1973). Intestinal transport of antibodies in the newborn rat. *J. Cell Biol.*, **58**, 189
2. de Jesus, C. H. and Smith, M. W. (1974). Sodium transport by the small intestine of newborn and suckling pigs. *J. Physiol. (Lond.)*, **243**, 211
3. Schultz, S. G., Curran, P. F., Chez, R. A. and Fuisz, R. E. (1967). Alanine and sodium fluxes across mucosal border of rabbit ileum. *J. Gen. Physiol.*, **50**, 1241
4. Smith, M. W. and Ellory, J. C. (1971). Sodium–amino acid interactions in the intestinal epithelium. *Phil. Trans. R. Soc. Lond. B.*, **262**, 131
5. Schultz, S. G. and Curran, P. F. (1970). Coupled transport of sodium and organic solutes. *Physiol. Rev.*, **50**, 637
6. Schaeffer, J. F., Preston, R. L. and Curran, P. F. (1973). Inhibition of amino acid transport in rabbit intestine by *p*-chloromercuriphenyl sulfonic acid. *J. Gen. Physiol.*, **62**, 131
7. de Jesus, C. H. and Smith, M. W. (1974). Protein and glucose-induced changes in sodium transport across the pig small intestine. *J. Physiol. (Lond.)*, **243**, 225
8. Porteous, J. N. (1968). The isolation of purified brush borders from rat small intestine. *FEBS. Lett.*, **1**, 46
9. Ferguson, D. R. and Twite, B. R. (1974). Effects of vasopressin on toad bladder membrane proteins: relationship to transport of sodium and water. *J. Endocr.*, **61**, 501
10. Smith, M. W., Ferguson, D. R. and Burton, K. A. (1975). Glucose and phlorrhizin protected thiol groups in pig intestinal brush-border membranes. *Biochem. J.*, **147**, 617
11. Tsan, M. F. and Berlin, R. D. (1971). Effect of phagocytosis on membrane transport of non-electrolytes. *J. Exp. Med.*, **134**, 1016
12. Bentley, P. J. and Smith, M. W. (1975). Transport of electrolytes across the helicoidal colon of the newborn pig. *J. Physiol. (Lond)*, **249**, 103
13. Munn, E. A. and Smith, M. W. (1974). Uptake of albumin by neonatal pig ileum incubated *in vitro*. *J. Physiol. (Lond.)*, **242**, 30P

Discussion 11

Armstrong: I have some difficulty with your model which invokes NaCl entry from the luminal side through the tight junction as an explanation for the enhanced net Na$^+$ flux following absorption of immunoglobulins. You postulate that this entry is caused by increased delivery of Na$^+$, via a transcellular route, to the intercellular spaces. This causes the spaces to swell and, as a result, the junctions become more leaky. My point is that, unless there is some kind of rectification for salt flow through the junctions, one could just as easily postulate an induced salt flow in the opposite direction, i.e. from the spaces to the lumen.

Smith: The immunoglobulin-dependent increase in net NaCl movement arises, I think, primarily from vesicles discharging into the intercellular space. These spaces swell and the conductance increases. This increase in conductance *could* be associated with an increased NaCl movement across the tight junction. If this were the case, I agree that there is no telling what this would do to net movement. If I were to bet, I should say that it probably results in a small net leak back to the lumen. The measured protein-dependent increase in net flux would then be underestimated by an unknown amount.

Case: Your model depends on an increase in intercellular volume, causing a 'spreading' of the tight junction. Is there any evidence that this 'spreading' takes place?

Smith: The increased conductance seen in the presence of immunoglobulin could be caused directly, if the vesicles were to constitute a transcellular low resistance pathway, or indirectly, if the tight junctions were to become more leaky due to swelling of the intercellular space. I have no means of distinguishing between these two possibilities at the present time. You cannot use markers such as inulin in this tissue to measure paracellular movements, since it is endocytosed by the cell. But I want to emphasise that the model, in describing how net Na$^+$ movement is increased, does not depend on whether tight junctions are open or not.

Levin: Have you checked whether the unstirred layers changed between the two conditions? This could cause the changes in 'apparent K_m'.

Smith: No. It is an interesting point that an increase in unstirred layer will show up kinetically as an increase in apparent K_m. The glycocalyx of the newborn pig ileum is less well developed than in the adult and one might suppose that unstirred layers are less of a problem here, but we have not carried out experiments to prove it.

Desjeux: Are the changes observed related to the characteristics of the protein?

Smith: Changes in mucosal morphology can be induced by both bovine immunoglobulin and bovine serum albumin, and both these proteins cause a rotenone-sensitive increase in oxygen consumption, so that these effects do not show specificity. Both bovine immunoglobulin and bovine serum albumin stimulate net Na$^+$ movement across everted sacs, but we have only used bovine immunoglobulin in the experiments reported here.

12
Role of Cyclic Nucleotides in the Regulation of Intestinal Ion Transport

MICHAEL FIELD, THOMAS A BRASITUS, HARLAND E. SHEERIN and DANIEL V. KIMBERG

Department of Medicine,
Harvard Medical School and Gastrointestinal Unit,
Department of Medicine,
Beth Israel Hospital, Boston, Massachusetts

The active absorption and secretion of Na^+, Cl^- and HCO_3^- by the small intestine can be regulated by hormones and agents such as cholera toxin that simulate the action of hormones. The role of cyclic 3',5'-adenosine monophosphate (cAMP) in secretion is generally acknowledged and has been the subject of many studies. Less attention has thus far been devoted to the oppositely directed effects of α-adrenergic agonists which, at least *in vitro*, are as large in magnitude as those of cAMP. Recent studies raise the possibility that cyclic 3',5'-guanosine monophosphate (cGMP) may be an intracellular effector for the α-adrenergic enhancement of active Na^+ and Cl^- absorption. Our understanding of the mechanisms involved in cAMP-mediated secretion and α-adrenergic-stimulated absorption is still very incomplete. Since both processes involve, in part at least, coupled movements of monovalent anion and Na^+, they may represent the two extremes of a single process. On the other hand, despite this particular similarity, the mechanisms involved may be quite different. This paper attempts to summarise present knowledge about these processes and attempts to define more clearly the role of cyclic nucleotides in regulating these processes. In particular, measurements of ion fluxes are related to measurements of tissue cyclic nucleotide levels and the problems involved in making such correlations are discussed.

cAMP-MEDIATED EFFECTS

Cyclic AMP (cAMP) and agents that increase its intracellular concentration stimulate or unmask an active secretory process for ions and water in the small intestine. This has been demonstrated *in vitro* for cAMP itself, dibutyryl cAMP, theophylline, prostaglandins, cholera and *E. coli* enterotoxins and vasoactive intestinal peptide (VIP)[1,2]. All of these agents except the first two have also been tested *in vivo* and found to elicit a secretory response.

Theophylline, the enterotoxins, PGE_1, and VIP have also been shown to increase cAMP concentration in small bowel mucosa, attesting to a close correlation between increases in mucosal cAMP concentration and the development of secretion. In the case of cholera toxin, the patterns of change in mucosal cAMP accumulation and in ion transport (initial lag period, 2 to 3 hour progression to maximal effect, prolonged persistence of the effect thereafter) are essentially identical[1]. There are several hormones, however, which have been shown to elicit small bowel secretion *in vivo* but which have not increased intestinal mucosal cAMP concentration or adenylate cyclase activity when tested *in vitro*. They include thyrocalcitonin, glucagon, pentagastrin and vasopressin[2-5]. It is certainly possible that some or all of these hormones, when administered *in vivo*, do not act directly on the intestinal epithelium but instead act indirectly by causing the release of another hormone. In the case of calcitonin, however, it has recently been shown (M. Walling, T. Brasitus and D. V. Kimberg, personal communication) that the addition of a very large amount (10 μg/ml) to rat ileum *in vitro* elicits a secretory effect (although a smaller one than the effect of theophylline) without increasing mucosal cAMP concentration. Possibly calcitonin elicits a secretory response not by affecting the synthesis or breakdown of cAMP but by acting at a more distal point in the chain of events leading to cAMP-dependent secretion. Alternatively, as indicated below, the pool of cAMP which is involved in secretion may be only a small fraction of total mucosal cAMP and measurements of the latter may not always accurately reflect changes in the former.

When theophylline, cholera toxin or VIP is added to short-circuited rabbit ileal mucosa *in vitro*, the short-circuit current (SCC) and electrical resistance increase, a large net secretion of Cl^- develops, net Na^+ absorption disappears and, in some instances, net Na^+ secretion also develops (see Figure 12.1). We have recently shown the development of Na^+ secretion in rabbit ileum to be a function of the HCO_3^- concentration (or pH) of the serosal bathing medium[6]: with serosal HCO_3^- set at 10 mM (pH 7.1), theophylline reduced net Na^+ flux from a high baseline rate of absorption to zero; with serosal HCO_3^- set at 50 mM (pH 7.8), however, theophylline shifted net Na^+ flux from a low baseline rate of absorption to a rather substantial rate of secretion. In both cases there were changes of approximately equal magnitude in the net fluxes of both Na^+ and Cl^-. Whether or not Na^+ secretion actually develops appears to be contingent upon the baseline rate of net Na^+ absorption.

There appears to be a discrepancy between *in vitro* and *in vivo* data with respect to HCO_3^- secretion: *in vitro*, net HCO_3^- secretion is unaffected by secretagogues in Cl^--containing Ringer solution, although it is increased moderately in Cl^--free sulphate Ringer[6]. *In vivo*, cholera toxin elicits a very substantial increase in net HCO_3^- secretion by the ileum[7,8]. This discrepancy suggests that there are factors other than cAMP which limit the rate of bicarbonate secretion *in vitro*. It is of interest in this regard that increasing serosal HCO_3^- concentration from 25 to 50 mM does not significantly increase the rate of net HCO_3^- secretion *in vitro*[6].

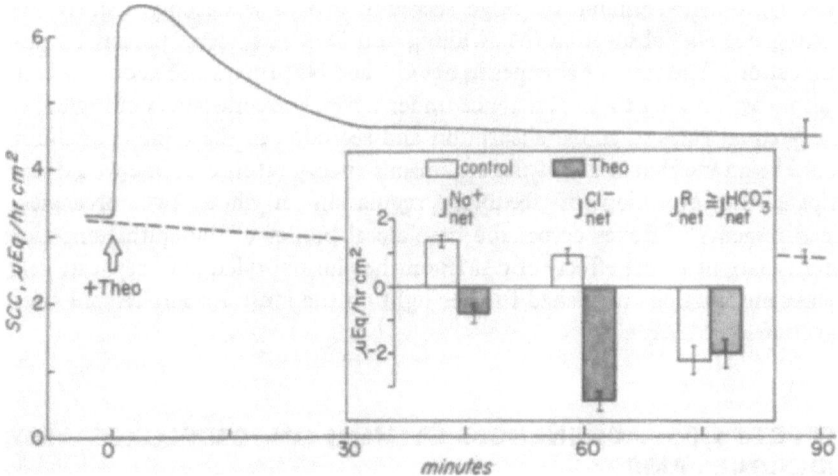

Figure 12.1 Effects of theophylline (Theo) on short-circuit current (SCC) and net ion fluxes. Results are means ±1 SE for 48 experiments with theophylline (5 to 10 mM) and 97 control experiments. The inset showing net Na^+ flux (J_{net}^{Na}), net Cl^- flux (J_{net}^{Cl}), and residual ion flux (J_{net}^{R}) corresponds to the actual time period over which fluxes were measured. All net fluxes are significantly different from zero ($P < 0.01$) (taken from reference 1)

The mechanism by which cAMP produces the ion transport changes cited above has been partly elucidated through the demonstration by Nellans, Frizzell and Schultz[9] that cAMP inhibits a one-for-one coupled influx process for Na^+ and Cl^- in the luminal border of the intestinal epithelium. Inhibition of NaCl influx can explain inhibition of net transmural absorption; however, it cannot in itself account for the development of net secretion. Either a preexisting and continuing active secretory process is unmasked when cAMP inhibits NaCl absorption or cAMP stimulates active secretion by interacting with a second membrane site. This possible second site for cAMP could be closely related to the first site: there could be cAMP-dependent active extrusion of NaCl from cell to lumen that shares the same molecular carrier system over which coupled influx of NaCl from lumen to cell occurs. Alternatively, cAMP could be acting at two separate loci: one in the luminal and the other in the basolateral border or one in villus cells and the other in crypt cells. The

235

NaCl influx that is inhibited by cAMP is about equal in magnitude to the changes caused by cAMP in net transmural fluxes of Na^+ and Cl^-[1,9]. Furthermore, the changes in net transmural fluxes of Na^+ and Cl^- caused by cAMP are about equal to one another in magnitude[1,6,10]. Thus, the stoichiometry of measured changes in influxes and transmural fluxes of Na^+ and Cl^- in rabbit ileum is entirely consistent with one site of action for cAMP. It should be pointed out, however, that the equivalence of cAMP-mediated changes in net transmural fluxes of Na^+ and Cl^- under short-circuit conditions may not apply to all mammalian intestinal preparations and incubation conditions. In rat ileum, for example, in the presence of glucose on the luminal side, dibutyryl cAMP stimulates a large secretion of Cl^- while only slightly inhibiting net Na^+ absorption (M. Walling and D. V. Kimberg, personal communication). The ratio of changes in net Cl^- and Na^+ fluxes was about 5 : 1. It is also worth noting that coexistence under normal circumstances of high and nearly equal rates of active absorption and secretion in the same epithelium would be an inefficient use of the organism's energy resources. One would anticipate the evolution of feedback regulation of these two processes. Measurements of fluxes across the basolateral border of the epithelium and determinations of the effects of cAMP on the phosphorylation of separate cell membrane fractions may shed further light on the ion transport-related sites of action of cAMP.

EFFECTS OF α-ADRENERGIC STIMULI ON ION FLUXES AND MUCOSAL cAMP

Ion transport alterations quite different from those produced by cAMP occur when epinephrine or norepinephrine are added to rabbit ileal mucosa *in vitro*; SCC and resistance decrease, net absorptions of Na^+ and Cl^- increase and net HCO_3^- secretion disappears (see Figure 12.2). When the mucosa is bathed with 25 mM HCO_3^-–Ringer, pH 7.4, the changes in net Na^+ and Cl^- fluxes are about equal in magnitude and therefore, the change in SCC is due largely to the inhibition of HCO_3^- secretion. These changes appear to be α-adrenergic in nature, although this has been specifically demonstrated only with respect to the change in SCC[11]. It is worth noting that the effect of epinephrine on SCC can be completely dissociated from its effect on Na^+ and Cl^- fluxes: ouabain, at a concentration of 3 μM, almost completely blocks stimulation by epinephrine of active Na^+ and Cl^- absorption but does not reduce baseline SCC and does not diminish the effect of epinephrine on SCC (100 μM ouabain is required to inhibit these latter functions by 50%). Thus stimulation by epinephrine of electrically neutral NaCl absorption is neither a cause nor a necessary consequence of the inhibitory effect of epinephrine on HCO_3^- secretion.

Alpha-adrenergic stimulation of active absorption or inhibition of active secretion of ions and water has been observed *in vivo* in canine proximal

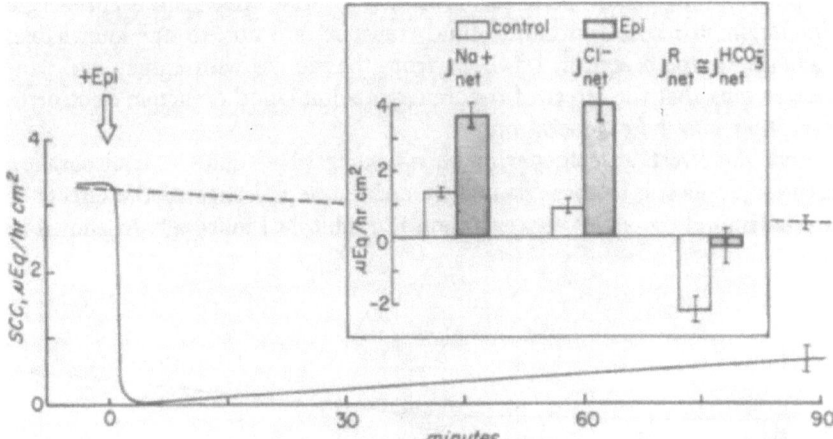

Figure 12.2 Effects of epinephrine (Epi) on short-circuit current (SCC) and net ion fluxes. Results are means ±1 SE for 37 experiments with epinephrine (0.05 mM) and 97 control experiments. The inset showing net fluxes corresponds to the actual time period over which fluxes were measured (taken from reference 1)

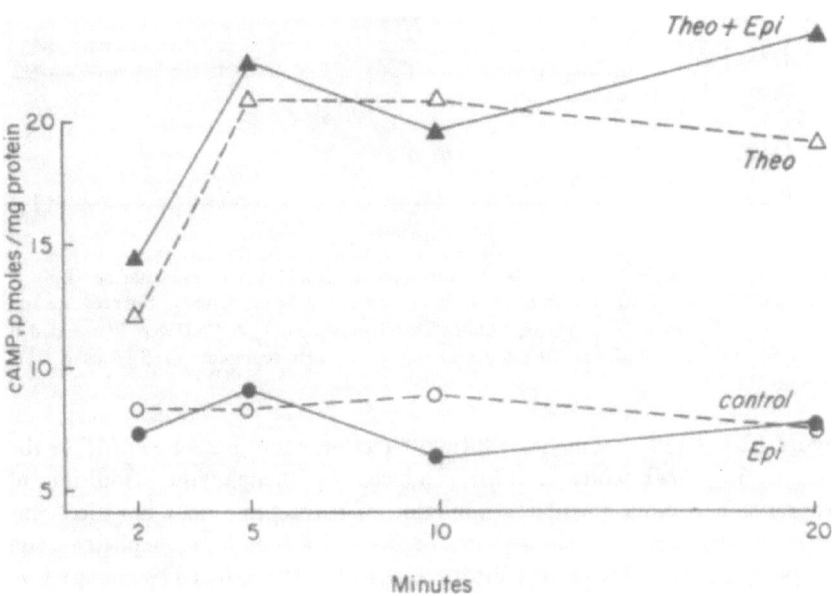

Figure 12.3 Variation of cAMP level with time after addition of epinephrine (Epi), theophylline (Theo), or both. All additions made at time zero. Concentrations of Epi and Theo were 50 μM and 5 mM respectively. Tissues were preincubated for 30 minutes prior to additions. Each point is the mean of results for three complete and separate experiments. Epinephrine did not significantly alter cAMP levels at any point in time (taken from reference 14)

tubule[12] and in rabbit pancreas[13]. Studies of the effects of α-adrenergic stimulation *in vivo* on intestinal fluid transport are not, to our knowledge, available. It would appear, however, from the studies with kidney and pancreas *in vivo* that the effect of α-adrenergic stimulation on active electrolyte absorption may be a general one.

Since the effects of epinephrine on transmural Na^+ and Cl^- transport are essentially opposite to those caused by cAMP, we investigated the effects of catecholamines on cAMP concentration in rabbit ileal mucosa[14]. As shown in

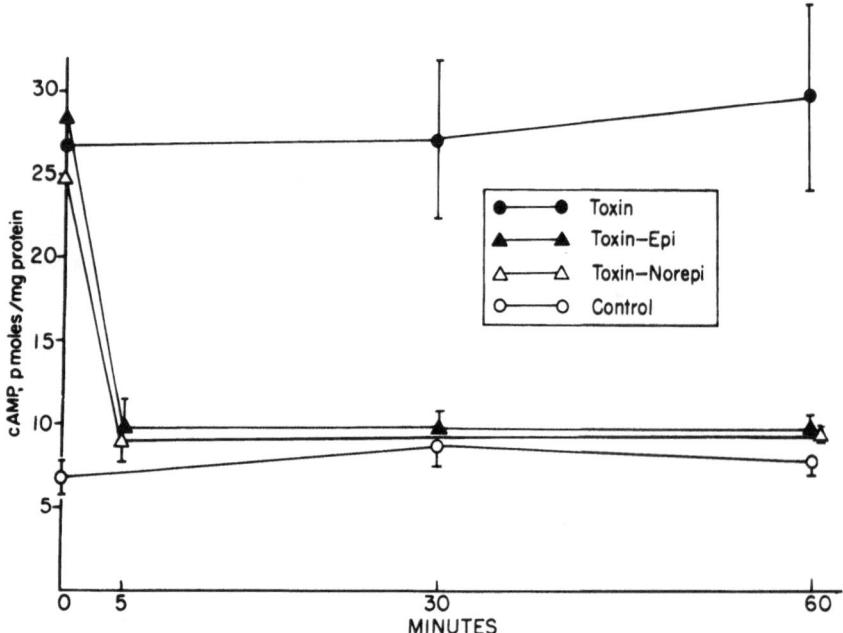

Figure 12.4 Variation of cAMP level with time after addition of epinephrine (Epi) or norepinephrine (Norepi) to cholera toxin-treated mucosa. Tissues incubated in the presence and absence of cholera toxin (2 $\mu g/ml$) for 3 hours. Catecholamines (50 nmol/ml) were then added at time zero and twice again at 20 minute intervals. Brackets represent ± 1 SE (taken from reference 14)

Figure 12.3, 50 μM epinephrine has no effect on either baseline cAMP or the increase in cAMP concentration produced by theophylline. Addition of propranolol to block possible stimulation of α-receptors does not alter this fact. In contrast, as shown in Figure 12.4, both epinephrine and norepinephrine quickly reverse the increase in cAMP produced by cholera toxin. Epinephrine also reduces the increment in cAMP concentration produced by PEG$_1$. Inhibitory effects of epinephrine or norepinephrine on hormone-augmented cAMP levels have also been observed in platelets[15,16], toad bladder[17] and kidney[18,19]. In renal medulla, as in ileum, norepinephrine does not decrease the baseline cAMP concentration[18].

There is little correlation between the effects of epinephrine on ileal mucosal cAMP concentrations and on ion transport. Under baseline conditions, there are marked changes in ion transport and no change in cAMP concentration. As shown in Table 12.1, this lack of correlation also extends to theophylline and cholera toxin-induced changes. Although epinephrine partially reverses the change in Cl⁻ flux produced by theophylline, it does not significantly alter the effect of theophylline on cAMP concentration. In contrast, despite the marked effect of epinephrine on the cholera toxin-augmented cAMP level, epinephrine did not significantly decrease toxin-induced Cl⁻ secretion. Epinephrine was not totally without effect on cholera toxin-treated mucosa, as there was some decrease in SCC and increase in conductance, but its effect on net Cl⁻ flux was clearly minimal. Although not shown in Table 12.1, this also proved to be the case for net Na⁺ flux.

Table 12.1 Epinephrine-induced changes in net Cl⁻ flux, SCC and conductance (G)

Condition	Δ Cl (μEq/h cm^2)	Δ SCC (μEq/h cm^2)	Δ G (mmho/cm^2)
Control (11)	4.1*	−2.0*	7.0*
Theophylline (8)	3.1*	−1.4*	9.2*
Cholera toxin (7)	1.2	−1.0	5.3*

Number of experiments in parentheses. *$p < 0.05$. Epinephrine changed (a) net Cl⁻ fluxes from 1.3 to 5.4 in control, from −4.1 to −1.0 in theophylline (theo)-treated and from −3.8 to −2.6 in cholera toxin (CT)-treated tissues; (b) SCC from 2.9 to 0.8 in control, from 4.3 to 2.9 in theo-treated and from 3.4 to 2.4 in CT-treated tissues; and (c) conductance from 29.0 to 36.0 in control, from 18.7 to 27.9 in theo-treated and from 17.5 to 22.8 in CT-treated tissues (data from reference 14).

The discrepancies between effects of epinephrine on cAMP concentration and on ion transport suggest that the pool of cAMP in the ileal mucosa that actually influences ion transport is only a small fraction of total mucosal cAMP. There may of course be other explanations for these discrepancies. Failure of epinephrine to reverse cholera toxin-induced secretion may indicate that cAMP-mediated secretion is only slowly reversible, that is, that cAMP, once bound to its effector site, is not readily released. Theophylline-induced secretion may reverse more rapidly than cholera toxin-induced secretion because there is less accumulation of cAMP and therefore perhaps less cAMP is bound to effector sites. It is also possible, as discussed below, that the effects of α-adrenergic stimulation on intestinal ion transport are not primarily the result of changes in cAMP accumulation.

Whatever the merits of these alternative considerations, however, we have confirmed in another way the presence in the mucosa of a large pool of cAMP that bears little or no relation to ion transport. Pieces of ileal mucosa clamped in Ussing chambers were exposed on either the mucosal, the serosal or both sides to cholera toxin. After 150 minutes, theophylline was added to all chambers and the resulting changes in SCC were recorded. Since the SCC response to theophylline is blunted by prior addition of another secretagogue[20,21], the magnitude of this SCC response provides a measure of

Table 12.2 Effects of serosally added cholera toxin on theophylline-augmented cAMP levels and SCC responses to theophylline

Cholera toxin added (5 μg/ml)	SCC, theophylline (μa/cm²)	cAMP (pmol/mg protein)
None	+87.9*	18.3*
to s only	+59.1	33.8
to m only	+15.9*	37.4
to m + s	+11.3*	56.7*

Tissues were incubated for 2.5 hour in vitro in the presence of cholera toxin on the mucosal (m), serosal (s), both or neither sides. Theophylline (5 μmol/ml) was then added to all tissues and the SCC responses recorded. Twenty minutes after adding theophylline, tissues were removed and assayed for cAMP. Results are means for ten experiments.
* Significantly different from 's only', $p < 0.05$

pre-existing secretion. Twenty minutes after adding theophylline, tissues were removed and assayed for cAMP. Results are summarized in Table 12.2. Whereas serosal toxin inhibited the SCC response to theophylline far less than did mucosal toxin, it increased cAMP to the same level. Furthermore, addition of toxin to both sides of the mucosa had an additive effect on cAMP levels. Thus, toxin added on the serosal side, while not entirely ineffective with respect to secretion, primarily affects a large pool of cAMP in the mucosa which has no bearing on secretion. Whether this cAMP pool exists in villus or crypt cells or in the lamina propria, where many mesenchymal cells (mostly lymphocytes) reside, remains to be determined. Poor correlation between changes in total tissue cAMP and presumed changes in cAMP level within the tissue compartment involved in a specific physiological response has also been observed with other tissues. In intact adipose tissue, PGE_1 increases cAMP level but does not stimulate lipolysis, whereas, in isolated adipocytes, PGE_1 decreases hormone-augmented cAMP levels[22]. In toad bladder, concentrations of PGE_1 and vasopressin that cause equal increases in cAMP level have unequal effects on Na^+ transport, the PGE_1 effect being considerably smaller[23].

INTESTINAL MUCOSAL cGMP: POSSIBLE ROLE IN ION TRANSPORT

Recent studies suggest that cGMP may be a mediator for the physiological effects of α-adrenergic stimulation. Intravenous infusion of epinephrine or norepinephrine together with propranolol has been shown to increase plasma cGMP in man[24]. Stimulation of α-receptors has been found to increase cGMP in smooth muscle[25] and in parotid gland[26]. Since the effects of α-adrenergic stimulation on intestinal ion transport cannot be simply explained in terms of associated changes in cAMP level, we investigated the effects of epinephrine and other hormones on cGMP levels in rabbit ileal mucosa *in vitro* and attempted to correlate some of these findings with effects on ion transport[27]. With respect to peptide hormones, we tested cholecystokinin octapeptide, glucagon-free insulin and secretin (1 μM); the first two hormones increased

Table 12.3 Effects of atropine on carbachol and epinephrine-induced increases in cGMP levels

Antagonist / Agonist	cGMP, (pmol/mg protein)			
	atropine (1 μM), N = 3		atropine (100 μM), n = 6	
	−atr	+atr	−atr	+atr
None	0.020 + 0.008	—	0.035 + 0.008	0.037 + 0.007
Carbachol (50 μM)	0.100 + 0.022*	0.020 + 0.009†	0.0138 + 0.012*	0.050 + 0.008†
Epinephrine (50 μM)	0.120 + 0.032*	0.119 + 0.34	0.172 + 0.014*	0.040 + 0.008†

Values are means ±1 SE. Atropine was added 5 minutes before and tissues were placed in TCA 2 minutes after additions of agonists.
* Greater than in the absence of agonist, $p < 0.01$
† p less than in the absence of atropine, $p < 0.05$

cGMP, secretin did not. Both carbachol (50 μM) and epinephrine (50 μM) caused a five-fold increase in cGMP concentration. With both agents, a peak effect developed within 2 minutes of addition and the effect disappeared within 30 minutes of addition. Further additions of carbachol and epinephrine at 30 minutes did not produce a second increase in cGMP level. Neither agent affected the cAMP level. The epinephrine effect on cGMP level is clearly α-adrenergic in nature: it was blocked by phenoxybenzamine (50 μM) but was unaffected by propranolol (50 μM); 50 μM isoproterenol (a β-agonist) had no effect on cGMP or cAMP levels; whereas 50 μM methoxamine (an α-agonist) increased cGMP. As shown in Table 12.3, 1 μM atropine blocked the increase in cGMP produced by carbachol but not that produced by epinephrine, whereas 100 μM atropine also blocked the increase in cGMP produced by epinephrine. The inhibitory effect of 100 μM atropine on the epinephrine-induced increase in cGMP has also recently been observed with rat parotid gland[26]. The mechanism involved is unclear, but since the carbachol effect is blocked by a far smaller concentration of atropine, the epinephrine-induced increase in cGMP is presumably not mediated by a muscarinic cholinergic mechanism.

Since 100 μM atropine blocked the increase in cGMP produced by epinephrine, we undertook experiments to determine what effect, if any, this concentration of atropine would have on epinephrine-induced alterations of ion transport. Addition of atropine (100 μmol/ml) to the serosal bathing solution had no effect on SCC and ion fluxes nor did it inhibit the normal electrical response to the addition of glucose to the luminal bathing solution. As shown in Figure 12.5, epinephrine decreased SCC to the same extent in the presence as in the absence of atropine. Therefore 100 μM atropine does not interfere with the inhibition of epinephrine of HCO_3^- secretion. However, as also shown in Figure 12.5, atropine almost completely inhibited the stimulatory effect of epinephrine on active Na^+ and Cl^- absorption. Thus 100 μM atropine, like 3 μM ouabain (see above), dissociated the effect of epinephrine on Na^+ and Cl^- transport from its effect on SCC and HCO_3^- transport. The

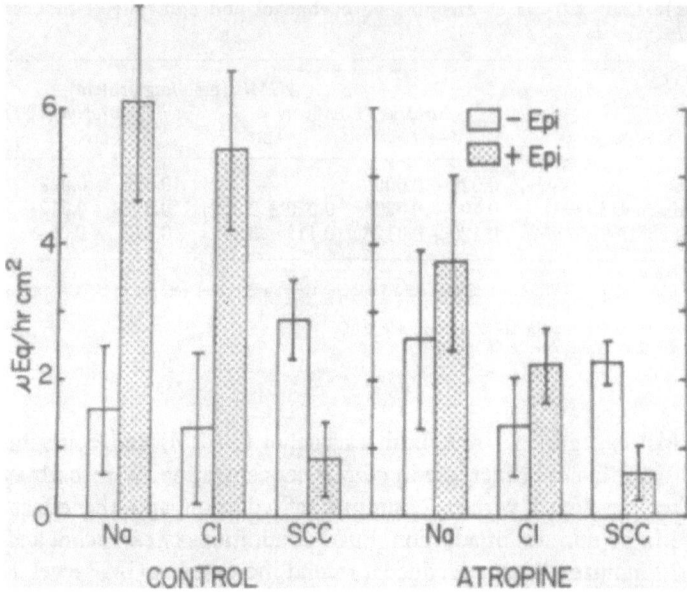

Figure 12.5 Inhibition by atropine of epinephrine-stimulated Na$^+$ and Cl$^-$ absorption. Unitional mucosa (m)-to-serosa (s) and s-to-m fluxes of Na$^+$ and Cl$^-$ across short-circuited rabbit ileal mucosa were measured in the presence and absence of atropine (100 μM). Epinephrine (50 μmol/ml) was then added to all chambers and fluxes were measured again. Epinephrine additions were repeated twice at 20-minute intervals. Values shown are net fluxes $\pm$1 SE for 11 experiments. Net Na$^+$ and Cl$^-$ fluxes in the presence of atropine and epinephrine were not significantly greater than in the presence of atropine alone and were significantly less than in the presence of epinephrine alone

atropine data suggest, therefore, that the effects of epinephrine on electrically neutral Na$^+$ and Cl$^-$ transport and on cGMP concentration are in some manner linked.

In order to examine this association more closely, we determined unidirectional mucosa-to-serosa Na$^+$ fluxes after adding 8-bromo-cGMP to the serosal bathing solution at concentrations of 40, 200, and 1000 nM. No effect of 8-bromo-cGMP was observed at any of these concentrations. Higher concentrations increased SCC, presumably producing a cAMP-like effect. Although a more exhaustive study needs to be done, these preliminary experiments suggest that it will not be possible to evaluate the physiological role of cGMP through addition of the nucleotide to the bathing medium. Low concentrations seem to be ineffective, and high concentrations mimic the action of cAMP. Therefore, whether cGMP does in fact mediate the action of epinephrine on NaCl transport or whether the increases in both are products of another more fundamental effect of α-adrenergic stimulation, such as an increase in Ca^{++} permeability, remains unresolved.

SUMMARY AND CONCLUSIONS

cAMP and agents that increase its intracellular concentration stimulate or unmask an active secretory process for ions and water in the small intestine. Although these changes can be attributed in part to inhibition of coupled NaCl influx at the luminal border, it seems likely that cAMP also acts to stimulate secretion at another as yet undefined site.

Alpha-adrenergic stimuli, when added *in vitro* to rabbit ileum, enhance active absorption of Na^+ and Cl^- and inhibit HCO_3^- secretion. The effect on NaCl transport can be dissociated from the effect on HCO_3^- transport by adding either 100 μM atropine or 3 μM ouabain. Both agents, at the concentrations used, inhibit the former without affecting the latter and also without affecting the baseline SCC, which is an approximate measure of the rate of HCO_3^- secretion.

Alpha-adrenergic stimulation does not reduce the baseline cAMP level, only marginally affects the theophylline-augmented cAMP level but almost completely reverses the cholera toxin-augmented cAMP level. In contrast, the relative effects of α-adrenergic stimuli on ion transport are in the reverse order: a large effect under baseline conditions, a moderate effect after theophylline and only a marginal effect after cholera toxin. This and other evidence (effects of serosally added cholera toxin) indicate that the ion transport-related pool of cAMP in rabbit ileal mucosa is only a small fraction of total mucosal cAMP. Thus, measurements of the latter may not always accurately reflect changes in the former.

Cyclic GMP may be an intracellular effector for the α-adrenergic influence on intestinal ion transport. Alpha-adrenergic stimulation by epinephrine and methoxamine increases cGMP in rabbit ileal mucosa. This increase can be completely blocked by atropine (100 μM), which also blocks the stimulation of Na^+ and Cl^- absorption. Whether the ion transport effects of epinephrine are due to the increase in cGMP or whether these actions are not related as cause and effect but are both consequences of a more fundamental influence of α-adrenergic stimulation remains to be resolved. We have thus far not been successful in reproducing the effects of epinephrine with exogenous 8-bromo cGMP.

Acknowledgements

The authors are indebted to Antonia Henderson, Philip L. Smith and E. Timothy O'Brien for invaluable technical assistance and to Dr Zvi Selinger of the Hebrew University of Jerusalem for a helpful discussion on the effects of atropine on α-adrenergic and cholinergic responses. This work was made possible by grants AI-09029 (US-Japan Cooperative Medical Science Program), AM-05114 and RR-05479 from the National Institutes of Health.

References

1. Field, M. (1974). Intestinal secretion. *Gastroenterology*, **66**, 1063
2. Schwartz, C. J. C., Kimberg, D. V., Sherrin, H. E., Field, M. and Said, S. I. (1974). Vasoactive intestinal peptide stimulation of adenylate cyclase and active electrolyte secretion in intestinal mucosa. *J. Clin. Invest.* **54**, 536
3. Barbezat, G. O. and Grossman, M. I. (1971). Intestinal secretion: Stimulation by peptides. *Science*, **174**, 422
4. Soergel, K. H., Whalen, G. E., Harris, J. A. and Geenen, J. A. (1968). Effect of antidiuretic hormone on human small intestinal water and solute transport. *J. Clin. Invest.*, **47**, 1071
5. Gray, T. K., Bieberdorf, F. A. and Fordtran, J. S. (1973). Thyrocalcitonin and the jejunal absorption of calcium, water and electrolytes in normal subjects. *J. Clin. Invest.*, **50**, 1218
6. Sheerin, H. E. and Field, M. (1975). Ileal HCO_3 secretion: Relationship to Na and Cl transport and effect of theophyline. *Amer. J. Physiol.*, **228**, 1065
7. Carpenter, C. C. J., Sack, R. B., Feeley, J. C. and Steenberg, R. W. (1968). Site and characteristics of electrolyte loss and effect of intraluminal glucose in experimental canine cholera. *J. Clin. Invest.*, **47**, 1210
8. Norris, H. T., Curran, P. F. and Schultz, S. G. (1969). Modification of intestinal secretion in experimental cholera. *J. Infect. Dis.*, **119**, 117
9. Nellans, H. N., Frizzell, R. A. and Schultz, S. G. (1973). Coupled sodium–chloride influxes across the brush border of rabbit ileum. *Amer. J. Physiol.*, **225**, 467
10. Nellans, H. N., Frizzell, R. A. and Schultz, S. G. (1974). Brush-border processes and transepithelial Na and Cl transport by rabbit ileum. *Amer. J. Physiol.*, **226**, 1131
11. Field, M. and McColl, I. (1973). Ion transport in rabbit ileal mucosa. III. Effects of catecholamines. *Amer. J. Physiol.*, **225**, 852
12. Gill, J. R. and Casper, A. G. T. (1972). Effect of renal alpha-adrenergic stimulation on proximal tubular sodium reabsorption. *Amer. J. Physiol.*, **223**, 1201
13. Hubel, K. A. (1970). Response of rabbit pancreas *in vitro* to adrenergic agonists and antagonists. *Amer. J. Physiol.*, **219**, 1590
14. Field, M., Sheerin, H. E., Henderson, A. and Smith, P. L. (1975). Catecholamine effects on cyclic AMP levels and ion secretion in rabbit ileal mucosa. *Amer. J. Physiol.*, **229**, 86
15. Marquis, N. R., Becker, J. A. and Vigdahl, R. C. (1970). Platelet aggregation. III. An epinephrine-induced decrease in cyclic AMP synthesis. *Biochem. Biophys. Res. Comm.*, **39**, 783
16. Moskowitz, J., Harwood, J. P., Reid, W. D. and Krishna, G. (1971). The interaction of norepinephrine and prostaglandin E_1 on the adenyl cyclase system of human and rabbit blood platelets. *Biochim. Biophys. Acta*, **230**, 279
17. Omachi, R. S., Robbie, D. E., Handler, J. S., and Orloff, J. (1974). Effects of ADH and other agents on cyclic AMP accumulation in toad bladder epithelium. *Amer. J. Physiol.*, **226**, 1152
18. Kurokawa, K. and Massry, S. G. (1973). Interaction between catecholamines and vasopressin on renal medullary cyclic AMP of rat. *Amer. J. Physiol.*, **225**, 825
19. Guder, W. G. and Rupprecht, A. (1975). Antagonism between parathyroid hormone and norepinephrine on cyclic adenosine-3',5'-monophosphate (cAMP) levels in isolated tubules from rat kidney cortex. *Pflügers Arch.*, **354**, 177
20. Field, M. (1971). Ion transport in rabbit ileal mucosa. II. Effects of cyclic 3',5'-AMP. *Amer. J. Physiol.*, **221**, 992
21. Field, M., Fromm, D., Al-Awqati, Q. and Greenough, W. B. (1972). Effect of cholera enterotoxin on ion transport across isolated ileal mucosa. *J. Clin. Invest.*, **51**, 796
22. Butcher, R. W. and Baird, C. E. (1968). Effects of prostaglandins on adenosine 3',5',-monophosphate levels in fat and other tissues. *J. Biol. Chem.*, **243**, 1713
23. Kaliner, M. A., Orange, R. P., Koopman, W. J., Austen, K. F. and LaRaia, P. J. (1971). Cyclic adenosine 3',5'-monophosphate in human lung. *Biochim. Biophys. Acta*, **252**, 160

24. Ball, J. H., Kaminsky, N. I., Hardman, J. G., Broadus, A. E., Sutherland, E. W. and Liddle, G. W. (1972). Effects of catecholamines and adrenergic-blocking agents on plasma and urinary cyclic nucleotides in man. *J. Clin. Invest.*, 51, 2124

25. Schultz, G. and Hardman, J. G. (1975). Regulation of cyclic GMP levels in the ductus deferens of the rat. In G. I. Drummond, P. Greengard and G. A. Robison (eds.) *Advances in Cyclic Nucleotide Research*, Vol. 5, p. 339 (New York: Raven Press)

26. Wojcik, J. D., Grand, R. J. and Kimberg, D. V. (1975) Amylase secretion by rabbit parotid gland: Role of cyclic AMP and cyclic GMP. *Biochim. Biophys. Acta* (in press)

27. Brasitus, T. A., Field, M. and Kimberg, D. V. (19**) Intestinal mucosal cyclic GMP: Regulation and possible role in ion transport. (Submitted for publication)

12

Discussion Paper on

Cyclic AMP Mediated Electrolyte Secretion in the Pancreas: Effect of Cholera Toxin

Pamela A. Smith and R. Maynard Case

Department of Physiology, University Medical School,
Newcastle upon Tyne

The exocrine pancreas is responsible both for the secretion of digestive enzymes, by a process of exocytosis, and for the elaboration of an isotonic electrolyte secretion rich in bicarbonate. The former takes place in the acinar cells (which comprise the bulk of the gland) following stimulation by cholecystokinin–pancreozymin (CCK–PZ) or acetylcholine (released from vagal nerve terminals), while the latter is thought to take place in the centro-acinar and duct cells following stimulation by secretin. Observations in some species suggests that this description is an oversimplification of the functional arrangement of the gland.

The role of cyclic AMP in mediating these secretory responses is still uncertain. Although few in number, most observations support a role for cyclic AMP in electrolyte secretion, whereas attempts to implicate cyclic AMP in enzyme secretion, though more numerous, are less convincing and the evidence remains equivocal[1]. Because cholera toxin has thus far been shown to have no other effect than that of stimulating adenylate cyclase, we have tested its actions on the isolated saline-perfused cat pancreas[2] in an attempt to clarify the role of cyclic AMP in these two pancreatic secretory processes.

Addition of purified cholera toxin (1.0 μg/ml) to the perfusate for 30 minute results in a biphasic secretory response from the gland (Figure *12.1*). The first, very small, phase of secretion began within 1 to 2 minutes of toxin application and was maintained as long as toxin was present in the perfusate. Because such an immediate effect of cholera toxin has not previously been described, it was investigated further and found to be an artefact due to the presence of sodium azide in the buffer in which cholera toxin is supplied by the US National Institutes of Health; it could be exactly reproduced by the addition of azide to the perfusate at the concentration present during toxin stimulation (6 × 10^{-7}). The fact that azide will stimulate pancreatic electrolyte secretion is itself of potential interest. The cause of this stimulation remains a mystery. It could be due to an effect on adenylate cyclase or phosphodiesterase (note the transitory rise in tissue cyclic AMP concentration in Figure 12.1) or a direct effect on the electrolyte transport mechanism; this will be investigated further.

The second, sustained phase of secretion, due to the action of the toxin proper, began after 30–60 minutes and increased in magnitude for many hours. It was accompanied by a parallel rise in the cyclic AMP concentration in pieces of tissue removed from the gland. The rise was not marked, but it is

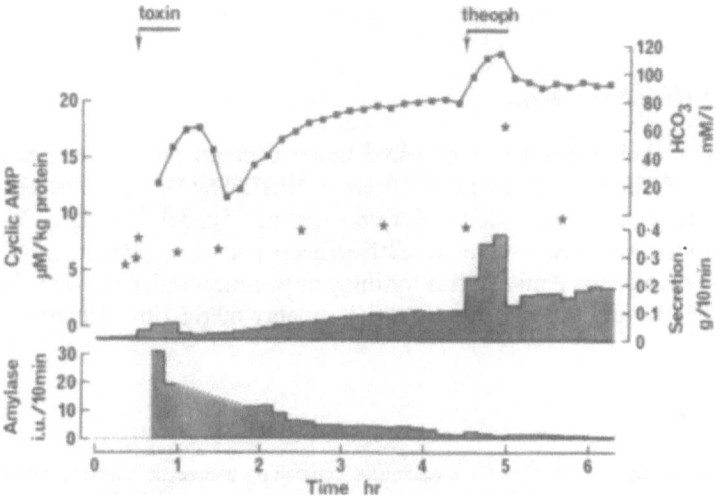

Figure 12.1 The effect of purified cholera toxin on the isolated saline-perfused cat pancreas. Cholera toxin (1.0 μg/ml) and theophylline (0.5 mM) were each added to the perfusate for 30 minutes as indicated by the horizontal bars. The upper curve illustrates the bicarbonate concentration of the secretion; the upper histogram illustrates the output of pancreatic juice; the lower histogram illustrates the amylase output in the juice (the dotted line on this histogram indicates instances where the volume of secretion was too small to allow amylase analysis). The stars indicate tissue cyclic AMP concentration; the third sample was taken half a minute after initial exposure to cholera toxin. The response to theophylline in this experiment was somewhat greater than average

not especially so at the higher secretory rates produced by secretin stimulation[3]. Secretion could be potentiated by theophylline at concentrations (5 × 10^{-4} M) which alone evoke only a very small electrolyte secretion in this preparation[4].

The composition of the secretion evoked by cholera toxin resembled that evoked by secretin in that it contained a high bicarbonate concentration but only basal amounts of enzymes (Figure 12.1). At a given secretory rate, the bicarbonate concentration was the same as that observed following secretin stimulation in this preparation[2]. It is true that an initial enzyme secretion is recorded in Figure 12.6. However, this can be attributed to a washout of enzymes which have accumulated in the duct during the pre-experimental period in the absence of electrolyte secretion. Thus most of the enzyme is contained in a volume of about 0.3 ml, which is the approximate volume of the duct space. In other experiments on incubated pieces of rat pancreas, cholera toxin also failed to stimulate enzyme secretion, despite large rises in tissue cyclic AMP concentration.

In conclusion, the action of cholera toxin supports a role for cyclic AMP in the electrolyte secretory response of the pancreas to secretin, but offers no evidence that cyclic AMP plays a similar role in the regulation of pancreatic enzyme secretion. A fuller report of this work is published elsewhere[5].

Acknowledgements

Purified cholera toxin was prepared under contract for the US National Institute of Allergy and Infectious Diseases (NIAID) by Dr R. A. Finkelstein, the University of Texas, Southwestern Medical School, Dallas, Texas and generously supplied by Drs R. S. Northrup and C. E. Miller.

We thank Miss Ann Mullins for diligent technical assistance and the Cystic Fibrosis Research Trust for financial support of this investigation.

References

1. Case, R. M. (1973). Cellular mechanisms controlling pancreatic exocrine secretion. *Acta Hepato-Gastroenterol.*, **20**, 435
2. Case, R. M., Harper, A. A. and Scratcherd, T. (1968). Water and electrolyte secretion by the perfused pancreas of the cat. *J. Physiol. (Lond.)*, **196**, 133
3. Case, R. M., Johnson, M., Scratcherd, T. and Sherratt, H. S. A. (1972). Cyclic adenosine 3',5'-monophosphate concentration in the pancreas following stimulation by secretin, cholecystokinin–pancreozymin and acetylcholine. *J. Physiol. (Lond.)*, **223**, 669
4. Case, R. M. and Scratcherd, T. (1972). The actions of dibutyryl adenosine 3',5'-monophosphate and methyl xanthines on pancreatic exocrine secretion. *J. Physiol. (Lond.)*, **223**, 649
5. Smith, P. A. and Case, R. M. (1975). Effects of cholera toxin on cyclic adenosine 3',5'-monophosphate concentration and secretory processes in the exocrine pancreas. *Biochim. Biophys. Acta*, **399**, 277

Discussion 12

Desjeux: Using the method of Frizzell and Schultz (*J. Gen. Physiol.*, **59**, 318, 1972) to discriminate between cellular and paracellular pathways, we obtained data suggesting that in rabbit ileum, purified cholera toxin acts on both cellular and paracellular pathways. The toxin stimulates an active Na^+ neutral secretion with preservation of the Na^+ active absorptive process. In addition it decreases the total tissue conductance with no change in partial sodium conductance.

Ellory: Dr Field, have you measured chloride uptake in the Schultz/Curran type apparatus (*J. Gen. Physiol.*, **50**, 1241, 1967) to see whether cholera toxin reduces this influx? We do not find any change in uptake of chloride in cholera-treated tissue.

Field: We have not made such measurements; perhaps Dr Frizzell has.

Frizzell: While we have not examined the effects of cholera toxin on Cl^- (or Na^+) influx across the brush border of rabbit ileum, the effects of the toxin, as Dr Field points out, are faithfully mimicked by cyclic AMP or theophylline. These agents, as I recounted yesterday, bring about significant decreases in both Cl^- and Na^+ influx which appear to simulate the effects of ion replacement. That is, maximal influx via the coupled mechanism is reduced by replacement of either Na^+ or Cl^- in the mucosal solution with non-transported ions. This effect is directly analogous to those of cAMP and theophylline (and presumably cholera toxin) which act as non-competitive inhibitors of neutral NaCl influx.

Desjeux: We measured the Na^+ influx in cholera toxin-treated tissue. There is a decrease in total Na^+ influx across the mucosal face of the rabbit ileum. The effect is more important on the paracellular than on the cellular pathway.

Turnberg: May I ask Dr Field whether he has measured cAMP levels during the first 2 minutes after addition of epinephrine or other agents, since I wonder whether early, rapid and short-lived changes in cAMP concentrations may have been missed? Is it conceivable that such changes could trigger off the alterations in ion transport which persist after cAMP levels return to normal?

Field: We have not measured cyclic AMP concentrations earlier than 5 minutes after epinephrine treatment. It is possible that we missed a transient decrease in cAMP. I cannot exclude the possibility that a transient decrease in cAMP might trigger off a prolonged change in ion transport, but this seems very unlikely. Why wouldn't the prior ion transport state return when the cAMP concentration increased back to normal?

Levin: Has anyone looked at the effect of cholera toxin, theophylline or adrenergic agents on cyclic AMP and GMP levels in isolated enterocytes rather than in intact tissue, which is necessarily heterogeneous? This would give us an important insight into whether the agents change the cyclic nucleotide levels in the enterocytes *per se*.

Field: We have observed that enterocytes removed from cholera toxin-pretreated mucosa have an increase in adenyl cyclase activity, but we have not measured the cAMP levels in these cells. I am not aware of such measurements by others.

Murer: We have tested the action of cholera toxin on basolateral membranes which contain adenyl cyclase. The enzyme levels are increased by the toxin.

13
Movements of Water and Ions Across Dog Ileal Mucosa Following Ischaemia or Occlusion

V. MIRKOVITCH AND H. MENGE*

Département de Chirurgie Expérimentale,
Hôpital Cantonal Universitaire,
Lausanne

Various degrees of ischaemia or occlusion are very frequent traumas in the pathology of the small intestine, with firmly acknowledged direct and significant repercussions upon the transmucosal movements of electrolytes and non-electrolytes. Certain aspects of these lesions, such as modifications in absorption and secretion of water, loss of sodium or potassium, disturbances in sugar or amino acid transport, or changes in epithelial structure, have generally been examined separately, and the authors concerned have almost always erroneously tried to correlate their own parameters with the depth of the mucosal damage and its subsequent evolution. The present multilateral studies in dogs represent an attempt simultaneously to trace in the same tissue sample the displacements of some ions and non-electrolytes, and to compare them with the morphology and enzyme content of ileal mucosa.

ISCHAEMIA

Methods

In mongrel dogs, weighing 10–15 kg, a loop of ileum, approximately 40 cm above the caecum, was subjected to one hour's arterial ischaemia, whereby the afferent artery and the intestinal wall were clamped and the efferent vein was

* On leave of absence from: Medizinische Universitäts–Klinik, Marburg-an-der-Lahn, Germany

left open. The morphology and function of the mucosa of these loops, and of contiguous controls were examined immediately or 1, 3 or 7 days after the trauma.

Tissue samples were fixed in 10% formalin, embedded in paraffin, cut (6 μm) and stained with haematoxylin–eosin. Morphometric evaluation was performed by measuring the villus height, villus width, crypt length and the epithelial cell height in the central part of a villus. Histochemical reactions were performed, using methods previously described in detail[1], to determine the activities of leucine–aminopeptidase and acid phosphatase. Optical density of the histochemical stains was evaluated in a Vickers M85 scanning microdensitometer, following detection of each absorption maximum. The results were corrected for the incubation time and the thickness of the tissues, and expressed as Extinction $\cdot$ min^{-1} $\cdot$ μm^{-1}. For each sample, 10–15 different determinations were made.

Intestinal function was assessed both *in vitro* and *in vivo*. Net movements of water, sodium, potassium, chloride and glucose were determined *in vivo* with the perfusion technique described in detail elsewhere[2]. After the perfusion, the loops were excised and dried overnight at 110 °C so that all values could be expressed in terms of dry tissue.

Determination of the transport capacity of slices of mucosa *in vitro* was carried out using methods detailed previously[3] and the results are expressed as the distribution ratio between intra- and extra cellular water.

Statistical evaluation was performed where possible by means of a random-block analysis of variance, considering each dog as one block. In addition, '*t*'-tests were applied to comparisons between groups of animals.

Results

The results concerning the ischaemic intestine are summarised in Table 13.1. Immediately after one hour's ischaemia, the enterocytes at the villus tips were desquamated into the lumen and bands of epithelial cells were detached from the sides of the villi. The single cells had shrunk. The lamina propria had disintegrated and sometimes also shed off towards the lumen. Interstitial oedema occurred frequently in the villus core. In the upper half of the crypts, there was also a serous exudate at the base of the cells, a dilatation of the blood vessels and slight interstitial oedema and haemorrhage, but the extent of these changes was much less pronounced than at the villus tips. One day after the ischaemia, the villi were again covered with a cylindrical epithelium, but the cells were smaller, and often diminished further towards the tips of the villi, and the villus height and the crypt length were both much less than in the control intestines. Synechia between neighbouring villi were often encountered. The vessels were still engorged with erythrocytes and the lamina propria was slightly oedematous; there was often a slight leucocytic infiltration at the tips of the villi. Three days after the insult, the mucosa appeared

Table 12.1 Data concerning intestines after ischaemia

Parameter	Control	Immediately after ischaemia	1 day after ischaemia	3 days after ischaemia	7 days after ischaemia
Morphometry (in μm)					
Villus height	749 + 17.3	—	397 ± 39**	729 ± 34	770 ± 40
Crypt length	553 ± 19.4	—	321 ± 27**	550 ± 27	618 ± 21
Epithelial cell height	30.5 ± 0.56	—	24.2 ± 1.14**	28.1 ± 0.60*	33.3 ± 0.72
Histochemistry (in E min^{-1} μm^{-1})					
Leucine–aminopeptidase	0.259 ± 0.009	0.158 ± 0.046**	0.191 ± 0.056**	0.253 ± 0.0130	—
Acid phosphatase	0.024 ± 0.002	0.016 ± 0.0017**	0.016 ± 0.012**	0.021 ± 0.0010	—
Uptake in vitro (DR)					
Phenylalanine	7.61 ± 0.32	1.34 ± 0.07**	8.18 ± 0.53	5.72 ± 0.44**	8.25 ± 1.16
β-methylglucoside	7.36 ± 0.37	1.57 ± 0.19**	5.53 ± 0.28*	5.05 ± 0.43*	6.33 ± 0.95
Net movement in vivo					
Water (in ml/h g dry tis.)	3.54 ± 0.37	-4.10 ± 1.35**	-0.23 ± 0.48**	2.08 ± 0.46**	2.20 ± 0.48
Sodium (in mmol/h g dry tis.)	0.54 ± 0.053	-0.54 ± 0.19**	-0.01 ± 0.07**	0.33 ± 0.06*	0.36 ± 0.07
Potassium (in mmol/h g dry tis.)	0.014 ± 0.0028	-0.076 ± 0.0156**	-0.0054 ± 0.0044**	0.003 ± 0.0054*	0.0056 ± 0.0039
Glucose (in mmol/h g dry tis.)	0.076 ± 0.0049	-0.005 ± 0.013**	0.028 ± 0.0038**	0.057 ± 0.0071*	0.055 ± 0.0086

Eight dogs were employed in each group, each dog providing a control and treated loop. Statistical analysis performed by comparing the ischemic loops with their own controls using a random-block analysis of variance (** = significant difference at 1% level; * = significant difference at 5% level). Control values represent means (± SEM) of all untreated loops. Values with negative signs imply net movement into the lumen. DR = distribution ratio.

almost normal. This was emphasised by the morphometric analysis which revealed that only the epithelial cell height remained significantly lower than the control values. Rare erythrocytes persisted in the lamina propria at the tips of some villi. Seven days after the ischaemia, there was no discernible morphological difference between the control and recuperated loops.

A brush-border enzyme, leucine–aminopeptidase, and a lysosomal enzyme, acid phosphatase, were studied with quantitative histochemical techniques. The levels of these enzymes were lower both immediately and 1 day after the ischaemia, but normal values were restored 3 days after the trauma. In addition, the levels of the brush-border enzyme were significantly lower immediately after the ischaemia than 1 day later. It should be stressed that even immediately after the insult, the enzymes were localised at their specific cytochemical sites and diffuse activity was not encountered.

Immediately after ischaemia, the mucosa was no longer capable of accumulating phenylalanine and β-methylglucoside *in vitro* against concentration gradients. One day later, the uptake of phenylalanine had normalised, whereas that of β-methylglucoside was still significantly reduced; the latter only attained normal values at the 7-day stage.

A considerable quantity of water and electrolytes appeared in the lumen *in vivo* immediately after the ischaemia, and no glucose absorption occurred. One day later, the loops were still unable to absorb water and ions. Glucose absorption was observed, though its level was significantly lower than normal. Absorption of all substrates, was still significantly lower than normal 3 days after the ischaemia, but had been restored to control levels 7 days after the trauma.

Discussion

Immediately after the ischaemia the histological examination revealed widespread damage to the epithelium with a decrease in histochemically determined enzymes in the individual enterocytes, and an abolition of all active transport measured *in vitro*. At the same time, the perfusion studies *in vivo* disclosed an abundant loss of water and electrolytes into the lumen.

One day after the ischaemia the intestinal surface was again covered with an intact epithelial lining, but morphometric analysis revealed that the villi were shorter and the epithelial cells smaller. In agreement with these observations, the enterocytes contained lower activities of various histochemically stainable enzymes. Similar reductions in enzyme levels have been reported in regenerating intestinal mucosa after irradiation, apparently as a result of the immaturity of the new cells originating from an increased proliferative activity and stimulated migration rate[4]. Although direct evidence has not been obtained, it could be assumed that a similar evolution occurs during recovery from ischaemia. The shortening of the crypts might be a result of the damage to these cells at the time of the ischaemia, just as the shortened villi could have resulted from previous ischaemic damage to the villus core. In this case, the proliferation of the epithelial cells and the fibroblasts of the lamina propria would be expected to occur in parallel, as demonstrated by others[5,6].

In agreement with the morphometric and histochemical findings, a partial recovery of β-methylglucoside transport *in vitro* was recorded, while phenylalanine uptake had completely normalised. It was observed in a previous study that the amino acid transport system recuperates more rapidly than that of monosaccharides[7]. One reason for the swift revival of the amino acid system may simply be the earlier development of this mechanism in comparison with that of monosaccharides during the early differentiation process of the enterocyte. Alternatively, there may be a precocious induction of amino acid transport to fulfil the needs of the rapidly regenerating cell.

Despite the active accumulation of sugars and amino acids *in vitro* at this stage, no net movement of water and ions could be detected *in vivo*. It is known[8] that the net absorption of water and electrolytes in the intestine *in vivo* is controlled by the delicate balance of two opposing fluxes, mediated by one absorptive and one secretory system. The lack of absorption may possibly be simply a further expression of the different rates of recovery of the various enzymatic mechanisms in the regenerating enterocytes, the secretory system being restored more rapidly than the absorptive one. On the other hand, the partial recovery of glucose absorption *in vivo* agrees with the measurements of sugar uptake *in vitro*, and apparently reflects the state of the villus epithelium.

All parameters indicate an almost complete recovery 3 days after the trauma; the outstanding function, which does not recuperate fully until the seventh day, is the absorption of water and ions *in vivo*. The results concerning absorption *in vivo* by the regenerating mucosa correlate well with findings in man during recovery from coeliac disease[9]. Both studies indicated that potassium absorption is always the last to recover fully, and that glucose absorption can co-exist with net sodium and water secretion.

OCCLUSION

Methods

The dog ileum was cut transversally 40 cm above the ileo-caecal valve, and a short piece of normal intestine was removed for control histological examination. The two ends of the intestine were sewn up and great care was taken to avoid impairing any blood supply. The animals, which received food and water *ad libitum* but no other treatment post-operatively, were re-examined under anaesthesia on the seventh day, and the loops above and below the occlusion were compared.

Before attempting any further manoeuvre, the intraluminal pressure above the occlusion was measured by a catheter attached to a water manometer. After the occluded loop had been drained of its contents, the net movement of water, sodium, potassium, chloride and glucose across the mucosa *in vivo* was studied by the above-mentioned perfusion technique. The tissue was then excised and subjected to the same examinations as in the case of the ischaemic loops.

Results

The dogs tolerated complete obstruction of the small bowel for up to 1 week, although there was progressive vomiting and evident loss of weight. The hydrostatic pressure within the intestine was low. After 4 days, the mean pressure was 3.9 ± 0.46 cmH$_2$O ($n = 20$), and after 7 days, it was 3.3 ± 0.39 cmH$_2$0 ($n = 15$). The highest recorded pressure in a loop was 8 cmH$_2$O. Bacteriological studies of the intestinal fluid revealed the presence of large quantities of *E. coli*, ranging between 3×10^7 and 6×10^9 organisms per ml of liquid.

Above the occlusion, a considerable reduction in the villus height and crypt length and an increase in the villus width was observed (Table 13.2). The individual epithelial cells were smaller, and in some cases transformed into irregular, flat cells. In the specimens where the transformation of the epithelium was most pronounced, the villus width was increased to the greatest extent. No ulceration was seen and the epithelial lining always

Table 13.2 Occluded intestines

Parameter	Control	Above occlusion	Below occlusion
Morphometry (in μm)			
Villus height	873 ± 35.7	$501 \pm 24.6^*$	$412 \pm 37.8^*$
Crypt length	632 ± 52.4	$422 \pm 33.6^*$	$249 \pm 16.8^*$
Epithelial cell height	27.7 ± 0.9	$24.5 \pm 1.3^*$	$23.7 \pm 0.8^*$
Histochemistry (in E min^{-1} μm^{-1})			
Leucine–aminopeptidase	0.279 ± 0.0095	$0.125 \pm 0.0098^*$	$0.200 \pm 0.0024^*$
Acid phosphatase	0.0190 ± 0.00027	$0.0226 \pm 0.00050^*$	$0.0137 \pm 0.00047^*$
Uptake in vitro (DR)			
Phenylalanine	7.61 ± 0.321	7.82 ± 0.940	$4.79 \pm 0.560^*$
β-methylglucoside	7.36 ± 0.366	$4.57 \pm 0.472^*$	5.58 ± 0.987
Net movement in vivo			
Water (in ml/h g dry tis.)	4.20 ± 0.45	$-1.84 \pm 0.39^*$	$2.18 \pm 0.79^*$
Sodium (in mmol/h g dry tis.)	0.64 ± 0.068	$-0.16 \pm 0.062^*$	0.46 ± 0.116
Potassium (in mmol/h g dry tis.)	0.022 ± 0.0022	$-0.074 \pm 0.0136^*$	$-0.080 \pm 0.0206^*$
Glucose (in mmol/h g dry tis.)	0.072 ± 0.0054	0.060 ± 0.0092	0.056 ± 0.0068

Intestinal loops examined 7 days after mechanical occlusion; results are means ± SEM of eight dogs. Control series concerns normal loops treated in an identical manner. * = significantly different from control, at least $P < 0.05$. Values with negative signs imply net movement into the lumen.

remained intact. There was often a moderate leucocytic infiltration of the lamina propria, and dilatation of the blood capillaries, but no evidence of oedema.

Below the occlusion, atrophy of the mucosa was evident: the villi were shorter and narrower, and the crypt length was reduced; there was also a reduction in the number of villi per mucosal length.

The activity of the brush-border enzyme, leucine–aminopeptidase, was reduced in both loops, though to a greater extent above the occlusion. On the other hand, the activity of acid phosphatase was reduced below the occlusion, but increased above it.

Phenylalanine transport by the mucosa of the occluded loop *in vitro* was always within the normal range, whereas transport of this amino acid by the mucosa of the intestine below the occlusion was significantly lower than the control values. The uptake of β-methylglucoside was reduced in the occluded loop.

The perfusion studies *in vivo* revealed a net loss of water, sodium and potassium, but not of chloride, into the lumen of the occluded intestine one week after the operation. Glucose continued to disappear from the perfusate; indeed this parameter was not significantly different from the control values. Below the occlusion, absorption of water and electrolytes occurred, except in the case of potassium, but the values for absorption were slightly lower than those of the control series.

Discussion

The epithelial covering of the occluded intestine remains intact, in strong contrast to the findings after one hour's ischaemia[3]. The structure is modified, insofar as the villi and crypts become shorter, but there are no important vascular changes and virtually no oedema. The reductions in transport *in vitro*, and in brush-border enzyme levels, studied histochemically, are relatively discrete, and may well be secondary to the structural alterations. One of the principal consequences of the intact epithelial layer might be that a mucosal permeability barrier exists to prevent toxins from reaching the blood stream. The most important misconception in the pathophysiology of intestinal occlusion involves the pressure build-up in the lumen of the occluded intestine and subsequent vascular stasis and ischaemia of the epithelium. We also showed in a previous study in rats that the pressure in the lumen did not surpass 5 mmHg, the epithelial covering of the villi was never destroyed, and no ischaemic damage was visible[10].

Furthermore, the collection of liquid in the intestinal lumen following the occlusion does not solely result from the piling up of gastric and pancreatic secretions that cannot be reabsorbed, but water and electrolytes are concomitantly secreted by the intestinal mucosa into the lumen. This finding indicates how a vicious circle is set up which prevents any spontaneous healing of the condition. The increased intraluminal pressure would be expected to favour absorption, rather than hinder it, as we have recently demonstrated[2]. Thus the secretory mechanism is working against a situation which would tend to neutralise it.

The question concerning the biochemical nature of the secretion mechanism is a very intriguing one. It is postulated but not proved that the intestinal epithelium possesses two mechanisms for pumping ions and water, which act in opposite directions[8]. Under normal conditions, the absorptive pump, which is apparently mediated by a Na^+–K^+-ATPase, removes more ions and water from the lumen than are exsorbed by the secretory pump, which is apparently mediated by a mechanism involving cyclic AMP[8]. However, the latter pump seems to be particularly delicately controlled, and could be stimulated by a number of agents, such as certain bacterial toxins which provoke intestinal secretion through an action on adenyl cyclase. The best known is the cholera enterotoxin, but it has been shown that some strains of E. coli are also capable of a stimulation of secretion[11–13]. The only conclusion that can be offered at the present stage is that a substance produced in the occluded intestine stimulates the loss of water and electrolytes across the mucosa in a similar way as enterotoxins act, and it is reasonable to suspect that this agent originates from the vast colony of E. coli. The presence of normal glucose absorption in vivo is a further indication that the balance of ion fluxes has simply been tipped in favour of secretion.

The tissue below the occlusion, ignored in most studies of intestinal obstruction, shows very important structural and functional modifications, though their nature is different from that occurring above the occlusion. Here we see a pronounced atrophy of the type that has been described by various authors studying blind loops[1,14]: reductions in villus height and width and in crypt length, normal epithelial cells of reduced size, reduced transport in vivo and in vitro, and decreased enzyme levels. It is most probable that in this case, as in other self-emptying blind loops, the diminished intraluminal nutrition is largely responsible for the changes observed[15,16]

COMMENTS

In the two experimental models, there was no parallelism among the various parameters studied. The normal amino acid uptake one day after ischaemia or after 7 days of occlusion could lead to the erroneous conclusion that the mucosa was functionally normal. Furthermore, the normal image of the epithelial lining 3 days after the ischaemia is totally misleading, because at that moment water, electrolytes, and sugar absorptions are far from being restored. The mechanisms controlling the movements of water and ions are therefore the most sensitive ones; they are very profoundly disturbed by ischaemia, and 7 days are required for complete recovery. Moreover, it was found in both experimental models that the movements of water and electrolytes could be reduced even when the morphology and the transport of non-electrolytes were normal. All these observations impose the conclusion that there is no single reliable parameter for assessing the functional capacity of the mucosa either during the first week after ischaemia or after prolonged occlusion, and therefore a multilateral approach to such problems is highly desirable. Finally, the fact that throughout the experiments the movements of water and sodium, potassium, sugar, and amino acids behaved independently of one another, suggests strongly that each of them might be controlled by a separate mechanism.

Acknowledgements

This study was supported in part by a grant from Zyma S. A., Nyon. The skilful technical assistance of Mmes H. Capt and P. Ganguillet and Mlles M. Augstburger, D. Mettraux, L. Schnell and J. Vouron, and the secretarial aid of Mlle W. Happee are gratefully acknowledged. We are indebted to Dr S. Neukomm, Institut de Médecine Sociale et Préventive, for the loan of the microdensitometer, and we are grateful to Prof. J. Frei and Dr J. Michod and the staff of the Laboratoire Central de l'Hôpital Cantonal for the analyses of ions and glucose.

References

1. Menge, H., Bloch, R., Schaumlöffel, E. and Riecken, E. O. (1970). Transportstudien, morphologische, morphometrische und histochemische Untersuchungen zum Verhalten der Dünndarmschleimhaut im operativ ausgeschalteten Jejunalabschnitt der Ratte. *Z. Ges. Exp. Med.*, **153**, 74
2. Mirkovitch, V., Menge, H. and Robinson, J. W. L. (1974). The effect of intraluminal hydrostatic pressure on intestinal absorption *in vivo*. *Experientia*, **30**, 912
3. Robinson, J. W. L. and Mirkovitch, V. (1972). The recovery of function and microcirculation in small intestinal loops following ischaemia. *Gut*, **13**, 784
4. De Both, N. J., Van Dongen, J. M., Van Hofwegen, B., Keukmans, J., Visser, W. J. and Galjaard, H. (1974). The influence of various cell kinetic conditions on functional differentiation in the small intestine of the rat. A study of enzymes bound to subcellular organelles. *Devel. Biol.*, **38**, 119
5. Marsh, M. N. and Trier, J. S. (1974). Morphology and cell proliferation of subepithelial fibroblasts in adult mouse jejunum. II. Radioautographic studies. *Gastroenterology*, **67**, 636
6. Parker, F. G., Barnes, E. N. and Kaye, G. I. (1974). Replication, migration, and differentiation of the subepithelial fibroblasts of the crypt and villus of the rabbit jejunum. *Gastroenterology*, **67**, 607
7. Robinson, J. W. L., Haroud, M., Winistörfer, B. and Mirkovitch, V. (1974). Recovery of function and structure of dog ileum and colon following two hours' acute ischaemia. *Europ. J. Clin. Invest.*, **4**, 443
8. Field, M. (1974). Intestinal secretion. *Gastroenterology*, **66**, 1063

9. Bloch, R., Menge, H., Lingelbach, B., Lorenz-Meyer, H., Haberich, F. J. and Riecken, E. O. (1973) The relationship between structure and function of small intestine in patients with a sprue syndrome and in healthy controls. *Klin. Wschr.*, **51**, 1151

10. Kubrová, J., Robinson, J. W. L. and Mirkovitch, V. (1973). La fonction de la muqueuse après une occlusion aiguë de l'intestin grêle du rat. *Res. Exp. Med.*, **160**, 321

11. Pierce, N. F. and Wallace, C. K. (1972). Stimulation of jejunal secretion by a crude *Escherichia coli* enterotoxin. *Gastroenterology*, **63**, 439

12. Guerrant, R. L., Ganguly, U., Caspar, A. G. T., Moore, E. J., Pierce, N. F. and Carpenter, C. C. J. (1973). Effect of *Escherichia coli* on fluid transport across canine small bowel. *J. Clin. Invest.*, **52**, 1707

13. Hynie, S., Rašková, H., Sechser, T., Vaněček, J., Matějovská, D., Matějovská, V., Treu, M. and Polák, L. (1974). Stimulation of intestinal and liver adenyl cyclase by enterotoxin from strains of *Escherichia coli* enteropathogenic for calves. *Toxicon*, **12**, 173

14. Gleeson, M. H., Cullen, J. and Dowling, R. H. (1972). Intestinal structure and function after small bowel bypass in the rat. *Clin. Sci.*, **43**, 731

15. Dowling, R. H. (1970). Small bowel resection and by-pass – recent developments and effects. *Mod. Trends Gastroent.*, **4**, 73

16. Menge, H., Müller, K., Lorenz-Meyer, H., and Riecken, E. O. (1975). Untersuchungen zum Einfluss von Methionin- und Methionin-Glucose-Lösungen auf Morphologie und Funktion der Schleimhaut selbstentleerender jejunaler Blindschlingen der Ratte. *Virchows Arch. Zellpath.*, **18**, 135

13

Discussion Paper on

Intestinal Blood Flow and Sodium Exchange

A. H. G. Love

Department of Medicine,
The Queen's University of Belfast

The diarrhoea associated with cholera is due to an imbalance between bidirectional fluid and electrolyte fluxes across the intestinal mucosa. It has been shown in man that net absorption or secretion in this disease is caused by a relatively small proportional change in large bidirectional fluxes. These fluxes

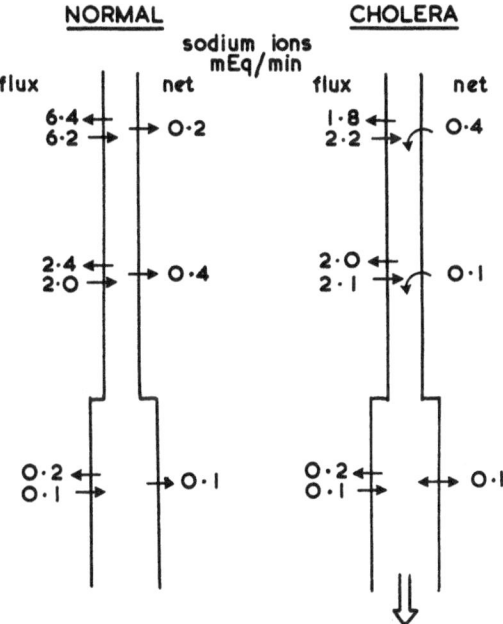

Figure *13.1* Sodium exchange across the human intestinal mucosa in cholera patients. Fluxes measured by double sodium label technique. Patients compared in acute and convalescent recovery periods

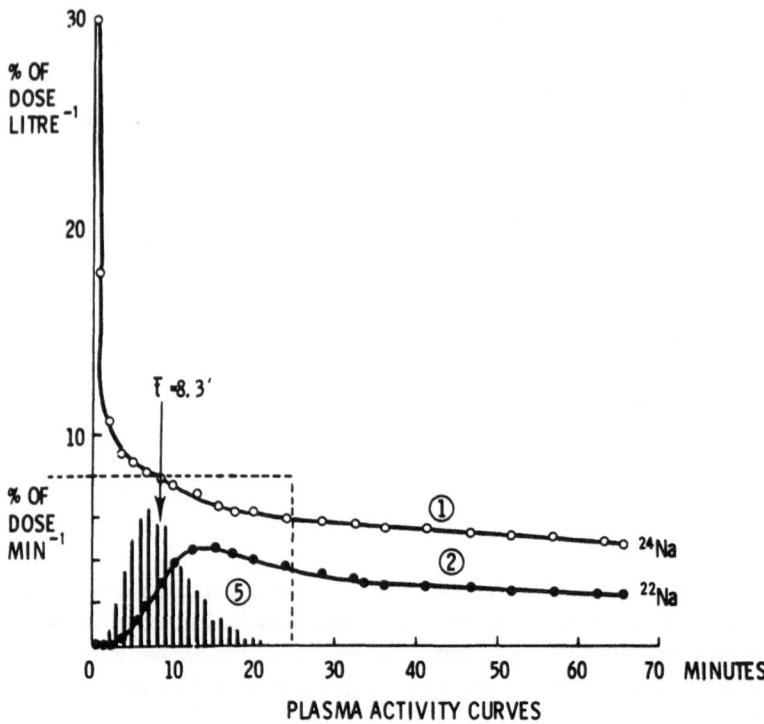

Figure *13.2* Plasma radioactivity as a function of time. Curve 1, ^{24}Na given intravenously; curve 2, ^{22}Na given orally. The calculated function is the single passage transfer rate from gut lumen to plasma. The mean transit time, $\bar{t}$, is shown

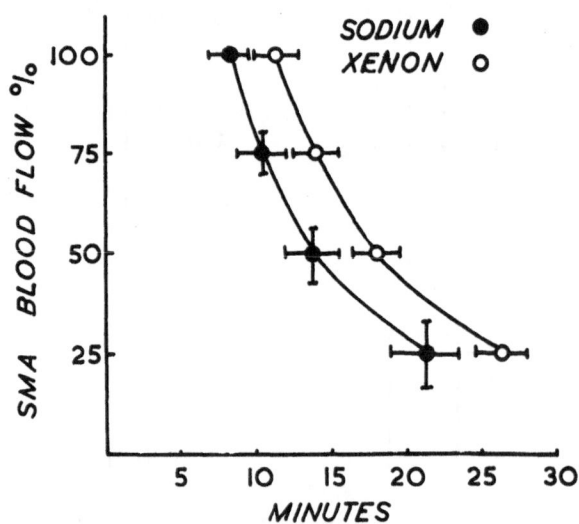

Figure *13.3* Sodium and xenon mean transit times from gut lumen to plasma in relation to alterations in total superior mesenteric artery blood flow

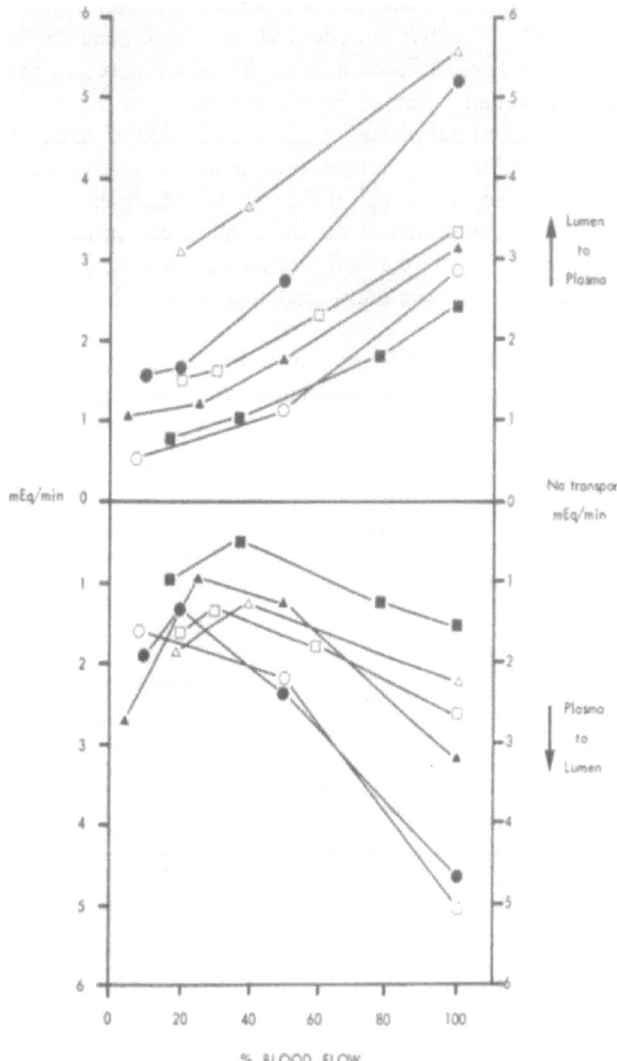

Figure *13.4* Bidirectional sodium ion movement across the total small intestinal mucosa. Fluxes measured by double sodium labels and superior mesenteric artery blood flow recorded by flow meter in the main artery

are also reduced in the acute disease[1]. Typical results comparing the diarrhoeal state with the normal convalescent intestine are shown in Figure *13.1*.

It is possible that intestinal blood flow is a determining factor in the exchange of fluid and electrolytes across the mucosa. Previous studies[2] have failed to demonstrate changes in total intestinal blood flow in cholera but these investigations did not take account of functional mucosal flow.

To test the hypothesis that functional mucosal flow may be important in determining mucosal absorptive function, studies have been carried out to compare exchange functions of sodium with that of an inert gas, xenon. This latter substance is exchange-limited by blood flow.

Using total small intestinal perfusion and the addition of radioactive labels to the bloodstream and intestinal lumen, it is possible to calculate functions of exchange across the mucosa[3]. A typical example of sodium exchange is shown in Figure 13.2. By deconvolution of the intravenous and intraluminal curves in plasma, it is possible to arrive at a figure for not only the quantity but also the mean transit time $(\bar{t})$ of sodium exchange across the small intestinal mucosa.

With dogs as the model, it has been shown that there is a close relationship between sodium transfer and xenon movement with varying degrees of blood

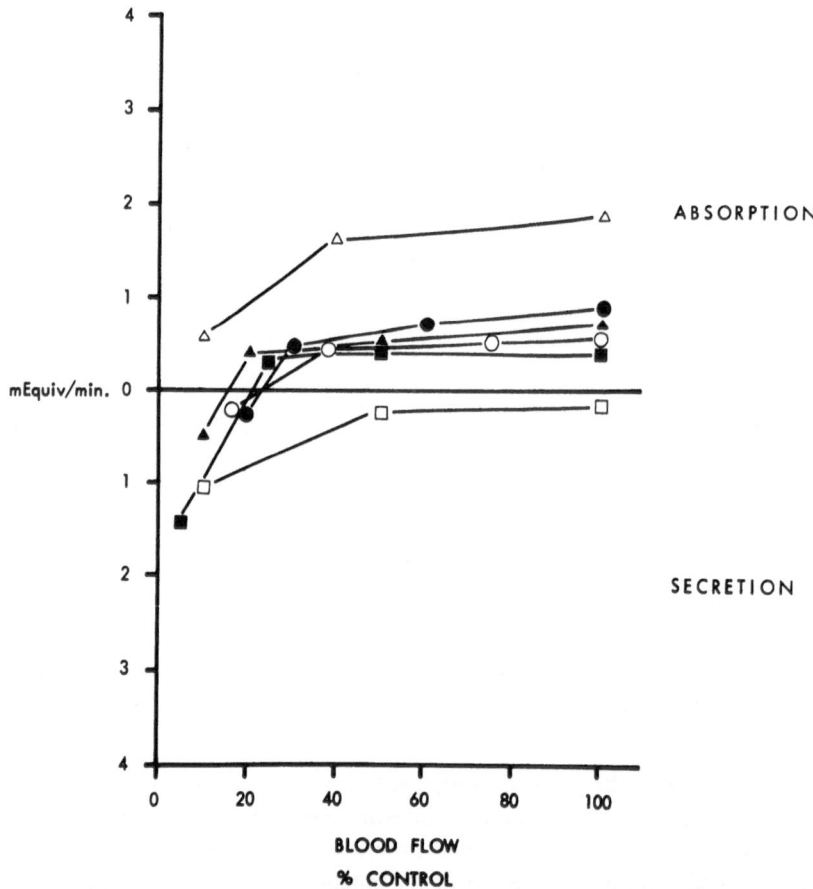

Figure *13.5* Net sodium transfer across the small intestine as a function of total intestinal blood flow

flow through the intestine (Fig. 13.3). Total flow was measured by an electromagnetic flow meter in the superior mesenteric artery. Xenon transfer was calculated from deconvolution of plasma (alveolar) concentration of isotope following intravenous and intraluminal injection of the label. It is interesting to note that sodium transfer (Na_t) is consistently faster than xenon and this may indicate the participation of active sodium transport.

The effects of blood flow restriction on sodium transfer are shown in Figures 13.4 and 13.5. Bidirectional fluxes are reduced with reduced flow and at low flow rates, the imbalance results in the occurrence of secretion rather than absorption.

In conclusion it has been demonstrated that alterations in blood flow produce changes in bidirectional sodium fluxes across the intestinal mucosa. It also appears that the relationship between 'functional mucosal flow' as measured by xenon transfer is very closely related to the magnitude and rate of sodium transfer. It is therefore likely that in various diarrhoeal states, changes in mucosal blood flow contribute to the deranged intestinal function in this state of secretory mucosal activity.

Acknowledgements

The author wishes to thank the Medical Research Council of Great Britain and the Royal Society for support in this work.

References

1. Love, A. H. G., Phillips, R. A., Rohde, J. E. and Veall, N. (1972). Sodium ion movement across intestinal mucosa in cholera patients. *Lancet*, **ii**, 151
2. Carpenter, C. C. J., Greenough, W. B. and Sack R. B. (1969). The relationship of superior mesenteric artery blood flow to gut electrolyte loss in experimental cholera. *J. Infect. Dis.*, **119**, 182
3. Love, A. H. G., Rohde, J. E., Abrams, M. E. and Veall, N. (1973). The measurement of bidirectional sodium fluxes across the intestinal wall in man using whole gut perfusion. *Clin. Sci.*, **44**, 267

Discussion 13

Armstrong: Your results show that, following ischaemia, glucose absorption recovers more rapidly than sodium absorption. How do you interpret this in terms of the well-known coupling between sodium and sugar transport in the intestine?

Mirkovitch: In the intestine 1 day after ischaemia, the surface is completely covered with a new, young epithelium. This mucosa recovered about half its absorptive power for monosaccharides (β-methylglucoside uptake *in vitro*, glucose absorption *in vivo*). However, the same mucosa reveals no net movement of water, sodium and chloride; this discrepancy suggests that in the young recovering mucosa, the transports of sodium and glucose may not be controlled by the same mechanism.

Whittembury: By analogy with cholera, it would appear that glucose feeding would be an effective therapy for patients with intestinal occlusion, since this would tend to reduce the secretion that you have demonstrated.

Dowling: Dr Menge, it was not clear from your slides whether the changes in enzyme activity were related to the varying masses of mucosa in the different experimental situations, or whether there were changes in specific activity.

Menge: The enzyme activities in the single cells were measured by histochemical techniques and quantitated with a Vickers microdensitometer.

Dowling: So the microdensitometer measures the concentration of enzyme per cell; in other words you are, in essence, measuring specific activity. May I also ask what you consider to be the mechanism for the mucosal hypoplasia distal to the site of occlusion?

Menge: We believe that the decreased enzyme activities below the mechanical occlusion are an indication of the atrophy of the single absorptive cell, due to diminished intraluminal nutrition in this condition.

Skadhauge: Dr Love, your main conclusion that blood flow to a large extent limits absorption rates is probably correct, as Prof. Winne has shown in several publications (e.g. *Z. Gastroent.*, **9**, 429, 1971). But I am in doubt as to how to interpret the similarity between xenon and sodium isotope appearances. When you are in steady state with changing specific activity, the sodium isotope appearance will indeed be blood-flow limited, but net sodium absorption may not.

Love: The problem with producing steady-state specific activities is that the label traverses the mucosa in both directions so quickly that the actual transfer measurements become uninterpretable. This is why we chose the bolus label method.

Dowling: You did not show a change in net ion fluxes until the total intestinal blood flow had been reduced to 20–25% of normal. This raises two questions: First, is there a reduction in blood flow in cholera comparable to this drastic change produced experimentally, and secondly, how do changes in mucosal blood flow vary in response to changes in total intestinal blood flow?

Love: I don't think that superior mesenteric flow changes necessarily reflect similar changes at the mucosal level. What I am suggesting is that the bidirectional dynamics of the sodium ion are affected to a major extent by 'functional mucosal flow'. This may alter in certain states without major changes being seen in the SMA flow. In the cholera situation, it may explain the general reduction in sodium ion movement, while the toxin effect on the mucosal cell is responsible for the final secretory state.

Levin: Do you think that the reversal of absorption into secretion that you find at low blood flow rates in the dog is due to a stimulation of chloride secretion in the anoxic mucosa, as suggested by Dr Armstrong's group for the frog intestine?

Love: Yes, I think that anoxia is an important factor in low flow rates.

Armstrong: Just to keep the record straight, what Drs Gerencser, Suh and I found (BBA 255, 647, 1972) was that, in Na^+-free media containing glucose, the mucosal-to-serosal movement of chloride under short-circuit conditions (that is, chloride absorption not secretion) was markedly increased by anoxia.

14
Effects of Aldosterone on the Colon

C. J. EDMONDS

Medical Research Council,
Clinical Research Centre,
Watford Road,
Harrow,
Middlesex

Principal emphasis has been laid on the actions of aldosterone on the kidney, but because of the complexity of the kidney and of its function, a precise delineation of the actions of aldosterone has been difficult to obtain. It has even been difficult to define the exact role that aldosterone plays in the sodium balance as controlled by the kidneys. Furthermore, when aldosterone is given to normal animals for a prolonged period, the renal sodium-retaining effect is only transitory and after a few days 'escape' occurs[1,2]. If however we turn to examining intestinal ionic transport, considerably more useful information about the mode of action of aldosterone can be obtained. Effects are demonstrable on both small intestinal and colonic mucosal epithelium[3-9]. In contrast to the kidney, there is little doubt that intestinal sodium conservation during periods of sodium depletion is largely if not entirely affected through the adrenal–aldosterone system[7,10]. Also when aldosterone is given for a prolonged period, there is no stimulation of 'escape' intestinal sodium absorption for as long as the administration is continued[11,12]. Despite the emphasis that has been laid upon the renal effects, therefore, it is quite conceivable that the primary role of aldosterone in sodium homeostasis may lie in the control of sodium transport across gut epithelia. In the present account, attention is only going to be devoted to colon, with a description of the results of some of our investigations in rat and in man by examining the way in which aldosterone modifies the ionic transport processes of the epithelium.

DIFFERENCES IN IONIC TRANSPORT PROCESSES OF THE EPITHELIUM

Most earlier studies have treated the colon as a single structure with relatively little attention being paid to possible variations along the length of the organ. The colon does however effect two principal operations with regard to salt and water conservation. First, its proximal part must absorb the main bulk of fluid and electrolytes presented to it by the ileum. Secondly, to complete sodium conservation, the ionic composition of the faecal fluid must be appropriately modified before excretion. This means that the distal part of the colon has to create, and maintain, considerable ionic gradients across its epithelium. Analyses of material taken from various regions of the colon demonstrate these different functions in operation[13]. Under normal conditions in the rat, nearly 85% of the fluid and 90% of the sodium presented by the ileum is absorbed in the proximal colon (Figure 14.1). Although the distal colon absorbs

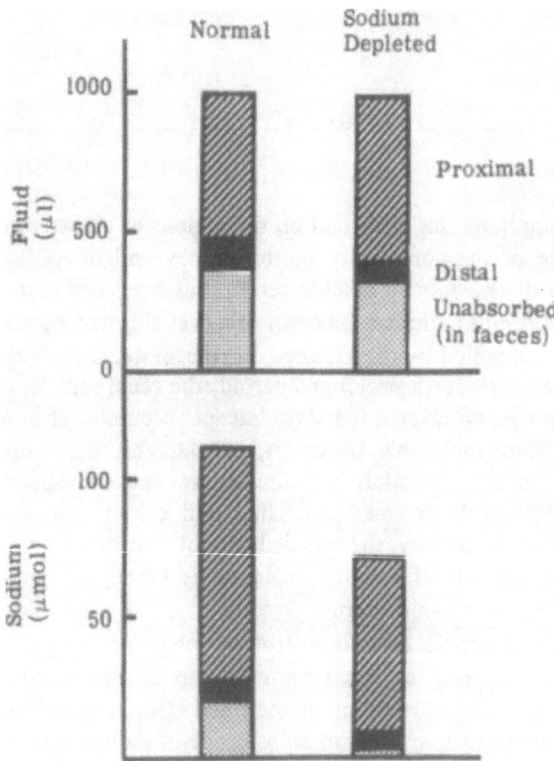

Figure 14.1 Water and sodium absorption by proximal and distal colon in normal and sodium-depleted rats based on analyses of material removed from various regions of the gut[13]. The figure shows the amounts of 1 ml of fluid delivered from the ileum absorbed and excreted in the faeces

relatively little of the sodium with regard to amount, it clearly has to do this against a considerably greater concentration gradient. Absorption studies on individual segments of the gut also show these differences in function[10,14]. In the proximal colon, there is considerable absorption of salts and water when the luminal sodium concentration is relatively high but when it falls below about 60 mmol/l in the rat, sodium and fluid absorptions cease. In the distal colon, absorption continues until a much lower sodium concentration is present in the luminal fluid.

EFFECT OF ALDOSTERONE ON IONIC TRANSPORT AND THE ELECTRICAL PROPERTIES OF PROXIMAL AND DISTAL COLON

Aldosterone stimulates the sodium absorption and potassium secretion mechanisms of both the proximal and distal colon[7,10] but in differing ways (Figure 14.2). Although sodium absorption is stimulated in the proximal colon

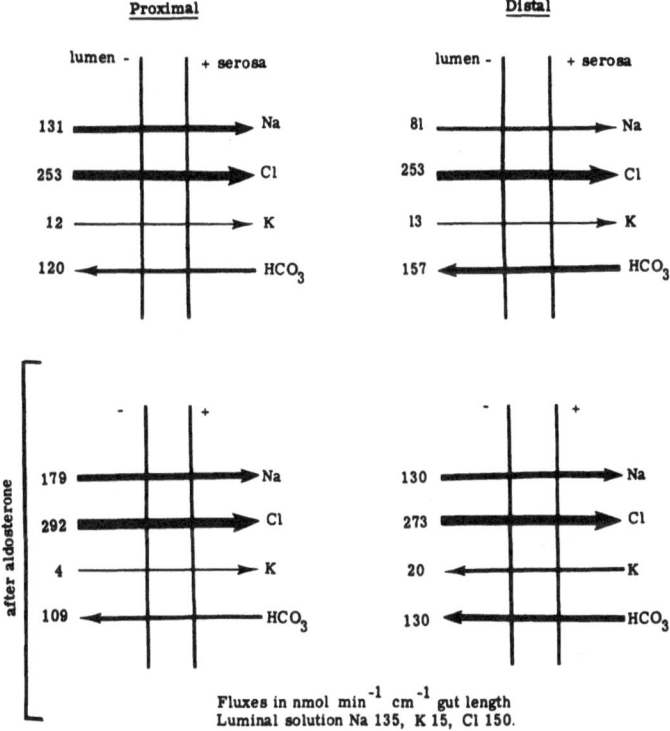

Fluxes in nmol min^{-1} cm^{-1} gut length
Luminal solution Na 135, K 15, Cl 150.

Figure 14.2 The absorption and secretion rates of the principle ions measured *in vivo* in proximal and distal colon of normal and aldosterone-treated rats[10]. In these and subsequent experiments aldosterone was infused at a rate of 50 ng min^{-1} kg^{-1} body weight intravenously for 6 hours

when the luminal sodium concentration is high, the increase in potassium secretion is relatively low, and the increased sodium absorption is largely accompanied by increased chloride absorption. In the distal colon, on the other hand, potassium secretion is stimulated to a much greater extent and, in addition, sodium absorption continues until a much lower luminal sodium concentration is attained. It is this change in epithelial function which is responsible for the very low sodium concentration which is found in the faecal fluid when aldosteronism is present.

The electrical properties of colonic epithelium are also altered by aldosterone and here again there is a difference between the proximal and distal colon[7,13]. Within two to three hours of giving aldosterone, the transepithelial electrical potential difference (PD) rises but the increase is much greater in the distal colon, especially towards its termination (Figure 14.3). Measurements *in vivo* on rat colon have demonstrated that a rise in the short-circuit current accompanies the rise of PD, but that the electrical conductance of colonic epithelium is unaltered by aldosterone[15].

It was mentioned above that aldosterone produces an increased chloride absorption, especially in the proximal colon. Chloride ions appear to move fairly freely across colonic epithelium and the increased chloride absorption associated with aldosterone stimulation may be the result of the increased electrical forces. Bicarbonate is the other principal anion transported by the

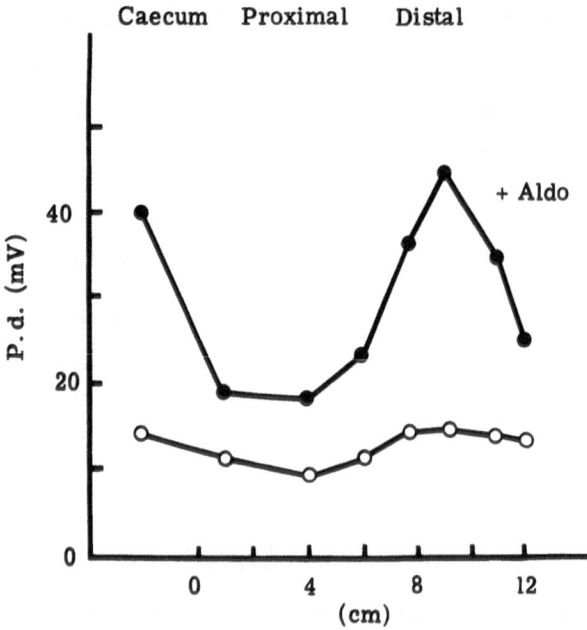

Figure 14.3 The effect of aldosterone on the transepithelial electrical potential difference of rat colon

epithelium, usually being secreted in even larger amounts than potassium, but aldosterone does not appear to have any effect on its secretion[10,14].

MECHANISM OF ACTION OF ALDOSTERONE ON COLONIC EPITHELIUM

Studies on amphibian tissues, such as toad bladder and frog skin, have suggested that the action of aldosterone depends on the production of some proteins (aldosterone-induced proteins, AIP) through an influence on the DNA–RNA–ribosomal system[16,17]. Both the nature of these hypothetical proteins and the way in which they modify the transport processes have not yet been determined. The action of AIP could be through some direct action on the active transport mechanism or indirectly on the mucosal membrane barrier, by increasing its permeability to sodium ions and so allowing greater access of these ions to the pump[18,19]. We have investigated some of these more fundamental aspects of aldosterone action as they occur in the mammalian colon and I shall now summarise some of the findings.

First, using a range of doses of inhibitors which act at various stages of protein synthesis, we were unable to demonstrate more than a minor effect on aldosterone action, as judged by the electrical responses (Figure 14.4). These results may be compared with similar findings for at least some of the effects

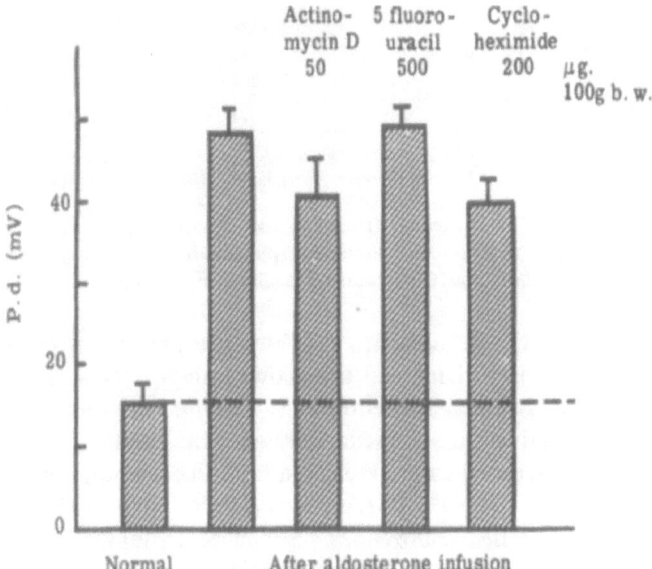

Figure 14.4 The effect of various inhibitors of protein synthesis on the stimulatory action of aldosterone on the transepithelial PD of rat distal colon. (Unpublished observations of Thompson and Edmonds)

of aldosterone which have been observed in studies on both kidney and salivary glands[20,21]. The experiments suggesting that the action of aldosterone is mediated through changes in protein synthesis have been carried out on amphibian tissues and the evidence remains indirect since no defined protein or proteins have been demonstrable. The apparent minor effect of protein synthesis inhibitors on aldosterone action in the mammalian gut does suggest that aldosterone may not here be acting by modulation of protein synthesis.

Secondly, since Na^+-K^+-sensitive ATPase appears generally to be intimately associated with the mechanisms of active sodium transport, one possible mechanism of aldosterone action could be through an increase in the pump

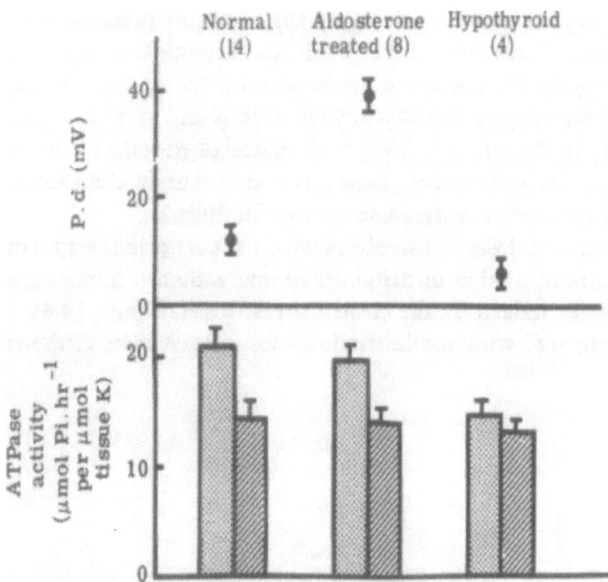

Figure 14.5 The effect of aldosterone treatment and hypothyroidism on the ouabain-sensitive, Na^+-K^+-ATPases of rat colonic epithelium. Epithelial ATPase activity was estimated both with (crosshatched) and without (stippled) the addition of ouabain[22]

ATPase. Certainly, Na^+-K^+-sensitive ATPases are present in colonic epithelium and both their activity and the active transport of sodium are inhibited by ouabain at similar concentrations. Enzyme activities and sodium transport were examined in epithelia derived from normal, aldosterone-treated and sodium-depleted rats[22]. We could find no evidence, however, that aldosterone influenced the Na^+-K^+-sensitive ATPase activity either in short-term experiments or when endogenously produced in longer term sodium depletion, despite demonstrable and considerable rises in sodium absorption (Figure 14.5). This failure to demonstrate an influence of aldosterone contrasted strikingly with the effect of thyroxine which both considerably modified the action of aldosterone on sodium transport and altered the epithelial Na^+–K^+-sensitive ATPase activity. We concluded, therefore, that although, for the stimulation of sodium transport, the epithelium must have adequate pump ATPase available, ordinarily the enzyme activity is more than sufficient to meet the requirements of the increased transport occasioned by aldosterone stimulation, a conclusion that is in general agreement with those reached for other epithelia[23,24,25].

Thirdly, we looked at the possibility that aldosterone increases the permeability of the luminal barrier, which could be the locus of action of the hormone if passage through this barrier was the rate-limiting step in sodium

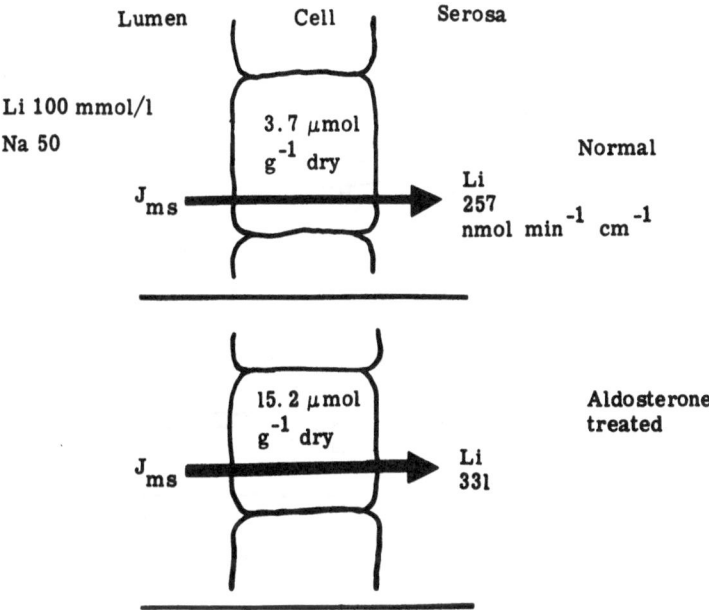

Figure 14.6 The epithelial lithium content and the lithium absorption rate in colonic epithelium of normal and aldosterone-treated rats. During the lithium exposure period of 15 minutes, the lumen contained LiCl 100 mmol/1, NaCl 50 mmol/1. Lithium inhibits sodium absorption by rat colon and the sodium absorption rates were similar in the two groups[27]

absorption. In this so-called 'permease' hypothesis, aldosterone or AIP is viewed as an agent interacting with and modifying the diffusion properties or carriers in the cell membranes on the luminal side of the epithelial cells. Some time ago, in studies on potassium kinetics in intestinal epithelium, we obtained results indicating that in sodium-depleted states, there is increased movement of potassium across the luminal barrier, suggestive of altered potassium permeability[26]. Recently we have carried out experiments using lithium as a probe ion to study permeability[27]. Lithium appears to enter many cells passively in a way similar to that of sodium, but because lithium is often poorly handled by the cation pump, it tends to accumulate in the epithelium[28,29,30]. Lithium absorption rate was measured when a lithium-containing solution was present in the lumen. Subsequently, the lithium content of the epithelial layer was determined after gentle scraping of the epithelium from the underlying muscular layers of the colon. Aldosterone treatment resulted in both a higher lithium absorption rate and a substantial increase in the lithium content of the epithelium (Figure 14.6). The results indicated that aldosterone considerably increased the cation permeability of the luminal barrier consistent with the 'permease' hypothesis.

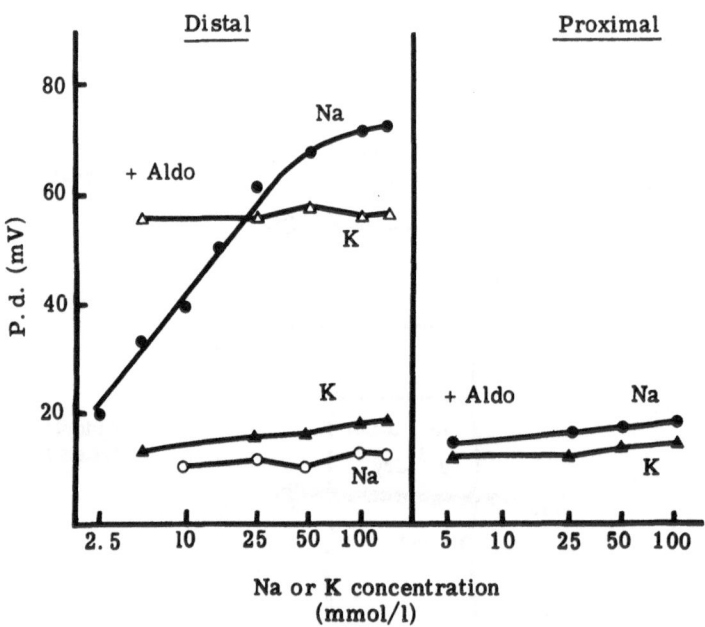

Figure 14.7 Changes of transepithelial PD related to luminal concentration of sodium and potassium in the colon of rats. The anion present was sulphate, mannitol was added to maintain iso-osmolality and the potassium solutions all contained sodium at a constant concentration of 50 mmol/1

Finally, observations on the changes of PD produced by altering the ionic composition of the solution in the gut lumen also provide evidence that some modification of the permeability of the luminal barrier is produced by aldosterone (Figure 14.7). Ordinarily, changing the sodium concentration of the solution has little effect on the transepithelial PD but when the PD is raised by aldosterone administration, the transepithelial PD becomes markedly sensitive to luminal sodium concentration, rapidly changing as the latter is altered[31,32]. Studies with isolated epithelium have shown that it is the mucosal side alone which is sodium-sensitive, since varying the sodium concentration on the serosal side of the epithelium has very little effect on the transepithelial PD[33]. The effect is most obvious in the distal colon where the

PD change with aldosterone is greatest, where the maximal lowering of luminal sodium concentration occurs and where there is the highest rate of potassium secretion.

Conclusion

Although other effects of aldosterone on colonic epithelium may occur, the present observations all suggest that an increase in cation permeability of the luminal barrier is provoked by the hormone. The change is probably of considerable importance for the observed actions of aldosterone on the colon in providing freer access of sodium to the pump and of potassium to the lumen. There are clear differences between the actions of aldosterone on the proximal and distal colon, particularly with regard to the transepithelial PD and potassium secretion but further studies are needed to elucidate these relationships.

SUMMARY

Changes in function of the colon in response to salt depletion are largely modulated through alterations in aldosterone secretion. Animal studies show that the colonic response is not uniform. In the proximal colon, aldosterone increases sodium and chloride absorption with a small increase of potassium secretion, while in the distal colon there is a greater effect on potsssium secretion associated with greater changes in the transmucosal electrical potential difference (PD). Inhibitors of protein synthesis, for example dactinomycin, have little effect on aldosterone action on the colon. Epithelial Na^+-K^+-activated ATPase activity although considerably influenced by thyroid hormones, is unaffected by aldosterone. Using lithium as a probe ion, evidence has been obtained to suggest that aldosterone makes the luminal membrane barrier more permeable to some cations. Such an effect would also be consistent with the behaviour of the transmucosal PD in response to mineralocorticoids, particularly when luminal ionic composition is varied. Present evidence suggests that changes in permeability of the luminal membrane barrier are largely responsible for the effects of aldosterone on the colon.

References

1. Relman, A. S. and Schwartz, W. B. (1952). The effect of DOCA on electrolyte balance in normal man and its relation to sodium chloride intake. *Yale J. Biol. Med.*, **24**, 540
2. August, J. T., Nelson, D. H. and Thorn, G. W. (1958). Response of normal subjects to large amounts of aldosterone. *J. Clin. Invest.*, **37**, 1549
3. Spät, A., Suligo, M., Sture, J. and Solyom, J. (1964). Effect of aldosterone on intestinal transport of sodium and potassium in rats. *Acta Physiol. Acad. Sci. Hung.*, **24**, 465

4. Levitan, R. and Ingelfinger, F. J. (1965). Effect of D-aldosterone on salt and water absorption from the intact human colon. *J. Clin. Invest.*, **44**, 801

5. Shields, R., Mulholland, A. T. and Elmslie, R. G. (1966). Action of aldosterone upon the intestinal transport of potassium, sodium and water. *Gut*, **7**, 686

6. Cofré, G. and Crabbé, J. (1967). Active sodium transport by the colon of Bufo marinus: stimulation by aldosterone and antidiuretic hormone. *J. Physiol. Lond.*, **188**, 177

7. Edmonds, C. J. and Marriott, J. C. (1967). Aldosterone and adrenalectomy on electrical PD of rat colon and on the transport of Na, K, Cl and bicarbonate. *J. Endocr.*, **39**, 517

8. Edmonds, C. J. and Godfrey, R. C. (1970). Electrical potentials of normal human rectum and colon; effect of aldosterone. *Gut*, **11**, 330

9. Noble, H. M. and Matty, A. J. (1971). Adrenal steroids and the electrical potential of rat small intestine *in vivo. J. Endocr.*, **49**, 377

10. Dolman, D. and Edmonds, C. J. (1975). The effect of aldosterone and the reinin–angiotensin system on sodium, potassium and chloride transport by proximal and distal rat colon *in vivo. J. Physiol. Lond.*, **250**, 597

11. Charron, R. C., Leme, C. E., Wilson, D. R., Ing, T. S. and Wrong, O. M. (1969). The effect of adrenal steroids on stool composition as revealed by *in vivo* dialysis of faeces. *Clin. Sci.*, **37**, 151

12. Thompson, B. D. and Edmonds, C. J. (1971). Effects of prolonged aldosterone administration on rat colon and renal electrolyte excretion. *J. Endocr.*, **50**, 163

13. Edmonds, C. J. (1967). Gradient of electrical PD and of sodium and potassium of the gut contents along the caecum and colon of normal and sodium-depleted rats. *J. Physiol. Lond.*, **193**, 571

14. Edmonds, C. J. (1967). Transport of sodium and secretion of potassium and bicarbonate by the colon of normal and sodium-depleted rats. *J. Physiol. Lond.*, **193**, 589

15. Edmonds, C. J. and Marriott, J. C. (1970). Sodium transport and short-circuit current in rat colon *in vivo*; effect of aldosterone. *J. Physiol. Lond.*, **210**, 1021

16. Edelman, I. S. and Fimognari, G. M. (1968). On the biochemical mechanism of action of aldosterone. *Recent Prog. Horm. Res.*, **24**, 1

17. Rousseau, G. and Crabbé, J. (1972). Effects of aldosterone on RNA and protein synthesis in the toad bladder. *Eur. J. Biochem.*, **25**, 550

18. Crabbé, J. (1963). Site of action of aldosterone on the bladder of the toad. *Nature, London*, **200**, 787

19. Sharp, G. W. G. and Leaf, A. (1966). Mechanism of action of aldosterone. *Physiol. Rev.*, **46**, 593

20. Gruber, W. D., Knauf, H. and Frömter, E. (1973). The action of aldosterone on Na^+ and K^+ transport in the rat submaxillary main duct. *Pflügers Arch.*, **344**, 33

21. Wiederholt, M., Schoormans, W., Hansen, L. and Behn, C. (1974). Sodium conductance changes by aldosterone in the rat kidney. *Pflügers Arch.*, **348**, 155

22. Thompson, B. D. and Edmonds, C. J. (1974). Aldosterone sodium depletion and hypothyroidism on the ATPase activity of rat colonic epithelium. *J. Endocr.*, **62**, 489

23. Landon, E. J., Jazab, N. and Forte, L. (1966). Aldosterone and sodium–potassium-dependent ATPase activity of rat kidney membranes. *Amer. J. Physiol.*, **211**, 1050

24. Jørgensen, P. L. (1972). The role of aldosterone in the regulation of $(Na^+ + K^+)$ ATPase in rat kidney. *J. Steroid. Biochem.*, **3**, 181

25. Hill, J. H., Cortas, N. and Walser, M. (1973). Aldosterone action and sodium- and potassium-activated adenosine triphosphatase in toad bladder. *J. Clin. Invest.*, **52**, 185

26. Barnaby, C. F. and Edmonds, C. J. (1969). A miniature GM counter and a whole body counter for the study of potassium kinetics by rat colon. *J. Physiol. Lond.*, **205**, 647

27. Dolman, D., Edmonds, C. J. and Salas-Coll, C. (1975). Effect of aldosterone on lithium permeability of rat colon mucosa. *J. Endocr.* (In press)

28. Zerahn, K. (1955). Studies on the active transport of lithium in the isolated frog skin. *Acta Physiol. Scand.*, **33**, 347

278

29. Skou, J. C. (1957). The influence of some cations on an adenosine triphosphatase from peripheral nerves. *Biochim. Biophys. Acta,* **23**, 394

30. Keynes, R. D. and Swan, R. C. (1959). The permeability of frog muscle fibres to lithium ions. *J. Physiol. Lond.,* **147**, 626

31. Edmonds, C. J. and Marriott, J. C. (1968). Factors influencing the electrical PD across the mucosa of rat colon. *J. Physiol. Lond.,* **194**, 457

32. Archampong, E. Q. and Edmonds, C. J. (1972). Effect of luminal ions on the transepithelial electrical potential difference of human rectum. *Gut,* **13**, 559

33. Edmonds, C. J. and Marriott, J. C. (1968). Electrical potential and short circuit current of an *in vitro* preparation of rat colon mucosa. *J. Physiol. Lond.,* **194**, 479

14

Discussion Paper on

The Effect of Angiotensin on Intestinal Fluid Transport

K. A. Munday and B. G. York

Department of Physiology and Biochemistry,
University of Southampton

Crocker and Munday[1] initially implicated the hormone angiotensin as possibly being involved in the control of salt and water metabolism by the intestine. It was further shown[2] using the everted sac preparation, that all areas of the intestine respond to angiotensin providing that the animals are sensitised to the hormone by prior adrenalectomy and nephrectomy. The response to angiotensin in the distal colon is quite distinct from that following aldosterone administration, since the former stimulates fluid transfer in the absence of any change in transmural PD or resistance[3], whereas aldosterone stimulates an electrogenic process[4]. The presence of a neutral sodium chloride transport process in the intestine has been suggested by Barry *et al.*[5] and more recently by Binder and Rawlins[6]. It is tempting to equate the angiotensin-stimulated process in the intestine with the angiotensin-stimulated second sodium pump of the kidney although the evidence for this is indirect. The work of Ude[7] and Binder and Rawlins[6] suggests that *in vitro*, the neutral sodium pumping process is very metabolically dependent and as the preparation ages, its contribution to the overall sodium transfer decreases. Thus it was of some considerable importance to confirm the angiotensin response in an intestinal preparation *in vivo*. Such a preparation was established and validated[8] and many of the experiments already performed with the preparation *in vitro* were repeated.

The closed sac *in vivo* preparation

Male 300 g Wistar rats were anaesthetised with sodium pentobarbitone. They were tracheotomised, and the right common carotid artery and both femoral veins were cannulated, the former for the measurement of blood pressure and the latter for the infusion of isotonic saline with or without angiotensin. A midline abdominal incision was made and 15 cm jejunum or 6 cm distal colon sacs were prepared, care being taken not to interfere with the intestinal blood vessels. The sacs were filled with Krebs bicarbonate saline, pH 7.4, containing [³H]inulin as a non-absorbable marker. Samples were removed with a syringe at appropriate intervals and assayed for tritium. The sacs were returned to the animals between sampling and isotonic saline was infused for the first time period, and saline with or without angiotensin for the second period. Thus each animal acted as its own control. The total fluid transport was measured by weight and also by the sum of the two infusion periods as measured by the increase in [³H]inulin concentration.

Results obtained with the *in vivo* preparation

Infusion of the hormone angiotensin at low subpressor doses (0.06–6 ng/kg min) stimulates fluid transport some 90% above control rates. As in the distal colon sac *in vitro* and in the kidney *in vivo*[9,10] the hormone showed a dose-dependent effect, in that low doses stimulate and higher pressor infusions inhibit fluid transport[11]. It had been inferred from the responses *in vitro* that the hormone was acting directly, not via a change in blood flow to the intestine. This possibility was tested *in vivo*. Two methods were used to measure blood flow, ^{86}Rb and macroaggregated serum albumin-^{131}I, and no measurable changes in either total blood flow or in the distribution of blood to the different layers of the intestine were observed with high or low doses of angiotensin[12].

The stimulatory response to low doses of angiotensin is prevented by injecting the animals with cycloheximide (2 mg/kg) 5 minutes prior to infusion of the hormone. This dose of cycloheximide inhibits protein synthesis by 94%. Actinomycin D, which inhibits the incorporation of [³H]uridine into RNA, was ineffective, indicating that as in the colon[2]and the kidney[13], some protein synthesis event at the translational level is necessary for the subsequent stimulatory response to angiotensin. It is of interest that the inhibitory response to pressor doses of angiotensin is not inhibited by cycloheximide, suggesting that this is not solely a reversal of the stimulatory response.

A study was also made of the changes in potential difference across the jejunum during the infusion of high and low doses of angiotensin, which demonstrated that both stimulatory and inhibitory responses occur in the absence of changes in transmural PD[14]. This result, together with those obtained from the colon *in vitro* suggests an involvement of an electroneutral Na⁺ transport process. However, as the jejunum is a low resistance tissue and the origin of the transmural PD is disputed, these studies were recently extended to the distal colon *in vivo*, which is a higher resistance tissue. Measurements of colon transmural PD, resistance and short-circuit current were made, while the response to the hormone was monitored by measurement of jejunal fluid transport in the same animals. The distal colon is also sensitive to angiotensin, low infusions stimulating fluid transfer some 180% above controls[15].

Electrical measurements

Transmural potential was measured using a mucosal 3 M KCl–4% agar mucosal electrode and an intraperitoneal agar–saline bridge serosal electrode. The electrodes were connected to a Vibron electrometer via calomel half cells. Short-circuit current (SCC) and resistance were monitored by passing 5-second pulses of direct current between two Ag/AgCl electrodes from a constant current supply in series with a microammeter (Sheffield construction)* to bring the potential to zero. The mucosal current electrode ran the length of the colon sac, and the serosal electrode consisted of a curved silver mesh which fitted round the sac. This arrangement was designed to provide a current field as uniform as possible across the gut wall. Resistance and SCC are quoted in relation to serosal surface area, which was measured by the method of Edmonds and Marriott[16].

Effect of angiotensin on SCC in distal colon *in vivo*

The results obtained are shown in Table *14.1*. Although there is a significant stimulation of jejunal fluid transfer in the presence of angiotensin, there is no change in PD, resistance, or SCC. This result confirms the suggestion that

Table *14.1* Effect of angiotensin on jejunal fluid transport and distal colon SCC, PD, and resistance

	1st period 0.9% saline	2nd period 0.9% saline	P
Fluid transport (ml/g wet wt 30 min)	0.72 ± 0.08	0.61 ± 0.05 (4)	NS
SCC ($\mu A/cm^2$)	100.3 ± 10.3	91.8 ± 10.4	NS
PD (mV)	24.3 ± 1.6	23.0 ± 1.6	NS
Resistance (Ω/cm^2)	242.5 ± 19.2	250.7 ± 20.1	NS
	0.9% saline	Angiotensin (7.0 ng/kg min)	
Fluid transport	0.58 ± 0.11	0.94 ± 0.09 (6)	<0.05
SCC	96.4 ± 8.7	112.4 ± 13.9	NS
PD	20.1 ± 2.0	22.5 ± 2.1	NS
Resistance	200.9 ± 15.3	199.7 ± 15.0	NS

Results are expressed as mean ± SEM; number of observations are in parentheses.

* We wish to thank Professor Smyth, Department of Physiology, University of Sheffield, for supplying the constant current supply and microammeter.

angiotensin stimulates an electroneutral Na^+ transport process. Thus the action of this hormone contrasts with that of aldosterone which stimulates electrogenic Na^+ transport[16]. It should be noted that resistance changes can be demonstrated by our method, since an expected rise in colon resistance *in vivo* with falling body temperature was observed in a series of experiments with hypothermic rats.

DISCUSSION

Angiotensin at physiological concentrations stimulates fluid transport across the rat jejunum and distal colon *in situ*. The action of the hormone appears to be direct, since no changes in intestinal blood flow have been observed under conditions which stimulate and inhibit fluid transport. However, angiotensin is known to cause the release of neurotransmitters from nerve endings and the possibility of this sort of indirect mechanism has not yet been investigated. It would seem that this explanation was improbable since the three most likely candidates, acetylcholine, noradrenaline and adrenaline have actions on the intestine which differ markedly from those of angiotensin. Acetylcholine stimulates electrogenic chloride secretion[17], whereas the stimulation of electrolyte absorption associated with catecholamines is characterised by a fall in SCC — a response which has never been observed with angiotensin[18].

In all of the preparations investigated, angiotensin stimulation of fluid transport is inhibited by cycloheximide, strongly suggesting that a protein synthesis event is a necessary part of the mechanism of the hormone action. It may be relevant that this antibiotic inhibits unidirectional fluxes of Na^+ and Cl^- across the brush border of the ileum[19]. The kinetic interpretation of this observation implicates an inhibition of the synthesis of proteins involved in carrier-mediated transport. One could thus speculate that angiotensin stimulates electroneutral transport via the synthesis of an Na–Cl carrier system. In order to explain the rapid inhibition of the angiotensin response by cycloheximide and also the rapid onset of the response itself, this carrier system would be expected to have a short half-life. James *et al.*[20] have shown that brush-border proteins do indeed show a rapid turnover, a fact that is not inconsistent with this hypothesis.

The absence of a change in SCC during stimulation of fluid movement by angiotensin can be explained either in terms of a second Na^+ pump in which Na^+ and anion movement is tightly coupled or by independent Na^+ and anion transport systems in which ion movements occur at approximately the same rate. The simplest model is coupled NaCl movement from mucosa to serosa. Replacement of Cl^- by SO_4^- abolishes the angiotensin stimulation across rat colon *in vitro* (Munday, Parsons and Evans, unpublished observations).

Furthermore a careful study of ion movements across the isolated rat colon by Binder and Rawlins[6] provides good evidence for the presence of such a neutral NaCl movement. This process is apparently highly dependent on exogenous substrate. Thus the metabolic status of the preparation could be of importance in determining the tissue responsiveness to angiotensin and this may partially explain the anomalous result that the response of the sac preparation *in vitro* to angiotensin is dependent on prior adrenalectomy and nephrectomy while the *in vivo* preparation is not.

The exact nature of the neutral process is uncertain. It may include two separate but related ion exchanges; Na–H and Cl–HCO_3. Such exchanges have also been proposed for the ileum[21]. The location of the process is open to speculation but coupled NaCl carrier transport across the brush border is well characterised[22]. However, our results, together with those of Binder[6], are consistent with the view that Na^+ absorption by the rat colon depends on (*a*) a high-affinity, low-capacity electrogenic pump which is aldosterone-sensitive, and (*b*) a low-affinity, high-capacity electroneutral process which is stimulated by angiotensin.

Acknowledgements

We are pleased to acknowledge the contributions of Miss Jennifer Bolton and Mr Nigel Levens to the experiments described in this article.

References

1. Crocker, A. D. and Munday, K. A. (1970). The effect of the renin–angiotensin system on mucosal water and sodium transfer in everted sacs of rat jejunum. *J. Physiol. Lond.*, **206**, 323
2. Davies, N. T. D., Munday, K. A. and Parsons, B. J. (1972). Studies on the mechanism of action of angiotensin on fluid transport by the mucosa of rat distal colon. *J. Endocr.*, **54**, 483
3. Munday, K. A. and Parsons, B. J. (1971). The action of angiotensin on sodium and fluid transport. In *Glaxo Symposium on Transport Across the Intestine* ed. Burland, W. L. and Samuel, P. D. p. 59 (Edinburgh and London: Churchill Livingstone)
4. Edmonds, C. J. and Marriott, J. C. (1967). The effect of aldosterone and adrenalectomy on the electrical potential difference of rat colon and on the transport of sodium, potassium, chloride and bicarbonate. *J. Endocr.*, **39**, 517
5. Barry, R. J. C., Smyth, D. H. and Wright, E. M. (1965). Short-circuit current and sodium transfer by rat jejunum. *J. Physiol. Lond.*, **181**, 410
6. Binder, H. J. and Rawlins, C. L. (1973). Electrolyte transport across isolated large intestinal mucosa. *Amer. J. Physiol.*, **225**, 1232
7. Ude, J. F. (1973). Relationships between fluid, sodium and non-electrolyte transfer in the rat small intestine. Ph.D. Thesis, Sheffield University
8. Bolton, J. E., Munday, K. A., Parsons, B. J. and York, B. (1975). Effects of angiotensin II on fluid transport, transmural potential difference and blood flow by rat jejunum *in vivo*. *J. Physiol. Lond.* (In press)
9. Bonjour, J. P. and Malvin, R. L. (1969). Renal extraction of PAH, GFR and $U_{Na}V$ in the rat during infusion of angiotensin. *Amer. J. Physiol.*, **216**, 554
10. Davies, N. T. D., Munday, K. A. and Parsons, B. J. (1970). The effect of angiotensin on rat intestinal fluid transfer. *J. Endocr.*, **48**, 39

11. Bolton, J. E., Munday, K. A., Parsons, B. J. and Poat, J. A. (1974). Effects of angiotensin on fluid transport by rat jejunum *in vivo*. *J. Physiol. Lond.*, **241**, 33P

12. Bolton, J. E., Munday, K. A. and Parsons, B. J. (1974). The effects of angiotensin on fluid transport and blood flow in rat jejunum. *J. Physiol. Lond.*, **244**, 27P

13. Munday, K. A., Parsons, B. J. and Poat, J. A. (1972). Studies on the mechanism of action of angiotensin on ion transport by kidney cortex slices. *J. Physiol. Lond.*, **224**, 195

14. Bolton, J. E., Munday, K. A., Parsons, B. J. and York, B. G. (1974). The non-electrogenic nature of angiotensin-stimulated sodium transport. *J. Endocr.*, **63**, 39P

15. Levens, N. R., Munday, K. A. and York, B. (1975). The effect of angiotensin II on fluid transport, transmural PD and resistance in the rat distal colon *in vivo*. *J. Endocr.* (In press)

16. Edmonds, C. J. and Marriott, J. (1970). Sodium transport and short-circuit current in rat colon *in vivo* and the effect of aldosterone. *J. Physiol. Lond.*, **210**, 1021

17. Turnberg, L. A., Isaacs, P. E. T., Corbett, C. L. and Riley, A. R. (1975). *In vitro* behaviour of human jejunum and ileum: response to theophylline and acetylcholine. This proceedings p. 339

18. McColl, I., Field, M. and Silen, W. (1968). Stimulation of electrical absorption from the ileum by epinephrine and norepinephrine. *Gastroenterology*, **54**, 1255

19. Frizzell, R. A., Nellans, H. N., Acheson, L. A. and Schultz, S. G. (1973). The effects of cycloheximide on influx across the brush border of rabbit small intestine. *Biochim. Biophys. Acta*, **291**, 302

20. James, W. P. T., Alpers, D. M., Gerber, J. E. and Isselbacher, K. J. (1971). The turnover of disaccharidases and brush-border proteins in rat intestine. *Biochim. Biophys. Acta*, **230**, 194

21. Turnberg, L. A., Bieberdorf, F. A., Morawski, S. G. and Fordtran, J. S. (1970). Interrelationships of chloride, bicarbonate, sodium and hydrogen transport in the human ileum. *J. Clin. Invest.*, **49**, 557

22. Nellans, H. N., Frizzell, R. A. and Schultz, S. G. (1973). Coupled sodium chloride influxes across brush border of rabbit ileum. *Amer. J. Physiol.*, **225**, 467

Discussion 14

Field: Do you feel that K^+ is actively secreted in the colon either normally or in response to aldosterone? Does aldosterone affect the permeability of the luminal border to K^+?

Edmonds: It is difficult to be sure whether active secretion of potassium is present in the colon and is provoked by aldosterone, as a considerable PD, with the lumen negative is present. It is evident from various studies that PD and K^+-secretion are closely related, but whether K^+-secretion depends on PD remains uncertain. Regarding the second point, we have measured ^{42}K movement from the lumen to the mucosa and this is increased by aldosterone, suggesting increased permeability to potassium also.

Sharp: I should like to make a comment on the results of your experiments which failed to demonstrate an effect of inhibitors of protein synthesis on aldosterone-induced changes in ion movement across the colon. In the absence of data on the effects of the inhibitors on protein synthesis in your preparations, your results cannot be interpreted to mean that aldosterone does not produce its effects on ion transport via the synthesis of a specific protein. The point is of importance, however, and worth following up, because of the fact that aldosterone has been shown to have effects on the handling of potassium which are apparently independent of protein synthesis. Thus the colon may be exhibiting a mechanism of this type. Do you have data on the effects of the inhibitors on protein synthesis and do you have any further comments on this part of your work?

Edmonds: I agree that what can be deduced from inhibitor studies is limited. All we can say is that our results are not what is expected from a nuclear action. They also apply to distal colon only, and this is the section intimately concerned with potassium secretion. Several studies on kidney and salivary glands have suggested that stimulation of potassium secretion by aldosterone is not inhibited by actinomycin, and may involve a different mechanism. Certainly, inhibition of protein production in the colon by our doses of inhibitors needs demonstrating.

Armstrong: In connection with the idea that aldosterone induces production of a permease which, *inter alia*, increases the Na^+ permeability of the brush border, have you tried looking at this with the mucosal uptake technique of Schultz and Curran? (*J. Gen. Physiol.*, **50**, 1241, 1967)

Edmonds: Agreed, the method of Schultz could be useful. Some preliminary experiments that we did on the kinetics of ^{24}Na uptake in the mucosa were not encouraging and so we switched to using lithium as the probe ion.

15
Inhibition of Transport Processes in the Dog Colon

J. W. L. ROBINSON

Département de Chirurgie Expérimentale,
Hôpital Cantonal Universitaire,
Lausanne

INTRODUCTION

The dog colon, unlike that of other mammalian species, is capable of accumulating amino acids and monosaccharides by saturable, Na^+-dependent
transport mechanisms, and of maintaining a significant net transport of these
substrates across isolated sheets of mucosa[1]. In addition, net ion fluxes across
the dog colon mucosa are large in contrast to the corresponding fluxes in the
ileum, where net movements are very small in comparison with the unidirectional fluxes[2]. These two properties render the tissue very amenable to the investigation of the different transport mechanisms in its mucosa.

It is known that the active accumulation of non-electrolytes by many
epithelial tissues[3], including the colon[1], is dependent on the maintenance of
the sodium gradient across the luminal membrane of the epithelial cell; when
this gradient is abolished by a metabolic poison or a specific sodium pump inhibitor, equilibrium uptake of the non-electrolytes is strongly inhibited,
whereas the initial velocity of entry of these substrates into the epithelial cell is
unimpeded, unless the inhibitor acts as the level of the brush-border
membrane[4,5]. This distinction, which we have employed in recent studies on
ion pumps in the small intestine[5] and the kidney[6,7], permits the delineation of
the locus of action of an inhibitor. In the present study, the actions of various
drugs which might be expected to influence ion transport have been examined
indirectly by monitoring their effects on sugar and amino acid accumulation
in strips of mucosa and directly by studying their effects on ion fluxes across
the tissue *in vitro*. The results obtained suggest that the dog colon mucosa
possesses a powerful sodium-pumping mechanism, represented by a $Na^+–K^+$-
ATPase located in the contraluminal membrane of the epithelial cell, which

pumps sodium towards the serosa, this movement being followed by chloride ions and water. The contribution of a hypothetical sodium + chloride secretory pump in the luminal membrane, as described for the colon of the rat[8,9], appears to be minimal in the tissue of the dog.

METHODS

Colons were obtained from healthy mongrel dogs, anaesthetised with pentobarbital. Immediately after removal, they were rinsed and then the mucosa was dissected free of its underlying muscular layers[10]. It was cut into strips for incubation in radioactive amino acid or sugar solutions or into squares for clamping in the flux chambers.

The accumulation of amino acid or sugar was determined exactly as described previously[1]. Mucosal strips were incubated for the desired period in a solution of ^{14}C-labelled L-phenylalanine or β-methyl-D-glucoside dissolved at the required concentration in Krebs bicarbonate buffer. After the incubation,

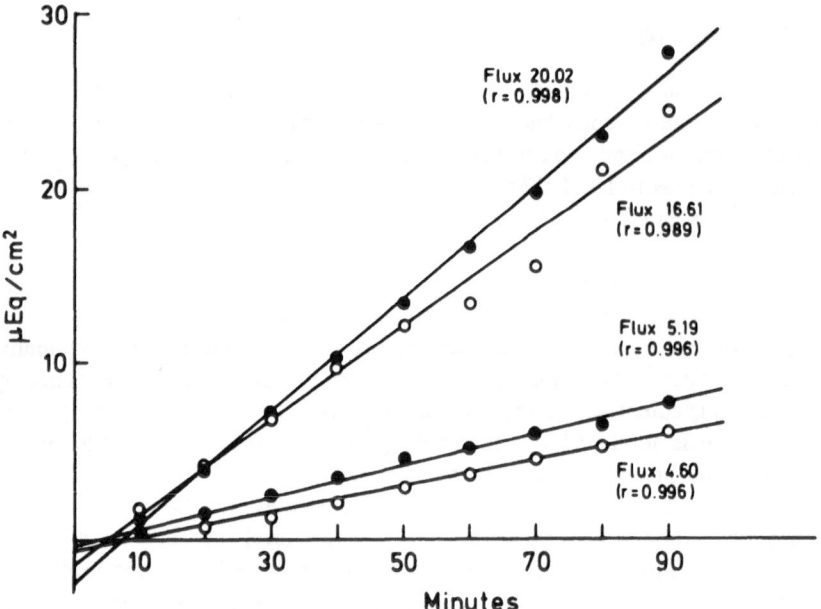

Figure 15.1 Unidirectional fluxes of sodium across sheets of dog colonic mucosa clamped in chambers of different sizes. The points represent the quantity of ion that has appeared in the opposing solution at the appropriate time, corrected for the area of the chamber. Closed circles refer to chambers of surface area 0.64 cm² and open circles to chambers of surface area 3.14 cm². The two upper lines represent the mucosal–serosal fluxes, and the two lower lines, the serosal–mucosal fluxes. The regression lines (with their correlation coefficients stated) have been drawn through the points, and the fluxes, calculated from the slopes, are expressed in μEq/cm² h

the strips were rinsed, blotted, weighed and dissolved in 30% KOH prior to counting in a liquid scintillation spectrometer, in accordance with previously described techniques[11]. Uptakes were expressed in μmoles per unit weight of fresh tissue or as distribution ratios, calculated on the basis of 79.3% (SE = 0.4; $n = 20$) tissue water and 8.6% (SE = 1.1; $n = 20$) extracellular space[1].

Ionic fluxes across sheets of colonic mucosa were studied using different labelling techniques under open-circuit conditions. Flux chambers of different sizes were constructed and compared, and the unidirectional fluxes of sodium were found to be proportional to the surface area of the apertures (Figure 15.1). Furthermore, the fluxes were steady for at least 90 minutes when Krebs bicarbonate buffer containing 0.2% glucose was used as the basic bathing medium. The media were thermostatically controlled with a water jacket and circulated by means of gas-lift system, using 95%/5% O_2/CO_2. For all experiments, except that illustrated in Figure 15.1, chambers of surface area 0.64 cm^2 were employed, and the volume of each compartment was 3.5 ml. The isotope was added to one side of the tissue and 50 μl samples were taken every 10 minutes from the opposite compartment. The flux was then determined from the slope of the regression line describing the rate of appearance of the isotope.

In preliminary experiments, tracer doses of ^{22}Na alone were used for the flux measurements. Later a triple-labelling technique was developed to enable the computation of each unidirectional flux of sodium, and one unidirectional flux of chloride across each individual tissue sample. ^{22}Na and ^{36}Cl were added to one side of the tissue, and ^{24}Na was introduced in the other compartment. Samples were taken over a period of one hour. The ^{24}Na was counted as β-radiation in a liquid scintillation spectrometer using Instagel solvent and a setting which eliminated a high proportion of the contaminating ^{22}Na and ^{36}Cl. The original specific activity of the ^{24}Na was ten times higher than that of the other two isotopes to permit a satisfactory separation. The samples were then allowed to decay for 10 days, and were recounted so that a correction for the contaminating radiation could be applied. The samples taken from the other chamber were counted, after decay of the ^{24}Na, in both β- and γ-counters; the chloride only emits β-radiation, and can thus be readily separated from the ^{22}Na.

The experimental design permitted six parallel chambers to be used in pairs; ^{24}Na was added to the mucosal side in one and to the serosal side in the other. One pair always served as control and so two pairs were then available for the study of the action of drugs. Factorial analyses of variance demonstrated that using this design, there was no bias concerning the flux measurements with the different isotopes of sodium, and that the largest variation was always due to the different tissues.

The preparation of Na$^+$–K$^+$-ATPase from homogenates of colonic mucosa, and its determination in microsomal suspensions were performed exactly as described previously[10].

Statistical evaluation of the uptake experiments was performed by a random block analysis of variance permitting the computation of 'D', the least significant difference between two means[6]. The comparisons of the fluxes were carried out by analyses of variance with replicates, the latter provided by the pairs of chambers, or by factorial analyses comparing the effects of the different variables within the system. Regression analysis was performed by the method of least squares.

RESULTS AND DISCUSSION

There is a net flux of 6–15 μEq/h cm^2 of sodium across isolated dog colonic mucosa (Figure 15.1), this being the difference between a relatively large m–s flux, and a much smaller flux in the opposite direction. Addition of the cardiac glycoside, ouabain, to the serosal medium abolished the net flux of sodium, by reducing the m–s flux to the level of the s–m flux (Table 15.1). This would appear to indicate that a ouabain-sensitive mechanism is solely responsible for the net flux of sodium across the tissue. The results with the triple-labelling experiments (Figure 15.2) confirm the fact that no residual net sodium flux remains in the presence of ouabain.

The uptake of phenylalanine by slices of dog colonic mucosa was strongly inhibited by ouabain; indeed the distribution ratio attained did not differ greatly from unity (Table 15.2). Since the initial velocity of uptake of this amino acid was not inhibited during an incubation of 2 minutes with ouabain (Table 15.3), this result suggests that the drug acts by dissipating the gradient of sodium necessary for the maintenance of active amino acid accumulation. Furthermore, the sensitivity of the phenylalanine transport system in the dog

Table 15.1 Inhibition of sodium unidirectional fluxes across the dog colon mucosa by ouabain, ethacrynic acid and n-butyl-biguanide

Condition	Experiment with ouabain ($n = 5$)	Experiment with ethacrynic acid ($n = 6$)	Experiment with n-butyl-biguanide ($n = 4$)
Control m–s flux	11.4 ± 1.15	11.0 ± 1.56	13.5 ± 0.85
Control s–m flux	5.0 ± 1.01	5.1 ± 0.92	3.9 ± 0.48
m–s flux in presence of inhibitor	5.8 ± 0.52	13.7 ± 1.23	13.8 ± 1.50

The unidirectional flux of sodium across dog colonic mucosa clamped in flux chambers and bathed with Krebs bicarbonate buffer containing 0.2% glucose was determined by following the movement of ^{22}Na. Three parallel measurements were made, namely the flux of sodium from mucosa to the serosa, the opposing unidirectional flux, and the flux from the mucosa to the serosa when the inhibitor (1 mM ouabain, 1 mM ethacrynic acid or 3 mM n-butyl-biguanide) was added to the serosal medium. The results are expressed in μEq/cm$^2 \cdot$ hr, and represent the means ± SEM of the number of experiments shown.

Table 15.2 Inhibition of the uptake of phenylalanine by slices of dog colonic mucosa

Inhibitor	Uptake (μmol/100 mg fresh tissue)	Distribution ratio
None	0.254	3.51
1 mM 2,4-dinitrophenol	0.096	1.33
1 mM ouabain	0.098	1.36
1 mM ethacrynic acid	0.152	2.09
3 mM n-butyl-biguanide	0.236	3.27
$D_{0.05}$	0.053	
$D_{0.01}$	0.073	
$D_{0.001}$	0.099	

Samples were incubated for 1 hour in a solution of 1 mM phenylalanine in Krebs bicarbonate buffer with or without inhibitors. The results are the means of six experiments. Statistical analysis by random-block analysis of variance with computation of 'D', the least significant difference at given probability levels.

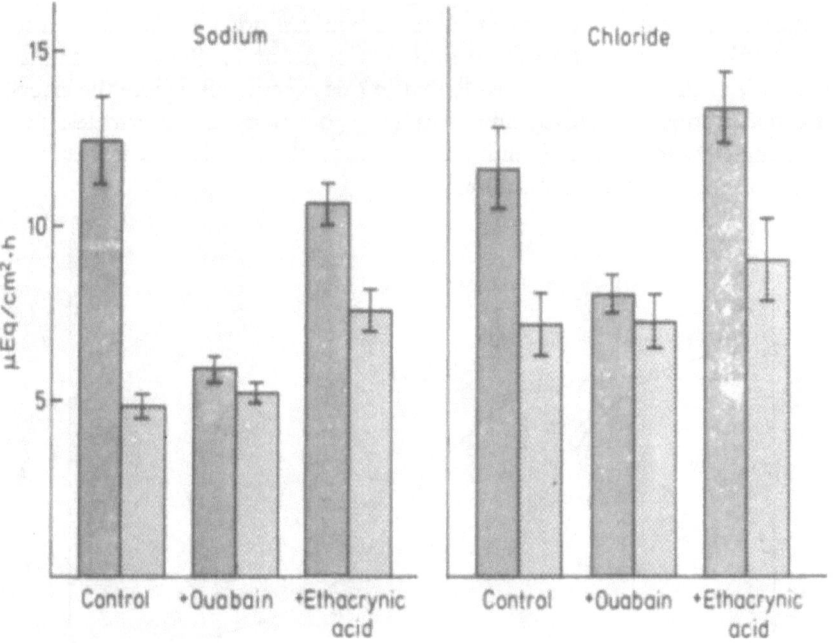

Figure 15.2 Influence of ouabain and ethacrynic acid on the fluxes of sodium and chloride across dog colonic mucosa. Hatched columns represent m–s fluxes and dotted columns s–m fluxes. The experimental design, involving three pairs of chambers, three conditions and three isotopes, is explained in the methodology. Each drug was added at a concentration of 1 mM on both sides of the tissue. The results are the means of nine different colons. In the presence of ouabain, there is no significant difference between the two unidirectional fluxes of either ion. Although ethacrynic acid does not significantly affect the m–s flux of sodium, it increases the s–m flux ($F_{1,24} = 25.5$ according to a factorial analysis of variance, comparing the effect of the drug and also the bias of the isotopes), and very significantly depresses the net flux of sodium ($F_{1,18} = 26.7$ according to a two-way analysis of variance with replicates). Ethacrynic acid also significantly increases the s–m flux of chloride ($F_{1,8} = 11.8$ according to a two-way analysis of variance)

Table 15.3   Lack of effect of ouabain and ethacrynic acid on the initial rate of uptake of phenylalanine by slices of dog colon mucosa

Inhibitor	Influx (μmoles/100 mg *fresh tissue*)
None	0.0229 ± 0.00195
1 mM ouabain	0.0259 ± 0.00386
1 mM ethacrynic acid	0.0259 ± 0.00277
$D_{0.05}$	0.0041
$D_{0.01}$	0.0058

Slices of mucosa, equilibrated with inhibitor-free buffer, incubated for 2 minutes in 1 mM phenylalanine in Krebs bicarbonate buffer. The results are the means of six experiments, presented $\pm$ SEM and with values of the least significant difference.

colon to ouabain is not very different from the sensitivity of its Na$^+$–K$^+$-ATPase to the drug (Figure 15.3); the slight difference encountered in the concentration required for semi-maximal inhibition can probably be ascribed to the difficulty of access of the drug to its site of action on the contraluminal membrane of the epithelial cell. Note that in this experiment, where the external concentration of phenylalanine was lower, ouabain was nevertheless unable completely to abolish all amino acid accumulation, a distribution ratio of two representing a maximal inhibition.

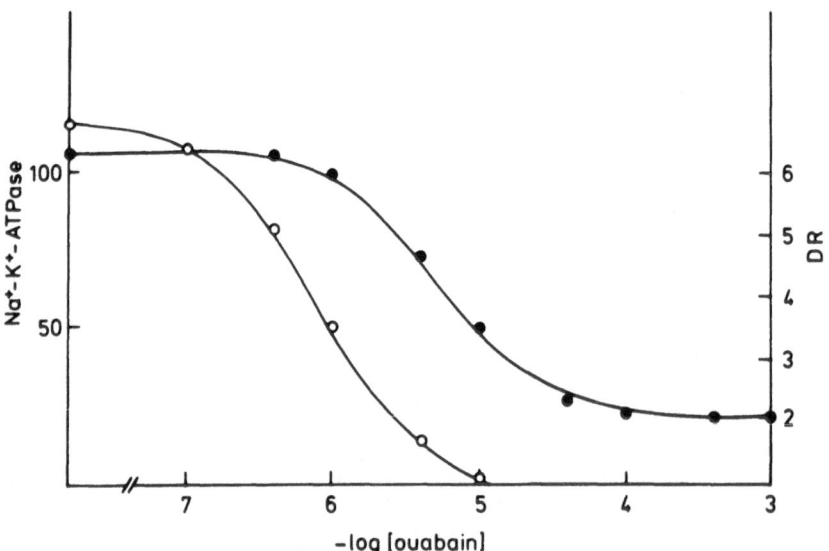

Figure 15.3 Sensitivity to ouabain of phenylalanine uptake by mucosal slices (closed circles) and of Na$^+$–K$^+$-ATPase of microsomal suspensions (open circles) from dog colonic mucosa. Uptake represented as distribution ratio established following one hour's incubation in 0.1 mM phenylalanine. The asymptote of the curve is a distribution ratio of approximately 2, and a 50% inhibition is obtained at a concentration of 5.10^{-6} M ouabain. Na$^+$–K$^+$-ATPase activity, expressed in nmoles phosphate liberated per min and per mg protein, is semi-maximally inhibited at a concentration of 8.10^{-7} M ouabain. Results are the means of six experiments in each case

The inhibitor of sodium movements in the kidney cortex[7], and of various transport systems in the small intestine[5,12], n-butyl-biguanide, does not inhibit either sodium movement across the mucosa (Table 15.1) or phenylalanine uptake in the tissue (Table 15.2). This result is surprising, since the drug is known to enter the cells of the colon[13], and indeed in our hands the ^{14}C-labelled product established a distribution ratio after one hour's incubation of 0.57 ± 0.06 (mean $\pm$SEM, $n = 5$), that is, much larger than the extracellular space of 8.6%. It should therefore be able to exert any general metabolic effects which have been ascribed to it in other tissues[12,14,15].

Ethacrynic acid had no effect on the m–s flux of sodium (Table 15.1), but it nevertheless significantly inhibited phenylalanine uptake by mucosal slices (Table 15.2) without influencing the initial velocity of uptake (Table 15.3). This finding was explained by the triple-labelling experiments, where it was revealed that ethacrynic acid reduced the net flux of sodium across the mucosa by increasing the s–m flux (Figure 15.2). Thus ethacrynic acid appears to increase the membrane permeability of this tissue; such an explanation has in fact been forwarded to explain the action of this drug in other systems[16,17]. If the permeability of a membrane is changed, then the apparent inhibition of phenylalanine uptake, observed in Table 15.2, may in fact be caused by increased efflux of phenylalanine that had already been accumulated in the cells, since the distribution ratio represents an equilibrium between influx and exit from the cells[18]. This point was investigated by preloading mucosal slices with radioactive phenylalanine, and then subjecting them to a second incubation in the presence and absence of ethacrynic acid. It is seen (Figure 15.4) that, as predicted, the efflux of the phenylalanine into the incubation medium is indeed greater in the presence of ethacrynic acid than in its absence. It is not certain which of the two membranes of the epithelial cells is affected by ethacrynic acid, though it is possible that the drug acts from an intracellular locus, since the ^{14}C-labelled compound rapidly equilibrates with the intracellular water.

The effect of other drugs known to affect sodium transport in the rat colon has also been investigated in the dog colonic mucosa using the triple-labelling technique (Figures 15.5 and 15.6). Oxyphenisatin, which increases the blood-lumen flux of sodium in the rat colon in vivo[19], has no effect on transmural sodium fluxes across the dog colon in vitro. Acetazolamide (Diamox), a potent inhibitor of sodium and chloride flux from the mucosa to the serosa in the rat colon in vitro[8], was inactive in the corresponding tissue of the dog. Dibutyryl-cyclic AMP has been shown to stimulate sodium and water transport across everted sacs of rat colon[20], but this substance is ineffective in the dog colon.

Finally, theophylline has been reported to stimulate chloride secretion and to abolish net sodium absorption in the rat colon[9]. In our experiments, there was still a significant net flux of both sodium and chloride in the m–s direction in the presence of theophylline, though this drug did induce a small but significant increase in the s–m flux of sodium and a consequent diminution of the net flux of this ion. This result suggests that there is an important species

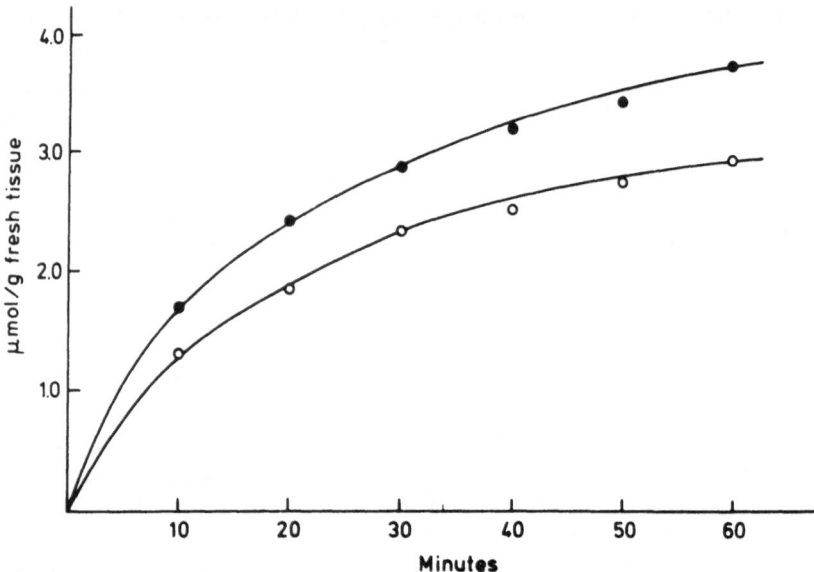

Figure 15.4 Influence of ethacrynic acid on the rate of efflux of phenylalanine from preloaded dog colonic mucosal slices. Tissues were preincubated for 1 hour in 2 mM phenylalanine, and were then transferred to an amino acid-free buffer with or without 1 mM ethacrynic acid. Results are the means of six animals. The efflux in presence of ethacrynic acid (upper curve) is significantly greater than the control ($F_{1,60} = 13.7$, according to a two-way analysis of variance with replicates, considering the times and the conditions as the two entries, and the different animals as the replicates)

difference between the rat on the one hand, and the dog and the human on the other; the latter two species possess colons that are also unaffected by cholera toxin[21-23], as would be expected in view of the lack of influence of dibutyryl-cyclic AMP and the minimal effect of theophylline. Binder and Rawlins[9] have argued that the mucosa of the rat colon possesses both absorptive and secretory sodium pumps, in analogy with the small intestine[24], the former being mediated by a Na^+–K^+-ATPase and the latter being dependent in some way on cyclic AMP and stimulated by theophylline and cholera toxin. The contribution of such a secretory pump in the regulation of ion transport in the colon of the dog appears to be minimal under the conditions of the present experiments.

It can be seen from the results presented in Figures 15.5 and 15.6 that wherever a sodium flux is affected by a drug, the corresponding chloride flux is altered concomitantly. In addition, there is a good correlation between sodium and chloride fluxes across the dog colon mucosa in both directions, the slope of the regression line being close to unity, and the intercept being near the origin (Figure 15.7). This correlation is also maintained in the presence of the inhibitors tested. Thus it would appear that the chloride ion follows the

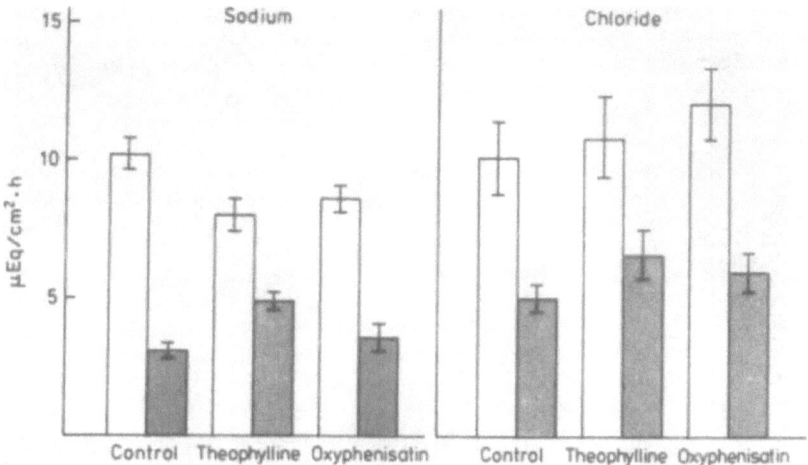

Figure 15.5 Influence of theophylline and oxyphenisatin on the fluxes of sodium and chloride across dog colonic mucosa. Triple-labelling experiment, open columns m–s flux; hatched columns s–m flux; means of seven experiments. Theophylline (10 mM) or oxyphenisatin (0.5 mM, dissolved first in ethanol and then diluted with buffer) added to both sides of the tissue. The only significant effect of either drug concerns the stimulation of the s–m flux of sodium by theophylline ($F_{1,14} = 16.6$ according to two-way analysis of variance with replicates), and the consequent reduction in net flux of sodium by this drug ($F_{1,14} = 14.6$)

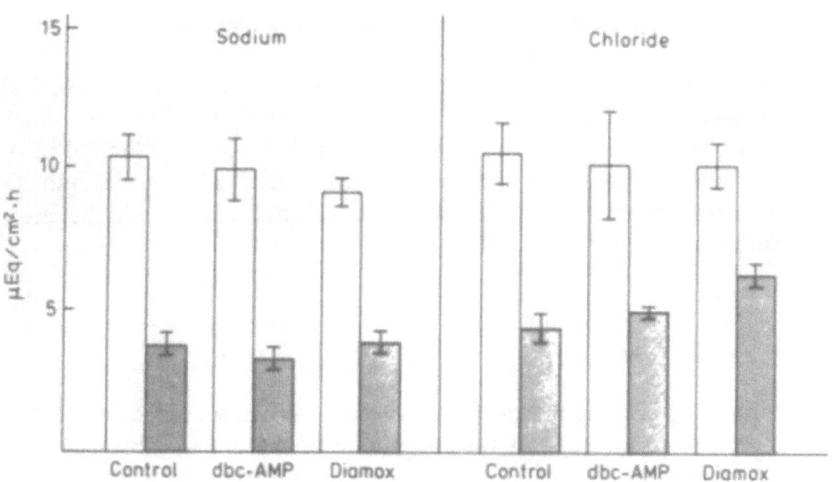

Figure 15.6 Influence of dibutyryl-cyclic AMP and diamox on the fluxes of sodium and chloride across dog colonic mucosa. Triple-labelling experiment, with representation as in Figure 15.5; means of nine experiments. Diamox (10 mM) or dbcAMP (1 mM) added to both sides of the tissue. No flux is significantly different from the control series

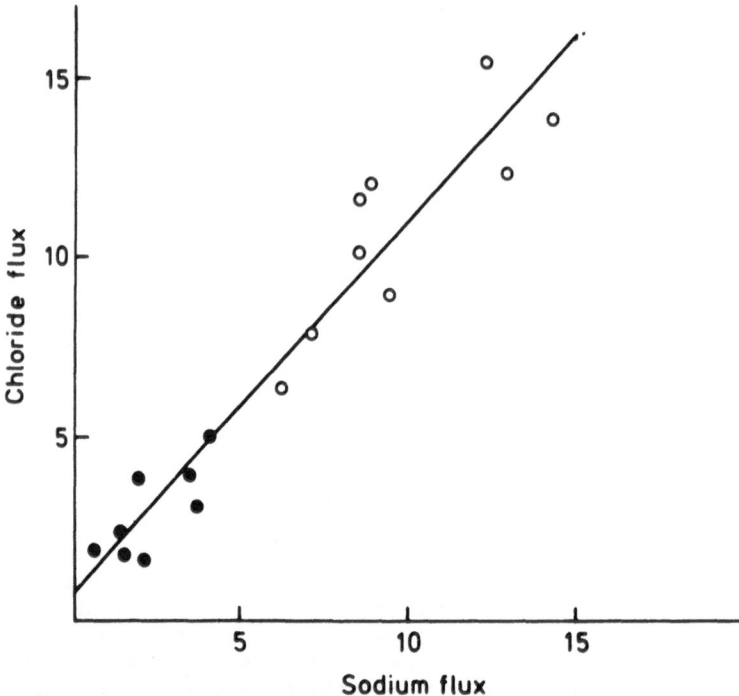

Figure 15.7 Correlation between the flux of sodium and the flux of chloride across dog colonic mucosa in a triple-labelling experiment. Open circles represent m–s fluxes and closed circles the s–m fluxes. The regression lines concerning the two separate fluxes do not differ significantly, and the correlation concerning the two series of fluxes together is highly significant ($r = 0.959$), with a slope of 1.03 and an intercept on the ordinate of 0.74

sodium ion passively in response to the active transport of the latter. This finding would agree with the premise that the dog colonic mucosa simply possesses one sodium pumping mechanism, a Na^+–K^+-ATPase located in the contraluminal membrane of the epithelial cell which exchanges sodium for potassium and induces a simultaneous flux of chloride and water in the serosal direction.

CONCLUSIONS

The existence of a sodium-dependent transport mechanism for amino acids in the dog colonic mucosa, and the magnitude of the net ion flux across its mucosa, permit the application of different tests to investigate the sodium-transporting systems of this tissue. The results agree that the vast majority of the sodium transport is mediated by means of a serosa-facing Na^+–K^+-ATPase, inhibited by ouabain. Two fragments of evidence testify to the existence of a small component of sodium extrusion which is independent of this enzyme, namely the establishment of a distribution ratio for the amino acid greater than unity despite the presence of concentrations of ouabain which would inhibit all $Na^+–K^+$-ATPase activity, and the slight stimulation of the sodium flux in the mucosal direction by theophylline. There is no evidence in favour of a second sodium pump, refractory to ouabain, but inhibited by ethacrynic acid and n-butyl-biguanide, analogous to that described in kidney cortex slices[6,7,25,26].

Acknowledgements

This work was supported by the Fonds National Suisse. The skilful technical assistance of Mme H. Capt and Mlles C. Brandt, D. Mettraux and U. Pässler is gratefully acknowledged. The [¹⁴C]n-butyl biguanide was kindly supplied by Dr R. Beckmann (Chemie Grünenthal) and the [¹⁴C]ethacrynic acid by Dr J. E. Baer (Merck, Sharp and Dohme).

References

1. Robinson, J. W. L., Luisier, A. -L. and Mirkovitch, V. (1973). Transport of amino acids and sugars by dog colonic mucosa. *Pflügers Arch. Europ. J. Physiol.*, **345**, 317
2. Powell, D. W., Binder, H. J. and Curran, P. F. (1972). Electrolyte secretion by the guinea-pig ileum *in vitro. Amer. J. Physiol.*, **223**, 531
3. Schultz, S. G. and Curran, P. F. (1970). Coupled transport of sodium and organic solutes. *Physiol. Revs.*, **50**, 637
4. Robinson, J. W. L. and Vannotti, A. (1966). Étude de l'absorption intestinale des acides aminés en physiopathologie. *Schweiz. Med. Wschr.*, **96**, 1002
5. Luisier, A. -L. and Robinson, J. W. L. (1973). Inhibition of intestinal sugar and amino acid transport by *n*-butyl-biguanide. In L. Bolis, K. Schmidt-Nielsen and S. H. P. Maddrell (eds). *Comparative Physiology*, pp. 465–475. (Amsterdam: North-Holland Publ. Co.)
6. Robinson, J. W. L. (1972). The inhibition of glycine and β-methylglucoside transport in dog kidney cortex slices by ouabain and ethacrynic acid: Contribution to the understanding of sodium-pumping mechanisms. *Comp. Gen. Pharmacol.*, **3**, 145
7. Robinson, J. W. L. and Luisier, A. -L. (1973). Inhibition of renal sugar and amino acid transport by *n*-butyl-biguanide. *Naunyn-Schmiedeberg's Arch. Pharmak.*, **278**, 23
8. Binder, H. J. and Rawlins, C. L. (1973). Electrolyte transport across isolated large intestinal mucosa. *Amer. J. Physiol.*, **225**, 1232
9. Binder, H. J. and Rawlins, C. L. (1973). Effect of conjugated dihydroxy bile salts on electrolyte transport in rat colon. *J. Clin. Invest.*, **52**, 1460
10. Robinson, J. W. L., Rausis, C., Basset, P. and Mirkovitch, V. (1972). Functional and morphological response of the dog colon to ischaemia. *Gut*, **13**, 775
11. Robinson, J. W. L. and Felber, J. -P. (1965). Compartments of the uptake of amino acids by intestinal fragments during *in vitro* incubation. *Gastroenterologia (Basel)*, **104**, 335
12. Caspary, W. F. and Creutzfeldt, W. (1973). Inhibition of intestinal amino acid transport by blood sugar lowering biguanides. *Diabetologia*, **9**, 6
13. Yoh, Y. -J. (1967). Distribution of *n*-butyl-biguanide-¹⁴C hydrochloride in mouse tissues. *Jap. J. Pharmacol.*, **17**, 439

14. Berger, W. (1969). Vues actuelles sur le mécanisme d'action des biguanides. *Méd. Hyg.* (*Genève*), **27**, 1034

15. Bloch, R., Menge, H., Schaarschmidt, W. D., Gottesbüren, H., Schaumlöffel, E. and Riecken, E. O. (1973). Biochemische, histochemische, histologische und funktionelle Untersuchungen zur Phenforminwirkung auf die Dünndarmschleimhaut bei Ratte und Mensch. *Klin. Wschr.*, **51**, 235

16. Chez, R. A., Horger, E. O. and Schultz, S. G. (1969). The effect of ethacrynic acid on sodium transport by isolated rabbit ileum. *J. Pharmacol. Exp. Therap.*, **168**, 1

17. Wolf, K., Bieg, A. and Fülgraff, G. (1969). On the mode of action of diuretics. II. Effects of ethacrynic acid on renal oxygen consumption and renal sodium reabsorption in dogs. *Europ. J. Pharmacol.*, **7**, 342

18. McNamara, P., Rea, C. and Segal, S. (1971). Sugar transport: Effect of temperature on concentrative uptake of α-methylglucoside by kidney cortex slices. *Science*, **172**, 1033

19. Nell, G., Overhoff, H., Forth, W. and Rummel, W. (1973). The influence of water gradients and oxyphenisatin on the net transfer of sodium and water in rat colon. *Naunyn-Schmiedeberg's Arch. Pharmak*, **277**, 363

20. Hornych, A., Meyer, P. and Milliez, P. (1973). Angiotensin, vasopressin and cyclic AMP: Effects on sodium and water fluxes in rat colon. *Amer. J. Physiol.*, **224**, 1223

21. Sack, R. B., Carpenter, C. C. J., Steenburg, R. W. and Pierce, N. F. (1966). Experimental cholera: A canine model. *Lancet*, **ii**, 206

22. Swallow, J. H., Code, C. F. and Freter, R. (1968). Effect of cholera toxin on water and ion fluxes in the canine bowel. *Gastroenterology*, **54**, 35

23. Love, A. H. G., Phillips, R. A., Rohde, J. E. and Veall, N. (1972). Sodium–ion movement across intestinal mucosa in cholera patients. *Lancet*, **ii**, 151

24. Field, M. (1974). Intestinal secretion. *Gastroenterology*, **66**, 1063

25. Herms, W. und Kersting, F. (1969). Die Wirkung von Diuretika auf Natrium- und Kaliumkonzentrationen sowie Sauerstoffverbrauch von kaliumverarmten Nierenrinderschnitten. *Z. Ges. Exp. Med.*, **149**, 13

26. Whittembury, G. and Proverbio, F. (1970). Two modes of Na extrusion in cells from guinea-pig cortex slices. *Pflügers Arch. Europ. J. Physiol.*, **316**, 1

Discussion 15

Smith: Does the presence of galactose or phenylalanine stimulate the transport of Na^+ and does it affect the bioelectric parameters of the dog colon?

Robinson: We have not yet measured the bioelectric parameters; as for the stimulation of Na^+ transport, we have shown no significant effect, but it might have been masked by the large variation between parallel chambers.

Field: How important quantitatively is amino acid absorption by canine colon when compared to absorption in canine small bowel?

Robinson: Net transmural phenylalanine flux is about 60 μmol cm^{-2} h in the colon and 300 μmol cm^{-2} h in the guinea-pig ileum, according to our own measurements. Distribution ratios of about six in the dog colon and 18 in the dog ileum are established following incubation of mucosal slices for one hour in 0.1 mM phenylalanine.

Matuchansky: You have shown on one hand that ethycrinic acid stimulates the serosal–to–mucosal flux across the dog colon; on the other hand, you have also shown that theophylline stimulates the same flux, though not to the same extent. Did you investigate the effect of ethacrynic acid on theophylline-induced flux, since ethacrynic acid has been shown *in vitro* to reverse the cAMP- and particularly the theophylline-stimulated secretion.

Robinson: No, the stimulation by theophylline was very small, and it would have been difficult to show an effect of an inhibitor on this small stimulation.

Caspary: Is the effect of ethacrynic acid on increasing efflux specific for the colon or can it also be observed in the small intestine?

Robinson: We have not tried it, but intuitively I suspect it is specific for the colon.

Parsons: I should like to know whether bicarbonate was present in your experiments. The colon secretes bicarbonate from blood to lumen if ammonium ion is not present in the lumen.

Robinson: Yes, we used bicarbonate buffer.

Binder: The failure to observe an effect of theophylline on colonic ion transport is reminiscent of the failure to see an effect of cyclic AMP on gastric secretion in the dog. Have you measured cyclic AMP levels after theophylline?

Robinson: No!

16
Adaptive Changes in Ion and Water Transport Mechanism in the Eel Intestine

T. HIRANO, M. MORISAWA, M. ANDO and S. UTIDA

Laboratory of Physiology, Ocean Research Institute,
University of Tokyo, Nakano, Tokyo

INTRODUCTION

Living in aquatic environments with a wide range of salt concentration, teleost fishes are known to maintain their osmotic pressure and electrolyte concentrations at levels largely independent of the salinity of their environment. Freshwater teleosts, which are hyperosmotic to the environment, tend to gain water by osmosis. They drink little water and the kidneys have the task of removing excess water. In contrast, seawater teleosts constantly face a pressing problem in water conservation because of their hypertonic environment. In order to replace the osmotic loss of water, they drink surrounding sea water and absorb water with monovalent ions from the intestine. The excess sodium and chloride ions are extruded by the gill, leaving osmotically free water in the body[1-4].

Most species of fish are stenohaline and have only a limited ability to move between fresh water and sea water, while others, euryhaline species, can adapt more readily to either type of solution. The osmotic adjustments by euryhaline fishes are particularly suitable to the study of adaptation of intestinal ion and water transport. We have been using mainly the Japanese cultured eel, *Anguilla japonica*, as experimental material. This fish is able to tolerate changes in the environment from fresh water to sea water or *vice versa*. In this paper, the functional changes in the intestine during the course of seawater adaptation of the eel are considered in relation to the process of ion and water absorption as well as the possible mode of actions of hormones.

CHANGES IN ION AND WATER ABSORPTION DURING SEAWATER ADAPTATION

During the course of seawater adaptation of the eel, Oide and Utida[5] observed a correlated change in the rate of water ingestion and of body weight loss. About 75% of the sea water that is imbibed is absorbed into the body fluid. The rate of drinking appears to relate directly to the need to replace the osmotic loss of water. In the European eel, *Anguilla anguilla*, Maetz and Skadhauge[6] similarly observed an increased rate of drinking with adaptation to higher external salinities. We have recently analysed internal and external factors affecting water ingestion in the eel and shown that drinking is regulated by the changes in extracellular fluid volume and plasma NaCl concentration, and by distension of the stomach and the intestine[7]. The eel is also known to drink immediately after transfer to sea water without any change in internal osmotic pressure or ion concentrations[8,9]. The chloride ion in sea water is responsible for this immediate drinking[7].

Since the ingested sea water is hypertonic to the body fluid, it is generally accepted that the sea water is first diluted and subsequent reabsorption of water follows as a consequence of ionic absorption[1]. When sea water is introduced into the isolated intestine of *A. japonica*, water first enters the gut lumen passively and then the flow of water is reversed. The ability of the intestine to reverse water flow and to start absorption is earlier in the intestine isolated from seawater eels than that from freshwater eels[10]. A similar observation was also made by Skadhauge[11] in the perfused intestine of *A. anguilla*, and the osmolality of the perfusion fluid which corresponds to zero net flow of water (the turning-point osmolality) is higher than plasma osmolality by 73 mosmol in freshwater eels and 126 mosmol in seawater fish. In the eel, however, the ingested sea water seems to be diluted before it reaches the intestine. In a recent report, Skadhauge[12] has shown that the osmolality of luminal fluid taken from the upper end of the anterior intestine is about 460 mosmol, corresponding to about half-strength sea water; the concentration of NaCl is about one-fourth that of sea water. According to Kirsch and Laurent[13], the swallowed sea water is already diluted to two-thirds or one-half during passage through the oesophagus. Further dilution seems to occur in the stomach. Our recent observation[14] indicates that the oesophagus of seawater eels is highly permeable to Na^+ and Cl^- ions but not to water, whereas that of freshwater eels is almost impermeable to both ions and water (Table 16.1). Thus the ingested sea water seems to be 'diluted' or desalted in the oesophagus and the stomach by simple diffusion of ions without causing any loss of body fluid. Considering the turning-point osmolality of the seawater eel intestine[11,12], which corresponds almost to 50% sea water, there may not be any inflow of water into the intestinal lumen.

However, the process of absorption of ions and water across the fish intestine has been studied only recently. The movement of ions and water from

Table 16.1 Effects of environmental salinity on permeability to ion and water in the isolated oesophagus of the eel

Adaptation	Net Na$^+$ flux (μEq/cm^2 h)	Net Cl$^-$ flux (μEq/cm^2 h)	Net H$_2$O flux (μEq/cm^2 h)
Fresh water	1.63 ± 0.135	4.51 ± 1.909	−1.31 ± 0.243
Sea water	20.56 ± 2.393†	24.57 ± 3.097†	−1.08 ± 0.643

(mean ± SE n = 5)

* Sea water was enclosed in the lumen, and the oesophagus was incubated in Ringer solution for 1 hour. Positive value indicates the movement from the lumen to serosa, and the negative flux from serosa to lumen.
† Significantly (p < 0.005) different from the freshwater value.

mucosa to serosa was first shown by House and Green[15,16] in the isolated intestine of the marine teleost, *Cottus scorpius*. The rate of intestinal salt and water absorption in goldfish[17] is several times lower than in *Cottus*, and the difference is ascribed to the need of marine teleosts to absorb more water in sea water. When the intestine is isolated from *A. japonica* and bathed on both sides with identical Ringer solution, net water movement is observed to occur from mucosa to serosa, and the rate of water absorption increases during seawater adaptation[18,19]. A similar augmentation of water absorption is observed in the everted intestine[20], and the amount of water absorbed from the everted preparation is almost identical to that of the normal sac. The increase in water absorption during seawater adaptation is accompanied by an increase in net movement of Na$^+$ and Cl$^-$ ions, and concentrations of these ions in the fluid passing through the membrane decrease as the absorption rates of the ions and water increase, although the concentrations are still higher than that of Ringer solution[4,18] (Table 16.2). This indicates that in the seawater eel intestine, more water is absorbed with the same quantity of the ions than in the freshwater eel, thus fulfilling one of the physiological requirements of the fish in sea water. Skadhauge and Maetz[21] and Skadhauge[11,12] also reported a similar augmentation of water absorption *in vivo* in the intestine of *A. anguilla* perfused with dilute sea water. Skadhauge[11,12] further showed an important role of solute (NaCl)-linked water flow in the process of water absorption in

Table 16.2 Effects of environmental salinity on ion and water movements in the isolated intestine of the eel*

Adaptation	No. of eels	Net influx (mucosa–serosa)			Conc. of the absorbate	
		H$_2$O (μl/cm^2 h)	Na$^+$ (μEq/cm^2 h)	Cl$^-$ (μEq/cm^2 h)	Na$^+$ (mEq/1)	Cl$^-$ (mEq/1)
Fresh water	7	6.3 ± 1.3	1.7 ± 0.40	2.0 ± 0.36	285 ± 24	332 ± 39
Sea water	6	39.6 ± 7.6†	7.2 ± 1.37†	6.7 ± 1.38†	181 ± 2†	168 ± 4†

(mean ± SE)

* The intestinal sac (not everted) was bathed on both sides with identical Ringer solution (Na$^+$, 151 mEq/1; Cl$^-$, 138 mEq/1).
† Significantly (p < 0.01) different from the freshwater value.

the eel intestine, although he did not find any difference in NaCl concentration of absorbate between the intestine of the seawater eel and that of the freshwater eel.

Under natural conditions, the Japanese yellow eel transforms into a silver eel in autumn and migrates to the sea. After transfer of these eels to sea water, the body weight decrease is significantly lower in silver eels than in yellow eels, indicating an increased tolerance of the silver eels to sea water[22]. A higher rate of intestinal water movement is observed in the migrating silver eel from the river as compared with the rates in yellow or cultured eels in fresh water[18,22]. Even in eels cultured in freshwater ponds, which do not turn silver in autumn, intestinal water movement tends to become higher in the migratory season than in other seasons[23]. Both the premigratory adaptive change in the silver eel intestine and the seasonal variation in the cultured eel suggest the presence of control mechanisms, probably by hormones, for intestinal absorption.

CHLORIDE PUMP AND WATER ABSORPTION IN THE SEAWATER EEL INTESTINE

In order to clarify the correlation between NaCl pumping ratio and water transfer, the electrical potential difference (PD) and short-circuit current (I_{sc}) were estimated in the eel intestine mounted in an Ussing chamber[24–26]. In freshwater eels, PD and I_{sc} across the intestine bathed on both sides with identical Ringer solution are nearly zero or slightly serosa-negative to the mucosa, the posterior half being more electronegative than the anterior half. When eels are adapted to sea water for a week, the negativity of the PD and I_{sc} increases markedly in the posterior intestine, suggesting the development of a Cl^- pump during seawater adaptation. The presence of a Cl^- pump was further confirmed by measuring unidirectional fluxes of ^{22}Na and ^{36}Cl in the posterior intestine under short-circuited conditions[25]. In freshwater eels influx from mucosa to serosa ($\mathcal{J}_{ms}$) and efflux ($\mathcal{J}_{sm}$) are both greater for Na^+ ions than for Cl^- ions, $\mathcal{J}_{ms}$ being always greater than $\mathcal{J}_{sm}$ for both ions. The net influxes of these ions are almost identical, corresponding to the near-zero values of PD and I_{sc} in the freshwater eel intestine. After transfer of the eel to sea water for a week, unidirectional fluxes of Na^+ and Cl^- ions increase considerably in both directions as compared with those of freshwater eels. The net influx of Cl^- ions also increases twofold, while that of Na^+ ions shows no appreciable change. The difference between the net fluxes of Cl^- and Na^+ ions is in agreement with the value calculated from I_{sc} in seawater eels (Table 16.3). This strongly suggests that seawater adaptation of the eel specifically induces the Cl^- pump, the Na^+ pump remaining unchanged.

The presence of a Cl^- pump in the seawater eel intestine was also confirmed by the reversal of the PD and I_{sc} after replacement of the NaCl Ringer

Table 16.3 Effect of environmental salinity on potential difference (PD), short-circuit current (I_{sc}) and sodium and chloride fluxes in the posterior intestine of the eel

Adaptation	PD (mV)	I_{sc} (μA/cm²)	Ion fluxes* (μEq/cm² h)						
			J^{Na}_{ms}	J^{Na}_{sm}	J^{Na}_{net}	J^{Cl}_{ms}	J^{Cl}_{sm}	J^{Cl}_{net}	J_{diff}
Fresh water	−0.53 ±0.25(15)	−4.2 ±2.2(15)	5.0 ±0.4(4)	3.7 ±0.3(5)	1.3	3.0 ±0.3(4)	1.2 ±0.4(5)	1.8	−0.5
Sea water	−2.46 ±0.28(14)†	−42.3 ±4.7(14)†	8.4 ±0.4(8)†	6.9 ±0.4(8)†	1.5	5.4 ±0.4(8)‡	2.3 ±0.2(8)‡	3.1	−1.6

(mean ± SE)

* J_{ms}, Mucosa-to-serosa flux; J_{sm}, serosa-to-mucosa flux; $J_{net} = J_{ms} - J_{sm}$; $J_{diff} = J^{Na}_{net} - J^{Cl}_{net}$
†,‡ Significantly different from the freshwater value at 0.1 and 5% levels, respectively

solution with Na_2SO_4–Ringer and by a high negative PD and I_{sc} after replacement with choline Cl-Ringer (Figure 16.1). Similar results were reported in the flounder intestine by Huang and Chen[27]. Another important change following seawater adaptation of the eel is a decrease in the tissue resistance. In accordance with the increased unidirectional fluxes of Na^+ and Cl^- ions, the tissue resistance of the intestine decreases from 88 Ωcm^2 in freshwater eels to 61 Ωcm^2 after 1 week in sea water and to 36 Ωcm^2 after 1 month[25].

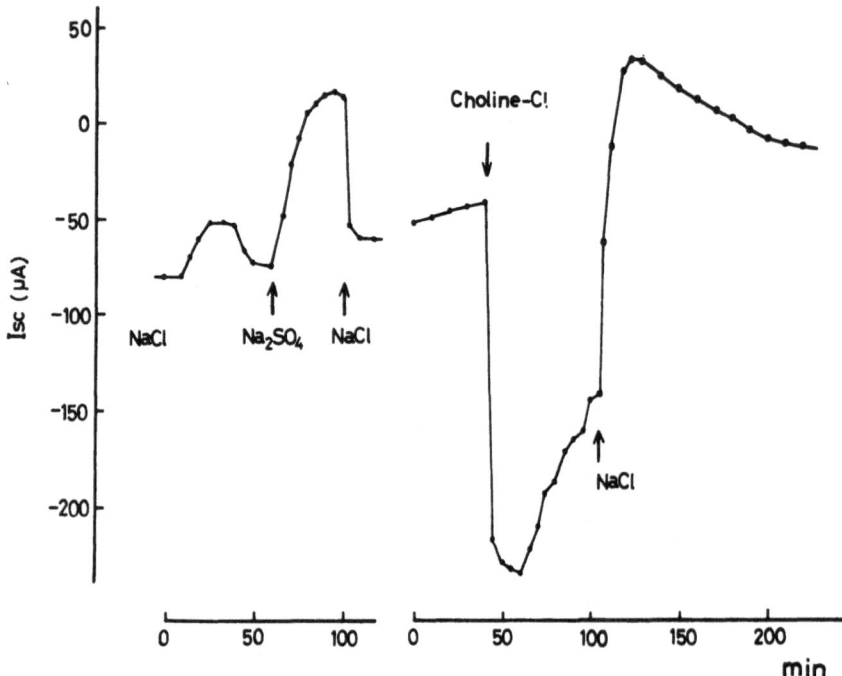

Figure 16.1 Effect of replacement of NaCl in Ringer solution to Na_2SO_4 or to choline–Cl on short-circuit current (I_{sc}) across the posterior intestine of a seawater eel (see reference 36)

The development of a serosa-negative PD or a Cl^- pump in the intestine is commonly observed after adaptation of euryhaline fishes to sea water and in stenohaline seawater fishes. A serosa-negative PD has been observed in flounders in sea water[27,28]. In our study, four out of five marine species showed a serosa-negative PD and one showed near-zero PD[25]. House and Green[16] reported a neutral pump in *C. scorpius*. On the other hand, freshwater species such as carp, Japanese catfish and rainbow trout in freshwater exhibited a slightly serosa-positive PD[25]. Serosa-positive PD was also observed in goldfish[17,29] and American catfish, *Ictalurus nebulosus*[30], although PD is serosa-negative in *Ictalurus punctatus*[31].

The role of a Cl^- pump in water absorption in seawater eel intestine was

306

further confirmed by measuring simultaneously the PD and net water flux in the everted intestine[26]. The intestine was not short-circuited in this experiment. When water flux of the individual eel is plotted against each PD, a highly significant correlation is seen in the seawater eel: the greater the serosal

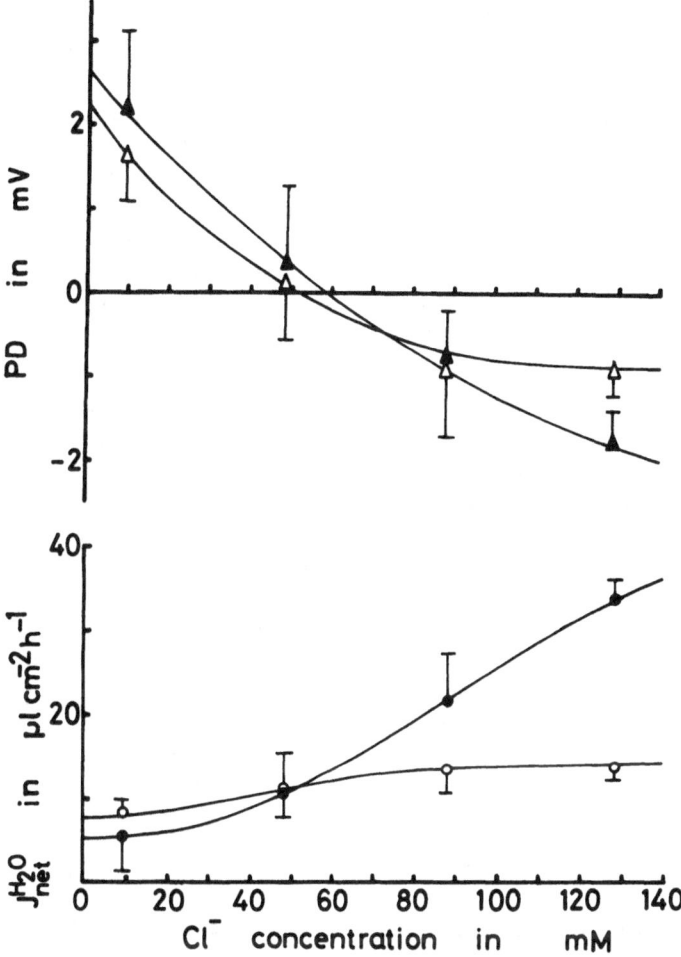

Figure 16.2 Effect of Cl^- concentration on potential difference (PD) and net water flux ($J_{net}^{H_2O}$) across the posterior intestine of the eel. Open triangles and circles indicate PD and $J_{net}^{H_2O}$ of freshwater eels, and closed, those of seawater eels. Vertical bars indicate standard errors of the means ($n = 5$ for freshwater eels, and $n = 6$ for seawater eels) (see reference 26)

negativity, the more the absorption of water. In contrast, no correlation is found between these parameters in freshwater eels. The rate of water absorption in the seawater eel intestine at zero PD obtained from the intercept of the regression line is almost equal to the rate in freshwater eels. A similar correlation between the serosa-negative PD and the rate of water absorption is observed in the conger eel, *Astroconger myriatus*, in sea water. In the freshwater goldfish, there is no correlation between the serosa-positive PD and the rate of water absorption.

When the Cl^- concentration of the bathing solution is reduced by replacing NaCl in the Ringer solution with Na_2SO_4, the water flux in seawater eels decreases in parallel with the decrease in Cl^- concentration and attains a freshwater level at < 50 mEq/1 [26]. In freshwater eels, however, the reduction in the Cl^- concentration has less effect on the water flux. On the other hand, the negative potentials observed in normal NaCl Ringer solution decreases in close association with the decrease in Cl^- concentration in both freshwater and seawater eels (Figure 16.2). The serosa-negative PD seems to be saturated at 90 mEq/1 Cl^- in freshwater eels, while the saturation is not attained at 130 mEq/1 in seawater eels. V_{max} and K_m calculated are 5.1 mV and 72 mM in freshwater eels and 9.7 mV and 143 mM in seawater eels respectively. These results clearly indicate that the serosa-negative potential due to the Cl^- pump is mostly responsible for the increment in the rate of water absorption in the seawater eel intestine.

The osmotic permeability coefficient (P_{os}) was also measured in the everted intestine by adding mannitol to the mucosal Ringer solution. It increases from 0.75×10^{-3} cm sec^{-1} in freshwater eels to 4.73×10^{-3} cm sec^{-1} in seawater eels [26]. Skadhauge[11] reported a two-fold increase in P_{os} during seawater adaptation of *A. anguilla*, although, in a more recent report[12] he did not find any difference. It is likely, therefore, that the low rate of water absorption in freshwater eel intestine is due to the neutral NaCl pump and to low osmotic permeability to water. On the other hand, the development of a Cl^- pump and the increase in P_{os} result in an increase in water absorption in the seawater eel intestine. The serosa-negative PD due to the Cl^- pump together with the increased permeability to Na^+ ions induces a passive movement of Na^+ ions following the electrochemical gradient. The important role of this passive Na^+ movement in facilitating water movement from mucosa to serosa has been discussed in detail by Ando[26].

Adaptive Changes in Enzymes Related to Ion Transport

Sodium–potassium-activated ATPase (Na^+-K^+-ATPase) is thought to play a key role in the active reciprocal transfer of Na^+ and K^+ ions across the cell membranes, and there is increasing evidence that it is intimately involved in the transport of Na^+ ions across epithelial membranes[32,33]. In the goldfish intestine, Smith[17] first identified the enzyme and confirmed the inhibition of Na^+ and water absorption by ouabain. In *A. japonica*, the activity of this enzyme is higher in eels adapted to sea water than in those in fresh water[34] (Figure 16.3). Ouabain inhibits the absorption of Na^+ ions and water, when added to the serosal side. According to Jampol and Epstein[35], the intestinal

Na⁺-K⁺-ATPase also increases during seawater adaptation of the American eel, *A. rostrata*. This enhancement of the enzyme activity in the seawater eel intestine parallels an increase in ion and water absorption capacity. As described above, however, there is no significant change in the Na⁺ pump or the net influx of Na⁺ ions in the short-circuited posterior half of the intestine during seawater adaptation of the eel[25]. Since net absorption of NaCl in the anterior intestine also increases without developing a Cl⁻ pump following seawater adaptation[36], the Na⁺-K⁺-ATPase activity may increase mainly in the anterior intestine. It is also possible that the increased activity is responsible for the increase in unidirectional flux of the ion, a part of which may be due to exchange diffusion. Our preliminary experiment indicates that the serosa-negative PD of the posterior intestine of both the freshwater and the seawater

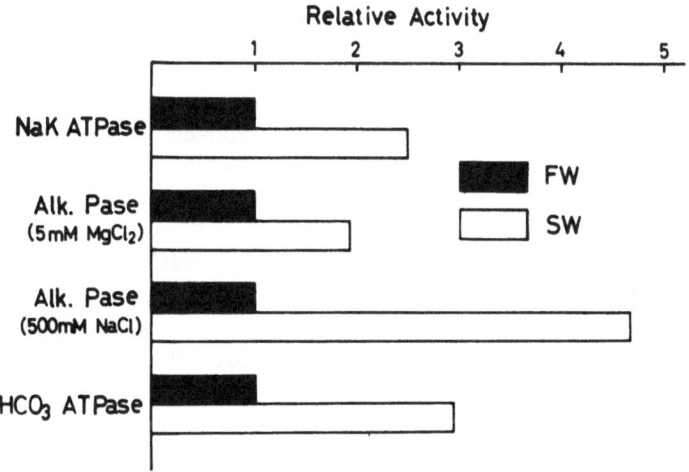

Figure 16.3 Relative activities of Na⁺-K⁺-ATPase, alkaline phosphatase and HCO₃⁻-ATPase in the intestinal mucosa of the eel. Eels were adapted to sea water (SW) for 7 days for Na⁺-K⁺-ATPase and phosphatase determination and for 5 days for HCO₃⁻-ATPase[34,47,65].

eels disappears after addition of ouabain to the serosal Ringer solution[36]. Skadhauge[12] reported that when hypertonic solutions of $MgCl_2$ and Na_2SO_4 are perfused into seawater eel intestine, the flow of Na⁺ or Cl⁻ ion is considerably reduced compared with that seen after NaCl perfusion, and that a solute-linked water flow is not observed unless both Na⁺ and Cl⁻ ions are absorbed. These observations indicate that Na⁺ pump and Cl⁻ pump are coupled, at least in part, in the eel intestine.

Alkaline phosphatase activity in the intestine also increases after seawater adaptation of the eel in parallel with the enhanced rate of ion and water absorption[37-39] (Figure 16.3). Inhibitors of alkaline phosphatase activity such as EDTA, sodium borate and L-cysteine reduce the net absorption of water when added to the mucosal surface[20]. Histochemical study revealed that the enzyme is localized at the luminal surface of the eel intestine[36]. The activity of this enzyme is enhanced by the addition of monovalent ions, especially Cl⁻ ions at high concentrations, and the degree of activation by NaCl is greater in the intestine of seawater eels than in freshwater eels[37,38]. When eels are transferred from fresh water to sea water, the concentration of Na⁺ ions in their plasma and intestinal tissue increases[18]; the intestinal alkaline phosphatase is then in an environment with higher NaCl concentrations in seawater eels. Similar elevations of the enzymatic activity after seawater adaptation and activation by NaCl are observed in the intestine and the gills of the rainbow trout, but not in the kidney and the liver[40]. Furthermore, the degree of activation of intestinal alkaline phosphatase by NaCl is greater in marine species than in freshwater species as in the case of serosa-negative PD[38]. The enzyme has been partially purified from the eel intestine, and total and specific activities are three times greater in seawater eels than in freshwater eels[39].

Since Kasbeker and Durbin[41] described a HCO_3^--activated, SCN-inhibited ATPase in the frog gastric mucosa, evidence has accumulated in favour of the suggestion that this enzyme is responsible for HCl secretion in the stomach[42] and for HCO_3^- secretion in the pancreas[43], accompanied by a Cl^-/HCO_3^- exchange. The occurrence of Cl^-/HCO_3^- exchange together with Na^+/H^+ or NH_4^+ exchange has been shown in the gills of the freshwater goldfish[44] and rainbow trout[45], and HCO_3^--ATPase activity occurs in the gills of the rainbow trout[46]. Huang and Chen[27] suggested the presence of Cl^-/HCO_3^- exchange in the flounder intestine. Recently Morisawa[47] has estimated HCO_3^--ATPase activity in the eel intestine and other tissues in relation to seawater adaptation. The enzyme activity is higher in osmoregulatory organs such as the gill, the kidney and the intestine of seawater eels than in those of freshwater eels (Figure 16.3). The enzyme is solubilised with Triton X-100 from the intestinal mucosa, and the specific activity is two times higher in seawater eels than in freshwater eels. The optimal pH of the intestinal HCO_3^--ATPase is 8.7, and the activity is completely inhibited by NaSCN at a concentration of 5 mM. Since the development of the enzyme in the seawater eel intestine is paralleled by the increase in ion and water absorption or in the Cl⁻ pump, it seems possible that this enzyme is also related to the ion pumping mechanism (especially for Cl⁻) in the eel intestine.

It is generally known that there is always a considerable quantity of clear, alkaline fluid in the intestine of teleosts living in sea water[1]. According to Oide[20], fluid in the intestine of the seawater eel is also alkaline (pH 8.7). In this respect, it is interesting to find a five- to six-fold increase in water movement in the everted eel intestine by raising the pH of the mucosal medium from 7.2 to 9.0 or 10.0[20]. Moreover, the serosa-negative PD and I_{sc} observed in the posterior intestine of seawater eels are also enhanced by raising the pH of the bathing solution[36] (Figure 16.4). Therefore, it is likely that alkaline phosphatase and HCO_3^--ATPase, possibly located at the mucosal surface, also play some role in the increased ion and water absorption in seawater eels.

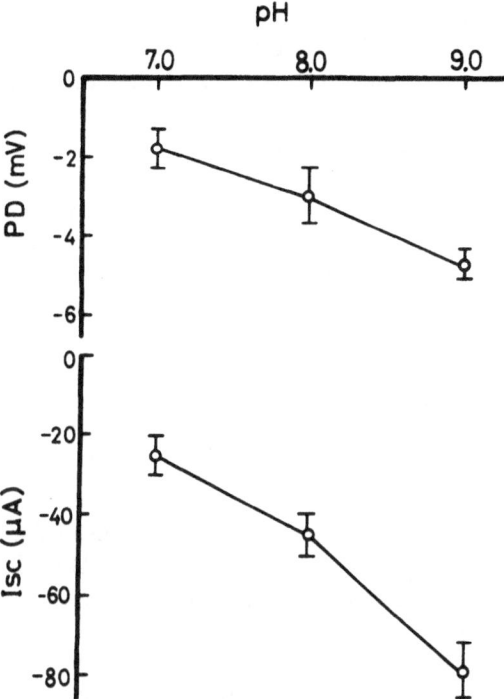

Figure 16.4 Effect of pH change in Ringer solution on potential difference (PD) and short-circuit current (I_{sc}) across the posterior intestine of seawater eels (see reference 36). Vertical bars indicate standard errors of the means ($n = 5$)

In relation to Cl^-/HCO_3^- exchange, Huang and Chen[27] observed an inhibitory effect of diamox, a specific inhibitor of carbonic anhydrase, on the serosa-negative PD of the flounder intestine. However, there seems to be no information on the occurrence of carbonic anhydrase activity in the intestinal mucosa of euryhaline teleosts. Although it is likely that Na^+-K^+-ATPase, alkaline phosphatase, HCO_3^--ATPase and possibly carbonic anhydrase are involved in ion and water transport mechanisms in teleost intestine, our understanding of how these enzymes work is still too limited to provide a molecular mechanism of the transport process.

HORMONAL CONTROL OF INTESTINAL ABSORPTION

In higher vertebrates, there is evidence that aldosterone is the typical mineralocorticoid acting on intestinal absorption. It stimulates ion and water absorption in the toad[48] and human[49] colon and in the rat jejunum[50]. The presence of aldosterone in fish blood has long been debated, and cortisol, the major corticosteroid in teleost fishes, including the eel, seems to have mineralocorticoid actions[24,51]. In our *in vitro* preparation[19,52], we have shown that when hypophysectomised eels are transferred from fresh water to sea water, the enhancement of water absorption is no longer observed. Injection of hormones into intact freshwater eels revealed that the pituitary-inter-renal axis is responsible for the adaptive changes to sea water[53]. Among the hypophysial hormones and corticosteroids tested, only ACTH and cortisol are effective in increasing the rate of ion and water transport in the freshwater eel intestine. Other corticosteroids such as aldosterone, deoxycorticosterone, cortisone and corticosterone have little effect. Ellory et al.[54], and Porthé-Nibelle and Lahlou[55] reported that hypophysectomy of goldfish markedly reduces serosal transfer of Na^+ and water and cortisol restores it to normal. In contrast to the eel intestine, the intestinal transport of Na^+ and water is greatly depressed in goldfish during NaCl adaptation, which is ascribed to reduction in mucosal permeability to Na^+ ions[54]. Cortisol is shown to stimulate the serosal Na^+ pump activity without modifying mucosal permeability to Na^+ ions[54]. On the other hand, our recent experiments[56,57] indicate that cortisol, when injected into freshwater eels, induces intestinal features similar to those of seawater-adapted eels such as an increase in net absorption of Na^+ and Cl^- ions and water, the development of serosa-negative PD (a Cl^--pump) and an increase in permeability to Na^+ and Cl^- ions and in osmotic permeability to water (Figure 16.5).

Mayer et al.[58] have shown that cortisol promotes Na^+ excretion by the eel gill. Cortisol appears to be physiologically important in the adaptation of intestinal as well as gill function to sea water, and an increased secretion of cortisol appears to occur during seawater adaptation. In A. japonica, we have observed only a short-term (2 to 4 hours) increase in circulating cortisol after transfer to sea water[59,60]. According to Ball et al.[61], an increase in plasma cortisol level is observed during the first 48 hours of seawater adaptation in A. anguilla. Transient increases in plasma cortisol are similarly observed in goldfish during NaCl adaptation[62]. As described above, however, the eel intestine maintains a significantly higher rate of ion and water movement as long as the eels are kept in sea water[53]. Essentially similar correlated changes in plasma cortisol level and intestinal function occur after treatment of the freshwater eel with a single injection of ACTH or cortisol: plasma cortisol increases during the first 2 to 4 hours and returns to its initial level after 24 hours, while the increase in intestinal water movement is observed after a latent period of about 10 hours and lasts for as much as a week or more[60]. The different time-course between the plasma cortisol level and ion and water absorption in the intestine may be explained by an increase both in secretion rate of cortisol from the interrenal and in consumption rate or disappearance from the blood in seawater eels[63].

The presence of a latent period in the response to cortisol suggests induction of some metabolic process basic to increased rate of ion and water absorption in the intestine. Epstein et al.[64] have reported that cortisol increases Na^+-K^+-ATPase activities of both gill and intestine of freshwater-adapted A.

rostrata. In *A. japonica,* an increase in intestinal alkaline phosphatase activity after seawater adaptation is not observed after hypophysectomy[65]. The effect of hypophysectomy on intestinal Na^+-K^+-ATPase and HCO_3^--ATPase activities has not been examined. In contrast to our results in the cultured Japanese eel, Gaitskell and Chester Jones[66] have recently observed that injection of a large dose of cortisol into the silver form of *A. anguilla* induces an

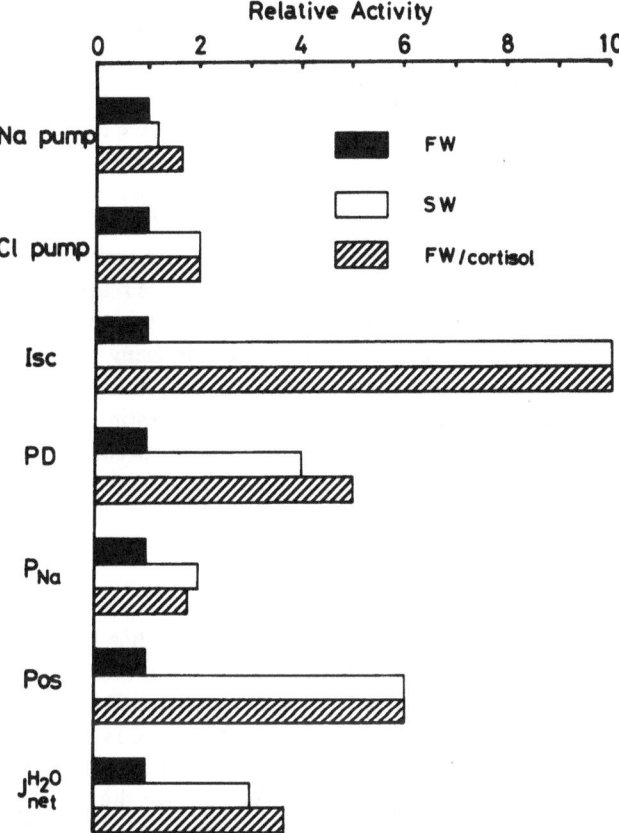

Figure 16.5 Effects of seawater (SW) adaptation and cortisol treatment of the freshwater fish (FW/cortisol) on the relative activity of Na^+ and Cl^- pumps (net movement of each ion under short-circuited condition), short-circuit current (I_{sc}), potential difference (PD), permeabilities to Na^+ (P_{Na}, serosa–mucosa) and to water (P_{os}), and net water movement ($J_{net}^{H_2O}$)[25,26,56,57]

increase in intestinal water absorption half-an-hour to 1 hour after the injection. Furthermore, the intestine of adrenalectomized freshwater eels is less permeable to water and cortisol administration restores the normal permeability: cortisol is also required for maintaining water absorption of the eel intestine in fresh water.

Prolactin has been recognized as essential for the survival of some euryhaline fishes in fresh water, and a high level of prolactin secretion is generally considered to occur in fresh water[24,51]. Although ovine prolactin has no effect on intestinal water absorption when injected into freshwater eels[53], injection into seawater eels decreases the rate of ion and water absorption in the isolated intestine[24,67]. The concentration of Na^+ and Cl^- ions in the fluid passing through the membrane is greater in the prolactin-treated fish than in the control seawater fish. Prolactin seems to decrease the rate of ion and water absorption in the intestine, probably by suppressing the Cl^- pump and lowering the permeability to water, and seems to act on the intestinal epithelium as an antagonist to cortisol. In the rat jejunum, prolactin is shown to increase Na^+ and water uptake[68,69].

In summary, the important increase in ion and water absorption observed in the eel intestine during seawater adaptation is due to the development of a Cl^- pump and resulting serosa-negative PD accompanied by an increased permeability to ions and water. Na^+-K^+-ATPase, alkaline phosphatase and HCO_3^--ATPase seem to be involved in the adaptive increase in ion pumping processes. Cortisol, a major corticosteroid in the eel, is responsible for the induction of the enhanced absorptive capacity in the seawater eel intestine, and prolactin seems to antagonise cortisol action by lowering the rate of ion and water absorption. Considering these adaptive changes in ion and water absorption capacity and its hormonal control, the eel intestine provides a model system for the study of ion and water absorption mechanism through the epithelium.

Acknowledgements

Work from our laboratory referred to in the paper has been supported by grants from the Ministry of Education, Japan and from the Japan Society for Promotion of Sciences (Co-operative Programme, Nos. 7114 and 73102). We are indebted to our former collaborators, Drs N. Isono, H. Oide and M. Oide for their considerable contributions. We are also grateful to Prof. Howard A. Bern, University of California, Berkeley, for reading the manuscript.

References

1. Smith, H. W. (1932). Water regulation and its evolution in the fishes. *Quart. Rev. Biol.*, 7, 1
2. Maetz, J. (1970). Mechanisms of salt and water transfer across membranes in teleosts in relation to the aquatic environment. *Mem. Soc. Endocrinol.*, 18, 3
3. Bentley, P. J. (1971). *Endocrine and Osmoregulation. A Comparative Account of the Regulation of Water and Salt in Vertebrates.* (Berlin, Heidelberg, New York: Springer Verlag)
4. Utida, S. and Hirano, T. (1973). Effects of changes in environmental salinity on salt and water movement in the intestine and gills of the eel, *Anguilla japonica*. In W. Chavin (ed.). *Responses of Fish to Environmental Changes*, p. 240. (Springfield, Ill: Charles C. Thomas)
5. Oide, H. and Utida, S. (1968). Changes in intestinal absorption and renal excretion of water during adaptation to seawater in the Japanese eel. *Marine Biol.*, 1, 172

6. Maetz, J. and Skadhauge, E. (1968). Drinking rates and gill ionic turnover in relation to external salinities in the eel. *Nature, London* **217**, 371

7. Hirano, T. (1974). Some factors regulating water intake by the eel, *Anguilla japonica. J. Exp. Biol.*, **61**, 737

8. Kirsch, R. (1972). The kinetics of peripheral exchanges of water and electrolytes in the silver eel (*Anguilla anguilla* L.) in fresh water and in sea water. *J. Exp. Biol.*, **57**, 489

9. Kirsch, R. and Mayer-Gostan, N. (1973). Kinetics of water and chloride exchanges during adaptation of the European eel to sea water. *J. Exp. Biol.*, **58**, 105

10. Utida, S., Isono, N. and Hirano, T. (1967). Water movement in isolated intestine of the eel adapted to fresh water or sea water. *Zool. Mag. Tokyo*, **76**, 203

11. Skadhauge, E. (1969). The mechanism of salt and water absorption in the intestine of the eel (*Anguilla anguilla*) adapted to waters of various salinities. *J. Physiol. Lond.*, **204**, 135

12. Skadhauge, E. (1974). Coupling of transmural flows of NaCl and water in the intestine of the eel (*Anguilla anguilla*). *J. Exp. Biol.*, **60**, 535

13. Kirsch, R. and Laurent, P. (1975). L'oesophage, organe effecteur de l'osmorégulation chez un téléostéen euryhalin (*Anguilla anguilla* L.), *C. R. Acad. Sci. D. Paris*, **280**, 2013

14. Hirano, T. and Mayer-Gostan, N. (1975). Adaptive changes in ion permeability in the eel oesophagus. (In preparation)

15. House, C. R. and Green, K. (1963). Sodium and water transport across isolated intestine of a marine teleost, *Nature, London*, **199**, 1293

16. House, C. R. and Green, K. (1965). Ion and water transport in isolated intestine of the marine teleost, *Cottus scorpius. J. Exp. Biol.*, **42**, 177

17. Smith, M. W. (1964). The *in vitro* absorption of water and solute from the intestine of goldfish, *Carassius auratus. J. Physiol. Lond.*, **175**, 38

18. Oide, M. and Utida, S. (1967). Changes in water and ion transport in isolated intestine of the eel during salt adaptation and migration. *Marine Biol.*, **1**, 102

19. Hirano, T. (1967). Effect of hypophysectomy on water transport in isolated intestine of the eel, *Anguilla japonica. Proc. Jap. Acad.*, **43**, 793

20. Oide, M. (1973). Role of alkaline phosphatase in intestinal water absorption by eels adapted to sea water. *Comp. Biochem. Physiol.*, **46A**, 639

21. Skadhauge, E. and Maetz, J. (1967). Étude *in vivo* de l'absorption intestinale d'eau et d'électrolytes chez *Anguilla anguilla* adapté à des milieux de salinités diverses. *C. R. Acad. Sci. D. Paris*, **265**, 347

22. Utida, S., Oide, M., Saishu, S. and Kamiya, M. (1967). Préétablissement du mécanisme d'adaptation à l'eau de mer dans l'intestin et les branchies isolés de l'anguille argentée au cours de sa migration catadrome. *C. R. Soc. Biol., Paris*, **161**, 1201

23. Utida, S., Hirano, T. and Kamiya, M. (1969). Seasonal variations in the adjustive responses to sea water in the intestine and gills of the Japanese cultured eel, *Anguilla japonica. Proc. Jap. Acad.*, **45**, 293

24. Utida, S., Hirano, T., Ando, M., Johnson, D. W. and Bern, H. A. (1972). Hormonal control of the intestine and urinary bladder in teleost osmoregulation. *Gen. Comp. Endocrinol.*, (**Suppl. 3**), 317

25. Ando, M., Utida, S. and Nagahama, H. (1975). Active transport of chloride in eel intestine with special reference to sea water adaptation. *Comp. Biochem. Physiol.*, **51A**, 27

26. Ando, M. (1975). Intestinal water transport and chloride pump in relation to sea-water adaptation of the eel, *Anguilla japonica. Comp. Biochem. Physiol.*, **52A**, 229

27. Huang, K. C. and Chen, T. S. T. (1971). Ion transport across intestinal mucosa of winter flounder, *Pseudopleuronectes americanus. Amer. J. Physiol.*, **220**, 1734

28. Lahlou, B., Smith, M. W. and Ellory, J. C. (1974). Le transport intestinal *in vitro* du sodium et du chlore chez le flet européen, *Platichthys flesus*, en eau de mer et en eau douce. *C. R. Acad. Sci. D. Paris*. **278**, 761

29. Smith, M. W. (1966). Sodium-glucose interaction in the goldfish intestine. *J. Physiol. Lond.*, **182**, 559

30. Datta, S. and Savage, N. B. (1968). Investigation of the electric potential of the isolated midgut of the freshwater teleost, *Ameiurus nebulosus*. *Experientia*, **24**, 572

31. Chen, T. S. T. and Huang, K. C. (1972). Structural specificity in the intestinal transport of hexoses, tyrosine derivatives and electrolytes in freshwater catfish. *J. Pharmacol. Exp. Therap.* **180**, 777

32. Schwartz, A., Lindenmayer, G. E. and Allen, J. C. (1972). The Na$^+$, K$^+$-ATPase membrane transport system: Importance in cellular function. In F. Bronner and A. Kleinzeller (eds.). *Current Topics in Membrane and Transport* 3, p. 1. (New York: Academic Press)

33. Dahl, J. L. and Hokin, L. E. (1974). The sodium–potassium adenosine triphosphatase. *Ann. Rev. Biochem.*, **43**, 327

34. Oide, M. (1967). Effects of inhibitors on transport of water and ion in isolated intestine and Na$^+$-K$^+$ ATPase in intestinal mucosa of the eel. *Annot. Zool. Japon.*, **40**, 130

35. Jampol, L. M. and Epstein, F. H. (1970). Sodium-potassium-activated adenosine triphosphatase and osmotic regulation by fishes. *Amer. J. Physiol.*, **218**, 607

36. Ando, M., Morisawa, M. and Hirano, T. (1975). (Unpublished observations)

37. Utida, S. and Isono, N. (1967). Alkaline phosphatase activity in intestinal mucosa of the eel adapted to fresh water or sea water. *Proc. Jap. Acad.*, **43**, 789

38. Utida, S., Oide, M. and Oide, H. (1968). Ionic effects on alkaline phosphatase activity in intestinal mucosa with special reference to sea water adaptation of the Japanese eel, *Anguilla japonica*. *Comp. Biochem. Physiol.*, **27**, 239

39. Oide, M. (1970). Purification and some properties of alkaline phosphatase from intestinal mucosa of the eel adapted to fresh water or sea water. *Comp. Biochem. Physiol.*, **36**, 241

40. Utida, S. (1967). Effect of sodium chloride on alkaline phosphatase activity in intestinal mucosa of the rainbow trout. *Proc. Jap. Acad.*, **43**, 783

41. Kasbeker, D. K. and Durbin, R. P. (1965). Adenosine triphosphatase from frog gastric mucosa. *Biochim. Biophys. Acta*, **105**, 472

42. Durbin, R. P. and Kasbekar, D. K. (1965). Adenosine triphosphatase and active transport by the stomach. *Fed. Proc.*, **24**, 1377

43. Simon, B., Kinne, R. and Sachs, G. (1972). The presence of a HCO$_3^-$-activated ATPase in pancreatic tissue. *Biochim. Biophys. Acta*, **282**, 293

44. Maetz, J. and Garcia-Romeu, F. (1964). The mechanism of sodium and chloride uptake by the gills of freshwater fish, *Carassius auratus*. II. Evidence for NH$_4^+$/Na$^+$ and HCO$_3^-$/Cl$^-$ exchanges. *J. Gen. Physiol.*, **47**, 1209

45. Kerstetter, T. H. and Kirschner, L. B. (1972). Active chloride transport by the gills of rainbow trout (*Salmo gairdneri*). *J. Exp. Biol.*, **56**, 263

46. Kerstetter, T. H. and Kirshner, L. B. (1974). HCO$_3^-$-dependent ATPase activity in the gills of rainbow trout (*Salmo gairdneri*). *Comp. Biochem. Physiol.*, **48B**, 581

47. Morisawa, M. (1975). HCO$_3^-$activated adenosine triphosphatase in intestinal mucosa of the eel (*Anguilla japonica*). (In preparation)

48. Cofré, G. and Crabbé, J. (1965). Stimulation by aldosterone of active sodium transport by the isolated colon of the toad, *Bufo marinus*. *Nature, London*, **207**, 1299

49. Levitan, R. and Ingelfinger, F. J. (1965). Effect of *d*-aldosterone on salt and water absorption from the intact human colon. *J. Clin. Invest.*, **44**, 801

50. Crocker, A. D. and Munday, K. A. (1969). Factors affecting mucosal water and sodium transfer in everted sacs of rat jejunum. *J. Physiol. Lond.*, **202**, 329

51. Johnson, D. W. (1973). Endocrine control of hydromineral balance in teleost. *Amer. Zool.*, **13**, 799

52. Hirano, T., Kamiya, M., Saishu, S. and Utida, S. (1967). Effects of hypophysectomy and urophysectomy on water and sodium transport in isolated intestine and gills of Japanese eel (*Anguilla japonica*). *Endocrinol. Japon.*, **14**, 182

53. Hirano, T. and Utida, S. (1968). Effects of ACTH and cortisol on water movement in isolated intestine of the eel, *Anguilla japonica*. *Gen. Comp. Endocrinol.*, **11**, 373

54. Ellory, J. C., Lahlou, B. and Smith, M. W. (1972). Changes in the intestinal transport of sodium induced by exposure of goldfish to a saline environment. *J. Physiol. Lond.*, **222**, 497

55. Porthé-Nibelle, J. and Lahlou, B. (1975). Effects of corticosteroid hormones and inhibitors of steroids on sodium and water transport by goldfish intestine. *Comp. Biochem. Physiol.*, **50A**, 801

56. Ando, M. (1974). Effects of cortisol on water transport across the eel intestine. *Endocrinol. Japon.*, **21**, 539

57. Chen, T. S. T., Ando, M., Utida, S. and Huang, K. C. (1975). Ion fluxes and permeabilities of Japanese cultured eel intestine. *Fed. Proc.* (In press)

58. Mayer, N., Maetz, J., Chan, D. K. O., Forster, M. and Chester Jones, I. (1967). Cortisol, a sodium excreting factor in the eel (*Anguilla anguilla* L.) adapted to sea water. *Nature London*, **214**, 1118

59. Hirano, T. (1969). Effects of hypophysectomy and salinity change on plasma cortisol concentration in the Japanese eel, *Anguilla japonica*. *Endocrinol. Japon.*, **16**, 557

60. Hirano, T. and Utida, S. (1971). Plasma cortisol concentration and the rate of intestinal water absorption in the eel, *Anguilla japonica*. *Endocrinol. Japon.*, **18**, 47

61. Ball, J. N., Chester, Jones. I., Forster, M. E., Hargreaves, G., Hawkins, E. F. and Milne, K. P. (1971). Measurement of plasma cortisol levels in the eel *Anguilla anguilla* in relation to osmotic adjustments. *J. Endocrinol.*, **50**, 75

62. Porthé-Nibelle, J. and Lahlou, B. (1974). Plasma concentrations of cortisol in hypophysectomized and sodium chloride-adapted goldfish (*Carassius auratus* L.). *J. Endocrinol.*, **63**, 377

63. Henderson, I. W., Sa'di, M. N. and Hargreaves, G. (1974). Studies on the production and metabolic clearance rates of cortisol in the European eel (*Anguilla anguilla* L.). *J. Steroid Biochem.*, **5**, 701

64. Epstein, F. H., Cynamon, M. and McKay, W. (1971). Endocrine control of Na-K-ATPase and sea-water adaptation in *Anguilla rostrata*. *Gen. Comp. Endocrinol.*, **16**, 323

65. Oide, M. (1973). Effects of hypophysectomy and environmental salts on intestinal alkaline phosphatase of the eel in relation to sea water adaptation. *Comp. Biochem. Physiol.*, **46A**, 647

66. Gaitskell, R. E. and Chester Jones, I. (1970). Effects of adrenalectomy and cortisol injection on the *in vitro* movement of water by the intestine of the freshwater European eel (*Anguilla anguilla* L.). *Gen. Comp. Endocrinol.*, **15**, 491

67. Hirano, T. and Bern, H. A. (1972). The teleost gall bladder as an osmoregulatory organ. *Endocrinol. Japon.*, **19**, 41

68. Ramsey, D. H. and Bern, H. A. (1972). Stimulation by ovine prolactin of fluid transfer in everted sacs of small intestine. *J. Endocrinol.*, **53**, 453

69. Mainoya, H. R., Bern, H. A. and Regan, J. W. (1974). Influence of ovine prolactin on transport of fluid and sodium chloride by the mammalian intestine and gall bladder. *J. Endocrinol.*, **63**, 311

16

Second Main Paper

Ionic Permeability of Fish Intestinal Mucosa in Relation to Hypophysectomy and Salt Adaptation

Brahim Lahlou

Laboratoire de Physiologie Comparée,
Faculté des Sciences (PCNI) de l'Université de Nice,
Parc Valrose, Nice

The ability of euryhaline teleosts to increase their intestinal absorption of salt and water in relation to the salinity of the external medium is an essential feature of their osmoregulatory adjustments. Freshwater (FW) animals drink only insignificant amounts of their surrounding medium and rely mainly upon their gills and kidneys to maintain their osmotic and ionic balance. By contrast, seawater (SW) fishes obtain water by drinking appreciable quantities of the medium and absorbing it across the gut wall. The excess salt thus introduced into the body is subsequently excreted via the gills. This pattern of osmoregulation was proposed by H. Smith[1] and shown to be valid for all euryhaline teleosts studied to date.

Stenohaline freshwater fishes, such as the goldfish, can adapt to a moderately concentrated medium (*ca* 400 mosmol), but plasma electrolyte concentrations are raised and become identical to or slightly higher than outside[2].

These contrasting behaviours may be expected to depend *pro parte* on differences in adjustment of intestinal function during salt adaptation and this may involve changes in passive permeability to ions and/or in pumping efficiency. The technique devised by Schultz *et al.*[3] may be useful to distinguish between these possibilities as it permits independent measurement of the rate of ionic entry through the apical membrane of intestinal cells.

Little is known about hormonal control of intestinal transport in fishes. The presence and possible role of aldosterone in these animals is still debated and it is assumed that the major circulating corticosteroid, cortisol, may replace it as a potent mineralocorticoid substance acting on the gill[4] and the gut[5,6]. The effects of aldosterone have been extensively studied in amphibian epithelia, but its site of action is still under discussion, as it may be apical[7,8] or basolateral[9], leading either to an increase in the overall permeability of the brush-border side to sodium ions or to a direct stimulation of the serosal ion pump. Here again, the technique of Schultz *et al.*[3] could help to separate these alternative interpretations when applied to the study of steroid actions on fish intestine.

The experiments reported below were carried out *in vitro* and deal with teleostean species differing from each other by their osmoregulatory capabilities. While the goldfish, *Carassius auratus*, is a stenohaline freshwater fish, the flounder, *Platichthys flesus*, is perfectly euryhaline, being directly transferable from fresh water to sea water and vice versa[10]. The trout, *Salmo irideus*, is intermediate: it stands a stepwise increase in external salinity until full sea water is attained[11].

METHODS

The animals were kept in the laboratory at a suitable constant temperature: 15 or 16 °C for goldfish and flounder, 11 °C for trout.

Hypophysectomy was performed by routine techniques on goldfish (by B. Lahlou) and flounder (by N. MacFarlane).

For incubations *in vitro* the tissue was bathed in a 280–300 mosmol medium made of Forster's Ringer[12] or Krebs–Henseleit[13] solution which both contained bicarbonate and 5 mM glucose and were gassed with a 95% O_2–5% CO_2 mixture. Where required, NaCl was replaced with mannitol, Na^+ with choline and Cl^- with sulphate.

Everted sacs were prepared according to Wilson and Wiseman[14]. Radioisotopes (^{24}Na or ^{22}Na; ^{36}Cl; ^{45}Ca) were incorporated into the sac serosal fluid in order to measure serosal–to–mucosal flux ($\mathcal{J}_{sm}$) in addition to net flux ($\mathcal{J}_n$) of the corresponding ion.

Short-circuit current (I_{sc}) was followed in Ussing-type chambers, in which the intestine was exposed as a flat sheet with an available area of 0.6 cm². Unidirectional fluxes were measured after an equilibration time of at least 30 minutes in presence of the isotope.

Mucosal uptake of ions was evaluated using the technique of Schultz *et al.*[3] as adapted for fish intestine[6,15]. The mucosal surface was in contact with the incubation solutions through six or eight circular ports presenting a sectional area of 0.25 and 0.07 cm² respectively. In addition to the radioactive ion(s), the test mucosal solution contained tritiated inulin or mannitol for the determination of the extracellular component of ion uptake. Exposure time to radioactivity was usually 45 seconds or 1 minute, being chosen in such a way as to yield an ionic entry linear with time, indicating a constant flux, $\mathcal{J}_{mc}$, from the external medium to the cells.

319

RESULTS AND DISCUSSION

Nature of the active ion transport

Kinetics and mechanisms of transport of water, inorganic ions and organic solutes have been well described for mammalian intestine. Active transfer of sodium at the serosal side of the cells is thought to provide the driving force necessary for water absorption, but a partial link between sodium and chloride movements and an energy-dependent passage of chloride through the apical brush border have also been suggested[16].

In fish intestine studied *in vitro* and bathed with Ringer solution on both sides, the transported fluid is essentially isotonic with respect to the mucosal medium, but it may become hyperosmotic, for example in *Cottus*[17]. In addition, the volume of water and the amount of sodium crossing the epithelium increase in parallel and in direct relation to the external salinity in euryhaline species such as the eel, the flounder and the trout[5,11,18,19]. The reverse is observed with the stenohaline freshwater fish, *Carassius auratus*. In this species, transfer to a hyperosmotic medium induces a 79% drop in water and sodium net fluxes across incubated sacs[6].

Table 16.1 Transepithelial potential difference in intestine of four teleosts adapted to various salinities (serosa with respect to mucosa; mean PD ± SE, in mV)

Medium	Carassius auratus	Salmo irideus	Platichthys flesus	Serranus sp.
Fresh water	+3.3 ± 0.2	+0.75 ± 0.15	−1.24 ± 0.14	
Intermediate salinity	+1.2			
Seawater		+1.12 ± 0.16	−1.91 ± 0.14	−0.5 to −4.0

Sources: Ellory *et al.*[20], Lahlou *et al.*[19], Crénesse[26] and unpublished data.

A significant point arises when one considers the transepithelial potential difference, PD (Table 16.1). After equilibration of isolated intestines in Ringer solution, this potential stabilizes at a low value (less than 4 mV in general), as usually observed with low resistance epithelia with large paracellular shunt pathways. It is serosa-positive in FW fishes, such as the goldfish, indicating that sodium is transported against its electrochemical gradient. Under short-circuit conditions, the I_{sc} corresponds to the current generated by sodium ions in this species[20]. The PD becomes negative in most seawater-adapted fishes, such as the American flounder[21], the Japanese eel[22], the European flounder[19] and the sea perch, *Serranus sp.*, a stenohaline marine animal. This provides evidence that active absorption of chloride may take place as well.

Bidirectional flux measurements under open or short-circuit conditions confirm the existence of a dual electrogenic pump[19,23,24]. These observations are consistent with the suggestion that the development of an intestinal chloride pump is a feature associated with permanent life in a marine environment (*loc. cit.*). The freshwater fish *Carassius* does not possess such a pump even in salt medium. The trout, *Salmo irideus*, which does not migrate to the sea, keeps a positive potential in all salinities. Conversely, the flounder, which normally lives in the sea, maintains a negative potential and a predominant chloride transport *in vitro* even in fresh water. A reasonable explanation for this situation is that the high levels of divalent cations in intestinal fluid of marine teleosts leave little space for sodium and that the fish shift to chloride transport as the driving-force for water absorption[19,24].

Mucosal entry of ions

This is measured over one minute or less on goldfish and flounder intestines which possess thin and flat epithelia.

With trout gut, uptake is linear with time over 3 minutes, but the regression line does not pass through the origin. This indicates that part of this uptake consists of a quick entry or retention of ions in a separate compartment which is not available to inulin. This initial component represents about 20% of the radioactivity entering within 3 minutes and a similar result is obtained with Na^+, Cl^- and Ca^{++}. It is not related to an anomalous behaviour of inulin as an extracellular marker since labelled mannitol yields similar data (unless of course both indicators are unsuitable for these experiments). Moreover, it is proportional to the external concentration. It is comparable to the fraction of calcium entry in rat duodenum described as Uptake 1 by O'Donnell and Smith[25]. We have not characterised it further but we believe it is related to the particular morphology of trout intestine which is thick and possesses heavy foldings[26].

When the corrected constant flux (expressed as nEq/cm^2 min) is plotted against the ion concentration of the incubation medium, a linear relationship is obtained for sodium in goldfish[6] (studied at 30 °C), and for sodium, chloride and calcium in trout[26] (at ambient temperature). The overall ionic permeability, expressed by the slope of the regression line, irrespective of the mechanism involved, is high, as the permeability coefficient, P (in cm per min), is about $2-3 \times 10^{-3}$ in all cases.

For sodium, these figures compare well with findings on rabbit ileum[27] as regards both the amplitude and the linearity of the uptake. By contrast, a curvilinear relationship and a lower rate of entry are observed in amphibian skin and bladder[28,29], for chloride in rabbit ileum[16], and for calcium in rat duodenum[35].

Thus a striking characteristic of goldfish and trout intestine is the high rate of penetration of ions into the mucosal cells. Despite its appearance of simple diffusion, this process does not necessarily mean that all the ions considered are driven into the cells down their electrochemical gradient. No more precise conclusions can be drawn regarding the mechanisms involved at the outer barrier of the cells as there are no available data concerning intracellular potential and chemical activities and the interactions of these ions with other permeating substances.

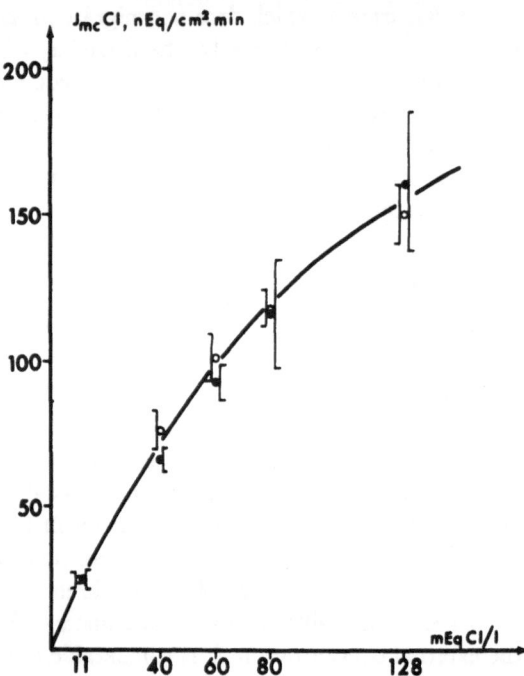

Figure 16.1 Mucosal uptake of chloride ($\mathcal{J}_{mc}$ Cl$^-$) in intestines isolated from seawater-adapted flounder, as a function of chloride concentration in the mucosal solution. Controls, O, and hypophysectomised fish, ●. (Unpublished data; in collaboration with N. A. A. MacFarlane)

A different situation is encountered with FW flounder intestine. Both sodium and chloride display saturation-type curves and reveal an ion uptake of about half that of goldfish or trout intestine at the concentration of Ringer solution (Figure 16.1). A double-reciprocal plot involves an extrapolation of the curves, as the observed fluxes are far below their maximum values. Figure 16.2 shows that $\mathcal{J}_{mc}^{max}$ Cl$^-$ is 312 nEq/cm^2 min: the apparent K_m (133 mM) indicates a low affinity of the carrier which possibly operates at the brush border. An almost identical $\mathcal{J}_{mc}^{max}$ Cl$^-$ but a much lower K_m (29 mM) have been reported for rabbit ileum[16].

The mucosal influxes are far higher than the corresponding net or bidirectional fluxes. With respect to the net flux, the ratio $\mathcal{J}_{mc}$ v. $\mathcal{J}_n$ varies between 10 (Cl$^-$ in flounder) to 25 (Ca^{++} in trout). With respect to $\mathcal{J}_{ms}$, the ratio is lower

Table 16.2 Changes in apical entry ($\mathcal{J}_{mc}$) and transepithelial transport ($\mathcal{J}_n$) of ions induced by adaptation to salt in three teleostean species

	Goldfish	Trout	Flounder
Apical entry	−	−	=
Serosal transport	−	+	+

(+ indicates an increase; − a decrease; = no change)
Sources: Ellory et al.[6]; Crénesse[26]; Smith et al.[24].

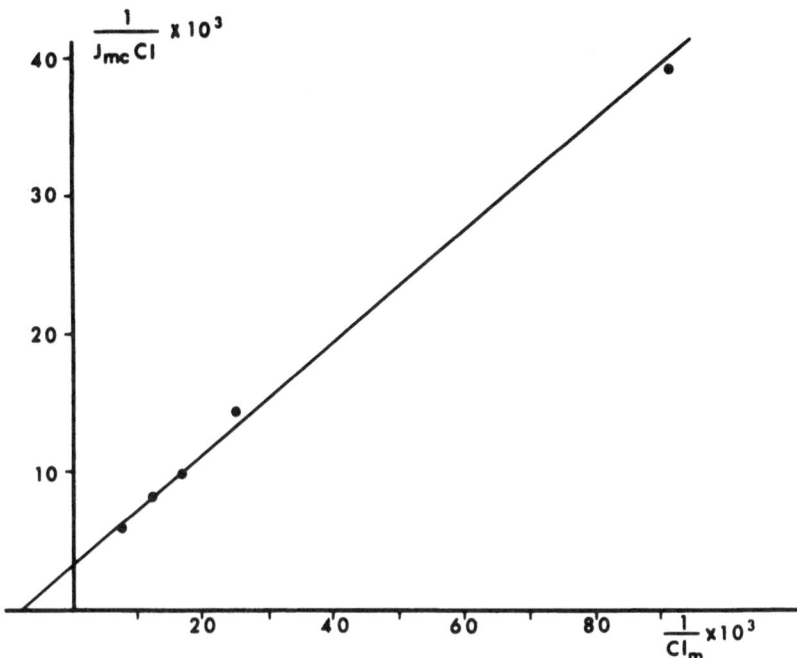

Figure 16.2 Lineweaver–Burk plot of $\mathcal{J}_{mc}$ Cl$^-$ against external chloride concentration in flounder intestine. Each ordinate value is calculated from the mean of the four average $\mathcal{J}_{mc}$ Cl$^-$, obtained from control and hypophysectomised flounder, both in fresh water and in sea water. (Unpublished data; in collaboration with N. A. A. MacFarlane)

but always higher than 3. As for mammalian intestine, this discrepancy may be explained either by an exchange–diffusion process or by an energy-dependent extrusion both of which would bring the excess of ions which had penetrated the cells back to the external medium through the brush border membrane[3].

Table 16.3 Water and chloride fluxes across everted sacs prepared from flounder intestine

		$\mathcal{J}_n H_2O$ $\mu l/h$ g	$\mathcal{J}_n Cl$ $\mu Eq/h$ g	$\mathcal{J}_{ms} Cl$ id.	$\mathcal{J}_{sm} Cl$ id.
Fresh water	Sham, $n = 8$	15.2 ± 4.7	4.7 ± 1.3	23.6 ± 2.9	18.9 ± 3.2
	Hypect, $n = 7$	0.6 ± 0.6	-0.55 ± 1.74	13.6 ± 2.4	14.2 ± 1.8
	t-test	$P < 0.01$	$P < 0.05$	$P < 0.02$	NS
Seawater	Sham, $n = 8$	182.9 ± 60.7	28.9 ± 6.1	68.4 ± 18.4	45.2 ± 13.9
	Hypect, $n = 6$	96.5 ± 28.2	18.7 ± 3.3	51.7 ± 7.4	33.0 ± 9.4
	t-test	NS	NS	NS	NS

Sham-operated (sham) and hypophysectomised (hypect) fish adapted to fresh water or to sea water.
Mean $\pm$ SE; number, n, of sacs.
NS indicates no statistically significant difference ($P > 0.05$) between sham and hypophysectomised animals. (In collaboration with N. A. A. MacFarlane.)

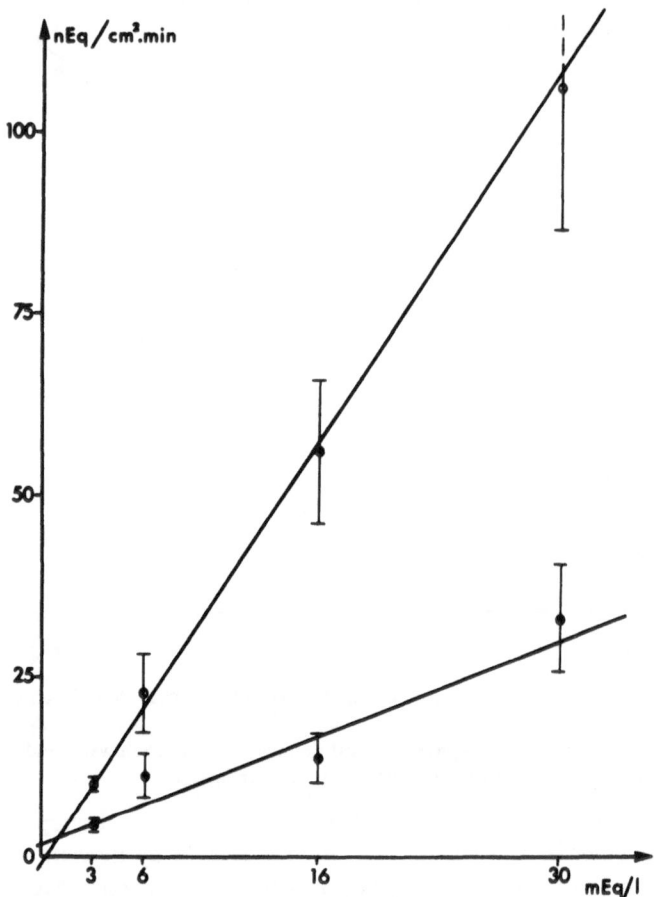

Figure 16.3 Mucosal uptake of calcium ($\mathcal{J}_{mc}$ Ca) by isolated trout intestine, as a function of calcium concentration in the mucosal solution. Trout adapted to freshwater, O, or to sea water, ●. (Data from Crénesse[26])

Salt adaptation results in various effects among these species (Table 16.2). In goldfish, transfer to 200 mM medium is followed by a 79% drop in transepithelial net flux of sodium. It also induces a 43% reduction in mucosal uptake[6]. In trout, the mucosal entry is also diminished in SW (by 39% for Na^+ and Cl^-, by 69% for calcium) as shown by Figure 16.3, while the transport of sodium across the anterior intestine is increased by about 200%[11]. Finally, the flounder intestine reveals a mucosal uptake which remains relatively high and does not change from FW to SW (Figure 16.2) while transport of water, Na^+ and Cl^- are greatly increased (Table 16.1).

These results show that apical entry and active serosal transport are modified separately in fish intestine during salt adaptation. Higher permeability in FW is likely to enhance the efficiency of the basolateral ion pumping and this is of adaptative value in a medium where gaining ions from outside is an absolute requirement. In SW, mucosal uptake diminishes in species which do not adapt readily to hypertonic media. This may be viewed as a compensatory mechanism by which intestinal absorption of salt is limited in presence of slow (as in trout) or poor (as in goldfish) development of gill extrusion of ions. In the perfectly euryhaline fish (flounder), mucosal entry may remain as high as when in FW, because the gills can cope immediately with increased absorption of sodium chloride which is also used by the animal as a means of conserving as much water as possible when in this hypertonic environment.

Hormonal control

Possible intervention of short-term acting hormones such as catecholamines, prostaglandins and other substances modifying adenyl-cyclase activity has not been analysed to date on fish intestine.

By contrast, steroid hormones have been well considered in view of their known effects in amphibians and mammals. Stimulatory action of the ACTH–cortisol system on transport by intestinal sacs has been established in *Anguilla japonica*[5], in *Anguilla anguilla*[30] and in *Carassius auratus*[6]. These hormones are ineffective if injected into intact animals, but are successful as replacement therapy in hypophysectomised animals. However, it has been reported recently[31] that the synthetic steroid, dexamethasone, which suppresses endogenous production of cortisol, is active even in normal goldfish, while the natural hormones, aldosterone, deoxycorticosterone, cortisone and corticosterone, have no effect even in hypophysectomised animals.

A more precise analysis of the effects of cortisol has been obtained on goldfish intestine[6], by measuring the short-term mucosal entry of sodium along with its net transport by incubated sacs. It was concluded that apical uptake is not controlled by cortisol which only stimulates the pump. Moreover, this uptake, which is largely depressed by salt adaptation, could be considered as a limiting factor for the subsequent serosal transport in goldfish, but this has not been confirmed for the other species.

In the flounder, as in goldfish, maintenance of high apical permeability in hypophysectomised animals (Figures 16.1 and 16.2) does not prevent a striking reduction in pumping, presumably due to cortisol shortage. Thus, in FW, transport of water and chloride by incubated sacs is abolished after hypophysectomy (Table 16.3). The transepithelial PD of posterior intestine drops from -3.62 ± 0.76 mV ($n = 5$) in sham controls to -1.44 ± 0.34 ($n = 4$) in operated animals. The corresponding short-circuit current, which is assumed to represent the net flux of chloride under these circumstances[19], drops from $-42.5 \pm 17.0 \, \mu A/cm^2$ to -10.8 ± 2.4. In SW-adapted flounder, the reduction is not statistically significant due to the scatter of data, but it is likely to attain about 50% following hypophysectomy (Table 16.3).

Augmentation of the transport in SW fish does not require a preliminary increase in mucosal permeability. Moreover, in salt-adapted trout, this augmentation even occurs while the apical uptake is diminished.

Again, these differences between species indicate that the two steps involved in transepithelial crossing by inorganic ions are in fact regulated separately in fish intestine.

An elevation or decrease in ion transport following salt adaptation is not paralleled by sustained changes in blood cortisol levels as shown in goldfish and in euryhaline teleosts[32]. Yet, in *Anguilla anguilla*, SW animals present significantly higher cortisol production and metabolic clearance rates than FW eels[33,34], indicating that the availability and usage of the hormone at the cellular level are different in the two media. Further work is needed to determine which parameter of cortisol metabolism is important for its action on transport. It is interesting to note that cortisol stimulates Na^+-K^+-ATPase activity in gill and intestine[35]. Whatever the mechanism, the above data demonstrate that the hypothesis presented for an interaction between aldosterone and carrier molecules located at the apical pole of the cells[7,8] is irrelevant for cortisol action on fish intestine.

Acknowledgements

This discussion results from joint research carried out in close collaboration with Drs M. W. Smith, J. C. Ellory, D. Crénesse, J. Porthé-Nibelle and N. A. A. MacFarlane. Supporting fellowships were provided by the University of Nice, the Centre National de la Recherche Scientifique, the European Molecular Biology Organization, the British Royal Society and Medical Research Council and the Commissariat à l'Énergie Atomique. The author is indebted to Dr J. Maetz for his continued interest, to Dr. G. P. Haywood for correcting the manuscript and to Mrs P. Saint-Marc for technical assistance.

References

1. Smith, H. W. (1930). The absorption and excretion of water and salt by marine fishes. *Amer. J. Physiol.*, **93**, 480
2. Lahlou, B., Henderson, I. W. and Sawyer, W. H. (1969). Sodium exchanges in goldfish (*Carassius auratus* L.) adapted to a hypertonic saline solution. *Comp. Biochem. Physiol.*, **28**, 1427
3. Schultz, S. G., Curran, P. F., Chez, R. A. and Fuisz, R. E. (1967). Alanine and sodium influx across mucosal border of rabbit ileum. *J. Gen. Physiol.*, **50**, 1241
4. Mayer, N., Maetz, J., Chan, D. K. O., Forster, M. and Chester-Jones, I. (1967). Cortisol, a sodium excreting factor in the eel (*Anguilla anguilla* L.) adapted to sea water. *Nature London*, **214**, 118
5. Hirano, T. and Utida, S. (1968). Effects of ACTH and cortisol on water movement in isolated intestine of the eel, *Anguilla japonica*. *Endocrinol. Jap.*, **16**, 557

6. Ellory, J. C., Lahlou, B. and Smith, M. W. (1972). Changes in the intestinal transport of sodium induced by exposure of goldfish to a saline environment. *J. Physiol. Lond.*, **222**, 549

7. Crabbé, J. and DeWeer, P. (1964). Action of aldosterone on the bladder and skin of the toad. *Nature London*, **202**, 298

8. Sharp, G. W. G. and Leaf, A. (1966). Mechanism of action of aldosterone. *Physiol. Rev.*, **46**, 593

9. Edelman, I. S. and Fimognari, G. M. (1968). On the biochemical mechanism of action of aldosterone. *Rec. Progr. Horm. Res.*, **24**, 1

10. Motais, R. (1967). Les mécanismes d'échanges ioniques branchiaux chez les téléostéens. *Ann. Inst. Océan. Monaco*, **45**, I

11. Bensahla-Talet, A., Porthé-Nibelle, J. et Lahlou, B. (1974). Le transport de l'eau et du sodium par l'intestin isolé de la truite *Salmo irideus* au cours de l'adaptation à l'eau de mer. *C. R. Acad. Sci. Paris*, **278**, 2541

12. Forster, R. P. (1948). Use of thin kidney slices and isolated renal tubules for direct study of cellular transport kinetics. *Science*, **108**, 65

13. Krebs, H. A. and Henseleit, K. (1932). Untersuchungen über die Harnstoffbildrung im Tierkörper. *Hoppe-Seyler's Z. Physiol. Chem.*, **210**, 33

14. Wilson, T. H. and Wiseman, G. (1954). The use of sacs of everted small intestine for the study of the transference of substances from the mucosal to the serosal surface. *J. Physiol. Lond.*, **123**, 116

15. Ellory, J. C. and Smith, M. W. (1970). Short-term measurements of amino acid and sodium fluxes across the mucosal border of goldfish intestine. *J. Physiol. Lond.*, **216**, 46

16. Nellans, H. N., Frizzell, R. A. and Schultz, S. G. (1973). Coupled sodium-chloride influx across the brush border of rabbit ileum. *Amer. J. Physiol.*, **225**, 467

17. House, C. R. and Green, K. (1965). Ion and water transport in isolated intestine of the marine teleost, *Cottus scorpius. J. Exp. Biol.*, **42**, 177

18. Maetz, J. and Skadhauge, E. (1968). Drinking rates and gill ionic turnover in relation to external salinities in the eel. *Nature London*, **217**, 371

19. Lahlou, B., Smith, M. W. and Ellory, J. C. (1974). Le transport intestinal *in vitro* du sodium et du chlore chez le flet européen, *Platichthys flesus*, en eau de mer et en eau douce. *C.R. Acad. Sci. Paris*, **278**, 761

20. Ellory, J. C., Nibelle, J. and Smith, M. W. (1973). The effect of salt adaptation on the permeability and cation selectivity of the goldfish intestinal epithelium. *J. Physiol. Lond.*, **231**, 105

21. Huang, K. C. and Chen, T. S. T. (1971). Ion transport across intestinal mucosa of winter flounder, *Pseudopleuronectes americanus. Amer. J. Physiol.*, **220**, 1734

22. Hirano, T. and Utida, S. (1972). In Japanese. *Seitai no kagaku*, **23**, 1

23. Ando, M., Utida, S. and Nagahama, H. (1975). Active transport of chloride in eel intestine with special reference to seawater adaptation. *Comp. Biochem. Physiol.*, **51A**, 27

24. Smith, M. W., Ellory, J. C. and Lahlou, B. (1975). Sodium and chloride transport by the intestine of the European flounder, *Platichthys flesus*, adapted to fresh or sea water. *Pflügers Arch.*, **357**, 303

25. O'Donnell, J. M. and Smith, M. W. (1973). Uptake of calcium and magnesium by rat duodenal mucosa analysed by means of competing metals. *J. Physiol. Lond.*, **229**, 733

26. Crénesse, D. (1974). Étude *in vitro* de la perméabilité aux ions minéraux de la face muqueuse de l'intestin isolé de la truite arc-en-ciel, *Salmo irideus*. Thèse 3ᵉ Cycle, Marseille

27. Curran, P. F., Schultz, S. G., Chez, R. A. and Fuisz, R. E. (1967). Kinetic relations of the Na-amino acid interactions at the mucosal border of intestine. *J. Gen. Physiol.*, **50**, 1261

28. Erlij, D. and Smith, M. W. (1973). Sodium uptake by the outside surface of frogskin. *J. Physiol. Lond.*, **218**, 33

29. Ferguson, D. R. and Smith, M. W. (1972). Direct measurement of sodium uptake by toad bladder mucosal cells. *J. Endocrinol.*, **55**, 195

30. Gaitskell, R. E. and Chester-Jones, I. (1970). Effects of adrenalectomy and cortisol injection on the *in vitro* movement of water by the intestine of the freshwater European eel (*Anguilla anguilla* L.). *Gen. Comp. Endocrinol.*, **15**, 491

31. Porthé-Nibelle, J. and Lahlou, B. (1975). Effects of corticosteroid hormones and inhibitors of steroids on sodium and water transport by goldfish intestine. *Comp. Biochem. Physiol.*, **50A**, 801

32. Porthé-Nibelle, J. and Lahlou, B. (1974). Plasma concentrations of cortisol in hypophysectomized and sodium chloride-adapted goldfish (*Carassius auratus* L.). *J. Endocrinol.* **63**, 377
33. Henderson, I. W., Sa'di, M. N. and Hargreaves, G. (1974). Studies on the production and metabolic clearance rates of cortisol in the European eel (*Anguilla anguilla* L.). *J. Steroid Biochem.*, **5**, 701
34. Leloup-Hatey, J. (1974). Influence de l'adaptation à l'eau de mer sur la fonction interrénalienne de l'anguille (*Anguilla anguilla* L.). *Gen. Comp. Endocrinol.*, **24**, 28
35. Epstein, F. H., Cynamon, M. and McKay, W. (1971). Endocrine control of Na-K-ATPase and seawater adaptation in *Anguilla rostrata*. *Gen. Comp. Endocrinol.* **16**, 323

16

Third Main Paper

Regulation of Drinking and Intestinal Water Absorption in Euryhaline Teleosts

E. Skadhauge

Institute of Medical Physiology A,
University of Copenhagen

Introduction

It should surprise no one that all three authors dealing with 'Adaptation of intestinal ion transport' turn to euryhaline teleosts as their experimental subjects. Euryhaline teleosts exposed to waters of various salinities can in hyperosmotic environments only gain water by drinking the surrounding fluid. Their intestinal salt and water transport system is, therefore, unique among vertebrates due to its crucial function in osmoregulation. Scientists interested in regulation of intestinal salt and water transport naturally become attracted to these fish. The three papers show different aspects of the efforts towards the understanding of adaptation. There is description of transport parameters, hormonal regulation, attempts to elucidate detailed cellular mechanisms, and — in my presentation — attempts to determine the role in osmoregulation of the integrated intestinal salt and water transport studied by means of a computer calculation. The papers here, therefore, reflect two recent trends in the development of the classical organ physiology. One is analytical: we go from cell, to membrane, to molecule. The other attempts to integrate the cells into organs, let organs function together, and by hormonal and nervous regulation become integrated to the organism. In these studies the concepts and models of servo-engineering are used.

I shall give here the physiological background for the interaction of drinking and interstitial transport in marine teleosts in sea water, present some of the data resulting from studies of adaptation and then develop a computer model of intestinal salt and water absorption, giving the results when the data of various fish are applied to that model.

PHYSIOLOGICAL BACKGROUND

Figure 16.1 shows the salt and water transport across surface and gills, excretion in urine and faeces, and drinking in a teleost in fresh water and in sea water.

When euryhaline teleosts live in waters of salinities higher than the osmolality of plasma they are threatened by dehydration. They can only gain water by drinking the surrounding media. They absorb NaCl and water through the intestinal wall, and excrete NaCl through the gills. Divalent ions are excreted through the anus and the kidney in isosmotic concentration. Thus they gain water to make up for the osmotic losses. The water being drunk is of course hyperosmotic to plasma. In the anterior end of the intestinal tract, the fluid is diluted by inflow of water from plasma, but before being

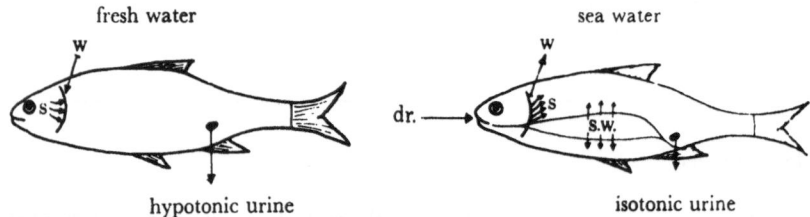

fresh water   sea water

hypotonic urine   isotonic urine

Figure 16.1 Exchange of salt and water with the surrounding medium in euryhaline teleosts. In fresh water, water flows into the fish. In sea water, water is lost to the surrounding medium. Water is gained by drinking of sea water followed by intestinal absorption of salt and water. NaCl is excreted through the gills (see reference 8)

isosmotic it is absorbed, proportional to the NaCl absorption, presumably caused by the NaCl absorption. This is called solute-linked water flow. It will appear from this that drinking rate is both a measure of intestinal NaCl absorption and osmotic water flow, provided the loss with faeces and urine is relatively small. It is also clear that if the fish is adapted to waters of even higher salinity, the new levels that the above-mentioned parameters reach must be closely correlated.

INTESTINAL TRANSPORT PARAMETERS

I shall now present some of the measurements of drinking rate and intestinal NaCl absorption and then develop a mathematical model to account quantitatively for the various data. The purpose is to elucidate the interaction of the parameters, their sensitivity and thus — hopefully — contribute to the understanding of the limiting factors in adaptation to high salinity.

The data are from my own work on the European eel[1,2] and from the little cyprinodont, *Aphanius dispar*, from Ein Fashkha at the Dead Sea, studied in collaboration with Dr Ruth Lotan from the Department of Zoology in Jerusalem[3]. In the calculations I have also used data from Shehadeh and Gordon[4] on the rainbow trout.

In the eel we first studied the gill sodium isotope turnover, and the drinking rate in animals adapted to fresh water, to sea water and to double strength sea water[5]. Both parameters went up as expected in waters of higher salinity.

I then measured the intestinal net absorption rates of NaCl in eels studied in a perfusion system *in vivo*. The Na^+ and Cl^- absorption rates ran parallel and went up in waters of higher salinity, as did the maximal osmolality difference against which the intestine could transport water[1].

The *Aphanius* were adapted to SW, to two times SW, and to three times SW, and at SW to three different temperatures. We measured plasma osmolality, drinking rate, and oxygen consumption. The plasma osmolality was remarkably stable in spite of severe osmotic stress. At stable temperature, oxygen consumption did not vary much. The most interesting observation was, however, that drinking rate was almost unchanged at the three salinities. What does that mean? It leads to the conclusion first that the intestinal NaCl absorption rate goes up in proportion to the salinity, and secondly that the gill osmotic permeability must be proportionally reduced. These findings prompted us to examine the relationship between drinking rate and NaCl absorption further on the computer model.

THE MODEL

The intestine is viewed as a straight, rigid tube where fluid flows into one end at an initial velocity — the drinking rate — with an osmolality made up of NaCl and $MgSO_4$ with appropriate osmotic coefficients. Water passes across the wall following the osmolality difference and the permeability coefficient, NaCl is absorbed according to saturation kinetics as measured *in vivo*, and H_2O follows NaCl as solute-linked water flow; $MgSO_4$ is not absorbed.

In the computer simulation, the concentrations along the length of the gut were calculated. The flow velocity is a measure of the integrated water movement across the walls. It is reciprocal to the concentration of unabsorbable ions. The model shows initial dilution in the anterior end and later absorption in the posterior end. The osmolality drops rapidly to plasma osmolality. In the three species of fish upon which the model is based, measurement of concentrations along the gut was in good agreement with the model, thus increasing its validity[6].

RESULTS OF THE MODEL

In the first simulation — in the eel — intestinal water absorption was calculated as a function of drinking rate (Figure 16.2). Drinking of SW and two times SW respectively was calculated at different intestinal NaCl absorption rates as multiples of the value found in SW-adapted fish. It was observed first that for each set of values, there is a narrow range of drinking rate which results in optimal water absorption. For the eel in SW the observed drinking rate was exactly at the optimum. This observation supports the concept that at steady state, drinking rate and therefore ability to survive in higher salinity is limited by the intestinal NaCl transport capacity. Second, in order to double the water absorption, the NaCl absorption must be doubled too. Third, to have double water absorption in two times SW, the NaCl absorption must be

Intestinal water absorption

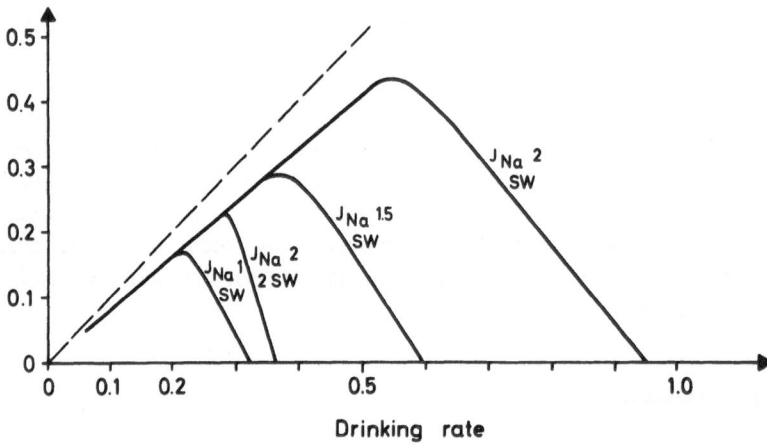

Drinking rate

Figure 16.2 A computer calculation of intestinal water absorption as a function of the drinking rate. The calculation is based upon values from the yellow european eel (see reference 6). The broken line indicates 100% absorption. J_{Na} stands for maximal intestinal NaCl absorption rate. '1' stands for the value determined in seawater (SW) adapted eels. For eels in SW the intestinal water absorption is proportional to the NaCl absorption. In double strength sea water (2 SW), the double NaCl absorption rate (J_{Na} 2) results in an only slightly higher water absorption

quadrupled. Our observations in nature showed somewhat lower values[5] suggesting a relatively smaller water loss. This comes out more clearly in the *Aphanius* simulation. But we will first turn to the rainbow trout data. We examined drinking rate and intestinal NaCl absorption rate as functions of the salinity of the medium. Values are only published up to full strength SW. The computer simulation was extended up to three times SW assuming proportional increase in NaCl absorption rates. The following was found: When NaCl absorption goes up proportionally in waters of higher salinity, the drinking rate will first increase proportionally as observed, then level off and eventually decrease.

This calculation, thus, makes it possible to understand why at lower salinities, an increase in drinking rate is found with higher salinity[4,5,7], whereas at higher salinities, as in *Aphanius*, drinking rate does not increase[3].

This leads to the last computation where drinking rate and intestinal NaCl absorption in *Aphanius* was examined in two hypothetical cases. First: NaCl absorption rate goes up proportional to salinity. This resulted in unchanged drinking rate. Second: Drinking rate goes up assuming unchanged osmotic permeability of the gills. This requires an exponential rise in NaCl absorption in the intestine. Since this is highly unlikely on energetic grounds[3], it is understandable that nature instead has chosen to reduce the osmotic permeability of the gills.

CLOSING WORDS

These computer calculations have thus brought agreement between various data which were at first sight conflicting. They have pinpointed the necessity of further studies into how (and by which mechanism) the osmotic permeability of the gills is reduced, and they have — finally — shown that increase in plasma osmolality is not only an error signal, but a useful part of the adaptation.

REFERENCES

1. Skadhauge, E. (1969). The mechanism of salt and water absorption in the intestine of the eel (*Anguilla anguilla*) adapted to waters of various salinities. *J. Physiol. Lond.*, **204**, 135
2. Skadhauge, E. (1974). Coupling of transmural flows of NaCl and water in the intestine of the eel (*Anguilla anguilla*). *J. Exp. Biol.*, **60**, 535
3. Skadhauge, E. and Lotan, R. (1974). Drinking rate and oxygen consumption in the euryhaline teleost *Aphanius dispar* in waters of high salinity. *J. Exp. Biol.*, **60**, 547
4. Shahadeh, Z. H. and Gordon, M. S. (1969). The role of the intestine in salinity adaptation of the rainbow trout, *Salmo gairdneri*. *Comp. Biochem. Physiol.*, **30**, 397
5. Maetz, J. and Skadhauge, E. (1968). Drinking rates and gill ionic turnover in relation to external salinities in the eel. *Nature, London*, **217**, 371
6. Kristensen, K. and Skadhauge, E. (1974). Flow along the gut, and intestinal absorption of salt and water in euryhaline teleosts. A theoretical analysis. *J. Exp. Biol.*, **60**, 557
7. Potts, W. T. W., Foster, M. A., Rudy, P. P. and Parry, G. H. (1967). Sodium and water balance in the cichlid teleost *Tilapia mossambica*. *J. Exp. Biol.*, **47**, 461
8. Maetz, J. (1970). Les mécanismes des échanges ioniques branchiaux chez les téléostéens. Études de cinétique isotopique. *Bull. Inf. Sci. Tech. C.E.A.*, **145**, 3

16
Discussion Paper on
Intestinal Ion and Water Transport in the Diamondback Terrapin Acclimatised Either to Sea Water or to Fresh Water

M. Gilles-Baillien

University of Liège
Laboratory of General and Comparative Biochemistry

The diamondback terrapin, *Malaclemys centrata centrata* (Latreille) is a euryhaline chelonian which can be acclimatised either to sea water or to fresh water. Survival of chelonians in sea water has often been attributed to the low permeability of the integument and to the presence of an orbital salt gland. However, there is no doubt they have to face important problems of water loss and salt gain. Indeed the Na^+ and Cl^- concentrations of the blood plasma are higher in seawater-acclimatised diamondback terrapins than in freshwater animals though the increase in osmotic pressure of the blood (from 270 to 430 mosmol/l) is mainly due to urea. The urine changes from hypo-osmotic in freshwater conditions to iso-osmotic[1]. But what is more striking is that animals with a 15 cm plastron length weigh 800 g when acclimatised to fresh water for several months and only 400 g when in sea water for the same period[2]. According to Bentley *et al.*[3] the diamondback terrapins completely stop drinking when in sea water in contrast to euryhaline teleosts.

In experiments *in vitro*, Na^+ fluxes have been measured across the jejunal mucosa of diamondback terrapins acclimatised either to sea water or to fresh

Table *16.1* Na^+ fluxes across the jejunal mucosa of the diamondback terrapin acclimatised either to sea water (SW) or to fresh water (FW)

	SW		FW	
	Influx	*Outflux*	*Influx*	*Outflux*
Na^+ 115 mEq/l	4.74 ± 1.20 (n = 6)	4.96 ± 0.85 (n = 6)	6.89 ± 1.22 (n = 6)	7.42 ± 0.71 (n = 6)
Na^+ 150 mEq/l	10.36 ± 1.49 (n = 3)	8.96 ± 1.36 (n = 3)	21.27 ± 2.16 (n = 3)	5.10 ± 0.38 (n = 3)

Results expressed in $\mu Eq\ cm^{-2}\ h^{-1}$

334

water. Table *16.1* shows the results obtained when the Na⁺ concentration of the incubating medium is similar to that of the plasma of freshwater animals (115 mEq/l), Na⁺ fluxes in both directions are higher in freshwater animals than in seawater ones and moreover within each group influx and outflux are not significantly different. When the Na⁺ concentration of the incubation medium is raised up to 150 mEq/l, both influx and outflux of Na⁺ are increased in seawater animals. In freshwater animals, the influx is highly significantly increased while the outflux is slightly but significantly decreased. Further experimentation is required before any conclusion can be drawn as to

Table *16.2* Net water flux measured across the mucosa of the colon and of the jejunum in the diamondback terrapin acclimatised either to sea water (SW) or to fresh water (FW)

		SW	FW
		(μl cm^{-2} h^{-1})	
Colon	FW gradient	20.6 ± 5.5 (5)	36.9 ± 14.3 (10)
	SW gradient	49.3 ± 8.2 (6)	69.4 ± 6.2 (5)
Jejunum	FW gradient	23.7 ± 2.9 (3)	16.3 ± 7.6 (4)
	SW gradient	48.4 ± 7.2 (4)	136.4 ± 27.5 (4)

FW gradient: the NaCl concentration is 115 mM in the serosal saline and 15 mM in the mucosal saline.
SW gradient: the NaCl concentration is 150 mM in the serosal saline and 50 mM in the mucosal saline.

the significance and origin of this net flux of Na⁺. These results however can be related to the permeability of the jejunal mucosa to water, measured in the presence of an osmotic gradient as shown in Table *16.2*. The water permeability is low in both seawater and freshwater animals when the NaCl concentration is only 115 mM in the serosal saline. But when this concentration is raised up to 150 mM, the water permeability, increased in seawater animals, appears to be much more enhanced in freshwater animals and could possibly be related to the important Na⁺ net flux observed at the same serosal Na⁺ concentration. At the level of the colon, the water permeability is significantly higher in freshwater-acclimatised terrapins at both serosal NaCl concentrations. These results are preliminary but already suggestive of changes occurring in intestinal transport during salt adaptation.

References

1. Gilles-Baillien, M. (1970). Urea and osmoregulation in the diamondback terrapin *Malaclemys centrata centrata* (Latreille). *J. Exp. Biol.*, **52**, 691
2. Gilles-Baillien, M. (1973). Hibernation and osmoregulation in the diamondback terrapin *Malaclemys centrata centrata* (Latreille). *J. Exp. Biol.*, **59**, 45
3. Bentley, P. J., Bretz, W. L. and Schmidt-Nielsen, K. (1967). Osmoregulation in the diamondback terrapin, *Malaclemys centrata centrata*. *J. Exp. Biol.*, **46**, 161

Discussion 16

Parsons: With regard to the chloride pump present in the seawater-adapted eels, does this operate on the basis of an exchange for bicarbonate?

Hirano: We have no information on Cl^-/HCO_3^- exchange in the eel intestine. Huang and Chen (reference 27 on p. 315) have suggested the presence of Cl^-/HCO_3^- exchange in the flounder intestine. Since HCO_3^--ATPase activity increases after seawater adaptation in parallel with the development of the chloride pump, it is likely that the Cl^- pump in the seawater eel intestine operates on the basis of an exchange for bicarbonate. However, experiments have yet to be done in the eel intestine.

Armstrong: Have you looked at chloride fluxes, PD and I_{sc} across seawater eel intestine in the absence of sodium? If so, can you tell us something about what you find in this situation? Our work with frog intestine shows that, in this system, there is a chloride pump which is independent of sodium and which is quite different in its metabolic dependence, sensitivity to inhibitors, etc. from the sodium pump.

Hirano: Serosa-negative PD and I_{sc} increase considerably after changing the bathing solution from NaCl–Ringer to choline–Cl–Ringer, indicating the presence of a Na^+-independent chloride pump in the eel intestine. This was shown in Figure 16.1 of the accompanying text. We have not measured chloride fluxes in choline–Cl–Ringer solution. However, part of the chloride pump in the seawater eel intestine may be coupled with a sodium pump, since ouabain abolishes the serosa-negative PD when added to the serosal Ringer solution.

Field: Are there morphological changes with saltwater adaptation that correspond to the observed changes in intestinal enzymes?

Hirano: We have only checked the ordinary histology of the eel intestine stained with haematoxylin and eosin. There is a reduction in the surface area or in the height of the villi after seawater adaptation. Note that there is no crypt in the eel intestine (reference 19 on p. 315).

Skadhauge: I wonder whether anyone can comment on the transient increase in blood cortisol level after transfer of eels from freshwater to seawater. Later the cortisol level returns to normal whilst the NaCl absorption is still high. Is the reason an increased turnover or is the target organ sensitivity changed?

Lahlou: In all species studied thus far, salinity changes induce only transient modifications in plasma cortisol levels. The rates of intestinal transport are not directly correlated with the actual blood cortisol concentration. Recent evidence (references 33 and 34, on p. 328) demonstrates that metabolic clearance rate of cortisol is largely increased in the eel following salt adaptation. Therefore it is the utilisation of the hormone by the target tissue which has to be considered and related to the amplitude of the transport.

Dowling: When the comparative physiologists talk about the effects of hypophysectomy on the intestinal adaptation of fish to changing conditions of salinity, have they considered the effects of nutrient intake on gut structure and function? In mammalian species, we and many others have shown that hypophysectomy leads to intestinal mucosal hypoplasia and hypofunction and that these changes are mainly due to the associated reduction in food intake. Is there a corresponding reduction in the nutrient intake of hypophysectomised fish and does this influence the ionic fluxes across the intestine? While talking about food intake, what happens to other migratory fish which move from sea to freshwater such as the Atlantic salmon and the sea trout which, as any angler knows, do not eat in freshwater? Do they show similar adaptational changes as do eels, goldfish and terrapins?

Lahlou: Suppression of the pituitary gland does not prevent food intake in the goldfish. Intestines from hypophysectomised or normal animals are therefore comparable as regards the presence of organic solutes in the lumen. In other species, starvation in laboratory conditions does not consistently alter the electrical or transport properties of the tissue, but in this case the operated animals are kept unfed as well. However, morphological changes are likely to occur if the fish are not fed for a protracted length of time, but this would not account for the large reduction in transport or mucosal ion permeability observed in the flounder or in the trout.

Maetz: I should like to make Dr Skadhauge aware of the limitations of his computerised model. In one of the slides, you studied the possibility of trout surviving in three times seawater. In fact, trouts cannot survive more than one times seawater. Your model should perhaps have predicted this!

Skadhauge: The computation was purely hypothetical showing what happens if net NaCl absorption rate goes up in proportion to the salinity. Since the gills can excrete more NaCl than the intestine can absorb (Mayer and Nibelle, *Comp. Biochem. Physiol.*, **35**, 553, 1970), the intestinal NaCl absorption rate will presumably limit the tolerance to high salinity. The rainbow trout can just stand full strength seawater because it cannot increase intestinal NaCl transport further than to match the osmotic water loss at this salinity. This aspect was not elucidated in the computation, but the original data of Shehadeh and Gordon (reference 4 on p. 333) may be interpreted to indicate saturation of NaCl absorption on seawater adaptation.

Wingate: Does the emphasis on drinking rates in fish reflect the fact that, in fish, endogenous secretions are unimportant in relation to oral intake, whereas in man the major part of the fluid load seen by the intestine is composed of endogenous secretions?

Maetz: I am not aware of any instance of endogenous fluid secretion in the intestinal tract of the fish. As discussed by Dr Skadhauge, however, when hypertonic saline is introduced into the gut of the seawater-adapted eel, water enters the gut lumen osmotically to dilute the fluid before absorption takes place. Now it is not even sure that the actually takes place in nature, as ingested seawater is diluted in the oesophagus by *salt loss* rather than *osmotic water entry*, in such a way that the fluid entering the intestine is iso-osmotic (reference 13 on p. 315).

Scharrer: Is there any information available as to whether non-electrolyte absorption is affected by adaptation to seawater?

Maetz: Michael Smith has studied glucose absorption in the freshwater goldfish (reference 29 on p. 315) and Huang and Rout have studied amino acid absorption in the seawater flounder (*Amer. J. Physiol.*, **212**, 799, 1967). Unfortunately, whether non-electrolyte absorption is affected by adaptation to sea water in a euryhaline fish has not been studied. This is an important problem to be investigated.

17
In vitro Behaviour of Human Jejunum and Ileum: Response to Theophylline and Acetyl choline

L. A. TURNBERG, P. E. T. ISAACS,
C. L. CORBETT and A. K. RILEY

Department of Medicine,
Manchester University

Using perfusion techniques *in vivo*, it has been possible during the last few years to demonstrate several characteristics of salt and water transport in the human intestine *in vivo*[1-4]. Information has been derived to suggest that the jejunum behaves differently from the ileum in several respects. For instance, permeability to sodium and water appears to be greater in the jejunum than in the ileum and this high permeability has made it difficult to demonstrate transport of sodium against electrochemical gradients in the jejunum *in vivo*. Transport of sodium and chloride against gradients has been more readily demonstrated in the ileum. There is also a major difference between jejunum and ileum *in vivo* in the handling of bicarbonate; in the jejunum, bicarbonate is removed from the lumen against considerable gradients, whereas it accumulates in the lumen of the ileum against considerable gradients.

Studies of the behaviour of human intestinal mucosa *in vitro* have been limited in number, but results do suggest that there are differences between *in vitro* and *in vivo* activity[5,6], which are difficult to explain on the basis simply of technical differences. The present investigations were undertaken to study the activity of the human jejunum and ileum *in vitro* and some comparisons are made with their activity *in vivo*.

Pieces of mucosa from fresh surgical specimens taken at laparotomy from patients with a variety of intestinal diseases were stripped of serosa and muscle coats and mounted rapidly between the two halves of a modified Ussing flux chamber and bathed on both sides with warmed, oxygenated and stirred

Table 17.1 Electrical characteristics of human jejunum and ileum *in vitro*

	Jejunum ($n = 14$)		*Ileum* ($n = 37$)	
	Control	*+ Glucose*	*Control*	*+ Glucose*
PD (mV)	4.8 ± 0.4	7.7 ± 0.3	3.5 ± 0.3	8.8 ± 0.4
SCC (μA.cm^{-2})	69 ± 5.7	182 ± 12.3	94 ± 7.0	237 ± 15.5
R (Ω cm^{-2})	75 ± 6.9	52.7 ± 4.3	40 ± 2.8	34.8 ± 1.8

isotonic solutions. All the mucosal specimens used in these experiments were shown subsequently to be histologically normal. Electrical potential was measured via two KCl-in-agar electrodes placed adjacent to the mucosa and a current was passed to nullify the potential through two saturated NaCl electrodes placed at opposite ends of the chamber. This short-circuit current was monitored and adjusted by hand every 3 to 5 minutes. Ionic fluxes across the mucosa were measured by adding isotopes of sodium and chloride to either side of paired tissues.

With glucose-free isotonic solutions, the electrical potential was significantly higher in the jejunum than in the ileum while short-circuit current was higher in the ileum than in the jejunum. The calculated tissue resistance was therefore higher in the jejunum than in the ileum (Table 17.1). Glucose caused a rise in PD and short-circuit current in both tissues, while it did not influence tissue resistance.

In both the jejunum and the ileum, it was possible to demonstrate a net absorptive flux of sodium, although this was small in the jejunum. Glucose stimulated sodium absorption in both regions and this accounted for the majority of the short-circuit current response. In the jejunum net chloride movement was indistinguishable from zero while there was a significant net absorption of chloride in the ileum. Glucose did not influence chloride movement in either tissue (Table 17.2). It is interesting to note that the unidirectional flux from serosa to mucosa, the presumably passive back flux, of sodium was

Table 17.2 Flux data in isolated jejunal and ileal tissues; response to glucose

	Na			*Cl*		
	ms	*sm*	*net*	*ms*	*sm*	*net*
Jejunum						
Control	6.5 ± 1.2	5.2 ± 1.1	$+1.3 \pm 0.4$	7.1 ± 1.2	6.6 ± 1.6	$+0.5 \pm 2.6$
D-Glucose	12.9 ± 1.5	7.1 ± 0.6	$+5.9 \pm 1.2$	7.9 ± 0.9	9.1 ± 0.8	-1.3 ± 0.8
Ileum						
Control	12.5 ± 0.8	10.3 ± 0.8	$+2.2 \pm 0.9$	11.5 ± 0.7	10.5 ± 0.5	$+1.0 \pm 1.0$
D-Glucose	20.2 ± 1.5	8.1 ± 0.5	$+12.1 \pm 1.4$	11.1 ± 0.6	9.5 ± 0.6	$+1.6 \pm 0.7$

smaller in the jejunum than in the ileum. This is an contradistinction to the permeability to sodium *in vivo* where the jejunum appears much more permeable than the ileum.

Residual ion fluxes were not distinguishable from zero in either tissue in the presence or absence of glucose. This is in contrast to the behaviour *in vivo* where bicarbonate transport, which would appear as a residual ion flux in these experiments *in vitro*, certainly represents a significant proportion of total net ion movement. The difference in bicarbonate handling by the intestine *in vitro* and *in vivo* has been noted many times, although explanations for this difference are somewhat unsatisfactory.

INFLUENCE OF THEOPHYLLINE

Theophylline, at a dose of 10^{-2} M, added to both sides of the mucosa, stimulated short-circuit current and PD in both the jejunum and the ileum. Tissue resistance also rose significantly. The increase in short-circuit current was due predominantly to a reversal of net chloride movement from absorption to secretion, due to a diminution of the mucosa-to-serosa unidirectional flux and also to an increase in the flux in the opposite direction. Net sodium absorption was also reduced. A similar response was observed in the jejunum and it is interesting to note that the jejunum is capable of secreting chloride against a gradient despite the fact that there is no net movement of chloride under control conditions.

The presence of glucose in the bathing medium caused a rather different effect on tissue resistance. As noted previously, resistance rose in the absence of glucose, while in its presence, resistance fell significantly. This observation was also noted in jejunal tissues. The response was observed when glucose was present on the mucosal but not on the serosal side of the tissue and was repeatable with 3-*O*-methyl glucose. This fall in resistance was also noted when glucose was added after theophylline, resistance rising first with theophylline and falling later on addition of the glucose.

RESPONSE TO ACETYL CHOLINE

Several pieces of evidence have suggested that the parasympathetic nervous system may influence intestinal ion transport[7-9], and histological sections stained with cholinesterase stain demonstrate probably cholinergic fibres in large numbers around the crypts and to some extent adjacent to the villous epithelial cells. It was conceivable, therefore, that these fibres may be concerned with transport processes. The response to acetyl choline was therefore investigated. Acetyl choline caused a rise in PD and short-circuit current which was not accompanied by a change in tissue resistance. The response was maximal at 10^{-4} M although some effect could be seen at 10^{-5} M. Neostigmine enhanced and atropine blocked the effect of acetyl choline suggesting that it was a true muscarinic response.

Ion flux measurements revealed that the short-circuit current response was almost entirely attributable to reversal of net chloride absorption to one of net chloride secretion, due predominantly to an increase in serosa-to-mucosa unidirectional flux. Sodium transport was not affected nor was the residual ion flux.

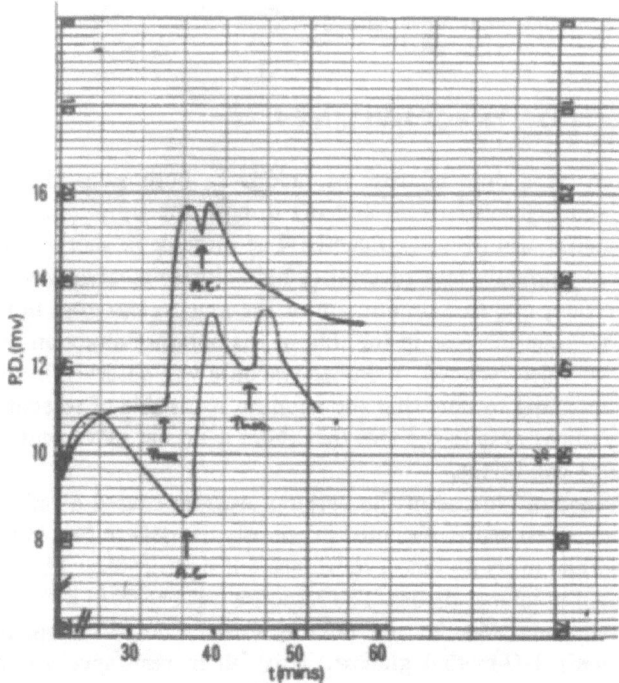

Figure 17.1 Ileal PD response to theophylline and acetyl choline given consecutively. There is no additive response to either of these agents given near the peak response of the other, suggesting activity via a common mechanism

In view of the similarities between the responses to theophylline and acetyl choline, the relationships between their responses was studied. Figure 17.1 demonstrates the PD response to each agent given shortly one after the other, and in both cases the response to one agent had no additive effect on the response to the other, suggesting that both agents acted through a similar mechanism, possibly cyclic AMP. Cyclic AMP levels were therefore measured in tissues incubated with acetyl choline or theophylline, using a competitive binding protein technique. Theophylline caused the expected rise in cyclic AMP but acetyl choline did not apparently influence cyclic AMP levels between 2 and 25 minutes.

342

These observations suggest that acetyl choline and theophylline, although invoking a similar mechanism, do not both act through cyclic AMP. The possibility exists that both theophylline and acetyl choline act through a common pathway which is not cyclic AMP. Since in other tissues acetyl choline stimulates cyclic GMP, the role played by this substance in the cholinergic response in intestinal mucosa is currently being investigated.

These observations do indicate a possible mechanism by which the parasympathetic nervous system could influence intestinal ion transport. Against it having a physiological role is the rather high dose of acetyl choline used in these experiments. However, it is recognised that there are very active cholinesterases present in sub-mucosal tissues and it is conceivable that the majority of the acetyl choline added to these tissues was inactivated before reaching receptors on epithelial cells. Thus the response could still be physiologically significant.

CONCLUSIONS

These studies demonstrate that some of the differences between the human jejunum and ileum *in vivo* may be observed *in vitro*. However, two *in vivo/in vitro* differences are clear: tissue conductance appears greater in the ileum than in the jejunum *in vitro* while the reverse is the case *in vivo*, and bicarbonate transport which forms a considerable proportion of total net ion transport *in vivo*, is apparently not significant *in vitro*. The observation too that theophylline can affect tissue resistance and ion transport in different ways according to whether glucose is present or absent is of interest and also emphasises the need for caution in transferring *in vitro* data to the situation *in vivo*.

The observation that acetyl choline can influence intestinal ion transport *in vitro* may or may not be physiologically important. Further studies are indicated on the effect of cholinergic mechanisms on transport *in vivo* before conclusions can be drawn.

References

1. Fordtran, J. S., Rector, F. C. and Carter, N. W. (1968). The mechanisms of sodium absorption in the human small intestine. *J. Clin. Invest.*, **47**, 884
2. Fordtran, J. S. and Ingelfinger, F. J. (1968). Absorption of water, electrolytes, and sugars from the human gut. *Handbook of Physiology*. American Physiological Society, Washington, (Section 6): 1457
3. Turnberg, L. A., Bieberdorf, F. A., Morawski, S. G. and Fordtran, J. S. (1970). Interrelationships of chloride, bicarbonate, sodium, and hydrogen transport in the human ileum. *J. Clin. Invest.*, **49**, 557
4. Turnberg, L. A., Fordtran, J. S., Carter, N. W. and Rector, F. C. (1970). Mechanism of bicarbonate absorption and its relationship to sodium transport in the human jejunum. *J. Clin. Invest.*, **49**, 548

5. Field, M. (1971). Intestinal secretion: effect of cyclic AMP and its role in cholera. *New Eng. J. Med.*, **284**, 1137

6. Al-Awqati, Q., Cameron, J. L. and Greenough, W. B. (1973). Electrolyte transport in human ileum: effect of purified cholera exotoxin. *Amer. J. Physiol.*, **224**, 818

7. Tidball, C. S., and Tidball, M. E. (1958). Changes in intestinal net absorption of a sodium chloride solution produced by atropine in normal and vagotomized dogs. *Amer. J. Physiol.*, **193**, 25

8. Tidball, C. S. (1961). Active chloride transport during intestinal secretion. *Amer. J. Physiol.*, **200**, 309

9. Caren, J. F., Meyer, J. H. and Grossman, M. I. (1974). Canine intestinal secretion during and after rapid distention of the small bowel. *Amer. J. Physiol.*, **227**, 183

17

Discussion Paper on

Intestinal Adaptation in Response to Chronic Glucagon Administration

W. F. Caspary and H. Lücke,

Division of Gastroenterology and Metabolism,
Department of Medicine, University of Göttingen

INTRODUCTION

Increased intestinal absorption of sugars[1-3], amino acids[2,3] and bile acids[4] has been observed in experimental diabetes mellitus[1-3], semistarvation[5] and in *ob/ob* mice[6]. Experimental diabetes mellitus is also associated with an increase in digestive brush-border enzymatic activity[2,7]. The mechanism responsible for these intestinal adaptive changes is not understood. Since endogenous glucagon levels are elevated in diabetes mellitus[7-9], as well as during starvation[9,11], glucagon may be considered as a candidate responsible for the adaptive changes of intestinal mucosal function under these conditions. The effect of exogenous glucagon administration on intestinal absorption of hexoses, water, and electrolytes was therefore examined by a perfusion technique in the rat small intestine *in vivo*.

METHODS

Female Wistar rats (180 ± 20 g) were injected intraperitoneally twice daily for 5 days with 10 or 100 μg of glucagon (Glukagon®, Eli Lilly GmbH, Giessen). Controls were injected with the phenol-containing commercial solvent. Rats received a standard laboratory chow diet and had free access to food and water. Intestinal absorption of 3-*O*-methyl-D-glucose was measured by an open perfusion technique after cannulation of a 30–35 cm jejunal gut segment beginning 15 cm beyond the pylorus in rats anaesthetised with pentobarbital. The perfusate consisted of Krebs–Henseleit phosphate buffer (pH 7.3) and 2 ×

10^{-2} M 3-O-methyl-D-glucose. The perfusion rate was 0.27 ml/min. Polyethylene glycol (PEG-4000) was used as a non-absorbable marker. [^{14}C]-3-O-methyl-D-glucose was added to the perfusate to give 5000 dpm/ml perfusion medium. Absorption of 3-O-methyl-D-glucose from the intestine was calculated by the following formula

$$S_R = I \, \frac{(S_i - S_a) \times \dfrac{PEG_i}{PEG_a} \times t}{g \ (or \ cm)}$$

S_R = Absorption of 3-O-methyl-D-glucose (μmole/t.g intestinal weight)
I = Perfusion rate (ml/min)
S_i = Initial substrate concentration in the perfusate
S_a = Final substrate concentration in the perfusate
PEG_i = Initial concentration of PEG in the perfusate
PEG_a = Final concentration of PEG in the medium
t = Time of perfusion (results expressed/30 minutes)

Transmural electrical potential difference (PD) was measured according to the method of Barry et al.[12] by a similar assembly described earlier for PD measurements in vitro[13]. Agar (1.5%)–KCl(3 M)–filled polyethylene tubing was used for salt bridges. The mucosal salt bridge was positioned 2 cm distal to the tip of the infusion inlet in the cannulated jejunal segment, and the serosal salt bridge was fixed in the peritoneal cavity moistened with physiological saline solution. Salt bridges were connected to beakers containing calibrated silver–silver chloride electrodes in saturated KCl. PD changes were detected by a Keithley 602 battery-operated voltmeter and documented by a recorder. Identical PD measurements were performed in the jejunum of streptozotocin-diabetic rats. Experimental diabetes was induced by injection of 75 mg/kg of streptozotocin 5 days prior to the experimental procedure as reported earlier[7].

Radioactivity of [^{14}C]3-O-methyl-D-glucose was assayed by a Packard liquid scintillation system using an automatic standardisation. PEG was measured by the turbidometric method of Hydén[14].

RESULTS

Treatment with 10 or 100 μg of glucagon twice daily for a period of 5 days did not have any significant effect on body weight, food intake or blood glucose levels, measured 3 hours after the last injection. Administration of 100 μg of glucagon resulted in increased absorption of 3-O-methyl-D-glucose and water, whereas administration of 10 μg of glucagon was without significant effect on these parameters (Figure 17.1). In addition, an increase in net sodium and potassium absorption could also be observed in the jejunum of rats treated with 100 μg of glucagon twice daily for 5 days. (Figure 17.2). The increased rate of absorption of 3-O-methyl-D-glucose and water could be observed, too,

346

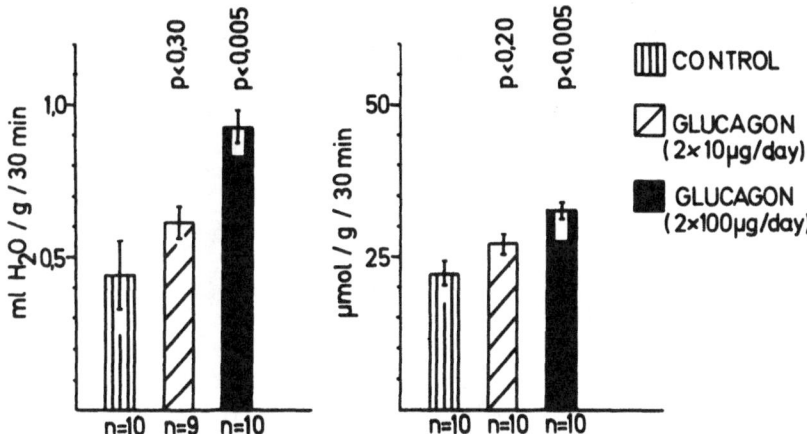

Figure 17.1 Effect of intraperitoneal glucagon administration (2 × 10 or 2 × 100 μg/day) for 4 days on intestinal absorption of water and 3-*O*-methyl-D-glucose. Results (means ± SEM) for water absorption (ml/g intestine · 30 min) are given on the left, and data for absorption of 3-*O*-methyl-D-glucose (μmol/g · 30 min) on the right

if the results were expressed per unit length of intestine, suggesting that the ratio of intestinal weight/unit length of intestine was not altered after 5 days of treatment with glucagon. Intravenous administration of glucagon (100 μg) by bolus injection did not affect the rate of intestinal absorption of 3-*O*-methyl-D-glucose, water, and electrolytes after a control perfusion period of 45 minutes (not shown). Measurements of the increase in transmural potential difference (PD) induced by D-glucose revealed a higher PD increment in glucagon-treated and streptozotocin diabetic rats compared with controls (Figure *17.3*). Significant increases in PD could be observed at 15 and 56 mM

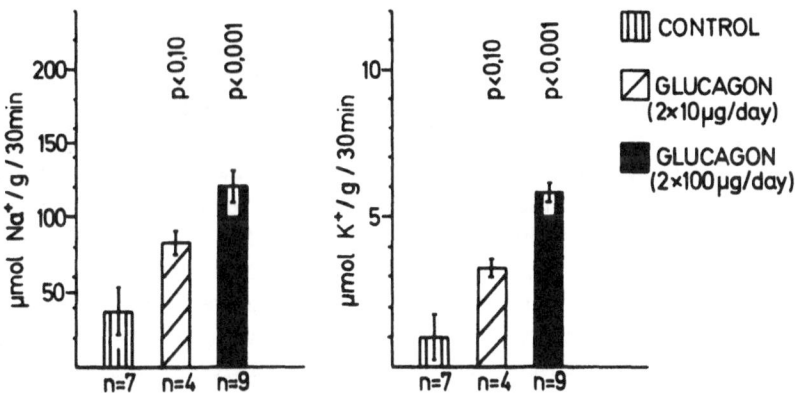

Figure 17.2 Effect of long-term glucagon administration on intestinal absorption of Na$^+$ and K$^+$. Results (means ± SEM) for Na$^+$-absorption are given on the left, and results for K$^+$-absorption are depicted on the right

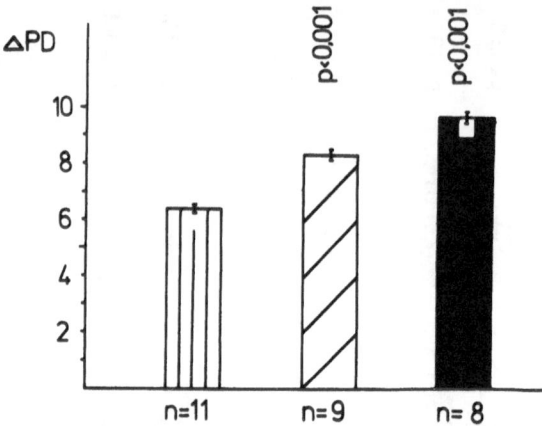

Figure *17.3* Effect of streptozotocin diabetes and chronic administration of glucagon on D-glucose-induced increments of transmural potential differences (PD); the graph contains the maximal PD increments induced by 56 mM D-glucose. Results are means ± SEM, vertically striped columns concern controls, diagonally striped columns the glucagon-treated rats (2 × 100 μg/day), and black columns the streptozotocin diabetic animals

D-glucose in the perfusion medium. PD increments were more marked in streptozotocin diabetic rat jejunum than in the glucagon-treated rats (Figure 17.3).

DISCUSSION

In agreement with recently reported results *in vitro*[15], the rate of absorption of the non-metabolisable sugar analogue, 3-O-methyl-D-glucose, and water, sodium and potassium by the rat jejunum *in vivo* was increased after chronic administration of glucagon for 5 days. These results were confirmed by measurements of D-glucose-induced transmural PD increases. Actively transported hexoses are able to induce, according to their carrier binding affinity and luminal substrate concentrations, an increase in transmural PD, that is most likely due to the hexose-coupled increase of Na^+-influx[16]. Since an increase in PD is achieved almost instantaneously in the presence of glucose, before a steady-state Na^+ absorption is obtained, we have to assume that an increase in Na^+ influx in the presence of D-glucose occurred in the jejunum of glucagon-treated and streptozotocin diabetic rats. The increase in PD was significantly greater in the treated rats at the highest concentration of D-glucose, 56 mM. Even though kinetic studies were not performed, these data are indicative of an increase in maximal transport rate (V_{max}) rather than in K_m. Maximal hexose transport rates (V_{max}) are also increased in experimental diabetes mellitus[23].

In contrast to chronic administration of glucagon, single bolus injection of the hormone had no effect on hexose, water, and electrolyte absorption under identical conditions as those applied to the study of the effect of chronic glucagon administration.

Our results are apparently in contradiction to the findings of other groups. Using a 'slow marker' intestinal perfusion technique, Ganeshappa et al.[17] observed a decrease in intestinal flow velocity in humans after continuous intravenous administration of glucagon (2.4 µg/min), but were unable to detect any change in the composition of the fasting intestinal contents. Endogenous hyperglucagonaemia induced by intravenous infusion of arginine decreased intestinal motor function, but did not alter intestinal net water and sodium transport[18].

Mekhjian et al.[19], however, found an inhibition of water and sodium absorption in humans after small doses of glucagon (2 µg/kg h) and a secretion of water and electrolytes into the intestinal lumen after higher doses (5 µg/kg h). A further increase in the dosage of glucagon (20 µg/kg h) reduced the intraluminal secretion of water and electrolytes again. These perfusion studies in vivo[17,18,19] were performed in the absence of glucose from the perfusion medium, and therefore are not directly comparable to the results presented in this paper. From perfusion experiments in the presence of cholera toxin in vivo, it is known that the secretion of water and electrolytes into the intestinal lumen may be stimulated, but transport of actively absorbed hexoses and hexose-stimulated Na^+ transport is not affected[20]. Indeed paradoxical effects of acute intravenous glucagon administration have been observed by Moore et al.[21,22] in rabbit and dog small intestine in the presence or absence of glucose. In the ileum of rabbits net water and Na^+-absorption could be observed, which was reduced by intravenous glucagon administration in the absence of glucose from the perfusate. The inhibitory effect of glucagon was completely reversed by D-glucose. In the dog, however, glucagon administration resulted in a significant increase in water secretion into the jejunum, whereas an increase in net water absorption was observed in the ileum, which was further increased in the presence of D-glucose. Data on the rate of glucose absorption were, however, not reported by these authors. Gottesbüren et al.[23] observed, in normal subjects after intravenous glucagon administration, a small increase in glucose absorption followed by a significant decrease, whereas in diabetics glucagon induced a significant increase in glucose absorption in the 15 minute sampling period immediately after bolus injection of glucagon. The authors explained the short-lasting rise in glucose absorption by an increase in serum insulin which subsequently reduced glucose absorption under their experimental intestinal perfusion conditions.

Intestinal responses to glucagon in experimental animals have also been observed after acute exposure. Ponz et al.[24] found a decrease in intestinal glucose absorption after glucagon treatment, whereas Varró et al.[25] reported that intra-arterial administration of glucagon during the perfusion had no effect on the transport of glucose from the lumen into intestinal tissue, but an increased rate of loss of glucose from the epithelial cells towards the serosa was observed. Recently Hubel[26] showed that glucagon, in contrast to secretin, caused an increase in net water and sodium absorption in rat small intestine in the absence of glucose from the perfusing medium.

Treatment with glucagon for 24 to 48 hours had no effect on transport of hexoses and amino acids *in vitro* nor did addition *in vitro* of glucagon to isolated small intestine (own unpublished results). Rudo and Rosenberg[15], however, observed that long-term administration of glucagon to rats (4 × 50 μg/day) resulted in increased intestinal transport of 3-O-methyl-D-glucose and 1-aminocyclopentane–1-carboxylic acid (ACPC) after 4 days of treatment. Under identical experimental conditions (everted intestinal rings), Rudo[27] found that starvation resulting in hyperglucagonaemia was associated with increased amino acid uptake in rat jejunum. Administration of an anti-glucagon antibody nearly normalised the increased absorption observed during starvation and hyperglucagonaemia. Rudo[27] concluded that hyperglucagonaemia in experimental diabetes mellitus and starvation is likely to be responsible for the increased transport capacity of amino acids in starved rats.

Our results *in vivo* confirm the findings *in vitro* of Rudo and Rosenberg[15], demonstrating that chronic intraperitoneal administration of high dosages of glucagon resulted in an increased absorption of hexoses, water and electrolytes, as well as an increase in D-glucose-induced transmural PD. Even higher D-glucose-induced PD increments could be observed in the jejunum of streptozotocin diabetic rats, thus complementing earlier observations on increased intestinal transport capacity for hexoses in experimental diabetes mellitus[1,2,3]. Glucagon therefore might be considered as a candidate for the increased absorption observed in experimental diabetes mellitus. The data of Rudo[27] and our own are, however, far from conclusive. Whether starvation leads to an increase in nutrient absorption is in dispute. In accordance with results of Levin[28], our own unpublished results both *in vitro* and *in vivo* suggest that starvation leads to a decrease in hexose absorption and does not significantly alter brush-border enzymatic activity. Since starvation has been reported to be associated with a decrease of digestive enzymatic activities[29], but experimental diabetes mellitus with a marked increase of brush-border enzymatic activity[3,7] and hexose absorption[1,2,3], it seems unlikely that glucagon may be responsible for both the increased absorptive and digestive functions in experimental diabetes mellitus. Brush-border enzymatic activities in total mucosal homogenates of glucagon-treated rats were not enhanced despite increased absorption of hexoses, water and electrolytes (own unpublished results).

The doses of glucagon used were large and for a period of time the plasma concentrations achieved after intraperitoneal injection were certainly higher than the physiological level. The mechanism responsible for the adaptive responses caused by glucagon in this study is not yet understood. A direct effect of glucagon or mediation by other hormonal or metabolic responses has to be considered.

Acknowledgements

This discussion has been supported by the Deutsche Forschungsgemeinschaft Ca 71/3.

References

1. Flores, P. and Schedl, H. S. (1968). Intestinal transport of 3-O-methyl-D-glucose in the normal and alloxan-diabetic rat. *Amer. J. Physiol.*, **214**, 725
2. Olson, W. A. and Rosenberg, I. H. (1970). Intestinal transport of sugars and amino acids in diabetic rats. *J. Clin. Invest.*, **49**, 96
3. Caspary, W. F. (1973). Effect of insulin and experimental diabetes mellitus on the digestive–absorptive surface of the small intestine. *Digestion*, **9**, 248
4. Caspary, W. F. (1973). Increase of active transport of conjugated bile salts in streptozotocin diabetic rat small intestine. *Gut*, **14**, 949
5. Kershaw, T. G., Neame, K. D. and Wiseman, G. (1960). The effect of semistarvation on absorption by the rat small intestine *in vitro* and *in vivo*. *J. Physiol. (Lond.)*, **152**, 182
6. Bihler, I. and Freund, N. (1975). Sugar transport in the small intestine of obese hyperglycemic, fed and fasted mice. *Diabetologia*. (In press)
7. Caspary, W. F., Rhein, A. M. and Creutzfeldt, W. (1972). Increase of intestinal brush border hydrolases in mucosa of streptozotocin diabetic rats. *Diabetologia*, **8**, 412
8. Müller, W. A., Faloona, G. R. and Unger, R. H. (1971). The effect of experimental insulin deficiency on glucagon secretion. *J. Clin. Invest.*, **50**, 1992
9. Unger, R. H. (1971). Glucagon physiology and pathophysiology. *New Engl. J. Med.*, **285**, 443
10. Unger, R. H., Aquilar-Parada, E. and Müller, W. A. (1970). Studies of pancreatic alpha-cell function in normal and diabetic subjects. *J. Clin. Invest.*, **49**, 837
11. Marliss, E. B., Aoki, T. T., Unger, R. H., Soeldner, J. S. and Cahill, G. F. (1970). Glucagon levels and metabolic effects in fasting man. *J. Clin. Invest.*, **49**, 2256
12. Barry, R. J. C., Dikstein, S., Matthews, J., Smyth, D. H. and Wright, E. M. (1964). Electrical potentials associated with intestinal sugar transfer. *J. Physiol. (Lond.)*, **171**, 316
13. Caspary, W. F., Stevenson, N. S. and Crane, R. K. (1969). Evidence for an intermediate step in carrier-mediated sugar translocation across the brush-border membrane of hamster small intestine. *Biochim. Biophys. Acta*, **193**, 168
14. Hydén, S. A. (1955). A turbidometric method for the determination of higher polyethylene glycols in biologic materials. *Ann. Roy. Agr. Coll.*, **22**, 139
15. Rudo, N. D. and Rosenberg, I. H. (1973). Chronic glucagon administration enhances intestinal transport in rats. *Proc. Soc. Exp. Biol. Med.*, **142**, 521
16. Lyon, I. and Crane, R. K. (1966). Studies on transmural potentials *in vitro* in relation to intestinal absorption. I. Apparent Michaelis constants for Na^+-dependent increment of transmural potential of rat small intestine. *Biochim. Biophys. Acta*, **112**, 146
17. Ganeshappa, K. P., Whalen, G. E. and Soergel, K. H. (1972). The effect of glucagon on small intestinal absorption in man. *Gastroenterology*, **62**, 750
18. Whalen, G. E., Wu, W. C., Ganeshappa, K. P., Wall, R. H., Kalkhoff, R. K. and Soergel, K. H. (1973). The effect of endogenous glucagon on human small bowel function. *Gastroenterology*, **64**, 822
19. Mekhjian, H., King, D., Sanzenbacher, L. and Zollinger, R. (1972). Glucagon (Gl) and secretin (Se) inhibit water and electrolyte transport in the human jejunum. *Gastroenterology*, **62**, 782
20. Field, M. (1974). Intestinal secretion. *Gastroenterology*, **66**, 1063

21. Moore, E. W. and Longacher, J. W. (1974). The effect of peptide hormones on simultaneous jejunal and ileal water and electrolyte transport in the rabbit: I. Glucagon: the nature of the effect. *Gastroenterology*, **66**, 748

22. Moore, E. W. and Tavano, R. J. (1974). The effect of peptide hormones on simultaneous jejunal and ileal water and electrolyte transport in the dog.: II. Glucagon: some paradoxical effects. *Gastroenterology*, **66**, 749

23. Gottesbüren, H., Menge, H., Lorenz-Meyer, H., Bloch, R. and Riecken, E. O. (1974). Effect of insulin and glucagon on intestinal absorption in man. In: R. H. Dowling and E. O. Riecken, (eds.). *Intestinal Adaptation*, p. 219. (Stuttgart, New York, F. K. Schattauer-Verlag)

24. Ponz, F., Lluch, M. and Planas, J. (1957). Efectos del glucagón sobre la absorción intestinal de glucosa. *Rev. Españ. Fisiol.*, **13**, 25

25. Varró, V. and Csernay, L. (1966). The effect of intra-arterial insulin and glucagon on glucose metabolism of the small intestine in the dog. *Scand. J. Gastroent.*, **1**, 232

26. Hubel, K. A. (1972). Effects of secretin and glucagon on intestinal transport of ions and water in the rat. *Proc. Soc. Exp. Biol. Med.*, **139**, 656

27. Rudo, N. D. (1973). Endogenous hyperglucagonemia as a mediator of increased intestinal transport in starvation: studies with anti-glucagon antibody. *Gastroenterology*, **64**, 686

28. Levin, R. J. (1974). A unified theory for the action of partial or complete reduction of food intake on jejunal hexose absorption *in vivo*. In R. H. Dowling and E. O. Riecken (eds.). *Intestinal Adaptation*, p. 125. (Stuttgart, New York: F. K. Schattauer-Verlag)

29. McNeill, L. K. and Hamilton, J. R. (1971). The effect of fasting on disaccharidase activity in the rat small intestine. *Pediatrics*, **47**, 65

Discussion 17

Simmonds: Do any of the manoeuvres *in vitro* affect the production or release of mucus?

Turnberg: We have not quantitated mucus release—this is difficult. But we have looked at histological sections of tissues after they have been clamped in flux chambers and exposed to theophyline or acetyl choline, and we have not seen any changes to suggest goblet cell discharge. However, one does notice mucus on the surface of the tissue when they are removed from the chambers.

Field: Your data on interactions between glucose and theophylline are fascinating. I was shown some results just before arriving here by a colleague, Marlin Walling, who determined the effect of dibutyryl–cyclic AMP on sodium and chloride fluxes across short-circuited rat ileum with glucose present on the luminal side. His data were remarkably similar to your own: in the presence of glucose, theophylline decreased electrical resistance, produced a net secretory chloride flux, and changed net sodium flux only slightly, the ratio of net Cl^- to Na^+ flux changes being 5:1. The differences from prior studies on the rabbit and guinea-pig, that you and he have observed, suggest either a species difference or an effect of glucose to uncouple the chloride flux changes produced by cAMP from sodium transport. I wonder what your thoughts are on this.

Turnberg: I did not show a slide of the effect of theophylline + glucose on *ileal* ion transport, but basically they are similar to the jejunal data in that the net Na^+ flux change was small compared to the Cl^- flux change. This may well be an example of the uncoupling of the $Na^+ + Cl^-$ serosa-to-mucosa flux mechanisms. It would be interesting to see whether the same phenomenon occurs in your rabbit ileal preparation.

Binder: These are very lovely studies. Two questions: (1) What is the concentration of bicarbonate in your incubation solution? (2) Would you speculate as to the differences between the results *in vivo* and *in vitro*?

Turnberg: The first question is somewhat easier than the second! The bicarbonate concentration was 25 mM. I am afraid I don't really know the basis of the *in vivo/in vitro* differences. Of course the tissue *in vitro* is short-circuited, the bathing media may be different and the tissue may be slowly dying, but I do not think that that is by any means the answer. I started the studies *in vitro* to try to understand more deeply our data *in vivo*, but I think we now have more questions than answers.

Armstrong: How did you measure resistances? I ask this because our analysis, in terms of an equivalent electrical circuit, of electrical events in the small intestine indicates that the steady-state PD/I_{sc} ratio does not give an unequivocal estimate of the transepithelial DC resistance.

Turnberg: We calculated resistances from the PD and I_{sc}, but I accept your point that we should have measured them by some other method.

Wingate: In my own experiments on isolated human ileum, PD was not a steady value but showed an initial overshoot followed by a steady decline. In plotting histograms of 'PD', when was the PD-value taken to be representative?

Turnberg: We took our 'steady' PD-values during the phase of steady decline.

Wingate: It is possible, from evidence recently published by Sanford, that the innervation of the mucosa is composed of afferent rather than efferent nerves. (Clothier *et al.*, *J. Physiol. Lond.*, **247**, 11P, 1975)

Turnberg: It is of course pure speculation at the moment as to the real function of the fibres that we have stained.

Lorenz-Meyer: We have investigated the influence on the intestinal function of chronically applied depot-glucagon (Novo) over a period of 10 or 20 days. We were indeed able to measure an increase in glucose absorption *in vivo* within the first 10 days of administration, which was not accompanied by alterations in villus height and food intake of the animals. But after 20 days' glucagon administration, there was a marked decrease in glucose absorption which was related to a decrease in daily food intake, in villus height and in mucosal disaccharidase activities. These results do not suggest that hyperglucagonaemia is the factor responsible for the alterations in intestinal function and structure in chronic alloxan-diabetes in the rat. Would Dr Caspary like to comment?

Caspary: We examined the effect of chronic glucagon administration for 5 days only, since the increases in the digestive–absorptive function caused by streptozotocin can be observed without increased food intake or intestinal weight only up to 5–8 days. The results presented show that, when looking at hormonal effects on transport changes, one has to differentiate between the acute and chronic effect of the hormones causing intestinal adaptation. Glucagon may therefore, like gastrin, have a trophic effect on the absorptive–digestive surface. Studies on the chronic hormonal effects may, however, be more relevant to explain intestinal function in patients with endocrine tumours.

18
Prostaglandins and Ion Transport in the Human Intestine: A Current Survey

C. MATUCHANSKY and J. J. BERNIER

*Unité de Recherches sur la Physiopathologie de la Digestion,
INSERM U54, Hôpital Saint-Lazare, Paris*

INTRODUCTION

Prostaglandins (PGs) of the E and F series have been found in the normal small intestine and colon of man and diverse animal species[1], although there is still little information on their occurrence in specific cell types within these organs. Local biosynthesis of PGs in the animal gut has also been demonstrated[1], as well as the rapid metabolism of PGE_1 by the small bowel[2]. Many studies have emphasised the influence of PGs on gastrointestinal muscle or gastric secretion; but, among the several extensive reviews which dealt over the past five years with the actions of PGs on the digestive system[1,3-6], none has been specifically devoted to the effects of these naturally occurring unsaturated fatty acids on intestinal fluid and ion transport. Recent advances obtained in this area seem now to warrant such a specific review.

The present paper is specially concerned with the effects of PGs on ion transport in the human intestine. Following a description of these effects in the different parts of the gut, special attention will be given to the possible mechanisms involved, since there is increasing evidence that PGs may provide a key to a better knowledge of intestinal transport processes.

EFFECTS OF PROSTAGLANDINS ON TRANSPORT OF WATER AND ELECTROLYTES IN THE HUMAN INTESTINE

Oral[7], intrajejunal[8,9] or parenteral administration[10,11] of PGs of the E and F series produces copious watery diarrhoea often accompanied by colicky pain.

355

In earlier reports, this effect was attributed primarily to PG-induced intestinal hypermotility and decreased transit time[7]. Recent studies, extending to humans the results previously obtained in other species, clearly indicate that PGs may directly act on transintestinal movements of water and ions[8,9,11].

Small intestine

In the human jejunum, studies *in vivo* from this laboratory[8,9] have shown that when administered into the jejunal lumen of normal volunteers in the course of small intestinal perfusion experiments, PGE_1:

(*1*) induces a profuse net secretion of water, sodium, chloride, potassium and bicarbonate (Figures 18.1 and 18.2), in cases where baseline net movements correspond to net absorption or to slight net secretion;

(*2*) slightly (by 25%) but significantly reduces glucose absorption; PGE_1 also results in a slower rate of glucose-stimulated sodium and water transport,

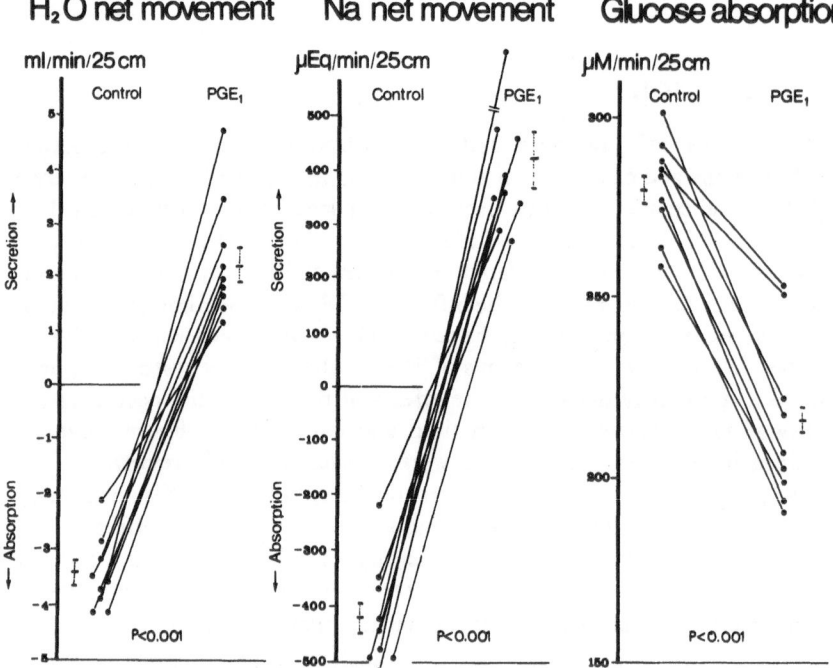

Figure 18.1 Effect of prostaglandin E_1 (PGE_1), delivered into the human jejunal lumen (0.9 μg/kg min), on net water, sodium and glucose absorption from a glucose–saline isotonic solution in nine subjects (intestinal perfusion technique, at a rate of 10 ml/min, with a proximal occluding balloon). Bars represent mean ± SEM; *P* from paired *t*-test applied to differences between PGE_1 and control values in the same subject. (From Matuchansky and Bernier[8], with permission of the publisher)

an effect which appears to be due both to decreased glucose absorption itself and to a decreased rate of sodium transport per micromole of glucose absorbed;

(3) strikingly increases the unidirectional flux rate of water and sodium from blood to lumen (exsorption), while decreasing the reverse flux (insorption).

It is of interest that in these studies, PGE_1 did not decrease jejunal transit time of luminal contents (Figure 18.3), and was accompanied by no clinical cardiovascular effects nor a significant rise in systemic plasma levels of PGE; furthermore, no significant changes in peripheral plasma levels of various hormones, capable of inducing net secretion or reducing net absorption in the jejunum, that is thyrocalcitonin, total glucagon, enteroglucagon, VIP, secretin, gastrin, were observed[12]. In these experiments, the secretory effect of PGE_1 was rapid in onset (less than 20 minutes), was maximal within 40 minutes, was sustained as long as PGE_1 was delivered into the lumen, and showed a decline towards baseline absorption rate less than 40 minutes following termination of the PGE_1 infusion. Moreover, the effect showed no tachyphylaxia and was entirely reproducible within 6 hours of perfusion (personal unpublished data). A

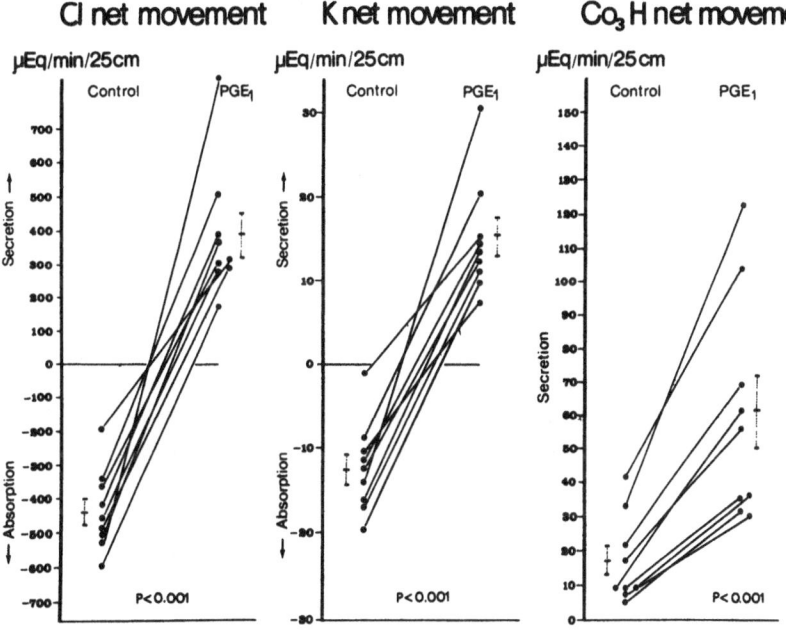

Figure 18.2 Effect of prostaglandin E_1 (PGE_1), delivered into the human jejunal lumen (0.9 μg/kg min), on net chloride, potassium and bicarbonate movements from a glucose–saline isotonic solution in nine subjects (intestinal perfusion technique, at a rate of 10 ml/min, with a proximal occluding balloon). Bars represent mean ± SEM; P from paired t-test. (From Matuchansky and Bernier[8], with permission of the publisher)

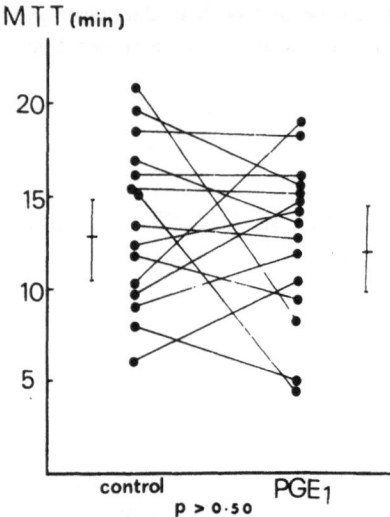

MTT(min)

Figure 18.3 Effect of prostaglandin E_1 (PGE$_1$), delivered into the human jejunal lumen (0.9 μg/kg min), on mean transit time (MTT) of luminal fluid along a 30 cm segment of jejunum perfused (10 ml/min) with a glucose–saline isotonic solution (intestinal perfusion technique using a triple-lumen tube without proximal occluding balloon). No significant change was observed in the 15 subjects tested. Bars indicate mean ± SEM; P from paired t-test

similar reversal of net jejunal absorption of water and electrolytes into secretion has been reported, during segmental perfusion studies in humans, after intraluminal administration of PGE$_2$[15]; the secretory effect appears to be dose-dependent and is accompanied by an increased transit time in most cases. Intravenous PGF$_{2\alpha}$ (0.81 to 0.85 μg/kg/min) also promotes net secretion of fluid in the human jejunum in a dose-dependent manner while not affecting the speed of transit through the experimental segment[11]. There is suggestive evidence from the above-mentioned studies that the fluid accumulation induced by PGs results, at least in part, from a true secretion into the lumen and not merely from a decreased absorption; however, the influence of PGs on spontaneous jejunal flow rate of fluid has not so far been evaluated and should be of interest.

In the human ileum, similar effects of PGs have been described, and, in terms of dose-action relationship, the distal intestine appears to be even more sensitive than the proximal one[11]. Intravenous infusion of PGF$_{2\alpha}$ (0.65 to 0.86 μg/kg/min) induces net secretion of both water and sodium from a saline-mannitol solution perfused at a rate of 10 ml per minute through a 30 cm segment[11]. Furthermore, both intravenous PGF$_{2\alpha}$ and PGE$_2$ increase significantly the spontaneous fasting ileal flow rate, from a mean of 1.69 ml/min to 4.63 ml/min; it is noteworthy that at the dose used in these studies no side effects were reported by any of the subjects tested[16].

Colon

To our knowledge, only one study has been reported on the effect of PGs on colonic transport of water and ions in man; Milton-Thompson et al.[16] have observed that colonic absorptive function, as evaluated by a perfusion technique in vivo at a flow rate of 10 ml/minute, was not significantly altered by either $PGF_{2\alpha}$ or PGE_2. This result is of special interest as regards the mechanism of PG-induced diarrhoea, suggesting that the small intestine is the only site of fluid and ion losses.

Inhibitors of prostaglandin actions

Among several substances which have been found to affect some actions of PGs, three principal types have revealed characteristics of specific competitive antagonism: 7-oxa-PG analogues (for example 7-oxa-13 prostynoic acid), dibenzoxazepine derivatives (for example SC 19220) and phosphorylated polymers of phloretin (for example polyphloretin phosphate, PPP)[17]. The influence of such inhibitors on PG-induced secretion in humans is unknown, but it is noteworthy that PPP selectively antagonises the response of human foetal intestine to PGE_2 and $PGF_{2\alpha}$[18], and that both PPP[19] and SC 19220[20] inhibit diarrhoea produced in mice by intraperitoneal injection of PGE_2. Whether this inhibition is primarily due to direct interaction with the movements of water and ions promoted by PGs remains to be determined.

We recently observed that PGE_1-induced jejunal secretion in man, which was not influenced by oral or intravenous administration of acetylsalicylic acid (an inhibitor of PG biosynthesis of which the possible direct effect on preformed PGs had not previously been investigated), is significantly decreased by ethacrynic acid[12] but not by other diuretic drugs such as furosemide (personal unpublished data). Data from these studies strongly suggest that the antisecretory effect of ethacrynic acid is not related to the drug-induced diuresis, systemic changes in hydration or hypovolaemia; such an inhibitory effect is of interest in view of the previous observation that ethacrynic acid reduces choleraic intestinal secretion in vivo in dogs[13] and cyclic-AMP mediated secretion in vitro[14]. The mechanism of the inhibitory effect of ethacrynic acid is discussed below.

PATHOGENESIS OF PROSTAGLANDIN ACTION ON INTESTINAL WATER AND ION TRANSPORT

Possible role of changes in intestinal motility, mucosal blood flow or intestinal morphology

PGs of the E and F series are known to affect the motility of the gastrointestinal tract[1] but there is now excellent evidence that their effects on intestinal ion transport are not mediated by changes in motility. While promoting fluid secretion into the jejunum or ileum, PGE_1, PGE_2 or $PGF_{2\alpha}$ do not decrease transit time of the luminal contents during segmental perfusion studies in man[8,9,11,15]; some slowing has even been observed in several experiments[9,11,15]. For E-type PGs, these findings *in vivo* agree with several experimental data: in the isolated small bowel of man and diverse animal species[1,21], PGE_1 and E_2 contract the longitudinal muscle but relax the circular one; furthermore PGE_1 decreases the peristaltic contractions and propulsion of fluid in the guinea-pig ileum[22] and reduces in cats[23] and dogs[24] intestinal motility and intraluminal pressures. In contrast to these results is the observation by Misiewicz *et al.*[7] that oral PGE_1 decreases in human volunteers transit time of radioactive chromium through the gut, especially the colon; but there is some evidence in this study (such as the passage of normally formed stools containing a quantity of clear fluid) suggesting that the increased propulsion was secondary to an increased bulk of luminal fluid along the whole length of the gut and perhaps to low segmental pressure activity. Concerning the effects of F type PGs, there are many more discrepancies between studies *in vivo* and *in vitro*. *In vitro*, PGFs have been shown to cause contraction of both the circular and longitudinal layers of the small intestine and the colon[1,4] and to increase intraluminal pressures in several species[1,24]. Conversely, *in vivo* in man, $PGF_{2\alpha}$ inhibits jejunal and ileal segmental contractions[11] and has no measurable effect on colonic segmental pressures[25].

E and F type PGs may influence mesenteric blood flow[26] and the possibility that PG-induced intestinal secretion is due to local changes in mucosal blood flow or capillary permeability cannot be definitively excluded. However, the observation *in vitro* that PGs inhibit net sodium absorption and stimulate net chloride secretion in isolated stripped ileal mucosa[27] supports the hypothesis that luminal loss of fluid is due to a direct effect upon the mucosa.

Very few data are available on the influence of PGs on intestinal morphology. In dogs, jejunal biopsies taken during high rate infusion (up to 100 μg/min) of PGE_1 and $PGF_{2\alpha}$ into the superior mesenteric artery showed a few alterations of the epithelium, consisting of necrosis and sloughing confined to the villus tips; no histological changes were observed at lower infusion rates (2 to 8 μg/min)[28]. Although there is so far no direct information in man, the rapid reversibility and reproducibility of the PG secretory effect, as observed during jejunal perfusion studies *in vivo*, strongly suggest that fluid and ion losses are not provoked by significant changes in small intestinal structures.

Adenylate cyclase–cyclic AMP system

Many recent observations have provided evidence that PGs may exert their effect on fluid and electrolyte transport through an interaction with the adenylate cyclase–cyclic AMP (cAMP) system:

(1) PGE_1 and PGE_2[29,30], like cholera toxin[29, 31, 32] and *E. coli* enterotoxin[32,33], stimulate intestinal mucosal adenylate cyclase activity in diverse animal species without affecting phosphodiesterase activity[29], and induce a measurable increase in cAMP concentration in intact mucosal cells[34,35]; recent findings also suggest that PGs and cholera toxin may release adenylate cyclase from an existing or preformed pool rather than causing synthesis of a new enzyme[36].

(2) PGs mimic *in vitro* the effect of cAMP and theophylline on short-circuit current and ion fluxes (inhibition of net sodium absorption and stimulation of net chloride secretion) when applied to the ileal serosal surface[27,34,37,38]; furthermore, changes in cAMP levels are in close temporal agreement with changes in short-circuit current[35], as shown by experiments performed on stripped ileal mucosa mounted in Ussing chambers; there is, *in vivo* in dogs, a significant linear relation between the magnitude of jejunal secretory response to cholera toxin and to either PGE_1 or $PGF_{2\alpha}$[28].

(3) The recent observation that ethacrynic acid reduces *in vivo* the PGE_1-[12] and cholera toxin-induced[13] intestinal secretion is an interesting finding, since ethacrynic acid may inhibit adenylate cyclase activity in several tissues including the intestine[39,40]; however, ethacrynic acid has also been recently shown to reverse cAMP-mediated intestinal secretion *in vitro* without reducing theophylline- and cholera toxin-augmented cAMP levels in rabbit ileal mucosa[14]. Although the latter study suggests that ethacrynic acid interacts with ion secretion at a step beyond generation of cAMP, the precise mechanism of the antisecretory effect of the drug *in vivo*, with special reference to the possible role of Na^+-K^+-ATPase or glycolysis inhibition[14], remains to be determined.

(4) It has been proposed by Bennett[41] that cholera toxin may activate the intestinal adenylate cyclase system by first stimulating the release or endogenous synthesis of PGs. This attractive hypothesis, apparently supported by the marked inhibition of the choleraic intestinal secretion promoted by aspirin and several other anti-inflammatory agents[42,43] (which are known inhibitors of PG endogenous biosynthesis[44]) should now be challenged. Kimberg *et al.*[29,35] have clearly shown that the effect on adenylate cyclase activity of preincubating the mucosa with cholera enterotoxin was additive to the effect of a maximally stimulating concentration of PGE_1, that PGs unlike cholera toxin affected intestinal mucosal adenylate cyclase upon direct addition to subcellular fragments without preincubation with the mucosa, and finally that indomethacin failed to reduce the magnitude of the cAMP response to cholera toxin. These observations strongly suggest that cholera toxin and PGs activate adenylate cyclase by independent means or by involving different receptors. Such a concept is in agreement with the striking differences between both substances with respect to the onset and time course of their secretory effect. Thus it is well established that the response to cholera toxin, contrary to the response to PGs[35], is associated with a significant delay in onset, followed by a

steadily increasing and prolonged secretion, even at low doses or if the toxin has been rapidly flushed out after contact with the gut[45,46]. However, in considering results of the studies *in vivo* with anti-inflammatory drugs, one cannot definitely exclude a cAMP-independent, prostaglandin-mediated effect of cholera toxin *in vivo*, as suggested by Kimberg *et al.*[30].

(5) Although some PG actions on the gastrointestinal tract may be accompanied by a release of hormones, for example a release of gastrin by PGE_1 in Heidenhain pouch dogs stimulated with food[47], several findings clearly suggest that the effect of PGs on intestinal ion transport is not mediated by release of hormones capable of inducing net secretion. No measurable increase in systemic blood levels of immunoreactive gastrin, total glucagon, entero-glucagon, vasoactive intestinal peptide, secretin or thyrocalcitonin has been observed in man during PG-induced fluid production[12]. It is noteworthy that none of these hormones, except vasoactive intestinal peptide, stimulates adenylate cyclase activity and/or cAMP levels in the intestinal mucosa[29,48].

Anatomical site and mechanisms of fluid and ion losses

The relative roles, in PG- as well as in cholera toxin-induced fluid production, of inhibition of an active absorptive process as opposed to enhanced movement toward the lumen, are not clearly defined. Studies *in vitro*, as recently reviewed by Field[38], have indicated that cAMP and cAMP-related stimuli inhibit the coupled influx of NaCl across the luminal membrane; whether cAMP might also increase the coupled efflux of NaCl and perhaps $NaHCO_3$ towards the lumen remains to be determined. However, there is some evidence from studies *in vivo*, such as the preservation in human and experimental cholera of the stimulating effect of glucose[49,50] and amino acids[51,52] on sodium absorption, suggesting that cholera toxin acts, at least in part, by causing a normal mechanism for fluid and ion secretion to function excessively; a similar suggestion holds true for fluid production induced *in vivo* by PGs, since these fatty acids leave unaffected a significant part of the glucose absorption and glucose-stimulated sodium transport[8]. One could reasonably emphasise that if the copious intestinal fluid accumulation found both in cholera or during PG administration was to be explained simply by inhibition of absorption (with subsequent unmasking of a pre-existing secretory process), then an almost complete suppression of all transport processes from the lumen would be implied.

Another fundamental question which arises concerns the precise anatomical site of action of PGs and cholera toxin within the intestinal mucosa. Once it has been accepted that both agents may interfere with a secretory mechanism, it remains to be determined whether such a secretion originates primarily from the crypt cells or from the villus cells. Evidence for both hypotheses, especially the former, derives from a variety of observations which have been recently reviewed[38]. Results of unidirectional flux measurements during studies *in vivo* with PGs or cholera toxin do not provide conclusions in this matter, since the precise physiological meaning of these fluxes is not clear. However, one can note that the PGE_1-induced changes in Na^+ mucosa-to-serosa flux (insorption) and serosa-to-mucosa flux (exsorption) closely resemble those observed in jejunal mucosa exposed *in vivo* to cholera toxin: both agents may increase exsorption[8,9,53–55], while insorption may be unchanged[53] or decreased[56,57]. The intimate mechanism of the stimulatory effect on Na^+ exsorption *in vivo* cannot be clearly elucidated, since this flux may result from various transport processes including passive or exchange diffusion, solvent drag and active transport. The inhibitory effect of cycloheximide, an inhibitor of protein synthesis interfering with the cell cycle of the crypts[58], on both Na^+ net secretion[59,60] and Na^+ exsorption[54] in cholera toxin-treated jejunal mucosa appears to be an attractive result; but, in turn, this finding is subject to diverse interpretations since cycloheximide, while observed by Serebro *et al.*[60] not to affect glucose absorption, has been shown to reduce markedly absorption of NaCl, alanine, 3-*O*-methyl-glucose and iron by the villus cells[61], at the same dose used to inhibit toxin-induced secretion. Thus one should consider whether the secretory process stimulated or unmasked by PGs and cholera toxin might not be limited to one cell (crypt or villus cell) population. Localisation by Parkinson *et al.*[62] of the action of cholera toxin on adenylate cyclase in the basolateral cell membranes of mucosal epithelial cells cannot be considered as an unequivocal conclusion, since the techniques of separation employed could not differentiate between basolateral and crypt cell luminal membranes. In that respect, special interest arises from the recent observations that cholera enterotoxin appears to bind to luminal membranes of both villus and crypt cells[63], and that both villus and crypt cells from rabbit and rat intestine contain a cholera toxin- and PGE_1-sensitive adenylate cyclase activity[64].

Whatever the intimate mechanism(s) of fluid secretion induced by PGs and cholera toxin in the small intestine, it is noteworthy that both agents do not seem to promote any significant secretory response in the colon, despite the apparent presence in this organ of a cAMP-mediated secretory process similar to that found in ileum[30,65]. This seems to be an interesting subject for investigation and additional studies in this area are required.

PATHOLOGICAL AND PHYSIOLOGICAL IMPLICATIONS OF PROSTAGLANDINS IN INTESTINAL ION TRANSPORT

High levels of PGs of the E and F series have been found in the blood and/or tumoural tissue of patients with medullary carcinoma of the thyroid[66], with amine-peptide secreting tumours of neural crest origin or deriving from foregut[67], and with Kaposi's sarcoma[68]. PGs were of course implicated as the agents responsible for the diarrhoea observed in some of these patients[66,67], but reasons why diarrhoea was absent in patients with similar plasma (or tumour) levels of PGs are not well understood. A surprising clinical observation made by Fanwell and Thompson[69] and Barrowman et al.[70] is that nutmeg might relieve diarrhoea associated with medullary carcinoma of the thyroid; it was suggested that nutmeg might antagonise PG synthesis or peripheral action, but whether it non-selectively depressed response to other secreted substances has not been determined[71]. Recently, serum elevation of $PGF_{2\alpha}$ was observed in a few cases of carcinoid tumours[72]; increased plasma levels of PGE_1 and $PGF_{2\alpha}$ were also noted in one recent patient with typical WDHA syndrome and with a very high level of vasoactive intestinal peptide in peripheral blood and a pancreatic tumour[73]. Excessive release of PGs has been implicated in the digestive symptoms, particularly diarrhoea, associated with abdominal exposure to penetrating radiation, on the basis that aspirin produced appreciable improvement in 12 of 15 patients with radiation-induced diarrhoea[74]; these preliminary results require confirmation by further studies, especially double-blind trials. Finally, the responsibility of PGs in diarrhoea occasionally associated with menstruation has been suggested from data showing that $PGF_{2\alpha}$ is found in menstrual fluid and may enter the circulation[1,75]. The possible relationship between PGs and choleraic diarrhoea has been discussed in another section of this paper; but it must be emphasised that the direct effects *in vivo* of bacterial toxins on local production and release of PGs in the small bowel are little known. In experimental models in dogs, there is some evidence suggesting that *Escherichia coli* enterotoxin may release PGs, and that intravenous administration of sodium acetylsalicylate significantly reduces the diarrhoea promoted by this toxin[76]. Human pathological conditions associated with selective or predominant hyperproduction of PGs remain to be discovered, but it is reasonable to assume that such conditions do exist.

The search for a role of PGs in intestinal physiology has been stimulated by their widespread distribution through the gut and by their effects in doses low enough to be consistent with a physiological action. In studies from our laboratory, the concentration of PGE_1 in the fluid delivered into the jejunal lumen approximated to 3 μg per ml, and, although the local tissue concentration obtained was unknown, it is evident that such a concentration is much higher than that proved to be active in some other non-digestive systems (0.01 ng/ml *in vitro*, 10 ng/kg *in vivo*[77]). It is at present impossible to translate the biological actions of PGs on intestinal ion transport into physiological significance; in that respect, the precise sites and mechanisms of PG biosynthesis, storage, release and metabolism within intestinal structures remain to be determined, as well as the threshold active concentration compared with the amount of material extracted from intestinal tissue. Nevertheless it is of special interest that PGs also influence the handling of water and ions in extradigestive tissues of diverse animal species, such as the frog skin[78], toad bladder[79,80], rabbit gallbladder[81], or kidney[82]; these findings are consistent with the hypothesis[78] that PGs might perform a physiological function in the regulation of ion fluxes across epithelial membranes. In the field of intestinal transport, PGs can reasonably be considered as providing one of the most convenient models for the study of secretion both *in vivo* in man and *in vitro*, in view of the rapid onset, reversibility and reproducibility of their striking action on ion transmucosal movements.

References

1. Bennett, A. and Fleshler, B. (1970). Prostaglandins and the gastrointestinal tract. *Gastroenterology*, **59**, 790
2. Parkinson, T. M. and Schneider, J. C. (1969). Absorption and metabolism of prostaglandin E_1 by perfused rat jejunum *in vitro*. *Biochim. Biophys. Acta*, **176**, 78
3. Waller, S. L. (1973). Prostaglandins and the gastrointestinal tract. *Gut*, **14**, 402
4. Matuchansky, C. and Bernier, J. J. (1973). Prostaglandines et appareil digestif. *Biol. Gastroenterol. (Paris)*, **6**, 251
5. Wilson, D. E. (1974). Prostaglandins. Their action on the gastrointestinal tract. *Arch. Int. Med.*, **133**, 112
6. Robert, A. (1973). Prostaglandins and the digestive system. In '*Les prostaglandines*', séminaire INSERM, p. 297 (Paris, INSERM)
7. Misiewicz, J. J., Waller, J. L., Kiley, N. and Horton, E. W. (1969). Effect of oral prostaglandin E_1 on intestinal transit in man. *Lancet*, **i**, 648
8. Matuchansky, C. and Bernier, J. J. (1973). Effect of prostaglandin E_1 on glucose, water and electrolyte absorption in the human jejunum. *Gastroenterology*, **64**, 1111
9. Matuchansky, C., Mary, J. Y. and Bernier, J. J. (1972). Effets de la prostaglandine E_1 sur le temps de transit et les mouvements nets et unidirectionnels de l'eau et des électrolytes dans le jéjunum humain. *Biol. Gastroenterol. (Paris)*, **5**, 175
10. Karim, S. M. M. and Filshie, G. M. (1970). Therapeutic abortion using prostaglandin $F_{2\alpha}$. *Lancet*, **i**, 157
11. Cummings, J. H., Newman, A., Misiewicz, J. J., Milton-Thompson, G. J. and Billings, J. A. (1973). Effect of intravenous prostaglandin $F_{2\alpha}$ on small intestinal function in man. *Nature, London*, **243**, 169
12. Matuchansky, C., Mary, J. Y. and Bernier, J. J. (1974). The influence of ethacrynic acid and aspirin on water and electrolyte secretion induced by prostaglandin E_1 in the human jejunum. *Gut*, **15**, 831
13. Carpenter, C. C. J., Curlin, G. T. and Greenough, W. B. (1969). Response of canine Thiry-Vella jejunal loops to cholera exotoxin and its modification by ethacrynic acid. *J. Infect. Dis.*, **120**, 332
14. Al-Awqati, Q., Field, M. and Greenough, W. B. (1974). Reversal of cyclic AMP-mediated intestinal secretion by ethacrynic acid. *J. Clin. Invest.*, **53**, 687
15. Mize, B. F., Wu, W. C. and Whalen, G. E. (1974). The effect of prostaglandin E_2 (PGE2) on net jejunal transport and mean transit time. *Gastroenterology*, **66**, 747
16. Milton-Thompson, G. J., Cummings, J. H., Newman, A., Billings, J. A. and Misiewicz, J. J. (1975). Colonic and small intestinal response to intravenous prostaglandin $F_{2\alpha}$ and E_2 in man. *Gut*, **16**, 42
17. Sanner, J. H. (1974). Substances that inhibit the actions of prostaglandins. *Arch. Int. Med.*, **133**, 133
18. Hart, S. L. (1974). The actions of prostaglandins E_2 and $F_{2\alpha}$ on human foetal intestine. *Brit. J. Pharmacol.*, **50**, 159
19. Eakins, K. E. (1971). Prostaglandin antagonism by polymeric phosphates of phloretin and related compounds. *Ann. N.Y. Acad. Sci.*, **180**, 386

20. Sanner, J. H. (1972). Dibenzoxazepine hydrazides as prostaglandin antagonists. *Intrascience Chem. Rept.*, **6**, 1

21. Bennett, A., Eley, K. G. and Scholes, G. B. (1968). Effects of prostaglandins E1 and E2 on human, guinea-pig, and rat isolated small intestine. *Brit. J. Pharmacol.*, **34**, 630

22. Bennett, A., Eley, K. G. and Scholes, G. B. (1968). Effects of prostaglandins E_1 and E_2 on intestinal motility in the guinea-pig and rat. *Brit. J. Pharmacol.*, **34**, 639

23. Turker, R. K. and Onur, R. (1971). Effect of prostaglandin E_1 on intestinal motility of the cat. *Arch. Int. Physiol. Biochim.*, **79**, 535

24. Shehadeh, Z., Price, W. E. and Jacobson, E. D. (1969). Effects of vasoactive agents on intestinal blood flow and motility in the dog. *Amer. J. Physiol.*, **216**, 386

25. Hunt, R. H., Dilawari, J. B. and Misiewicz, J. J. (1975). The effect of intravenous prostaglandin $F_{2\alpha}$, and E_2 on the motility of the sigmoid colon. *Gut*, **16**, 47

26. Nakano, J. and Cole, B. (1969). Effect of prostaglandins E_1 and $F_{2\alpha}$ on systemic, pulmonary and splanchnic circulation in dogs. *Amer. J. Physiol.*, **217**, 222

27. Al-Awqati, Q. and Greenough, W. B. (1972). Prostaglandins inhibit intestinal sodium transport. *Nature New Biol.*, **238**, 26

28. Pierce, N. F., Carpenter, C. C. J., Elliot, H. L. and Greenough, W. B. (1971). Effects of prostaglandins, theophylline and cholera exotoxin upon transmucosal water and electrolyte movement in the canine jejunum. *Gastroenterology*, **60**, 22

29. Kimberg, D. V., Field, M., Johnson, J., Henderson, A. and Gershon, E. (1971). Stimulation of intestinal mucosal adenyl cyclase by cholera enterotoxin and prostaglandins. *J. Clin. Invest.*, **50**, 1218

30. Kimberg, D. V. (1974). Cyclic nucleotides and their role in gastrointestinal secretion. *Gastroenterology*, **67**, 1023

31. Sharp, G. W. G. and Hynie, S. (1971). Stimulation of intestinal adenyl cyclase by cholera toxin. *Nature, London*, **229**, 266

32. Banwell, J. G. and Sherr, H. (1973). Effect of bacterial enterotoxins on the gastrointestinal tract. *Gastroenterology*, **65**, 467

33. Evans, D. J. Jr., Chen, L. C., Curlin, G. T. and Evans, D. G. (1972). Stimulation of adenyl cyclase by *Escherichia coli* enterotoxin. *Nature, London*, **236**, 137

34. Field, M. (1971). Intestinal secretion: effect of cyclic AMP and its role in cholera. *N. Engl. J. Med.*, **284**, 1137

35. Kimberg, D. V., Field, M., Gershon, E. and Henderson, A. (1974). Effects of prostaglandins and cholera enterotoxin on intestinal mucosal cyclic AMP accumulation. Evidence against an essential role for prostaglandins in the action of the toxin. *J. Clin. Invest.*, **53**, 941

36. Kimberg, D. V., Field, M., Gershon, E. Schooley, R. T. and Henderson, A. (1973). Effects of cycloheximide on the response of intestinal mucosa to cholera enterotoxin. *J. Clin. Invest.*, **52**, 1376

37. Al-Awqati, Q., Cameron J. L., Field, M. and Greenough, W. B. (1970). Response of human ileal mucosa to choleragen and theophylline. *J. Clin. Invest.*, **49**, 2a

38. Field, M. (1974). Intestinal secretion. *Gastroenterology*, **66**, 1063

39. Ebel, H. (1974). Effect of diuretics on renal Na-K-ATPase and adenyl cyclase. *Naunyn-Schmiedeberg's Arch. Pharmacol.*, **281**, 301

40. Sharp, G. W. G., Hynie, S., Lipson, L. C. and Parkinson, D. K. (1971). Action of cholera toxin to stimulate adenyl cyclase. *Trans. Assoc. Amer. Phys.*, **84**, 200

41. Bennett, A. (1971). Cholera and prostaglandins. *Nature, London*, **231**, 536

42. Finck, A. D. and Katz, R. L. (1972). Prevention of cholera-induced intestinal secretion in the cat by aspirin. *Nature, London*, **238**, 273

43. Jacoby, H. I. and Marshall, C. H. (1972). Antagonism of cholera enterotoxin by anti-inflammatory agents in the rat. *Nature, London*, **235**, 163

44. Flower, R., Gryglewski, R., Herbaczynskacedro, K. and Vane, J. R. (1972). Effects of anti-inflammatory drugs on prostaglandin biosynthesis. *Nature, New Biol.*, **238**, 104

45. Greenough, W. B., Carpenter, C. C. J., Bayless, T. M. and Hendrix, T. R. (1970). The role of cholera exotoxin in the study of intestinal water and electrolyte transport. In G. B. Jerzy-Glass (Ed). *Progress in Gastroenterology*, vol. 2, p. 236. (New York: Grune and Stratton)

46. Carpenter, C. C. J. (1971). Cholera enterotoxin. Recent investigations yield insights into transport processes. *Amer. J. Med.*, 50, 1

47. Reeder, D. D., Becker, H. D. and Thompson, J. C. (1972). Effect of prostaglandin E_1 on food-stimulated gastrin and gastric secretion in dogs. *Physiologist*, 15, 246

48. Schwartz, C. J., Kimberg, D. V., Sheerin, H. E., Field, M. and Said, S. I. (1974). Vasoactive intestinal peptide stimulation of adenylate cyclase and active electrolyte secretion in intestinal mucosa. *J. Clin. Invest.*, 54, 536

49. Pierce, N. F., Sack, R. B., Mitra, R. C., Banwell, J. G., Brigham, K. L., Fedson, D. S. and Mondal, A. (1969). Replacement of water and electrolyte losses in cholera by an oral glucose–electrolyte solution. *Ann. Int. Med.*, 70, 1173

50. Carpenter, C. C. J., Sack, R. B., Feeley, J. C. and Steenberg, R. W. (1968). Site and characteristics of electrolyte loss and effect of intraluminal glucose in experimental canine cholera. *J. Clin. Invest.*, 47, 1210

51. Nalin, D. R., Cash, R. A., Rahman, M. and Yunus, M. (1970). Effect of glycine and glucose on sodium and water absorption in patients with cholera. *Gut*, 11, 768

52. Rohde, J. E. and Cash, R. A. (1973). Transport of glucose and amino acids in human jejunum during asiatic cholera. *J. Infect. Dis.*, 127, 190

53. Iber, F. L., McGonagle, T., Serebro, H. A., Webbers, E., Bayless, T. M. and Hendrix, T. R. (1969). Unidirectional sodium flux in small intestine in experimental canine cholera. *Amer. J. Med. Sci.*, 258, 340

54. Grayer, D. T., Serebro, H. A., Iber, F. L. and Hendrix, T. R. (1970). Effect of cycloheximide on unidirectional fluxes in the jejunum after cholera exotoxin exposure. *Gastroenterology*, 58, 815

55. Banwell, J. G., Shepherd, R., Thomas, J., Pierce, N. F., Mitra, R. P., Gorbach, S. L., Brigham, K. L., Fedson, D. S. and Mondal, A. (1972). Net and unidirectional transmucosal flux of sodium and water in acute human diarrheal disease. *J. Lab. Clin. Med.*, 80, 686

56. Phillips, R. A. (1968). Asiatic cholera. *Ann. Rev. Med.*, 19, 69

57. Swallow, J. H., Code, C. F. and Freter, R. (1968). Effect of cholera toxin on water and ion fluxes in the canine bowel. *Gastroenterology*, 54, 35

58. Verbin, R. S. and Farber, E. (1967). Effect of cycloheximide on the cell cycle of the crypts of the small intestine of the rat. *J. Cell Biol.*, 35, 649

59. Moritz, M., Iber, F. L. and Moore, E. W. (1972). Rabbit cholera: effects of cycloheximide on net water and ion fluxes and transmucosal electric potentials. *Gastroenterology*, 63, 76

60. Serebro, H. A., Iber, F. L., Yardley, J. H. and Hendrix, T. R. (1969). Inhibition of cholera toxin action in the rabbit by cycloheximide. *Gastroenterology*, 56, 506

61. Frizzell, R. A., Nellans, H. N., Acheson, L. S. and Schultz, S. G. (1973). Effects of cycloheximide on influx across the brush border of rabbit small intestine. *Biochim. Biophys. Acta*, 291, 302

62. Parkinson, D. K., Ebel, H., Dibona, D. R., Sharp, G. W. G. (1972). Localization of the action of cholera toxin on adenyl cyclase in mucosal epithelial cells of rabbit intestine. *J. Clin. Invest.*, 51, 2292

63. Peterson, J. W., Lospalluto, J. J. and Finkelstein, R. A. (1972). Localization of cholera toxin *in vivo*. *J. Infect. Dis.*, 126, 617

64. Schwartz, C. J., Kimberg, D. V. and Ware, P. (1975). Adenylate cyclase in intestinal crypt and villus cells: stimulation by cholera enterotoxin and prostaglandin E_1. *Gastroenterology*, 68, 478

65. Binder, H. J. and Rawlins, C. L. (1973). Effect of conjugated dihydroxy bile salts on electrolyte transport in rat colon. *J. Clin. Invest.*, 52, 1460

66. Williams, E. D., Karim, S. M. M. and Sandler, M. (1968). Prostaglandin secretion by medullary carcinoma of the thyroid. A possible cause of the associated diarrhoea. *Lancet*, i, 22

67. Sandler, M., Karim, S. M. M. and Williams, E. D. (1968). Prostaglandins in amine-peptide-secreting tumours. *Lancet*, ii, 1053

68. Bhana, D., Hillier, K. and Karim, S. M. M. (1971). Vasoactive substances in Kaposi's sarcoma. *Cancer*, **27**, 233

69. Fanwell, W. N. and Thompson, G. (1973). Nutmeg for diarrhea of medullary carcinoma of the thyroid. *N. Engl. J. Med.*, **289**, 108

70. Barrowman, J. A., Hillenbrand, P., Rolles, K. and Wright, J. T. (1974). Nutmeg for diarrhea. *N. Engl. J. Med.*, **290**, 810

71. Bennett, A., Gradidge, C. F. and Stamford, I. F. (1974). Prostaglandins, nutmeg and diarrhea. *N. Engl. J. Med.*, **290**, 110

72. Feldman, J. M., Plonk, J. M. and Cornette, J. C. (1974). Serum prostaglandin $F_{2\alpha}$ concentration in the carcinoid syndrome. *Prostaglandins*, **7**, 501

73. Rambaud, J. C., Modigliani, R., Matuchansky, C., Bloom, S., Said, S., Pessayre, D. and Bernier, J. J. (1975). Pancreatic cholera: studies on tumoral secretions and pathophysiology of diarrhea. *Gastroenterology*. (In press)

74. Mennie, A. T. and Dalley, V. (1973). Aspirin in radiation-induced diarrhoea. *Lancet*, i, 1131

75. McCance, R. A. and Pickles, V. R. (1960). Cyclical variation in intestinal activity in women. *J. Endocrinol.*, **20**, 27

76. Collier, H. O. J. (1974). Prostaglandin synthetase inhibitors and the gut. In H. J. Robinson and J. R. Vane (eds.), *The Prostaglandin Synthetase Inhibitors*, p. 121. (New York: Raven Press)

77. Bergström, S., Carlson, L. A. and Weeks, J. R. (1968). The prostaglandins: a family of biologically active lipids. *Pharmacol. Rev.*, **20**, 1

78. Hinman, J. W. (1972). Prostaglandins. *Ann. Rev. Biochem.*, **41**, 161

79. Orloff, J., Handler, J. S. and Bergström, S. (1965). Effect of prostaglandin (PGE₁) on the permeability response of the toad bladder to vasopressin, theophylline and adenosine 3′,5′-monophosphate. *Nature, London*, **205**, 397

80. Lipson, L. C. and Sharp, G. W. G. (1971). Effects of prostaglandin E₁ on sodium transport and osmotic water flow in the toad bladder. *Amer. J. Physiol.*, **220**, 1046

81. Leyssac, P. P., Bukhave, K. and Frederiksen, O. (1974). Inhibitory effect of prostaglandins on iso-osmotic fluid transport by rabbit gallbladder *in vitro*, and its modification by blockade of endogenous PGE-biosynthesis with indomethacin. *Acta Physiol. Scand.*, **92**, 496

82. McGiff, J. C., Crowshaw, K. and Itskovitz, H. D. (1974). Prostaglandins and renal function. *Fed. Proc.*, **33**, 39

Addendum

Observations of potential importance with respect to the relationship between PGs and cholera toxin have been published since submission of this manuscript: Bedwani and Okpako (*Prostaglandins*, **10**, 117, 1975) have reported that pure cholera toxin, unlike crude toxin, did not influence the release of PG-like material by perfused rabbit ileum *in vivo*. These results are consistent with those of Hudson *et al.* (*Clin. Res.* **22**, 604A, 1974), who showed that pure cholera toxin was without effect on PG levels in rabbit ileal mucosa, and with those of Kimberg *et al.* reported in reference 35.

Discussion 18

Sharp: I should like to ask Dr Matuchansky whether he has tried to confirm the reports that aspirin or indomethacin can reverse or lessen the fluid secretion due to cholera toxin. I ask this because there seems to be no reason why prostaglandin synthesis should be involved in the response to cholera toxin.

Matuchansky: I thank Dr Sharp for his question, but unfortunately I have no personal data on the subject. I agree that recent data suggest that prostaglandin synthesis may not be involved in choleraic secretion; however, those data are derived from studies with the adenyl cyclase–cyclic AMP system. In view of the effects of aspirin on choleraic secretion *in vivo*, one cannot definitely exclude the possibility that cholera secretion may have something to do with a prostaglandin-mediated, cAMP-independent mechanism. This has been admitted in a recent progress report on cyclic nucleotides by Kimberg (reference 30 on p. 366).

Binder: At the recent American Gastroenterological Association meeting, Dr Powell reported that aspirin could reverse cholera enterotoxin-induced secretion in the rabbit ileum *in vitro*. He provided evidence to suggest that aspirin increased Na^+ and Cl^- absorption.

Matuchansky: I thank Dr Binder for this comment. This work of Powell is in agreement with studies published in *Nature*, particularly by Finck, indicating that aspirin inhibits cholera-toxin-induced secretion *in vivo* (reference 42 on p. 366).

Dowling: There is some evidence that transit in the small bowel may be increased by PGE. Can you be sure that you can measure transit adequately between two points on a segmental perfusion tube? It has also been suggested that the diarrhoea seen in association with excess prostaglandins may be due to CCK release. Have you any comments?

Matuchansky: Recent studies performed *in vivo* in man with prostaglandins have all clearly shown that these fatty acids do not decrease and may even increase segmental transit time, despite their secretory effect (see references 15 and 16 on p. 365). The only evidence of an increased transit time *in vivo* in man, due to PGE, was provided in a preliminary study by Misiewicz *et al.* with oral prostaglandin E_1. But in this study, transit time was specially increased in the colon, and there is some evidence that this was due to a primary increase in the bulk of fluid entering the colon. Anyway, the observed effect of PGE_1 on intestinal transit may fit with the known influence of PGE_1 on intestinal muscle, namely a contraction of the longitudinal layer but relaxation of the circular one. I have no personal information on the relationship between prostaglandins and CCK-release.

Levin: The various measured levels of the gastrointestinal hormones that you show before and during infusion of PGE_1 are interesting, but one always has to beware of over-interpreting their importance, as it is possible that

369

the immunoassays measure material apart from the active GI hormone principles (in other words, PGE_1 infusion may have some indirect actions via changes in bioactive agents).

Matuchansky: I agree with the comment of Dr Levin, but this is a general problem of interpretation of radioimmunoassays.

Robinson: It is rather surprising that you had such a large reduction in glucose absorption, whereas those who work with cholera toxin find little or no reduction in glucose absorption *in vivo* with this agent. Could you comment?

Matuchansky: First, in human cholera, normal absorption of glucose has not, to my knowledge, been proved by the intestinal perfusion technique. The only studies of which I um aware concerned oral or intraluminal administration of glucose and the subsequent observation of a reduced rate of faecal losses. Secondly, the reduction in glucose absorption that I observed during PGE_1 administration was only 20% and may simply be explained by the decrease in luminal glucose concentration due to dilution by secreted fluid.

Love: Why did you choose to use a bicarbonate-free solution for perfusion? This surely creates a highly abnormal situation in the intestinal lumen.

Matuchansky: The test solution used, which induces an important basal absorption, is similar to that employed in numerous other studies. It is suitable for testing the effect of a given drug on water and sodium absorption, which was the purpose of the present study.

Love: Secondly, I was confused by the glucagon figures; the total values were less than the pancreatic values. This would appear to give, by subtraction, a negative quantity for enteroglucagon.

Matuchansky: Immunoassays for total and pancreatic glucagon were not always performed in the same subject, and when performed in the same subject, were done on different plasma samples obtained during the course of the perfusion experiments. This may undoubtedly account for the differences in means, which are not different from the sensitivity of the assay methods.

19
Relationship Between Structure and Function in the Human Intestine

E. O RIECKEN, H. LORENZ-MEYER, M. SAHLFELD and R. BLOCH

Medizinische Universitätsklinik, Marburg/Lahn

In the past, we have been interested in the study of mucosal structure in the small intestine and in the dynamics of its alterations in different diseases in man and also in the experimental animal[1]. In continuation of these investigations, we have explored the relationship between function and mucosal structure in healthy controls and in patients with the sprue syndrome[2]. This condition is characterised by mucosal alterations, which include a decrease in villus height, an increase in crypt length and a flattening of the surface epithelial cells, together with a generalised decrease in enzyme activities[3]. Investigations in which adequate histological studies have been used[4,5] are few, but no precise morphometric data have hitherto been presented. Three-dimensional studies of the mucosa in conjunction with absorptive function are completely lacking.

In a first series of experiments, jejunal biopsies from ten healthy controls and nine patients with the sprue syndrome were obtained just below the ligament of Treitz. The tissue was fixed in formalin and paraffin sections were prepared by cutting the material parallel to the villus–crypt axis. Villus length was measured under the microscope using a graded eye piece. The number of villus cells was counted after projection on graph paper and expressed per 1 mm length of mucosa. In addition, absorption of glucose, electrolytes and water was determined within a jejunal segment, 30 cm in length, from which the biopsies had been taken. A triple lumen tube was used and polyethyleneglycol (PEG) served as non-absorbable marker to correct the test solution for water absorption[6].

371

Table 19.1 Morphometric data and surface cell counts.

	Controls	Sprue syndrome (total number)	Treated sprue syndrome	Untreated sprue syndrome
Villus height (in μm)	504 ± 54 (10)	155 ± 155 (9) *	174 ± 117 (4)	49 ± 29 (5)
Number of epithelial cells (per mm intestine)	1401 ± 341 (9)	528 ± 445 (9) *	937 ± 327 (4)	282 ± 60 (5)

Mean values with standard deviation are given. N is given in brackets. *Statistically significant on comparison with controls ($p < 0.05$).

The morphometric data and the counts of the surface cells are given in Table 19.1. As one would expect, the lowest values were obtained in the untreated patients while those of the treated ones were distinctly higher but lower than the controls.

The values of glucose, sodium, potassium and water absorption are given in Table 19.2. Glucose absorption in untreated sprue was less than 20% of the controls while the treated group amounts to around 60%. It can further be seen that the movement of sodium, potassium and water in the untreated group is reversed. In the treated group net movement of sodium is around zero whereas potassium is still secreted.

There is a close correlation between the net fluxes of sodium and water ($r = 0.98$; $N = 19$; $2\alpha < 0.001$) with a constant movement rate of 130 mval sodium per litre water in either direction. Furthermore, a close linear relationship exists between glucose and sodium absorption ($r = 0.9$; $N = 19$; $2\alpha < 0.001$). Finally, opposing net fluxes of sodium and glucose may occur under the conditions of malabsorption of the sprue type.

In order to recognise possible relationships between these values, correlations between functional and structural data were calculated[2] and these were found to be linear and highly significant for villus height and villus circumference on the one hand and absorption of glucose, sodium, potassium and water on the other ($2\alpha < 0.001$). When there was a complete lack of villi, glucose was still absorbed while water and electrolytes were secreted. Counts

Table 19.2 Glucose, electrolyte and water absorption from the upper jejunum as obtained by triple lumen perfusion technique.

Absorption	Controls	Sprue syndrome (total number)	Treated sprue syndrome	Untreated sprue syndrome
Glucose (mg cm^{-1} h^{-1})	59.7 ± 5 (10)	21.7 ± 13.4 (9)*	34 ± 9.2 (4)	11.8 ± 5 (5)
Na$^+$ (mEq cm^{-1} h^{-1})	0.69 ± 0.013 (10)	−0.06 ± 0.18 (9)*	0.029 ± 0.01 (4)	−0.13 ± 0.02 (5)
K$^+$ (mEq cm^{-1} h^{-1})	0.0173 ± 0.0062 (10)	−0.0133 ± 0.0109 (9)*	−0.0137 ± 0.013 (4)	−0.013 ± 0.015 (5)
H$_2$O (ml cm^{-1} h^{-1})	6.37 ± 1.1 (10)	−0.88 ± 0.13 (9)*	0.15 ± 0.093 (4)	−1.7 ± 0.92 (5)

N is given in brackets. *Statistically significant on comparison with controls ($p < 0.05$).

of epithelial surface cells per mm length mucosa were also linearly correlated with glucose absorption ($N = 18$; $r = 0.8$; $2\alpha < 0.001$).

The evidence suggested by these findings is that villus height in the healthy small intestine and in situations with mucosal alterations of the sprue type may be considered as a reasonable structural parameter from which information on the absorptive function may be obtained. In addition, the single epithelial cell in mucosal alterations of the sprue type does seem to absorb relatively more glucose than normal mucosa. This is surprising in view of the decrease in enzyme activities which has been measured biochemically in this condition using mucosal homogenates[7] and has also been described from cytochemical studies[3,8]. To explore these results further, a second series of experiments was carried out in healthy controls and in seven patients with the

Table 19.3 Morphological and functional data as obtained from the upper jejunum in second series (ten healthy controls, seven patients with the sprue syndrome).

Parameter investigated	Controls	Sprue syndrome (total number)	Treated sprue syndrome	Untreated sprue syndrome
Mucosal surface per mm² intestine	8.3 ± 1.1 (10)	2.4 ± 1.8 (7) *	3.4 ± 1.8 (4)	1 ± 0 (3)
Villus height (μm)	529 ± 107 (10)	73.7 98.6 (7)*	128.3 ± 101 (4)	0 (3)
Glucose absorption (mg cm⁻¹ h⁻¹)	51.14 ± 10.5 (10)	14.2 ± 9.1 (7)*	18.94 ± 9.39 (4)	7.95 ± 3.27 (3)
Sucrase (U/g protein)	98.2 ± 40.3 (10)	41.7 ± 20.35 (6)*	47.95 ± 22.88 (4)	28.8 ± 3.25 (2)
Leucine aminopeptidase in surface c cells E min⁻¹ μm⁻¹	0.0989 ± 0.0145 (8)	—	0.128 ± 0.0468 (4)	—

Mean values are given ± SD. *N* is given in brackets. * Statistically significant on comparison with controls ($p < 0.05$).

sprue syndrome. In this study, the three-dimensional structure of jejunal biopsies was investigated using the microdissection technique according to Clarke[9]. Furthermore, leucine-aminopeptidase and alkaline phosphatase activities were measured microdensitometrically using cytochemical techniques. In addition, sucrase activity was determined biochemically in mucosal homogenates to serve as a marker of mucosal surface. These data were correlated with the absorption of glucose, sodium, potassium and water which had been studied in the same way as described above. There was a decrease (Table 19.3) in mucosal absorptive surface and in villus height in the sprue syndrome. Simultaneously, there was an increase in crypt height and mitotic counts. Absorptive data corresponded to those of the previous series.

When the correlation between villus height and mucosal surface was calculated, there was a close linear relationship between these two parameters. Correspondingly the mucosal surface correlated linearly with absorption of glucose, sodium, potassium and water ($2\alpha < 0.05$). The correlation between glucose absorption and mucosal surface could be further improved

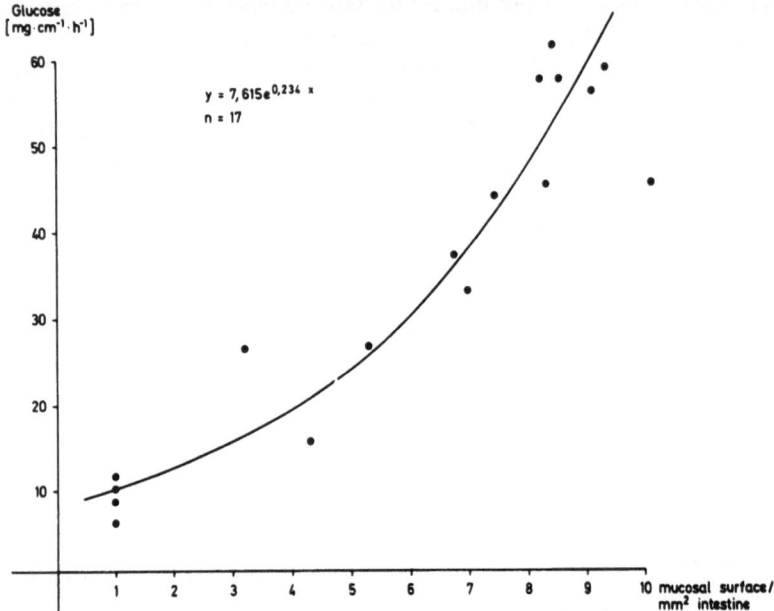

Figure 19.1   Correlation between glucose absorption and mucosal surface. Regression analysis reveals the closest fit with an exponential curve

when the least squares of a given exponential curve were calculated (Figure 19.1).

The activities of leucine aminopeptidase and alkaline phosphatase in the surface cells were generally found to be higher in patients with treated sprue syndrome as compared with the controls (Table 19.3). Only one specimen from a case which did not respond to a gluten-free diet showed reduced activity of leucine-aminopeptidase. For technical reasons, no measurements could be obtained in the untreated patients.

Sucrase activity was reduced to about half the activity (47%) in patients with treated sprue syndrome and to less than a third (28%) in those with untreated sprue syndrome (Table 19.3). These values correlated rather loosely and in decreasing order with mucosal surface, villus height, glucose and water

Table 19.4   Statistical significance of correlation coefficients (r) between saccharase activity and some variables measured (second series). $n =$ number of persons studied; $p =$ probability

Sucrase activity correlated with	r	n	p
Mucosal surface	0.59	16	< 0.05
Villus height	0.58	16	< 0.05
Glucose absorption	0.55	16	< 0.05
Water absorption	0.51	16	< 0.05
Sodium absorption	0.47	16	> 0.05

absorption respectively (Table 19.4). No significant correlation could be demonstrated between sucrase activity and sodium absorption.

On the basis of these findings it may be concluded:

(1) In the healthy small intestine and in mucosal alterations of the sprue type villus height and mucosal surface correlate well with absorption of glucose, sodium and water. Villus height therefore may be used as a valuable diagnostic parameter for absorptive function in the conditions studied.

(2) The decrease in mucosal surface is proportionally more pronounced than the reduction in sucrase activity as measured biochemically in mucosal homogenates. This is true — though to a varying degree — for the treated as well as for the untreated condition (47% and 28% respectively as compared with 41% and 11.9%).

(3) Leucine-aminopeptidase and alkaline phosphatase activities are increased in the single absorptive cell in treated sprue in spite of the still reduced mucosal surface. This increase is considered to compensate partially for the reduced mucosal surface.

Acknowledgements

This discussion has been supported by grants Ri 136/9 and 10 of the Deutsche Forschungsgemeinschaft.

References

1. Riecken, E. O. and Martini, G. A. (1973). Die Klassifizierung pathologischer Dünndarm-schleimhautbilder. Morphologie, Funktion und diagnostische Bedeutung. *Dtsch. Med. Wschr.*, **98**, 998

2. Bloch, R., Menge, H., Lingelbach, B., Lorenz-Meyer, H., Haberich, F. J. and Riecken, E. O. (1973). The relationship between structure and function of small intestine in patients with a sprue syndrome and in healthy controls. *Klin. Wschr.*, **51**, 1151

3. Riecken, E. O. (1970). Die normale Dünndarmschleimhaut und ihre Veränderungen bei einheimischer Sprue. *Dtsch. Med. Wschr.*, **95**, 2295

4. Holdsworth, C. D. and Dawson, A. M. (1965). Glucose and fructose absorption in idiopathic steatorrhoea. *Gut*, **6**, 387

5. Silk, D. B. A., Kumar, P. J., Webb, J. P. W., Lane, A. E., Clarke, M. L. and Dawson, A. M. (1975). Ileal function in patients with untreated adult coeliac disease. *Gut*, **16**, 261

6. Bloch, R., Menge, H., Lorenz-Meyer, H. and Riecken, E. O. (1971). Automatisierte segmentale Dünndarmperfusion. Eine Methode zur Messung der intestinalen Resorption. *Klin. Wschr.*, **49**, 1218

7. Plotkin, G. R. and Isselbacher, K. J. (1969). Secondary disaccharidase deficiency in adult celiac disease (non-tropical sprue) and other malabsorption states. *New Engl. J. Med.*, **271**, 1033

8. Padykula, H. A., Strauss, E. W., Ladman, A. J. and Gardner, F. H. (1961). A morphologic and histochemical analysis of the human jejunal epithelium in non-tropical sprue. *Gastroenterology*, **40**, 735

9. Clarke, R. M. (1970). Mucosal architecture and epithelial cell production rate in the small intestine of the albino rat. *J. Anat. (Lond.)*, **107**, 519

Discussion Paper on

Possible Coupling Between Na+ and D-Glucose Absorptions in Normal Jejunal Mucosa of Children

J.-F. Desjeux

Department of Paediatrics,
Université Paris VII and INSERM U83,
Hôpital Hérold, 75019 Paris

The Na+ gradient hypothesis has been widely invoked to explain the dependence on luminal Na+ concentration of accumulative sugar transfer across the brush border of epithelial cells of small intestine (for review, see reference 1). According to this hypothesis, sodium and actively transported sugars share a coupled transport system. The chemical or electrochemical Na+ potential gradient is the driving force for the transport of sugars. On the other hand, sugars increase sodium absorption. This hypothesis has received much support from experiments performed on animal tissues, but very little is known about the intestinal mucosa of children. The possibility of a coupling between Na+ and glucose absorptions in the jejunal epithelium of children was therefore investigated.

Pieces of jejunal epithelium (weighing 3 to 10 mg and normal according to light microscopic criteria) were obtained by peroral biopsies performed for diagnostic purposes. The steady-state accumulation of glucose by the tissue was measured as a function of the Na+ concentration gradient as previously described[2]. In brief, the tissue was divided into two or three pieces and placed in Ringer (Na+ : 140 mM) or in Ringer plus 10^{-4} M ouabain, or in Na+-free solution. Different glucose concentrations (1 mM and 10 mM), [^{14}C]glucose, ^{22}Na, and [^{3}H]inulin as extracellular marker, were added to the solutions (pH = 7.3, $T = 37$ °C, gassed with 95% O_2 and 5% CO_2). After a 60-minute incubation period, the tissue was dipped in cold mannitol (0.3 M), gently blotted, weighed, and placed in 2 ml N/10 nitric acid for extraction. The intracellular concentrations of glucose and Na+ were estimated assuming that the specific

Table *19.1* Intracellular steady-state accumulation of glucose (mean ± SEM) as a function of Na⁺ concentration gradient in normal jejunum of children.

	$Glucose_M$	$Glucose_C$	Na_C
Ringer (6)	10	42 ± 6.3	28 ± 14.9
Ringer (8)	10	18 ± 3.4	78 ± 20.0
+ 10⁻⁴ M Ouabain Na⁺-free (5)	10	9 ± 3.1	4 ± 1.4
Ringer (2)	1	25	29
Ringer (2)	1	6	82
+ 10⁻⁴ M Ouabain Na⁺-free (2)	1	1.9	3.7

M and C refer to medium and cellular concentration in mM. Numbers given in parentheses are number of observations. The Na⁺ concentration in Ringer solution was 140 mEq/1 and 3 mEq/1 in 'Na⁺-free' solution

activity in the tissue was equal to the specific activity in the incubation solution. The results appear in Table *19.1*. In Ringer solution there is intracellular accumulation of glucose; the intracellular Na⁺-concentration is low. When the Na⁺ gradient is decreased (in the presence of ouabain), or in the absence of a Na⁺ gradient (in Na⁺-free solution), there is a marked decrease in glucose accumulation. These results are qualitatively in agreement wth the Na⁺ gradient hypothesis. However, in these experiments, the tissue could in principle accumulate glucose or Na⁺ from the brush-border membrane or the basolateral membrane, or both. Furthermore, the tissues are very small and the numbers may not be very accurate. However, the calculation of the energy required to accumulate glucose was attempted. The assumptions involved in the calculation are (*a*) the specific activity of intracellular glucose is equal to the specific activity of extracellular glucose; (*b*) the intracellular Na⁺ activity is 50 per cent[3], and (*c*) the potential difference across the cellular membrane is 40 mV, intracellular negative[3,4]. In the presence of 10 mM glucose in the bathing solution, the energy required to accumulate 42 mM into the cell is 980 cal/mol. On the other hand, the Na⁺ electrochemical gradient may provide 2200 cal/equivalent. Therefore, a coupling between Na⁺ electrochemical potential and sugar accumulation is possible; the coupling efficiency would be 45%. These values are very similar to those obtained by Armstrong *et al.*[3] for the coupling between the Na⁺ electrochemical potential and galactose absorption in bullfrog intestine. In the presence of 1 mM glucose, the coupling is still possible, but the efficiency required would have to be 85%. In these calculations, a metabolic degradation of glucose by tissue would strongly affect the results. No attempt was made to measure metabolism in these experiments; however, Elsas *et al.*[5] were unable to find significant glucose metabolites under similar conditions. Clearly, further studies are required to establish the concept of an energetic coupling between the Na⁺ electrochemical gradient and glucose absorption across the brush-border membrane.

The second aspect of the Na⁺ gradient hypothesis is provided by the stimulation of Na^+ absorption in the presence of glucose. This situation is particularly interesting to the paediatrician. It was studied in the following way: Three normal jejunal biopsies were mounted in Ussing chambers (aperture: 12 mm^2) with Ringer solution on both sides (pH 7.3, oxygenated, circulated and maintained at 37 °C). After a 30-minute period in Ringer solution, the short-circuit current, I_{sc} was 2.7 μEq/h cm^2, the PD was 2.6 mV, serosa positive, and the conductance was approximately 30 mmho/cm^2. The effect of glucose on Na^+ absorption was estimated by reading the I_{sc}. Indeed, in the guinea-pig[6] and rabbit[7] ileum, it has been suggested that the I_{sc} is a measure of the Na^+ absorptive (electrogenic) process as opposed to the Na^+ secretory (neutral) process. The addition of glucose to the solutions on both sides of the tissue was followed immediately by an increase in the I_{sc}. Furthermore, I_{sc} appears to be a saturable function of glucose concentration. The plateau (I_{sc}: 5.93 μEq/h cm^2) was reached with 30 mM glucose; at the same time, the conductance increased to 40 mmho/cm^2. Although kinetic studies are probably unreliable on such a small number of studies, the apparent affinity constant for glucose and the maximal I_{sc} appear to be of the same order of magnitude in rabbit ileum[1] and in the jejunum of children. The stimulation of the I_{sc} by glucose does not appear to be related to a metabolic effect since 3-O-methyl glucose (30 mM) increased I_{sc} from 3.56 μEq/h cm^2 to 6.53 μEq/h cm^2 on one piece of tissue. Finally, in all the reported studies, ouabain reduced I_{sc} and PD to zero.

In conclusion, these preliminary results support the concept of a coupling between Na^+ and glucose absorptions in normal jejunal mucosa of children.

References

1. Schultz, S. G. and Curran, P. F. (1970). Coupled transport of sodium and organic solutes. *Physiol. Rev.*, **50**, 637

2. Desjeux, J.-F., Sassier, P., Tichet, J., Sarrut, S. and Lestradet, H. (1973). Sugar absorption by flat jejunal mucosa. *Acta Paediat. Scand.*, **62**, 531

3. Armstrong, W. McD., Byrd, B. J. and Hamang, P. M. (1973). The Na^+ gradient and D-galactose accumulation in epithelial cells of bullfrog small intestine. *Biochim. Biophys. Acta*, **330**, 237

4. Rose, R. C. and Schultz, S. G. (1971). Studies on electrical potential profile across rabbit ileum. *J. Gen. Physiol.*, **57**, 639

5. Elsas, L. J., Hillman, R. E., Patterson, J. M. and Rosenberg, L. E. (1970). Renal and intestinal hexose transport in familial glucose–galactose malabsorption. *J. Clin. Invest.*, **49**, 576

6. Powell, D. W., Binder, H. J. and Curran, P. F. (1972). Electrolyte secretion by the guinea-pig ileum *in vitro*. *Amer. J. Physiol.*, **223**, 531

7. Binder, H. J., Powell, D. W., Tai, Y. H. and Curran, P. F. (1973). Electrolyte transport in rabbit ileum. *Amer. J. Physiol.*, **225**, 776

Discussion 19

Levin: May I congratulate Dr Riecken and his colleagues on doing all the hard work in measuring and correlating villus height with mucosal surface area and absorption? The problem of quantifying absorption *in vivo* has always been difficult when one needs to place the data on some structural basis. His work now permits us to use villus height as an index for absorption. But one thing worries me, did you measure your absorption at just one single concentration? It would have been better to correlate the V_{max} with the villus height, enterocyte numbers, surface area, etc., rather than the absorption at a single concentration. One can get K_m changes as well as alterations in V_{max}.

Riecken: I am aware of the problems of quantifying absorption without having recourse to kinetic studies. However, Holdsworth *et al.* (reference 4 on p. 375) have carried out kinetic studies in sprue patients using different glucose concentrations, and, as far as I recall, they did not find alterations in the kinetics.

Matuchansky: Did Dr Riecken mention whether the patients he studied had proximal or diffuse coeliac disease? If these patients only had proximal coeliac disease, did he investigate the movements of water and ions below the damaged area? I ask this question because it has recently been shown by Silk *et al.* (presented to the British Society of Gastroenterology in 1974) that an increased absorption of glucose and ions may occur in the ileum of a patient with solely proximal coeliac disease.

Riecken: I know the work of Dr Silk and his collaborators, which has just appeared in reference 5 on p. 375, where they showed that the distal small intestine may compensate for the reduced function of the proximal gut by increasing its sodium and chloride absorption. In our studies, we have simply assessed the sprue-like lesions in the proximal small intestine by taking biopsies, and the extent of the alterations was only crudely explored by radiological studies. I don't think, however, that the question of the extent of the disease is relevant to the problem that we set ourselves.

Menge: Returning to the question of Dr Matuchansky, may I point out that the perfusions in the patients with coeliac disease were performed about 50 cm below the ligament of Treitz? The biopsies showing typical lesions were taken from the same region. So the biopsies showed that the perfused part of the intestine was involved in the disease. I should also like to underline that Dr Riecken found in the human small intestine recovering from coeliac disease a similar functional behaviour as Dr Mirkovitch and I encountered in the small intestine of the dog which was regenerating after one hour's ischaemia. In both cases, there was a net absorption of glucose, water and sodium, but still a net movement of potassium towards the lumen. Is there any explanation available for this discrepancy?

Murer: The potassium secretion might be attributed to a loss of cells from the villi in the ischaemic intestine. On your slides, the intestinal epithelium looked rather damaged.

Menge: No, the movement of potassium towards the lumen still occurred during the regeneration phase, when there is no longer any desquamation of the epithelial cells. The latter can only be observed immediately after the ischaemic trauma.

Riecken In sprue, it is known that there is increased shedding of the surface cells, and this could contribute to the increased intraluminal potassium concentrations. However, there may be other factors involved, for example, the possible secretory function of the enlarged crypts observed in these conditions.

Dowling: Could I just clarify one small point about one of your slides where you correlated glucose absorption with the number of epithelial cells per mm intestine? How did you measure this?

Riecken: As I pointed out in my paper, only two-dimensional studies were carried out on the histological sections in the first series of our experiments. In the latest series, the number of surface cells was not counted.

Armstrong: Dr Desjeux, have you attempted to calculate the energetic adequacy of sodium gradient in the human intestine in the situation where $(Na)_o/(Na)_i = 140/29$ and $(Glucose)_o/(Glucose)_i = 1/25$? You could make reasonable assumptions concerning the internal Na^+ activity and the mucosal membrane potential from published values for these parameters in other systems.

Desjeux: The energy available from the electrochemical gradient of Na^+ is theoretically adequate. However we have no direct measurement available of the transmucosal PD and of the intracellular Na^+ activity.

20
Functional Alterations in Ulcerative Colitis

JØRGEN RASK-MADSEN

Glostrup Hospital
Copenhagen

INTRODUCTION

Until the early 1960s, little attention was paid to the mechanisms responsible for transepithelial ionic transport in man. Studies on human colonic absorption were based mainly on modifications of the classic balance procedure, that is, the comparison of ileostomy discharges versus normal faecal output[1]. However, the calculations are based on the assumption that ileostomy discharge is representative of the chymus which normally enters the caecum, but in the case of HCO_3^- the technique yields inconclusive results because this ion reacts chemically with organic acids in the faeces.

The interest in colonic absorption in intact man increased after Levitan *et al.*[2] in 1962 had demonstrated that continuous perfusion of whole colon *in vivo* permits a direct quantification of water and ionic transport. Later on, compelling evidence was presented that the colon may play an important role in the pathogenesis of diarrhoea — which further stimulated interest in this organ[3–9].

Since conservation of salt and water is the principal function of the colon[10] and rectum[8,11], both of which generate substantial transmural potential differences (PD)[7,9,12–18], the human large bowel is well suited — even in intact man — for studies on epithelial ionic transport mechanisms. The inflamed colon provides a useful model for the study of solute–solvent flow relationships in greatly differing bulk flow conditions, and — most important — offers a unique opportunity to investigate electrical changes in relation to ionic transport *in vivo*. The study of functional alterations in ulcerative colitis is, therefore, of special interest not only from the standpoint of gastrointestinal pathophysiology, but also for a better understanding of normal human physiology.

The purpose of this communication is to describe some characteristics of water-electrolyte transport, mucosal polarization, and permeability in ulcerative colitis, and to discuss how transport data and bioelectrical parameters reflect the relationship between membrane structure and cellular function. Methodological possibilities and limitations of studies *in vivo* and some properties of normal colonic mucosa seem relevant, however, to the present discussion, and will be briefly reviewed, but references to literature will, of necessity, be selective rather than exhaustive.

METHODOLOGICAL POSSIBILITIES AND LIMITATIONS OF STUDIES *IN VIVO*

Steady-state perfusion

Measurements of colonic and rectal absorption during continuous perfusion with the aid of non-absorbable markers have until now yielded the most informative and accurate results[2,5–8,10,19,20]. Besides offering information about colonic transport capacity, the technique is well suited for describing mucosal permeability under the specific experimental conditions employed[7,8]. Furthermore, simultaneous measurements of bidirectional ionic fluxes and the transmural PD during steady-state perfusion makes it possible to define the actual electrochemical forces in the gut lumen, and thus the ability of the epithelial cells to transport charged particles actively[7,17] (see Figure 20.1).

However, it is important to consider the limitations inherent in this technique. First, the composition of the interstitial fluid at the contraluminal

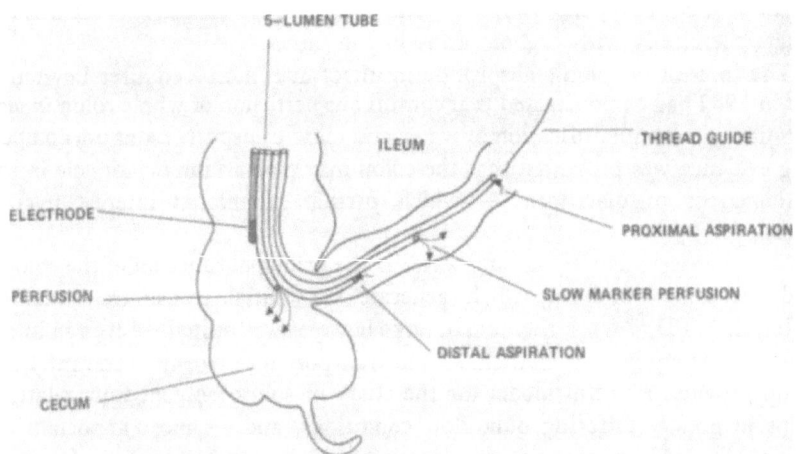

Figure 20.1 Technique for perfusion of colon in intact man. A 5-luminal perfusion tube has been pulled from the anus into the ileum by a thread guide. One of the lumina is a KCl electrode for measuring the transmural electrical potential difference (PD). The three proximal lumina are for slow marker perfusion of the ileum, permitting correction for reflux and intestinal contents entering the colon

membrane can neither be controlled nor precisely determined. Second, the permeability of mucosa to hydrophilic charged and uncharged particles can be evaluated only in the direction lumen-plasma by means of osmotic gradients[19] and in the opposite direction by means of diffusion gradients[8]. Third, in the case of charged particles, the evaluation of mucosal permeability is further compromised by the effect of the transepithelial PD imposed on the unidirectional fluxes across the two limiting membranes of the epithelium, which cannot be short-circuited *in vivo*. Fourth, the influence of solute–solvent flow interactions cannot be anticipated under normal conditions.

In studies of the permeability characteristics of inflamed mucosa some aspects of the problems are solved. Even in mild ulcerative colitis, low resistance pathways seem to permit electrical coupling between the electromotive forces across the two limiting membranes of the diseased epithelium, which is essentially short-circuited in severe inflammation[17]. Since also net volume flow is reduced or abolished in acute inflammation[3,5–8], the solvent drag effect need not be considered, and the plasma–lumen fluxes can be used for calculations of permeability coefficients[17]. However, perfusion of the colon at rates of 10–20 ml/min establishes highly unphysiological conditions. Moreover, the effects of, for example, endogenous bile acids, hydroxy fatty acids, and possible cathartics derived from bacteria cannot be observed during 'steady-state' perfusion, since the colonic contents are washed out[20].

Dialysis *in vivo*

The use of non-equilibrium dialysis[11] in the study of transepithelial ionic transport *in vivo* has, therefore, both theoretical and practical implications[9,11,20,21,22]. Although the theory of non-equilibrium dialysis rests on several assumptions which cannot be tested satisfactorily in intact man, the analysis of faecal dialysates has several advantages. Most important, the method is very sensitive, and it leaves the physicochemical environments in the gut lumen unaffected by the procedures of measurement[20]. Therefore, non-equilibrium dialysis permits evaluation of absorptive function under physiological conditions, that is, the influence of biochemical regulators in the gut lumen included. The method has proved useful for clinical research, and in unanaesthetized man it offers the only practical way of assessing ionic fluxes simultaneously with the transmural PD in a defined segment of the gut[9,11,20,22] since the application of occlusive balloons in colon is not only unreliable, but also disagreeable for the patient.

Electrical measurements

A substantial electrical PD exists across the wall of the large intestine. This PD may be considered as the result of an electric current through an ohmic resistance. However, this interpretation implies that the epithelial tissue is considered as a single homogeneous membrane, although the transepithelial PD appears to be the sum of two PDs arranged in series — one across the mucosal membrane, and the other, opposite in direction, across the serosal membrane. In the human colon and rectum, the active absorption of Na^+ is thought to be responsible for the transepithelial PD, which can be used as a simple index of mucosal integrity, reflecting both the activity of the Na^+ pump and the resistance of the tissue to the flow of ions.

In intact man the transmural colonic PD can easily be measured by means of a high impedance electrometer or a high impedance recorder and two symmetrical electrodes — calomel[7,9] or Ag–AgCl electrodes[15]. Disturbing junction potentials are reduced most effectively by use of flowing KCl salt bridges[7,9] (Figure 20.2). The terminal porous plug of the probe electrode may be placed in the luminal fluids when the PD is measured during continuous perfusion or directly in contact with the mucosa if a dialysis tube is used for

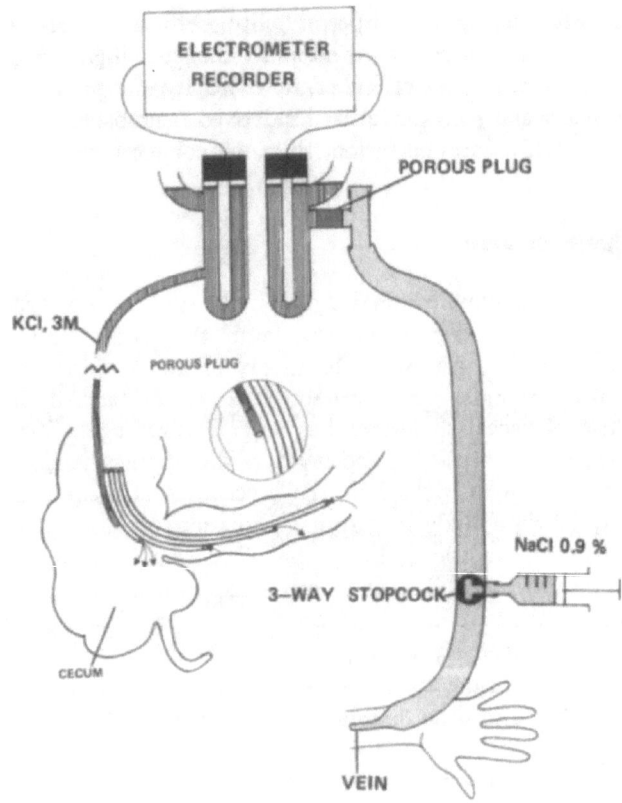

Figure 20.2 Intracolonic and reference electrodes used to measure the transmural potential difference (PD) simultaneously with transport of water and electrolytes in the human colon. For further explanation see text of Figure 20.1

the assessment of transepithelial ionic movements. As a reference an intravenous electrode is most suited, since peripheral blood is equipotential to the serosa[12,13], but for security reasons it is necessary to insert a bridge of KCl in agar[12], or more simply, a bridge of isotonic NaCl[7,9] (Figure 20.2) between the electrode and systemic blood. On the contrary, intact skin has a potential of minus 20–30 mV relative to blood[18], and although use of intradermal saline eliminates the electrical charge of the skin[16], the method seems unreliable.

FUNCTIONAL PROPERTIES OF NORMAL HUMAN COLON

Electrical polarization and permeability characteristics of normal colonic mucosa

In contrast to other gut epithelia, that of normal human colon is characterised by a high transepithelial electrical PD[7,9,12–16,18,20], a relatively high transepithelial resistance[23,24], a low passive permeability to monovalent ions[17,24], and hypertonic absorbates[7,8,19]. These properties may be explained by a high resistance to the diffusion of ions through extracellular pathways, which is in accordance with the observation that the colonic epithelium is impermeable to molecules with a diameter of more than 4 Å (urea)[19].

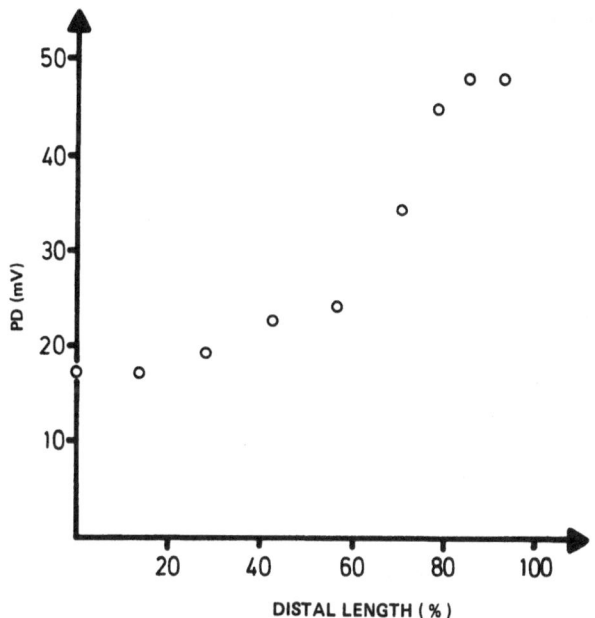

Figure 20.3 Profile of the transmural electrical potential difference (PD) along the length of normal human colon during perfusion with isotonic saline (four experiments; data from reference 1)

It is apparent from Figure 20.3 that the transmural PD increases along the length of colon to reach its maximum value in the rectum[7]. Since also the absorptive tendency — judged by the Na$^+$ flux ratio — increases along the length of colon, regional differences in colonic absorptive capacity may be explained by differences in mucosal permeabilty, which fits a characteristic general pattern in the ultrastructure of the gut, in other words, decreasing pore size from duodenum to colon[7,25].

By altering the composition of the luminal fluids, Archampong and Edmonds[16] showed that Na$^+$ is the only cation which influences the magnitude of the PD. However, they observed only a small reduction in the PD when luminal NaCl was changed from 100 to 10 mEq/l. Dalmark[14] also observed large PDs when luminal Na$^+$ was reduced almost to zero. By altering the anion accompanying Na$^+$, Archampong and Edmonds[16] were furthermore able to demonstrate a small effect on the PD, which had its greatest value when the radius of the hydrated anion exceeded 3.5 Å. Since the permeability to Na$^+$, K$^+$, and Cl$^-$ seems to differ little, and since the establishment of osmotic gradients has no effect on the PD, it seems most reasonable to interpret the observations that neither diffusion potentials nor streaming potentials participate in maintaining the electrical PD of colon[16]. Assuming that the plasma-to-lumen flux of Na$^+$ is entirely due to free diffusion, when the luminal Na$^+$ concentration approximates zero, the passive diffusional permeability coefficients of Na$^+$ is less than 5×10^{-6} cm/sec[17]. This finding is consistent with the notion that the colonic epithelium constitutes an extremely effective diffusional barrier.

Transepithelial transport of water and monovalent ions by the normal colon

Water

In the human colon, water absorption reaches a maximum when water activities in perfusate and plasma are identical, but absorption may occur against an osmotic difference of 50 mosmol/kg[19]. For this reason it is not necessary to postulate an active process for the transport of water since the observation can be explained by the simple physical forces arising as a consequence of active ion transport. The flow of water is proportional not only to the luminal NaCl concentration, but also to the rate of NaCl absorption, which continues in the absence of water transport[19]. Recent studies *in vivo*[7] indicate that Na$^+$ is the fundamental determinant of fluid absorption, since the relation between Cl$^-$ and water, but not that between Na$^+$ and water, varies with the composition of the perfusate (Figure 20.4).

Figure 20.5 illustrates an oversimplified model for ionic transport by human colon, relating transepithelial transport to hypothetical carrier processes at the mucosal border.

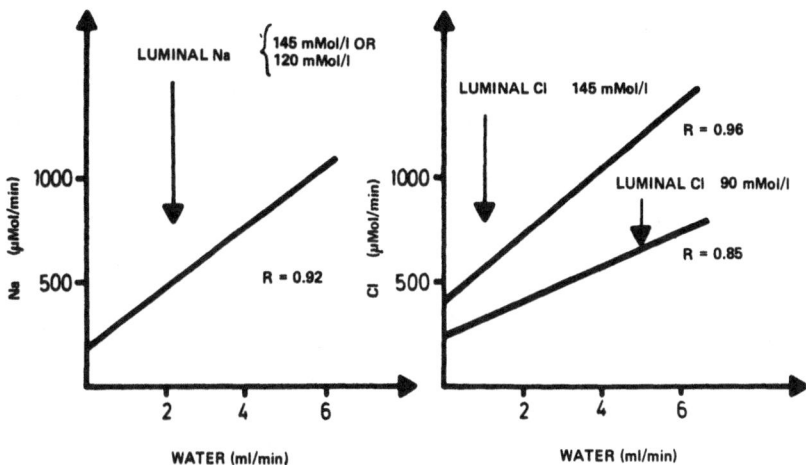

Figure 20.4 Relations between net transport of Na⁺ and water and net transport of Cl⁻ and water in the normal colon during perfusion with isotonic saline and an isotonic test solution simulating ileal output (Na⁺ 120 mEq/l, Cl⁻ 90 mEq/l, K⁺ 25 mEq/l and HCO₃⁻ 53 mEq/l) (data from reference 7)

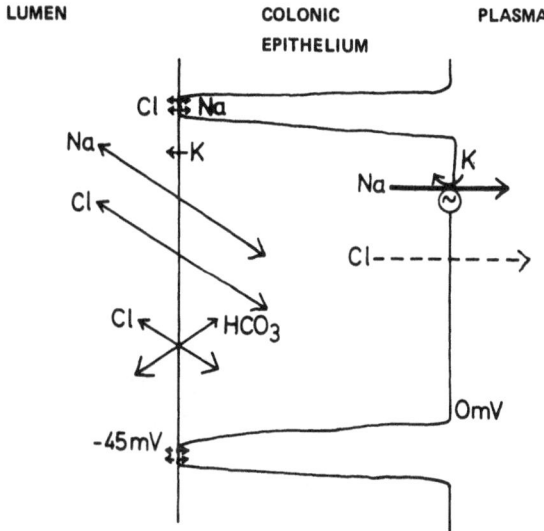

Figure 20.5 Model for Na⁺, Cl⁻, K⁺, and HCO₃⁻ transport by human colon. The oblique arrows designate passive, though highly specific, carrier-mediated transport, while the dashed arrows illustrate passive diffusion. The circle in the upper right corner symbolizes the active pump mechanism exchanging Na⁺ for K⁺ at a ratio different from one to one. Inasmuch as neither Cl⁻ entry nor Cl⁻ extrusion are directly linked to metabolic energy, active Na⁺ absorption may provide the electrochemical driving force for the downhill diffusion of Cl⁻ from lumen to plasma. On the contrary, secreted HCO₃⁻ may be derived from endogenous oxidative metabolism. The size of the arrows indicate the fluxes, which are taken from references 17 and 20

387

Na^+

Na^+ absorption works against both chemical and electrical gradients[7,9]. Experimental determinations of the Na^+ flux ratio simultaneously with the electrical PD during colonic perfusion shows flux ratios which are 8 to 55 times greater than the predicted values, suggesting the presence of an active Na^+ transport mechanism[7]. In addition, evidence has been presented for the idea that a carrier-mediated process accelerates the bidirectional Na^+ fluxes across the epithelium. This concept is based on the observation that a marked fall in the plasma-to-lumen flux of Na^+ occurs if the Na^+ concentration of isotonic perfusates is reduced, in spite of the fact that a greater electrochemical gradient is established[17] (Table 20.1). Since large bidirectional fluxes of both Na^+ and Cl^- are observed during perfusion with isotonic NaCl, the carrier-mediated transport process might be coupled to Cl^-, but this hypothesis requires further studies.

Table 20.1 Mean rates ($\pm$SEM) of bidirectional Na^+ fluxes in the normal human colon during perfusion with isotonic NaCl and mannitol solutions (perfusion rate 15 ml/min)

Perfusate	Subjects	Collection periods	Na^+ ($\mu mol/min$)	
			J_{m-s}	J_{s-m}
NaCl (145 mmol, 290 mosmol)	9	32	864 ± 140	234 ± 73
Mannitol (290 mosmol)	3	11	6 ± 1	41 ± 9

K^+

K^+ is secreted into the colonic lumen along its electrical gradient, which may be sufficient to account for passive transport. Since K^+ secretion seems unaffected by the luminal Na^+ concentration in perfusion studies, Devroede and Phillips[10] concluded that an interaction between cation movements was most unlikely; but non-equilibrium dialysis experiments[9] suggest a coupling between Na^+ and K^+, the latter being secreted *in vitro* in the absence of an electrochemical gradient[24,26]. These observations favour the concept of an electrogenic Na^+–K^+ exchange mechanism with a coupling coefficient different from 1.

Cl^- and HCO_3^-

As regards net transport of Cl^-, this ion is absorbed in excess of Na^+ against its chemical gradient, but along a sufficient electrical gradient to account for passive transport[7,20]. Thus, net transfer of Cl^- may be driven by the electrochemical gradients set up by the electrogenic Na^+ pump which is supposed to be working at the basolateral membranes. But anion transport also seems to be a complex phenomenon. HCO_3^- secretion equals Cl^- absorption[7,8,10], while HCO_3^- is absorbed from isotonic solutions of mannitol with 25 mEq $NaHCO_3$, and secreted if NaCl is added to the perfusate[10]. It is possible, therefore, that a specific mechanism without the expenditure of metabolic energy couples the absorption of Cl^- to the secretion of HCO_3^-.

FUNCTIONAL ALTERATIONS IN ULCERATIVE COLITIS

Although the human colon can compensate for failing intestinal absorption, it plays a minor role in body homeostasis. However, disruption of its functional integrity — as is seen in inflammatory conditions — may result in excessive fluid loss and severe electrolyte disturbances. In acute ulcerative colitis, exudation of protein, blood, and mucus may occur, but it is seldom that exudation explains the diarrhoea, and evidence is accumulating that transport of water and monovalent ions is abnormal in all stages of ulcerative colitis and Crohn's disease localized to the colonic wall[3,5-9,17,18,22,26,27].

Electrical polarization and permeability characteristics of inflamed colonic mucosa

In ulcerative colitis, the colonic mucosa is characterized by reduced or even abolished transepithelial PDs[7,9,15,17-18,22], low transepithelial resistances[24], increasing permeabilities to monovalent ions[17,26,27] and small non-electrolytes[8], and slightly hypertonic to isotonic absorbates[8].

Recent studies on functional changes in ulcerative colitis have presented electrophysiological evidence for the presence of low-resistance shunt pathways in the diseased epithelium. Edmonds[15] was the first to show that the inflamed mucosa is abnormally polarized. However, the interpretation of the results are complicated by the fact that lumen was registered positively charged during acute exacerbations of ulcerative colitis. A reversed PD would imply the existence of unknown transport mechanisms, even if defective active ion transport and/or changed mucosal permeability characteristics were postulated. Results from similar investigations[18] of patients with ulcerative colitis suggest that Edmonds's results represent the sum of the PDs across the skin and the rectal mucosa. Thus the transepithelial PD may approach zero in severe cases, while its polarity is never reversed (Figure 20.6). Other studies have disclosed the relationship between bioelectrical properties and transepithelial ionic transport in the inflamed rectum. This is illustrated by rectal perfusions in normal individuals and in patients who have undergone colectomy for inflamatory bowel disease, but preserved a rectal stump[17]. Analysis of the data shows a positive linear correlation between the logarithm of the Na^+-flux ratio and the transepithelial PD with a Na^+-flux ratio of unity

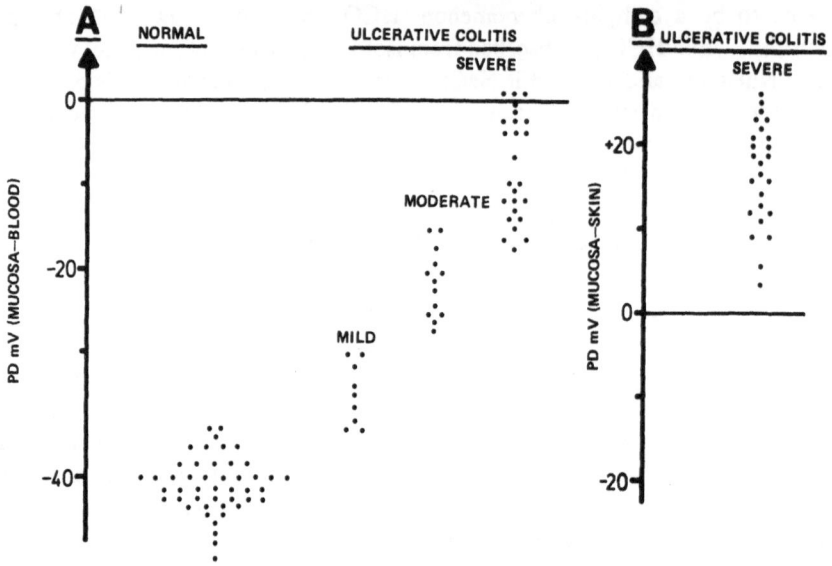

Figure 20.6 **A** is the transmural potential difference (PD) of human rectum in the normal condition and in different stages of ulcerative colitis. **B** is the electrical potential of rectal lumen relative to skin in severe ulcerative colitis

at zero PD in the absence of transepithelial ionic gradients (Figure 20.7). The reduction of Na$^+$-flux ratio — and of Na$^+$ net transport — with decreasing PD is the result of an increase in the plasma-to-lumen flux with no significant

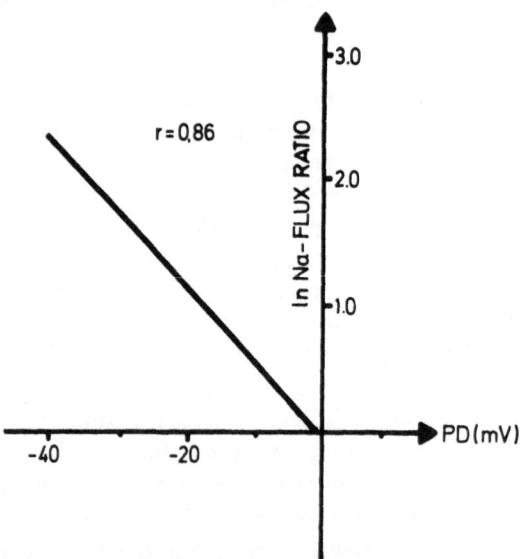

Figure 20.7 Relation between the natural logarithm of Na$^+$ flux ratio and the transmural potential difference (PD) in the inflamed human rectum (from reference 17)

change in the opposite flux. This may be interpreted as (a) the development of low resistance shunt pathways which attenuate the difference between the electromotive forces across the epithelial membranes, so that the transepithelial PD decreases. In the absence of Na^+ net transport, no PD is generated, and ionic fluxes may have essentially short-circuited the epithelial membranes. Accordingly, the permeability coefficient is in the range of 10^{-2} to 10^{-3} cm/sec — a factor 10^3 greater than in the normal colon. An alternative explanation is that (b) PDs between zero and normal values represent, in part at least, Na^+ diffusion potentials — notwithstanding an electrogenic Na^+ transport from lumen to plasma. If the mucosa is inflamed or contains increased interstitial fluid, the hydrostatic pressure may be increased, promoting bulk flow of water and ions into the lumen — particularly if high hydraulic conductivities are present. This may result in artefacts in the system with regard to isotopic measurements of bidirectional fluxes, for example (c) if it is assumed that Na^+ is actively transported into the lateral intercellular space, it exists — on the standing gradient hypothesis[28] — as an isotonic or slightly hypertonic solution. Here, abnormal bulk flow occurring in the direction plasma to lumen might sweep isotopic Na^+ (already pumped into the lateral interspace) back into the lumen. The return of isotopic Na^+ to the lumen would result in (i) generation of falsely low lumen-to-plasma fluxes, and therefore falsely high plasma-to-lumen fluxes with falsely low flux ratios, (ii) creation of an osmotic gradient favourable to bulk flow of water into the lumen, and (iii) generation of a Na^+ diffusion potential due to higher Na^+ activity at the mucosal border depending on the relative mobilities of the accompanying anions. However, it seems most reasonable to attribute the observed changes in Na^+ transport and electrical polarisation to the presence of a high conductance shunt pathway, which offers a possible explanation of the observations made in permeability studies. In addition, the fact that the curve in Figure 20.7 passes through zero suggests that the active Na^+ transport mechanism is responsible for the generation of the colonic transepithelial PD. This notion is supported by the dissociation between the rectal PD observed and that predicted from the luminal and contraluminal equilibrium concentrations of Na^+ by the Nernst equation — and by the fact that the predicted value equals zero in the absence of a transmural PD[24] (Figure 20.8). On the contrary, the PD of inflamed rectum can be described adequately by the Nernst equation over a wide range of luminal Cl^- concentrations. In the case of K^+, the dissociation between observed and predicted values may be attributed to increased K^+ permeability of the mucosal membrane, whether an active Na^+–K^+ exchange mechanism is working at the basolateral membrane or not.

From a physiological as well as a pathophysiological standpoint, it seems important to decide whether leaking ions cross the two membranes in series at opposite faces of the epithelium, or bypass the cells either through intercellular pathways or through gross lesions in the epithelial layer. In order to

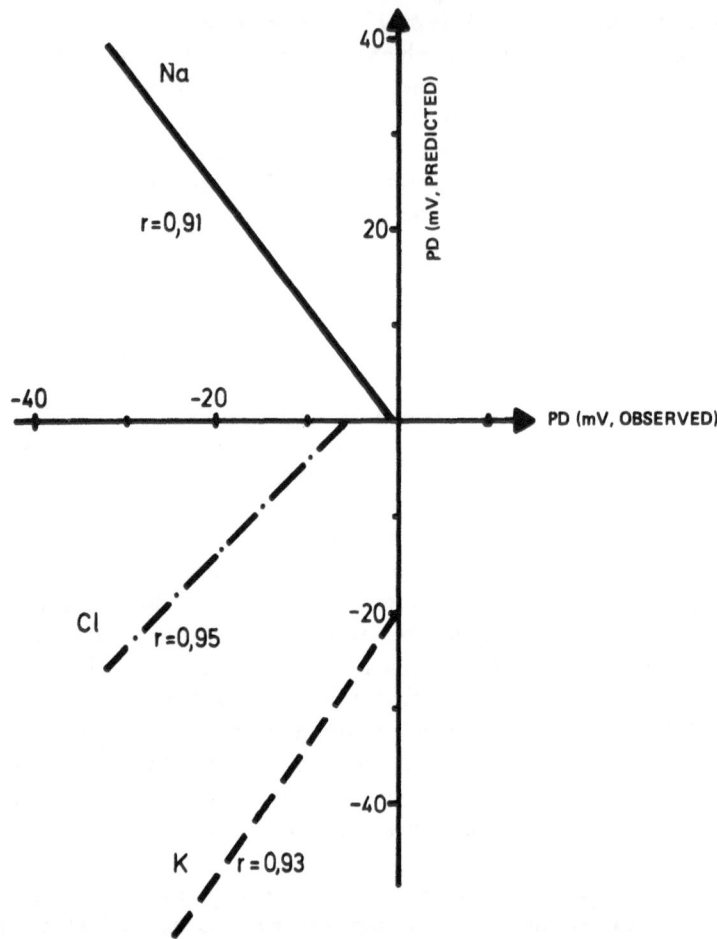

Figure 20.8 Relations between transmural potential difference (PD) observed in acute ulcerative colitis and that predicted from the luminal and contraluminal equilibrium concentrations of Na^+, Cl^-, and K^+ by the Nernst equation $[PD = (RT/zF) \times \ln (C_{plasma}/C_{lumen})]$

distinguish between shunt pathways and gross mucosal lesions, the inflamed rectal stump of the patients mentioned above was perfused with normally impermeant non-electrolytes[8]. Table 20.2 shows that the estimated permeability coefficients are proportional to the corresponding coefficients of free diffusion, suggesting that theoretical leaks in chronically inflamed epithelium cause no hindrance to the diffusion of the named test molecules. Consequently, the equivalent radius of such leaks is larger than the radius of vitamin B_{12}, or the pore size and number are inversely related. However, another approach to the problem permits the conclusion that the defective absorption in ulcerative colitis may be ascribed to ultrastructural changes in the passive diffusional barrier between the gut lumen and the blood[29]. Following

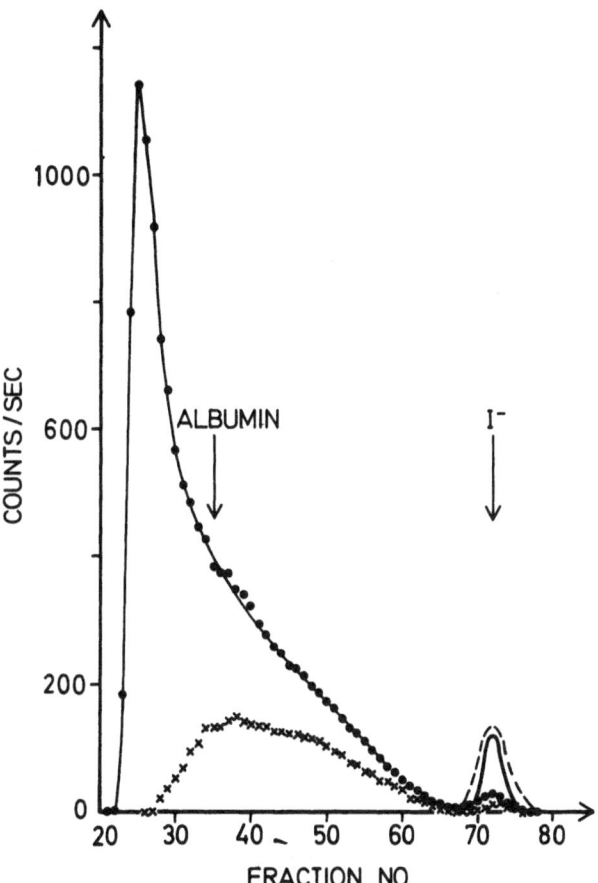

Figure 20.9 Elution curves for [^{125}I]polyvinylpyrrolidone (PVP) in the test solution (●————●), urine after intravenous injection (×————×), and urine 5 hours after rectal instillation of [^{125}I]PVP in a normal individual (————), and in a patient with ulcerative colitis (—————). The molecular weight distribution analysis of [^{125}I]PVP present in test solution and urine samples was performed in Sephadex G-200 + G-100 columns. The protein content was determined by measuring optical density at 280 nm (from reference 29)

Table 20.2 Permeability coefficient (P_D) (mean $\pm$ SEM) of the inflamed rectal mucosa compared to the free diffusion coefficient ($D_{25°}$)

No. of tests	Substance	$D_{25°} \times 10^5$ (cm^2/sec)	$P \times 10^5$ (cm/sec)	$P/D_{25°}$
10	Urea	1.38	14.0 $\pm$ 5.2	10
7	Fructose	0.69	4.3 $\pm$ 2.3	6.2
10	[^{51}Cr]EDTA	0.52	3.7 $\pm$ 1.0	7.1
10	[^{57}Co]vitamin B$_{12}$	0.30	2.4 $\pm$ 0.15	8.0
9	[^{125}I]PVP	?	1.2 $\pm$ 0.26	—

rectal instillation of ^{125}I-polyvinyl-pyrrolidone in patients with acute proctosigmoiditis, only the low molecular fractions are absorbed and excreted in the urine (Figure 20.9). On the contrary, fractions with molecular weights up to 60 000-70 000 are found in the urine following intravenous injection which means that the equivalent pore size of the inflamed epithelium is considerably smaller than that of normal renal glomeruli. Thus, gross lesions in the epithelial layer are unlikely to provide the transepithelial route. However, evaluation of these 'black box' properties of a membrane with unknown structure cannot give rise to more definite conclusions concerning the permeation mechanism.

Transepithelial transport of water and monovalent ions by the inflamed colon

In spite of greatly differing bulk flow conditions in ulcerative colitis, the flow of water is proportional to the rate of NaCl absorption[6,7,8]. Since the close correlation between water and Na^+ movements is preserved, water transport may be considered linked to transepithelial Na^+ transfer, but the absorbates are less hypertonic than in the normal condition[8,9].

Severe ulcerative colitis causes a marked decrease in the absorption of water, Na^+, and Cl^-[3,6-9,22,26] — and HCO_3^- secretion is proportionally reduced[7,8] (Figure 20.10). Thus, the normal reciprocal relationship between net transfer of Cl^- and HCO_3^- is preserved — despite malabsorption of water and Na^+. Secretion rates of K^+ are not different from normal[3,7,8,22], even if bulk flow of water is in the direction plasma to lumen; but normal net

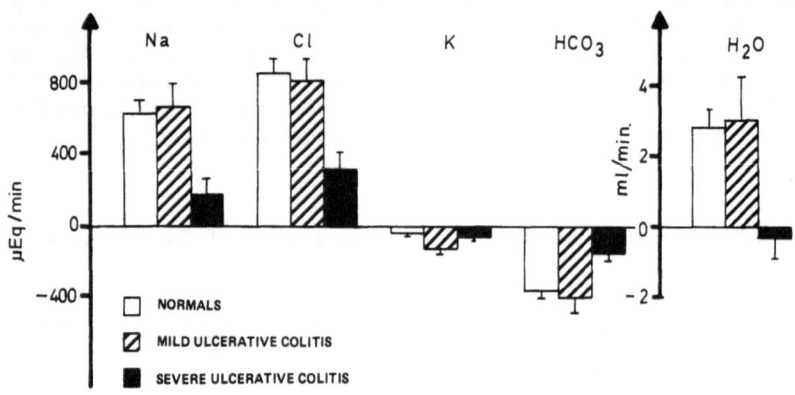

Figure 20.10 Net transport rates of electrolytes and water during steady state perfusion (15 ml/min) of the normal and the inflamed human colon with isotonic saline (data from reference 7)

movements of K^+ in the absence of large transepithelial PDs suggest that the transfer of this ion is abnormal as well. Unlike diffuse ulcerative colitis, mild proctosigmoiditis does not affect the transport of water, Na^+, Cl^-, and HCO_3^- by whole colon, but it brings about a significant increase in K^+ secretion[6,7,26] (Figure 20.10). These net effects may be attributed primarily to an increase in the plasma-to-lumen fluxes of water, Na^+, and K^+, but also a decrease in the opposite fluxes contributes to secretion[6–9,22,26] while a reduction in the lumen-to-plasma fluxes is responsible for the impairment of net Cl^- absorption[9].

The functional alterations referred to may all be explained by the presence of low-resistance shunt pathways in the otherwise tight epithelial barrier between lumen and plasma. Characteristically, observed Na^+ flux ratios approach those predicted by the flux ratio equation, indicating that colon loses its ability to transport Na^+ actively from lumen to plasma in progressive inflammation[7,9,17,22]. Consequently, an osmotic gradient for the movement of water in the direction lumen to plasma cannot be created, and net fluid transport is reduced or reversed, resulting in diarrhoea. The fact that only the flux from lumen to plasma affects net transfer of Cl^- is consistent with the observation that the transepithelial PD — which normally accelerates Cl^- absorption — is reduced or abolished[9].

Similar findings of preferential secretory processes in the perfused rectal stump of patients having undergone colectomy for inflammatory bowel disease[8] argue against the theory that increased production of endogenous vasopressin and aldosterone may be responsible for the abnormal absorptive pattern. Neither can contamination of the perfusates by K^+, derived from desquamated epithelial cells account for the high rates of K^+ secretion found in perfusion experiments. However, some properties of inflamed mucosa seem relevant to the distinction between artefacts in the perfusion system and abnormalities in the diseased epithelium. First, Archampong et al.[26] found increased net transfer of K^+ from the plasma-to-lumen side of colonic mucosa short-circuited in vitro. Second, Lockwood et al.[27] observed that intracellular K^+ concentrations are much reduced in ulcerative colitis. They also demonstrated that the epithelial cells continue to leak K^+ after artificial K^+ depletion in vitro, while normal mucosal cells rapidly regain K^+ when they are reincubated in Ringer's solution. Therefore the route for abnormal ion permeation may, in part at least, be via leaks in the cellular membranes themselves. A conceivable interpretation would be that preferential K^+ permeation occurs via the mucosal membrane of the diseased epithelial cell, resulting in diffuse leakage and subsequent cellular destruction if an accelerated Na^+/K^+ exchange can no longer preserve the intracellular environment. These predictions are in agreement with the experimental findings cited — but are still premature. New experiments are required specifically designed to evaluate the permselective properties of the inflamed epithelium, and to define the anatomic counterpart of the shunt pathways of colonic mucosa in preclinical stages of ulcerative colitis.

References

1. Fordtran, J. S. and Ingelfinger, F. J. (1968). Absorption of water, electrolytes, and sugars from the human gut. In C. F. Code (ed). *Handbook of Physiology, Section 6: Alimentary Canal, vol. III. Intestinal Absorption*, p. 1457 (Washington, DC: American Physiological Society)

2. Levitan, R., Fordtran, J. S., Burrows, B. A. and Ingelfinger, F. J. (1962). Water and salt absorption in the human colon. *J. Clin. Invest.*, 41, 1754

3. Duthie, H. L., Watts, J. M., deDomball, F. T. and Goligher, C. M. (1964). Serum electrolytes and colonic transfer of water and electrolytes in chronic ulcerative colitis. *Gastroenterology*, 47, 525

4. Hofmann, A. F. (1967). The syndrome of ileal disease and the broken enterohepatic circulation: cholerheic enteropathy. *Gastroenterology*, 52, 752

5. Head, L. H., Heaton, Jr., J. W. and Kivel, R. M. (1969). Absorption of water and electrolytes in Crohn's disease of the colon. *Gastroenterology*, 56, 571

6. Harris, J. and Shields, R. (1970). Absorption and secretion of water and electrolytes by the intact human colon in diffuse untreated proctocolitis. *Gut*, 11, 27

7. Rask-Madsen, J. (1973). Simultaneous measurement of electrical polarization and electrolyte transport by the entire normal and inflamed human colon during in vivo perfusion. *Scand. J. Gastroent.*, 8, 327

8. Rask-Madsen, J., Hammersgaard, E. A. and Knudsen, E. (1973). Rectal electrolyte transport and mucosal permeability in ulcerative colitis and Crohn's disease. *J. Lab. Clin. Med.*, 81, 342

9. Rask-Madsen, J. and Jensen, P. B. (1973). Electrolyte transport capacity and electrical potentials of the normal and the inflamed human rectum *in vivo*. *Scand. J. Gastroent.*, 8, 169

10. Devroede, G. J. and Phillips, S. F. (1969). Conservation of sodium, chloride, and water by the human colon. *Gastroenterology*, 56, 101

11. Edmonds, C. J. (1971). Absorption of sodium and water by human rectum measured by a dialysis method. *Gut*, 12, 356

12. Geall, M. G., Code, C. F., McIlrath, D. C. and Summerskill, W. H. J. (1970). Measurement of gastrointestinal transmural electric potential difference in man. *Gut*, 11, 34

13. Dalmark, M. (1970). The transmucosal electrical potential difference of rectum in the unanesthetized man. *Scand. J. Gastroent.*, 5, 277

14. Dalmark, M. (1970). The transmucosal electrical potential difference across the human rectum *in vivo* following perfusion of different electrolyte solutions. *Scand. J. Gastroent.*, 5, 421

15. Edmonds, C. J. (1970). Electrical potentials of the sigmoid colon and rectum in irritable bowel syndrome and ulcerative colitis. *Gut*, 11, 867

16. Archampong, E. Q. and Edmonds, C. J. (1972). Effect of luminal ions on the transepithelial electrical potential difference of human rectum. *Gut*, 13, 559

17. Rask-Madsen, J. (1973). The relationship between sodium fluxes and electrical potentials across the normal and inflamed human rectal wall *in vivo*. *Acta Med. Scand.*, 194, 311

18. Rask-Madsen, J. and Dalmark, M. (1973). Decreased transmural potential difference across the human rectum in ulcerative colitis. *Scand. J. Gastroent.*, 8, 321

19. Billich, C. O. and Levitan, R. (1969). Effects of sodium concentration and osmolality on water and electrolyte absorption from the intact human colon. *J. Clin. Invest.*, 48, 1336.

20. Rask-Madsen, J., Bruusgaard, A., Munck, O., Nielsen, M. D. and Worning, H. (1974). The significance of bile acids and aldosterone for the electrical hyperpolarization of human rectum in obese patients treated with intestinal bypass operation. *Scand. J. Gastroent.*, 9, 417

21. Wrong, O., Metcalfe-Gibson, A., Morrison, R. B. I., Ng, S. T. and Howard, A. V. (1965). *In vivo* dialysis of faeces as a method of stool analysis. I. Technique and results in normal subjects. *Clin. Sci.*, 28, 357

22. Edmonds, C. J. and Pilcher, D. (1973). Electrical potential difference and sodium and potassium fluxes across rectal mucosa in ulcerative colitis. *Gut*, **14**, 784

23. Grady, G. F., Duhamel, R. C. and Moore, E. W. (1970). Active transport of sodium by human colon *in vitro*. *Gastroenterology*, **59**, 583

24. Rask-Madsen, J. (1975). Transepithelial ionic transport by human colon and rectum *in vivo* and *in vitro*. (In preparation)

25. Fordtran, J. S., Rector, Jr., F. C., Ewton, M. F., Soter, N. and Kinney, J. (1965). Permeability characteristics of the human small intestine. *J. Clin. Invest.*, **44**, 1935

26. Archampong, E. Q., Harris, J. and Clark, C. G. (1972). Absorption and secretion of water and electrolytes across the healthy and the diseased human colonic mucosa measured *in vitro*. *Gut*, **13**, 880

27. Lockwood, C. M., Harris, J. and Clark, C. G. (1971). Intracellular potassium in diffuse proctocolitis. *Lancet*, **i**, 889

28. Diamond, J. M. (1964). The mechanism of isotonic water transport. *J. Gen. Physiol.*, **48**, 15

29. Rask-Madsen, J. (1973). Sieving characteristics of inflamed rectal mucosa. *Gut*, **14**, 988

Discussion Paper on

Effect of Diet on Mucosal Water and Solute Transfer by Rat Colon

E. Scharrer and Ö. Katona

Institut für Tierphysiologie
München

INTRODUCTION

Water intake of adult rats fed a diet high in protein (73.5% protein) is about twice as high as in rats fed a low-protein diet (11% protein)[1]. This is probably connected with the excretion of large amounts of urea formed under this condition.

Since to our knowledge nobody has yet investigated whether dietary-induced changes in water requirement are associated with changes in intestinal water transport, we have investigated net transfer of water by rat colon as affected by feeding a high-protein diet. Because water transport is closely linked to sodium and total solute transport[2], net transfer of sodium and net osmolar transfer was also studied.

METHODS

Adult male Sprague–Dawley rats were fed for about 3 weeks either a diet with 11% protein (group LP) or a diet with 73.5% protein (group HP). At this time the respective average body weights were 350 g (group LP) and 331 g (group HP). The animals could drink water *ad libitum*. The first 10 cm of the colon was removed from the anaesthetised animals and flushed with ice-cold Krebs–Henseleit bicarbonate buffer, and then stripped of serosa and external muscle layers by the method of Parsons and Patterson[3]. The mucosal tube was then everted; one end was tied off, 1.0 ml of Krebs–Henseleit bicarbonate buffer containing 16.7×10^{-3} M glucose was placed in the serosal compartment and the remaining end was tied off. The preparation was weighed rapidly and placed in a 100 ml Erlenmeyer flask containing 20 ml of Krebs–Henseleit bicarbonate buffer (glucose concentration: 16.7×10^{-3} M).

The flasks were filled with the appropriate gaseous phase ($O_2 : CO_2 = 95 : 5$) and then closed and agitated (120 oscillations/min) for 60 minutes at 37 °C. Net water flux (net F_{H_2O}) was measured gravimetrically at the end of the incubation. Net sodium flux (net F_{Na}) was calculated from the water flux and the increase in Na^+ concentration (Δ Na) in the serosal fluid during the incubation. Similarly net osmolar flux was obtained from net water flux and the increase of osmolality (Δ Osm) in the serosal fluid. Na^+ was determined with a flame photometer. Osmolality was measured by the freezing-point depression method using a Knauer osmometer.

RESULTS AND DISCUSSION

An increase in sodium concentration and osmolality was observed in the serosal fluid of the everted sacs of colonic mucosa when compared with the initial sodium concentration and osmolality of the Krebs–Henseleit solution introduced. These gradients were significantly higher in group LP than in group HP (Figure *20.1*).

This group difference appears to be attributable to the much higher (95%) net water flux (net F_{H_2O}) in group HP as compared to group LP (Figure *20.2*).

Yet net flux of sodium (net F_{Na}) and net osmolar flux (net F_{Osm}) in group HP also exceeded those in group LP (Figure *20.2*). However, the group

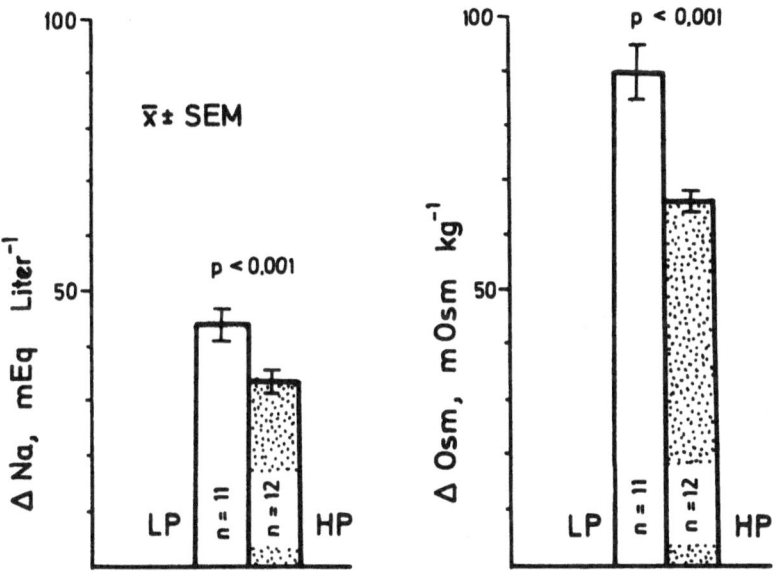

Figure 20.1 Increase in sodium concentration ($= \Delta$ Na) and osmolality ($= \Delta$ Osm) of the serosal fluid in everted sacs of colonic mucosa from rats fed either a diet low (11% protein, group LP) or high (73.5% protein, group HP) in protein

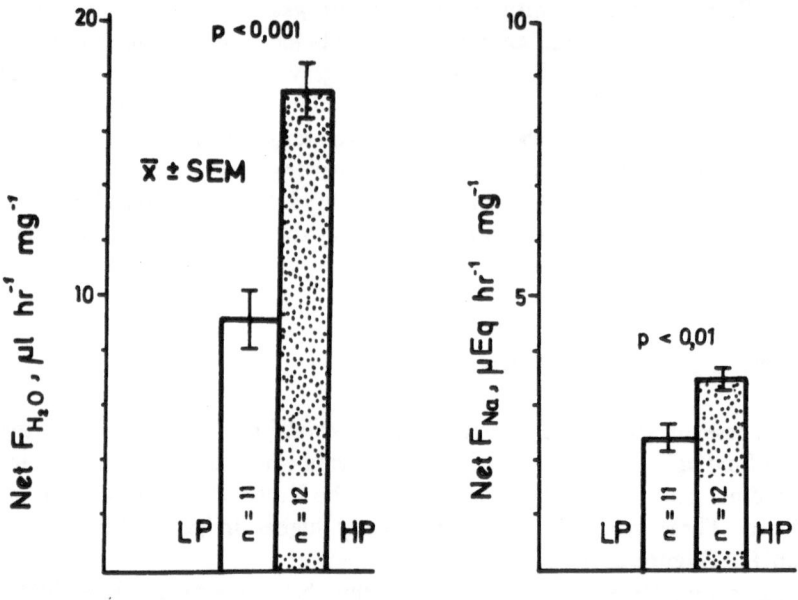

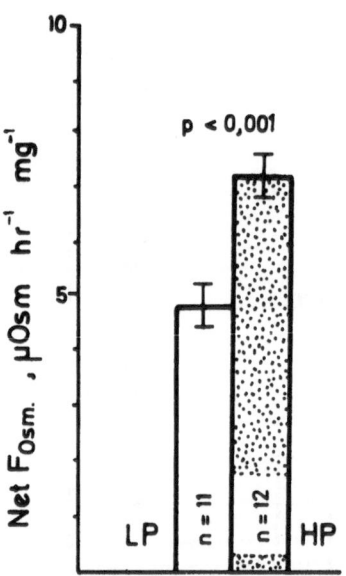

Figure 20.2   Net fluxes of water (= Net F_{H_2O}) and sodium (= Net F_{Na}) and net osmolar flux (= Net F_{Osm}) in everted sacs of colonic mucosa from LP and HP rats. Values are related to 1 mg dry weight

differences were much smaller (45% and 49% respectively), and therefore the ratio between both net fluxes of water and sodium and net fluxes of water and total solutes were higher in group HP than in group LP (Figure 20.3). Thus the fluid transported was less hypertonic in group HP than in group LP. Similar results have been obtained with rat colon, in which the serosa and external muscle layers had not been removed[1].

Curran's theory of passive water transport requires a primary step of solute transfer resulting in an osmotic gradient to which water passively responds, presumably by bulk flow through pores[2,4]. According to this theory, the

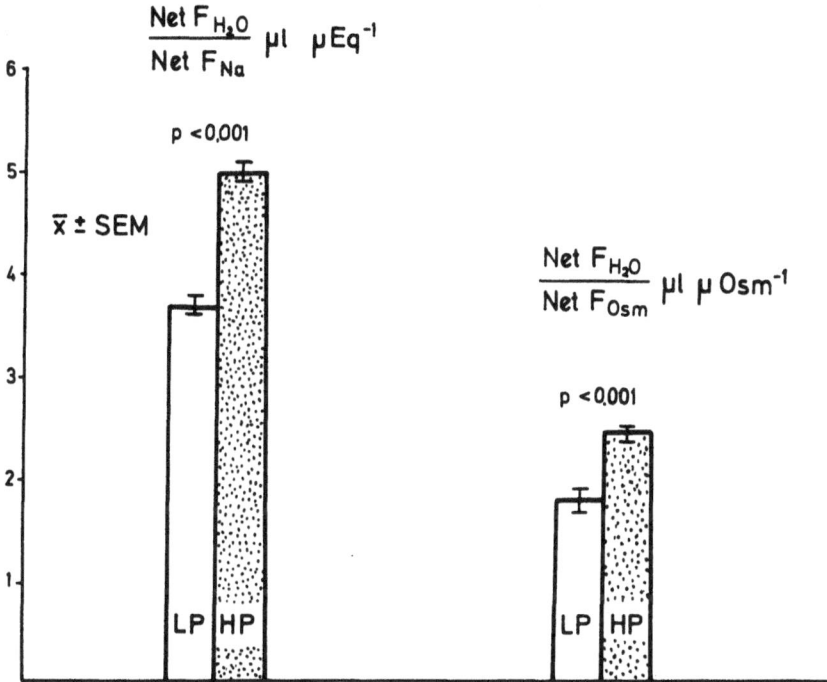

Figure 20.3 Ratio between net fluxes of water and sodium (= Net F_{H_2O}/Net F_{Na}) or total solutes (= Net F_{H_2O}/Net F_{Osm}) in everted sacs of colonic mucosa from LP and HP rats

degree of hypertonicity of the serosal fluid of everted sacs of colonic mucosa would depend on the efficiency with which water could move in response to the osmotic gradient developed. Thus an increase in the efficiency of the water movement in response to the osmotic gradient developed could account for the lower hypertonicity of the serosal fluid in everted sacs of colonic mucosa from HP rats as compared to LP rats.

To summarise: our results indicate that the ratio between net water and solute transport of rat colon can be changed by diet (Figure 20.3). This possibly represents a regulatory mechanism for water absorption, which might come into action when the water requirement of the animal changes.

References

1. Scharrer, E., Lutz, J. and Boehncke, E. (1971). Ernährungsbedingte Veränderungen der intestinalen Natrium- und Wasserresorption. *Ernährungs-Umschau*, **18**, 248
2. Curran, P. F. and Schwartz, G. F. (1960). Na, Cl, and water transport by rat colon. *J. Gen. Physiol.*, **43**, 555
3. Parsons, D. S. and Patterson, C. R. (1965). Fluid and solute transport across rat colonic mucosa. *Quart. J. Exptl. Physiol.*, **50**, 220
4. Curran, P. F. (1960). Na, Cl, and water transport by rat ileum *in vitro*. *J. Gen. Physiol.*, **43**, 1137

Discussion 20

Parsons: I wonder whether you have studied ion fluxes in your cases under conditions when NH_4^+ is present in the luminal fluid. NH_4^+ is a normal constituent of the mammalian colon and if it is present, the bicarbonate secretion which occurs into NaCl solutions is abolished and bicarbonate, if present, is absorbed.

Rask-Madsen: No, I have not yet done studies with ammonium present in the luminal fluid, but such experiments should be done in the future.

Nell: How do you measure the permeability coefficients? Did you administer the molecules from the luminal or the blood side?

Rask-Madsen: All test molecules were administered from the luminal side, since there was no bulk flow of water and the solvent drag effect could consequently be ignored. Only the permeability coefficients of the small non-electrolytes, urea, fructose, and [^{51}Cr]EDTA, were calculated directly from the concentration changes of the substances relative to those of the high molecular weight marker, [^{125}I]PVP. In order to calculate the permeability coefficient of the poorly absorbed [^{57}Co]vitamin B_{12} and the marker, [^{125}I]PVP itself, as well, the fraction of the [^{51}Cr]EDTA absorbed was also calculated from the appearance of radio-chromium in the urine; then a factor, X, was evaluated in order to reduce the result to the absolute value of $P_D^{51Cr-EDTA}$ measured. Finally, the fractions of ^{57}Co and ^{125}I appearing in the urine were corrected to 100% recovery and then reduced by the factor, X, to provide the absolute values of $P_D^{Vit. B_{12}}$ and P_D^{PVP}.

Edmonds: Our findings in ulcerative colitis, based on studies of the distal colon, have given essentially similar results to those described by Dr Rask-Madsen. Regarding the PD, we would agree that this appears to be reversed in severe colitis only when a skin reference is used. If an intravenous electrode is employed, then we do not observe reversal. I should like to ask Dr Rask-Madsen if he thinks the interesting excess potassium secretion that occurs in colitis might be due to excess mucus secretion.

Rask-Madsen: I cannot exclude the possibility of mucus production being responsible for at least some of the excess potassium secretion, but since the colon was perfused several hours before the period of measurement, this should represent freshly secreted potassium. Neither albumin nor haemoglobin could be detected in the perfusates, a fact that speaks against the possibility that transudation or exudation might be responsible for the excess potassium secretion in the patients with mild ulcerative colitis. Finally, the inflammatory changes in the patients were localised in the distal sigmoid and rectum, so that mucus secretion can hardly account for the extremely high net potassium secretion rates in these individuals.

Caspary: I have a question addressed to the two rectal PD experts: Measurement of rectal PD has been reported as the cheapest and perhaps the most reliable method for the diagnosis of hyperaldosteronism. Is this still considered to be so? Has it been confirmed or were further results disappointing?

Rask-Madsen: I do not think that measurements of rectal PD can be used as a reliable screening test for primary hyperaldosteronism at least. I have measured the rectal PD in eight of these patients and found a significantly increased potential in only three of them. The maximum value reported was −66 mV which is also the largest of all previous measurements with the exception of the patient with congenital chloridorrhoea, to whom I have previously referred at this meeting, who recorded a rectal PD of −116 mV and a serum aldosterone concentration that was four times higher than the normal upper limit!

Edmonds: My comment on the use of rectal PD as a guide to hyperaldosteronism is that, as a simple screening test, it is not satisfactory. We have now observed several false negatives, the PD being within the normal range. The explanation is still uncertain. Normal individuals given aldosterone show a rise in PD which persists for several days, if aldosterone administration is continued; there seems to be no escape, which agrees with faecal electrolyte studies. But in primary hyperaldosteronism, when the tissue will have been exposed to aldosterone for a very long period, the PD does not always seem to remain elevated. The PD is probably closely linked to the sodium–potassium exchange with the rectal lumen and disturbances of potassium metabolism in hyperaldosteronism may be responsible for the subsequent fall in PD despite the fact that the aldosterone levels remain high.

Rask-Madsen: I can confirm the results to Dr Edmonds insofar as exogenous aldosterone caused a considerable rise in the rectal PD of normal individuals.

Dowling: This must be a very difficult procedure, especially in sick patients. I have three points: (a) How did your patients tolerate the investigation? (b) How did you classify your patients as having mild, moderate, or severe colitis? (c) Have you had the chance to study any patients for a second time after treatment?

Rask-Madsen: To the first question, I should say that it was no greater strain to the patient than a barium enema in connection with radiological examinations of the colon, but it was certainly of longer duration. To the second question, the patients were classified according to the criteria of Truelove and Witts (*Brit. Med. J.*, ii, 1041, 1955) as regards the severity of the disease, while the local appearance of the mucosa was graded as described by Baron, Connell and Lennard-Jones (*Brit. Med. J.*, i, 89, 1964), since this classification had previously been used by Edmonds. Thirdly, the patients with mild proctosigmoiditis have been studied up to 1.5 years after the first investigation and in accordance to Dr Edmonds's experiences, the PD is seldom normalised in patients with relapses. This is consequently of prognostic significance, and the PD can be abnormally low even if there are no obvious morphological changes.

Skadhauge: May I ask Dr Scharrer whether the increased water intake might be due to a fairly constant renal concentrating ceiling, since rats only drink the amount of water necessary to be close to the maximal renal concentrating ability?

Scharrer: Yes, this is probable.

Skadhauge: In your study, did you measure the V_{max} or the K_m for sodium transport? In the sheep for example, a threefold larger food load results in the same fractional colonic salt and water absorption (Grovum and Williams, *Brit. J. Nutr.*, **29**, 13, 1973). This can simply be due to the sodium transport being fairly complete.

Scharrer: Sodium transport was only measured at one sodium concentration in the incubation medium. Therefore it is not clear whether the higher net sodium transfer by the colonic mucosa of high-protein-fed rats is due to an increase in V_{max} or decrease in K_m.

Skadhauge: Since the solute-linked water flow had a lower osmolality in the high-protein animals, was the percentage of water in the faeces lower?

Scharrer: The faeces looked normal; the water content was not determined.

Simmonds: Were the rats pair-fed? Was casein the protein supplement — this alters many aspects of gastrointestinal function? Finally, were the electrolyte intakes comparable in the two groups?

Scharrer: Because feeding the high-protein diet resulted in a slight (10%) chronic depression of food intake, both *ad libitum* and pair-fed animals were used for the experiments, but the mode of feeding did not influence the results obtained. The protein component of the diets was purified casein, and lastly the mineral contents of the diets were identical.

21
Closing Summary*

D. S. PARSONS

Department of Biochemistry,
University of Oxford

INTRODUCTION

In this Conference we have been discussing Intestinal Ion Transport. The word 'transport' means to carry, convey or remove from one place to another; discussion of transportation therefore requires consideration of the nature and location of the starting place and of the final destination. I should like to remind you that the starting place here in the intestine is within the fluid present in the intestinal lumen while the destination *in vivo* is the microcirculation in the intestinal wall. This microcirculation will include the capillaries of the mucosal epithelium and also the lymphatic capillaries. Properly speaking the consideration of intestinal transport must therefore include a discussion of three steps: (*a*) delivery to the epithelium; (*b*) epithelial transport, and (*c*) clearance away from the epithelium. Although in this conference most attention has naturally been paid to the second event, and the phenomena of epithelial transport have been the dominant theme of our discussion, the interactions of the three steps cannot be forgotten.

You will recall that *in vivo*, delivery of substrate to the mucosal epithelium is achieved by gastrointestinal motility and by diffusion. *In vitro*, diffusion from some compartment mixed by mechanical means is the usual process of delivery. *In vivo*, the clearance from the epithelium is by bulk flow and diffusion into the blood and across a region which is well stirred by the microcirculation in the intestinal wall. *In vitro*, the clearance from the epithelium is by bulk flow and diffusion through the whole intestinal wall, or in cases where the muscle layers are removed, through the submucosal region, and the destination is the fluid bathing the serosal surface.

* Note that in this text, references to presentations at the symposium are given by printing the names in capitals.

Table 21.1 Summary of techniques reported to be employed for studying intestinal ion transport

Procedure	Number of papers
Absorption studies using whole animal	3
Absorption studies using whole intestinal segments	
(a) in vivo	8
(b) surviving in vitro	7
Net and unidirectional flux measurements including short-circuit current, using sheets of mucosa	13
Other procedures	
(a) Subcellular fractionation, enzyme assay, etc.	5
(b) Histochemistry and morphometry	2

Note: some papers reported the use of more than one procedure

Epithelial transport must not be confused with membrane transport. Membrane transport plays a major role in epithelial transport, but the architecture of epithelia endows them with unique properties that are not possessed by the elements that compose the epithelium.

Before discussing the major aspects of intestinal ion transport that have been descried during the two days of our deliberations, I should like to draw your attention to the variety of techniques used to study intestinal absorption that have been reported here (see Table 21.1)[1]. It is to be noted that some authors reported the use of more than one procedure.

With studies on the kidney, two papers dealt with findings from subcellular fractionation procedures and one with perfused isolated tubules.

A wide variety of techniques have been described at the Conference, ranging from studies on the rate of drinking by fishes to quantitative morphological studies in the human intestine. Clearly the most popular procedures appear to be those involving the use of sheets of mucosa, usually stripped of the extrinsic muscle coats and mounted in a chamber of the Ussing type. The use of techniques of subcellular fractionation and the assay of enzymes and substrates should also be noted. The everted sac, popular since 1954, although still usefully employed, seems to be less prominent.

Table 21.2 Summary of animal species reported to be employed for studying intestinal ion transport

Animal	Number of papers
Human	9
Rat	7
Guinea-pig	6
Rabbit	6
Fish	4
Dog	2
Frog	1
Pig	1
Tortoise	1
Terrapin	1

From Table 21.2 it is seen that the rat does not appear to be an especially popular animal for the current investigation of intestinal salt transport. The use of clinical material is interesting, and no work has been reported in which hamsters were used.

There are some striking omissions from Table 21.1. No one has reported observations using the intestine surviving *in vitro* and perfused artificially through the vascular bed. There is no report of experiments on water and electrolyte exchanges in isolated intestinal cells and there are no experiments in which artificial membranes are employed to throw light on ionic transport. It will be interesting to see what techniques will be popular in ten years' time.

MEMBRANE TRANSPORT

By membrane transport I mean transport across the membranes that separate the cell interior from its environment. Usually this transport is via special systems located within these membranes.

Why membrane transport?

Membrane transport is a necessity of cell life. Cells that have membranes permeable to water and small electrolytes such as Na^+, K^+, Cl^-, HCO_3^- and the like, will not be in osmotic equilibrium with their environment unless they are furnished with functioning membrane transport systems for some of the ions. This follows because an osmotic burden is imposed upon the cells by the presence within them of impermeant molecules including polyelectrolytes (see Figure 21.1). The cell interior tends to become hypertonic with respect to the environment and unless the cell interior is maintained isotonic with respect to the environment, the cell will swell up (see Appendix 1). In animal cells, osmotic compensation is achieved by regulating the concentrations of the small diffusible ions within the cell; it is usually the cations that are controlled. The regulation is achieved by two sorts of transport system acting in concert. In the steady state, the flux in one direction through one system is exactly equal to that in the opposite direction through the other system.

One sort, the 'pump', transports ions (usually Na^+ and K^+) through the membrane in a direction which is independent of and usually against the electrochemical gradient of the ion. Pumping operations require energy which is supplied directly by the hydrolysis of ATP, so that the functioning of the pumps is related to membrane-bound ATPases. The other sort of system, the 'leak', is a different separate membrane transport system through which the direction of movement is determined by the transmembrane electrochemical potential of the ion in question.

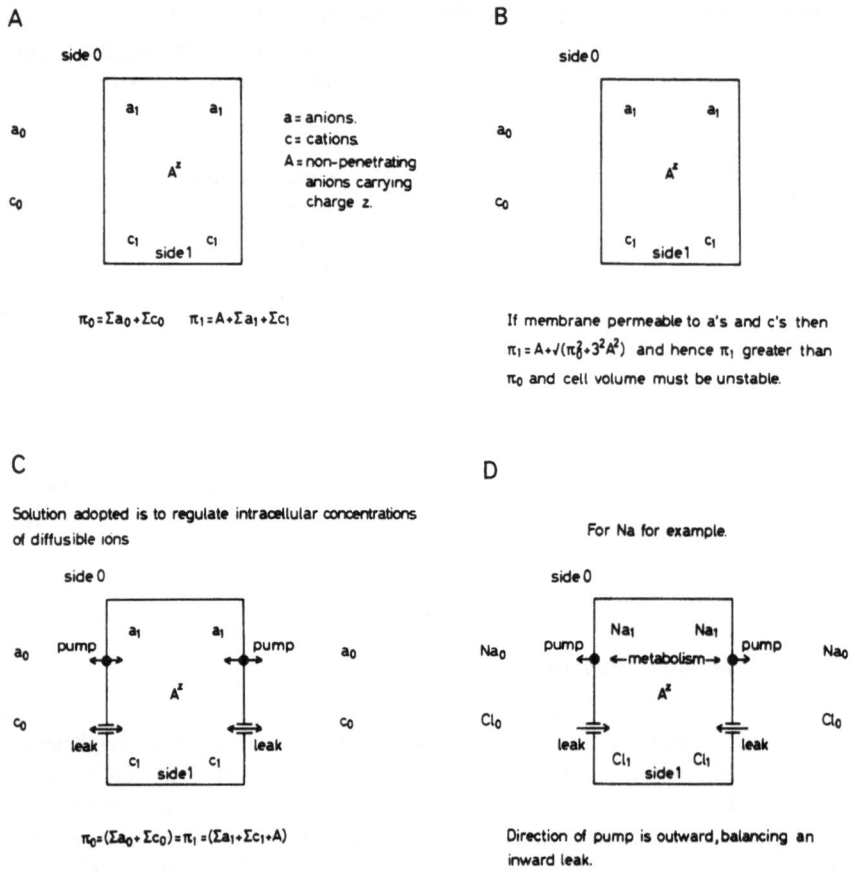

Figure 21.1 Membrane transport necessary for regulation of cell volume. Cell permeable to water and to small anions and cations, a and c; a_o, c_o = concentration outside cell; a_1 and c_1 = concentration inside cell. A = concentration of non-penetrating ('fixed') anions carrying charge z, see also Appendix 1

Sorts of Na⁺ pump

The classical Na⁺-K⁺-ATPase represents the biochemical basis of one sort of pump[1], and this is inhibited by ouabain. There is increasing evidence that in many cells, volume regulation may be maintained in the presence of ouabain and in the absence of the external potassium that the classical Na⁺ pump requires (see, for example, Macknight *et al.*[2] for a discussion of this point). We have now heard WHITTEMBURY and PROVERBIO tell us that in the proximal tubular cells of the kidney, there may be a pump that is ouabain-insensitive and sensitive to ethacrynic acid.

Two questions arise. Is there really only one sort of molecular system underlying these pumps, which can operate in either of two modes? And do either or both of these pumps play any role in salt pumping in the intestine? You will remember that ROBINSON has shown that salt transport in dog colon is inhibited by ouabain. As yet, we have no final answer to these problems. Indeed, so far no one has demonstrated the presence in intestinal mucosal cells of a metabolically dependent, potassium-independent, ouabain-insensitive mechanism related to salt pumping towards the blood. It should certainly be looked for.

Leaks

A leak is a distinct specific membrane transport system for substrate. It differs from the pump in that it is not equipped with a power supply and the flow of substrate through the system is therefore always in the downhill direction of the electrochemical gradient for the substrate across the membrane, the rate of flux being determined by the magnitude of this gradient. However, we have heard good evidence that the potential energy otherwise dissipated by, for example, Na^+ moving down its own electrochemical gradient can be used to drive another substrate, for example monosaccharide or amino acid, uphill, in other words, to drive a 'secondary pump'.

Secondary pumps

The primary pumping systems for Na^+ and K^+ utilise directly the free energy of hydrolysis of ATP as the power supply. However, when an ion, for example, Na^+, passes into the cell down an electrochemical gradient via its 'leak' system for membrane transport, the possibility arises that the energy otherwise dissipated in its passage down the electrochemical gradient may be captured and used as a source of power for a pump for another substrate. Such a system could be called a secondary pump. The energy for driving the pump for the second substrate is derived only secondarily from the hydrolysis of ATP. The exceedingly elegant experiments of KINNE and MURER have shown such a secondary pump to be present in the brush-border membranes. The pump drives glucose and amino acids in the inward direction, the source of power being the movement of Na^+ down the electrochemical gradient.

Membrane flow and vesiculation

It must not be forgotten that another important mode of membrane transport is one in which the transport of substrate is associated with the actual movement of the membrane itself. Membrane flow and vesiculation play an important part in intestinal transport. SMITH has pointed out that suckling in the newborn pig is associated with the formation of vacuoles in the cytoplasm of the ileum and colon. Associated with this vacuolation, the Na⁺ influx decreases in the ileum, but in the colon it increases, findings that raise interesting questions with respect to the processes of vacuolation and of Na⁺ uptake by the epithelium.

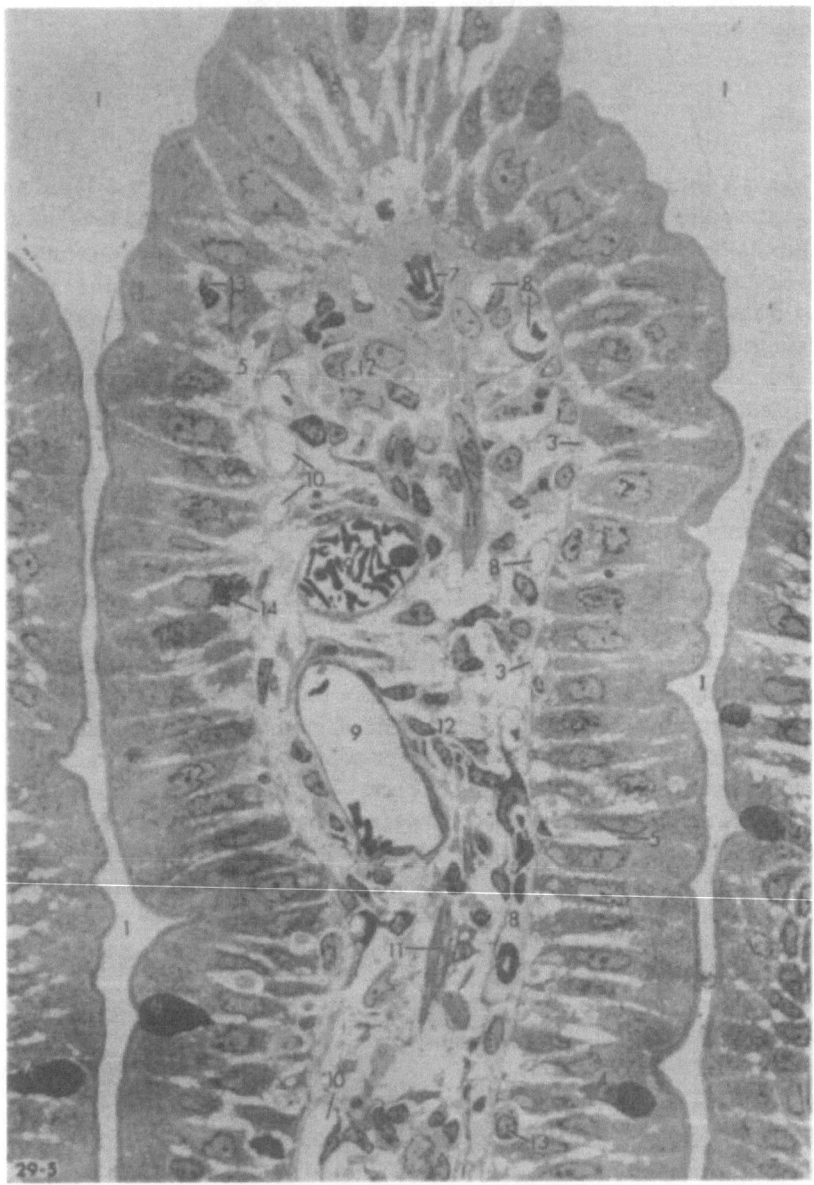

Figure 21.2 Intestinal villus of rat ×800; 1 Intestinal lumen; 2 nuclei of mucosal cells; 3 basement membrane; 7, 8, 9 blood vessels; 10 lacteal; 14 endocrine cells (data from Rhodin[4])

A question related to that of membrane foldings and invaginations is that of the water permeability of membranes, which is inversely related to the radius of curvature of the membrane, the more curved the membrane, the smaller the radius of curvature and the greater the water permeability[3]. This fact has interesting implications on the influence of invaginations, and convolutions of the plasma membrane and the presence of microvilli on the water permeability (see also the remarks by WRIGHT in discussion following WINGATE's paper).

I do not propose to deal here with the role of diffusion in transmembrane transport, but I would like to point out that lateral diffusion of membrane constituents in the plane of the membrane is now well recognised[4]. There are

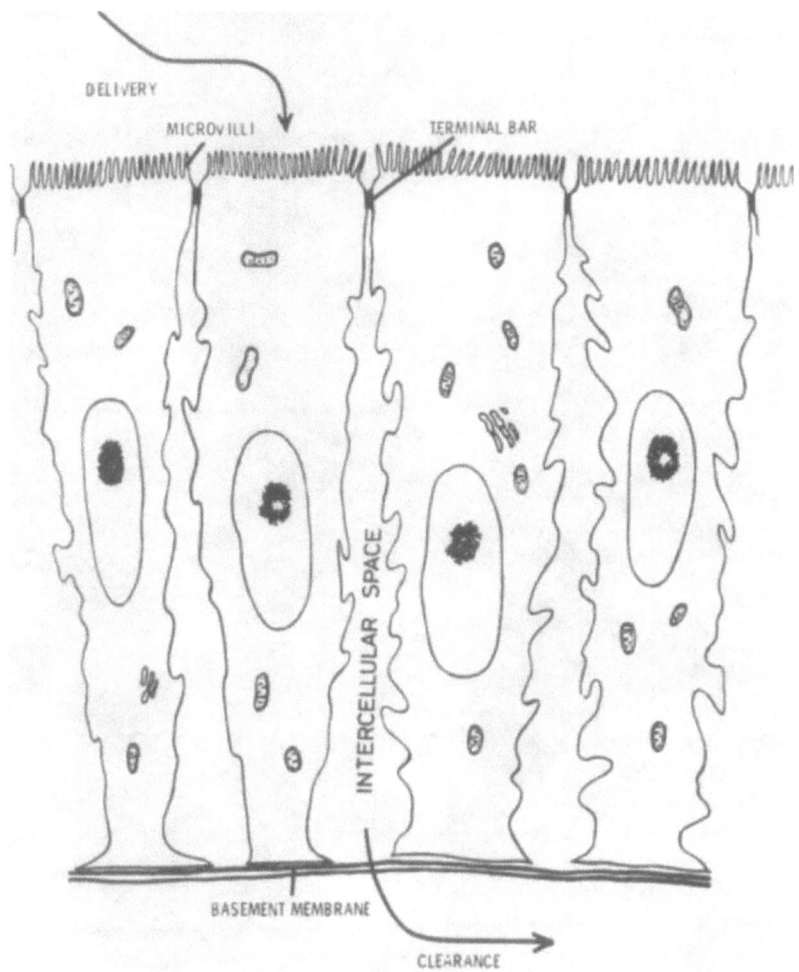

Figure 21.3 Diagram showing relationships of mucosal epithelial cells to intercellular space and basement membrane

evidently some interesting implications for this phenomenon in connection with access of substrate to channels for transmembrane transport. I will deal later with the role of diffusion in epithelial transport (page 424).

EPITHELIAL TRANSPORT

There are two routes across the intestinal epithelium, the cellular route and the paracellular route.

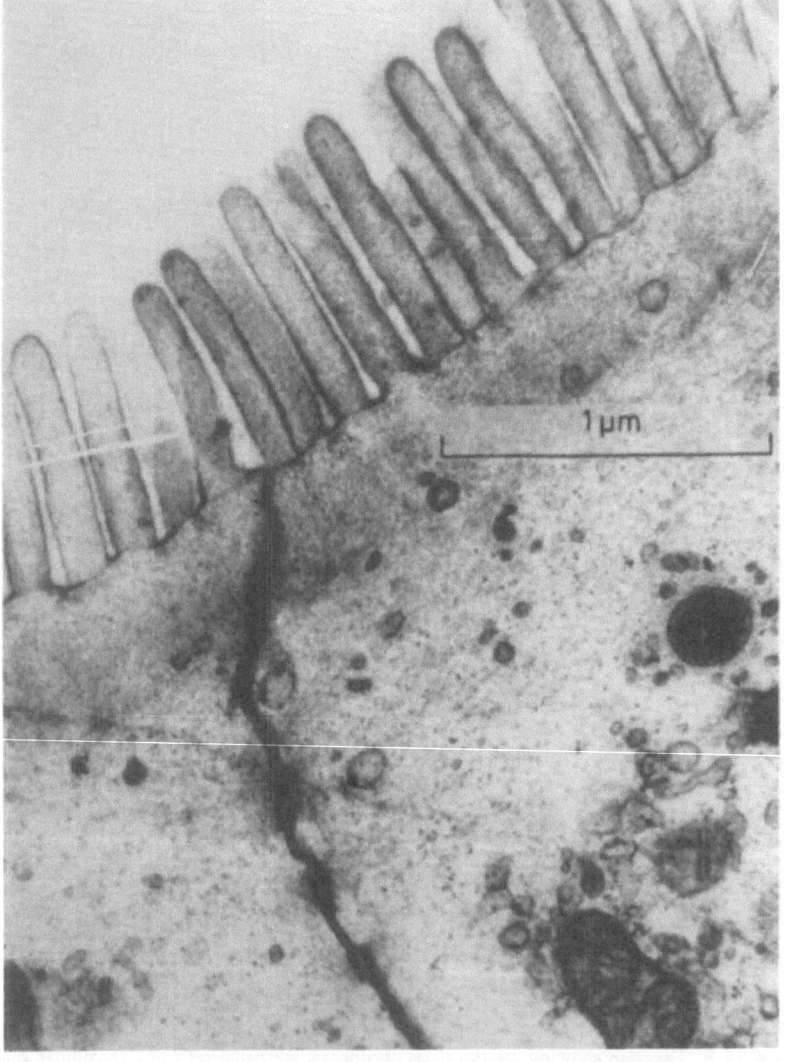

Figure 21.4 Junctional region between two adjacent epithelial cells of frog small intestine

An important structural feature of the intestinal epithelium is that the individual cells that form the palisade are packed in a hexagonal array and are separated by a long and complicated pericellular sleeve. It seems that the output from the cells occurs into this intercellular space, which is bounded by the so-called basolateral membranes of the cell. The space is bounded at the luminal end by the zonula occludens (tight junction) and at its distal end by the basement membrane.

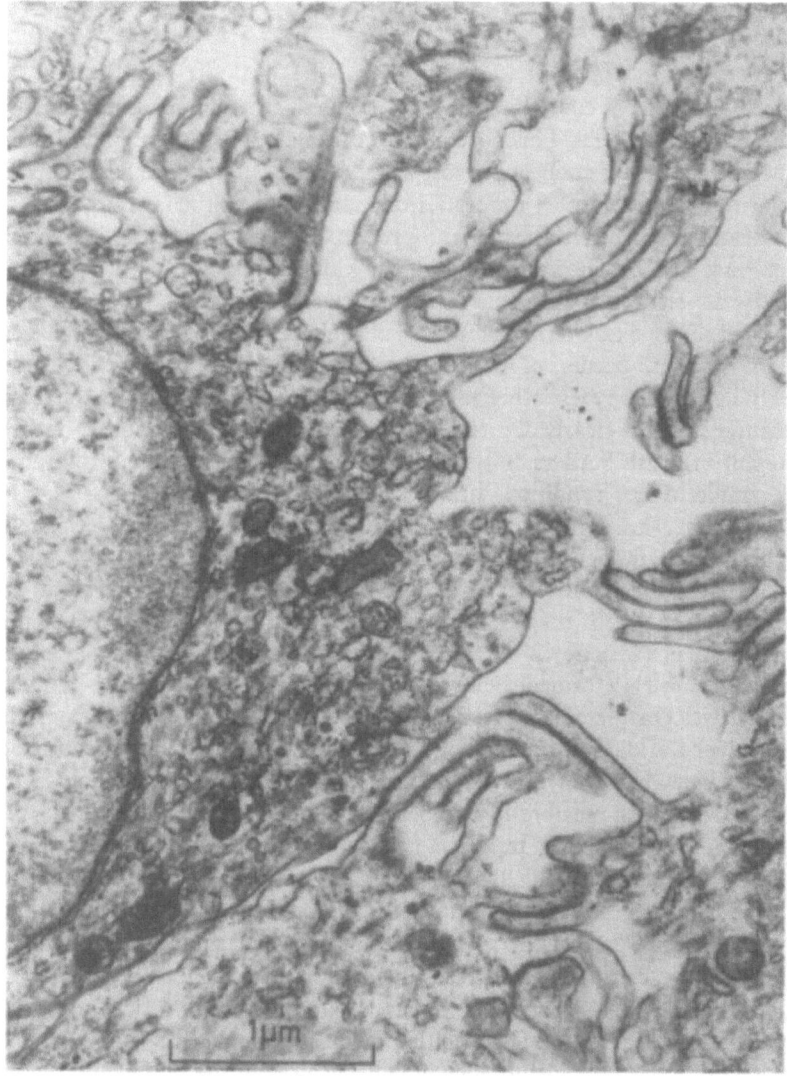

Figure 21.5 Intercellular space in intestinal mucosa of frog; plane of section is approximately parallel to epithelial surface at level of nuclei of mucosal cells

The intercellular space represents a highly specialised microenvironment within which local gradients of solute concentration and of hydrostatic and osmotic pressure are established. Some of the features of epithelial structure are shown in Figures 21.2–21.5.

I now propose to consider some of the features of the cellular and the paracellular routes of epithelial transport.

CELLULAR TRANSPORT

The cellular mode of epithelial transport seems to depend upon a fundamental asymmetry of the cells. This is related to differences in the functions of the epithelial cell. In this connection, just as KINNE and MURER have demonstrated a polarity in the transport properties of kidney and epithelial cells, so EBEL has demonstrated differences in the protein composition of the basolateral membranes and brush borders of the rat kidney.

As far as salt transport is concerned, the classical Na^+-K^+-ATPase seems to be located in the basolateral membranes of the mucosal cells and is not present at all in the brush borders of mouse or rat epithelial cells. However, as we have already heard, there exist other sorts of ATPases, some of which are ouabain-insensitive and it is clearly of interest to discover whether one or other of these is present in brush borders or is capable of being induced in the membranes, for example, under conditions under which secretion is induced.

Two points arise in connection with the notion that the basolateral membranes are the site of an outward Na^+ pump.

The first is the implication that these membranes are impermeable in the passive sense to salt. If the salt is pumped into the intercellular space, then in the interests of efficiency it would be expected not to leak back! Such an impermeability to Na^+ formed the basis of the prototype model of Na^+-pumping cells that was postulated by Ussing[5] to account for salt transport in frog skin. The evidence to date, for frog skin and also for other epithelia, is consistent with that view. However, it does not necessarily follow that the whole of the complex basolateral membrane is impermeable in the passive sense to Na^+. If, under secretory conditions, there is a translation of NaCl from blood to lumen by passage through the epithelial cells, then either the direction of the classical Na^+ pump must be reversed or Na^+ must enter the cells passively, perhaps through a special part of the plasma membrane, for example, that bounding the foot of the cell and which rests upon the basement membrane.

The second point is that evidence is now accumulating that Na^+ secretion from cells may occur by processes situated in the endoplasmic reticulum or in some related system of membranes in continuity with the basolateral plasma membrane. The evidence for this view is derived from work on frog skin[6,7] and also on the frog oocyte[8]. By looking at electron micrographs of intestinal epithelia, the complexity of the internal membrane system becomes readily apparent. It should be noted that, according to current views of lipid absorption, the endoplasmic reticulum is assigned a major role in the excretion of triglyceride and lipoprotein from the intestinal mucosal cell. If, in fact, the endoplasmic reticulum is in continuity with the plasma membrane, then procedures for the isolation of basolateral membranes must at the same time yield 'internal' membranes. Such membranes may be the locus of the Na^+-K^+-ATPase activity to which I have already referred.

KINNE and MURER have told us that the movement of sugars and of amino acids across the basolateral membranes, although stereospecific, is independent of Na^+. In contrast, it is the Na^+ movement down its electrochemical potential gradient that drives these organic molecules uphill across the brush border. Across the basolateral membrane there may be no downhill movement of Na^+, so a comparable coupling to sugar and amino acid transport need not be expected. However, it is of interest to know whether the movement of sugars and of amino acids across the basolateral membranes is in any way coupled to the hydrolysis of ATP, and to that extent influenced by Na^+ and K^+.

Acid-base changes and transport

I would like to point out a feature of intestinal absorption that has been somewhat neglected although it was considered by BINDER and by TURNBERG. Salt transport is not an isohydric process in the intestine, so that pH changes occur in the lumen during absorption.

Solutions of NaCl, isotonic with normal extracellular fluid and buffered with HCO_3^- and CO_2 are absorbed approximately isotonically. However, the rates of absorption of Na^+ and Cl^- differ, and in the rat, dog and in man, the relative rates of absorption of these two ions also differ according to whether the jejunum, the ileum or the colon is investigated[9,10]. FRIZZELL has suggested that a coupled NaCl influx occurs across the brush border of rabbit ileum. This suggestion is, of course, entirely consistent with the presence of independent, but separate processes of Na^+-H^+ exchange and Cl^--HCO_3^- exchange that seem to be present in many intestinal epithelia. In the rat jejunum, HCO_3^- has a stimulatory effect on salt absorption in vitro, but this effect is not found in the ileum, and it may be that there is a secretion of $NaHCO_3$ in the direction lumen to serosa in the presence of CO_2-containing buffers. In the rat colon, it appears that there is a $NaHCO_3$ secretion from blood to lumen[11], a finding that is of interest in connection with the data of FIELD that Na^+ secretion is only seen when HCO_3^- is present in the serosal fluids. In other words, there appears to be a secretion of HCO_3^- as well as of Cl^- under secretory conditions.

Control of cellular transport

It is of interest that HIRANO has shown that the Cl⁻-pump, which appears in eels that are adapted to sea water, is associated with the secretion of HCO_3^-. It is thus possible that this pump is driven by a downhill movement of Na^+ into the cells. Conceivably therefore, in mammalian intestine, the Cl⁻-HCO_3^- exchange across the brush-border membranes could be driven in either direction by a movement of Na^+ in the same direction as the Cl⁻. Under secretory conditions, the movement of Na^+ into the lumen is induced by something else, perhaps the formation of a new protein of which depends upon the presence of some cyclical nucleotide. According to FIELD, the ion-transport-related pool of cAMP is only a small fraction of the total mucosal cAMP, while cGMP may be an intracellular effector for NaCl absorption.

In connection with the induction of the secretory states, it must be remembered that there are close connections between the gastrointestinal hormones and the induction of intestinal secretion. Thus both the gastric inhibitory peptide (GIP) and the vasoactive intestinal peptide (VIP) and also glucagon can produce watery diarrhoea in patients and also in experimental animals. At the same time it appears that the cholera toxin, as CASE has shown, can exert a secretin-like action on the pancreas. Evidently all these agents operate via intracellular effectors which may be cyclic nucleotides.

What does not yet seem to be clear is the extent to which the entry of Na^+ across the brush border that is associated with the uptake of sugars and of amino acids is related to the postulated neutral NaCl uptake and to the Na^+-H^+ exchange. It appears from the work of SEPÚLVEDA and ROBINSON that the powerfully hallucinogenic drug, harmaline, inhibits the influx of amino acids and monosaccharides across the brush border by acting at the sodium site of the uptake processes for these substances.

The possibility, suggested by FIELD, of an adrenergic influence in the direction of stimulation of salt transport is of interest. It may be recalled that many years ago Florey and his co-workers pointed out how common was the occurrence of a paralytic secretion from the small intestine when the extrinsic sympathetic nerves were divided[12]. It is possible that this paralytic secretion follows the removal of transmitters that act via α-adrenergic receptors. However, the doses of adrenaline and noradrenaline that are required to produce effects on absorption *in vitro* are so large as to require an investigation under *in vivo* conditions when physiological doses can be delivered directly to the epithelium.

MUNDAY has produced evidence to show that in kidney cortex and in rat jejunum and distal colon, physiological concentrations of angiotensin appear to stimulate a neutral NaCl transport system, possibly similar to that of WHITTEMBURY. The effect does not seem to be mimicked by cAMP but it is prevented by substances that inhibit the translational stage of protein synthesis. An interesting point is that in the jejunum the effects of angiotensin appear to be dose-dependent; low doses stimulate the induction of salt absorption while high doses are inhibitory.

PARACELLULAR TRANSPORT

It is now well recognised that in the mucosal epithelium of the intestinal tract, there is a low resistance shunt pathway which has important implications for the interpretation of electrical phenomena in the tissue. Extracellular shunt pathways appear in all epithelia and the pathways appear to depend upon the zonula occludens (tight junction) and the associated intercellular space. Staehelin[13] has recently shown that the basis of the junction that forms the zonula occludens is a system of fibres connecting adjacent cells in the epithelium. The fibres run from one membrane to the next and the number of fibres appears to be related directly to the electrical resistance of the epithelium (see Table 21.3). In this conference ALVARADO, ARMSTRONG, MUNCK and NELL, in particular, have considered the paracellular route.

The high ionic conductivity of the zonula occludens together with the fact that the intercellular space contains modified extracellular fluid lends strong support to the suggestion of ARMSTRONG that a liquid junction potential may exist across the zonula occludens. The presence of such a potential will have further profound implications with respect to comprehension of the electrical properties of the intestine mucosa.

Although the intercellular region is clearly a path of low electrical resistance, to what extent does it represent a path for solute and water movement? There is no doubt that the paracellular route is important for solutes. Indeed as has been mentioned earlier, the epithelial cells evidently discharge salts directly into the intercellular space, so that the clearance of salt transported by the cellular route in fact occurs via the paracellular pathway. However, is there a significant ionic flux through the zonula occludens? The answer would appear to be 'yes'. It is characteristic of epithelia that the influx of Na^+ is always very much greater than the influx measured across the plasma membrane, and this generalisation appears to obtain in every case that has been investigated, a fact first pointed out by Cereijido and Rotunno[14] (see Table 21.3).

The possibility of movement of solutes across the zonula occludens seems real, especially for substances with molecular weights below about 200. ALVARADO has also suggested that Na^+ may pass back from the intercellular spaces to the lumen (Figure 21.6). Clearly, very different conditions obtain *in vivo* and *in vitro*. Under the latter conditions, the clearance away from the epithelium across the basement membrane depends upon a movement across the submucosal tissues, including the muscle layers. *In vivo*, the clearance is directly into the blood so that the feasibility of a direct route from the intestine lumen via the paracellular pathway would then be entirely dependent

Table 21.3 Relationship between epithelial conductance and structure of zonula occludens; data from Staehelin[13]

Epithelium	Epithelial resistance $\Omega\ cm^{-2}$	Number of strands in zonula occludens (mean ± SE)
Mammalian proximal convoluted tubule	6	1.2 ± 0.1
Necturus proximal convoluted tubule	70	3.3 ± 0.2
Rabbit gall bladder	30	4.1 ± 0.1
Necturus gall bladder	300	6.2 ± 0.2
Rat, mouse jejunum	300+	5.3 ± 0.2
Distal convoluted tubule	300–600	
Necturus		4.8 ± 0.4
Mouse		5.8 ± 0.2
Gastric mucosa		
Mouse	—	8.1 ± 0.3
Anuran urinary bladder	1000–2000	
Toad		8.1 ± 0.9
Frog		7.9 ± 0.4

upon the extent to which the zonula occludens region is permeable to the substance in question.

The hydraulic properties of the epithelium are interesting because the intestine exhibits the phenomenon of rectification of hydraulic flow. The extent to which fluid can be caused to filter across the epithelium under an imposed gradient of hydrostatic pressure depends upon the direction of that gradient.

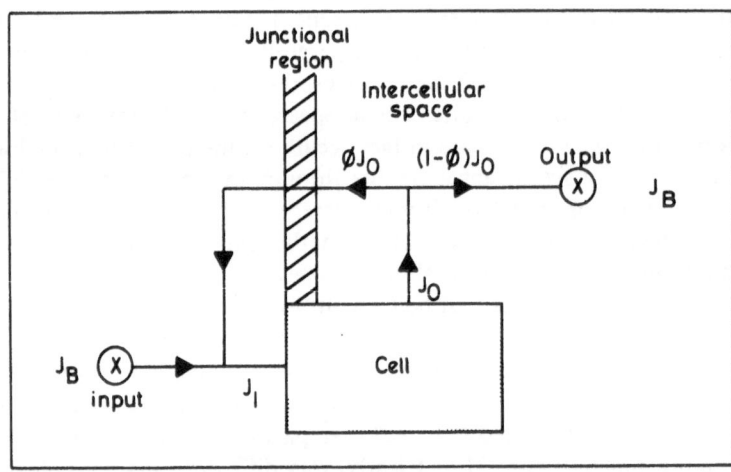

Figure 21.6 Effects of shunt pathway between intercellular space and lumen *in vitro*. In the steady state of absorption, input to mucosa from bulk phase in lumen = output across serosa = J_B, and input to cells from lumen J_1 = output into the intercellular space J_o for non metabolised substrate, e.g. Na^+. If flux through shunt to lumen = ϕJ_o, $J_B = (1-\phi)J_o$ and shunt has effect of reducing apparent V_{max} of cellular route. See also articles by ALVARADO AND ARMSTRONG. *In vivo* flux may be from left to right, in which case $J_B = (1 + \phi)J_1$

It has been known for many years, in the case of intestine surviving under optimum conditions *in vivo*, that distension of the lumen with hydrostatic pressures in the range of 5–50 cm saline is without influence on the rate of net transfer of fluid. It therefore appears that the hydraulic conductivity of the epithelium and the shunt pathway and, in particular, of the zonula occludens, is very low in the case with hydrostatic pressure gradients positive in the direction lumen–serosa (that is, with lumen P > serosa P). On the other hand, if the intestine, arranged as a sac or as a diaphragm of mucosa, is subjected to an hydrostatic pressure gradient in which the pressure in the lumen is lower than on the serosal face, then it exhibits different properties. Under these conditions it is found that with serosal pressures 2–5 cm positive to that in the lumen, a substantial filtration of fluid will occur into the lumen (for references see Parsons[16]; see also Loeschke *et al.*[17]). This phenomenon of rectification of hydraulic flow may be related to the architecture of the epithelium and to the presence of the long convoluted intercellular channels bounded at the luminal end by the fibrous bridges that constitute the zonula occludens. These considerations raise the possibility of secretion into the lumen by a process of filtration through junctional regions *in vivo*. This could occur when the tissue pressure in the epithelium is abnormally high.

However, it has certainly not yet been proved that this rectification of hydraulic flow across the mucosa is a property of the paracellular route. It may simply be that access to the cells occurs more readily under the influence of an hydrostatic pressure, for example, via 'scalloped sacs'[6,7] from the serosal faces than from the mucosal face (see also Figure 21.5, reference 17). The remarks made by WRIGHT during the discussion of WINGATE'S paper are very pertinent in this connection.

The findings of MUNCK indicate that in rat jejunum *in vitro*, in the presence of glucose, there is a net volume flow directed towards the mucosal solution through the paracellular route. MUNCK terms this process a 'fluid circuit' and shows that it profoundly affects amino acid transport. But does such a 'fluid circuit' occur *in vivo* when transport forward into the blood is so much easier? A question that is obscure is whether the effects of increased hydrostatic pressure on the serosal face are reversible, or whether permanent damage is caused during the process of filtration into the lumen. So far none of these questions appear to have been fully answered.

EFFECTS OF BILE

The physiological effects of bile with respect to fat digestion and absorption are now fairly well understood. Yet it is a remarkable fact that the digestion and absorption of lipid is a function of the upper small intestine and this is a region where the bile salts are not reabsorbed. Bile salt reabsorption is a function of highly specific systems located in the ileum; in fact not all bile salts are absorbed in the ileum for some remain to enter the colon.

The fact that bile has purgative effects has been known for many years (Figure 21.7 shows a reference from the nineteenth century[18]), but it was not until 1962 that the effects of bile acids on transport were discovered by Rummel[19-21] (see also Pope et al.[22]). Experiments with bile acids are complicated by the fact that each species, including man, secretes characteristic bile acids that recycle through an enterohepatic circulation[23]. Some bile acids are of primary origin and others are produced secondarily by microbial action[23]. For each species, different bile acids have differing inhibitory effects on transport.

The findings presented by NELL show clearly that in the rat deoxycholate (and oxyphenisatin) increase the salt and water flux from blood to lumen and that this is achieved by an action on the paracellular pathway. The findings of WINGATE can also be similarly explained and it is of interest that the effects of bile acids in WINGATE's experiments are completely reversible. It seems likely

> Another use that has been assigned to the bile is, that it exerts a stimulating action on the intestinal walls, and thus acts as a natural purgative; and in support of this view, it may be mentioned that jaundice (in which the bile does not flow into the intestine) is often accompanied by extreme constipation, and that purified ox-gall, taken either in the form of pill or enema, produces an undoubted purgative action.

Figure 21.7 Reference to influence of bile on intestinal transport from Chambers Encyclopaedia[18], 1860

that the situation is complicated by the fact that bile salts are detergents. Thus if they are used at high concentrations other direct, and perhaps irreversible, effects may be induced on brush-border membranes and at the junctional region.

The influence of bile may be related to an important question. What is there to prevent the water and salt contained in the lumen of the small intestine from being completely absorbed by the time the contents have reached the ileum or the descending colon? Why are the intestinal contents not completely desiccated before the lower intestine is reached? Is there a system that controls the quantity of fluid that passes through the ileocaecal valve each day? Perhaps the answers may lie in the actions of the bile salts. If this is so, then factors that increase gallbladder emptying might also influence the fluidity of the intestinal contents.

A detailed study of caecal-fermenting herbivores, such as the rabbit and the guinea-pig, might provide useful data. In these species an appreciable proportion of the body water is present in the intestinal contents[24], and the small intestine appears to go through phases of secretion.

SECRETION

Various aspects of secretion have been dealt with in this conference and I have already referred to many of these. I wish now to point out some other features of small intestinal secretion.

It has not yet been decided whether secretion by the small intestine is function of specialised cells, say those in the crypts of Lieberkühn, or whether it is the result of a change in functioning of cells that usually absorb.

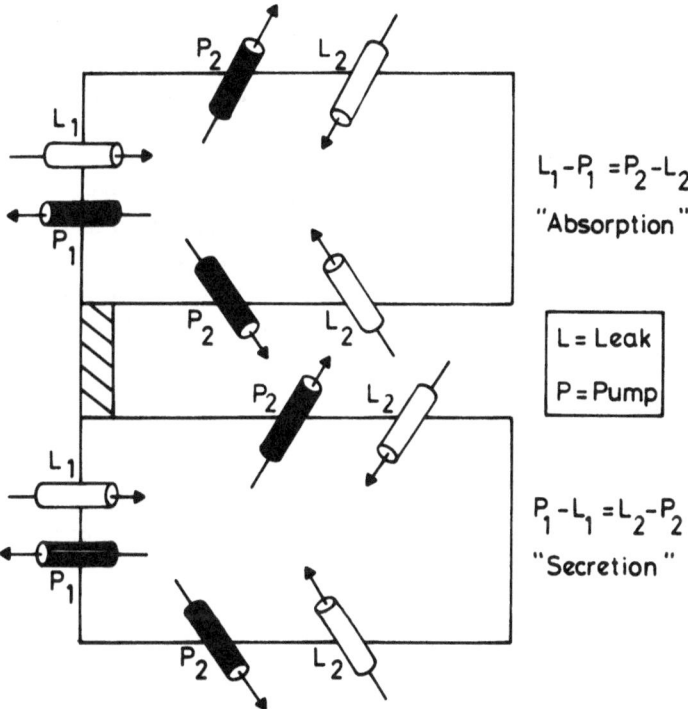

$$L_1 - P_1 = P_2 - L_2$$

"Absorption"

L = Leak

P = Pump

$$P_1 - L_1 = L_2 - P_2$$

"Secretion"

Figure 21.8 Two adjacent intestinal mucosal cells separated by intercellular space. Brush borders of each cell are furnished with both 'pumps' and leaks (P_1 and L_1) as are the basolateral membranes (P_2 and L_2). The upper cell is operating in the 'absorption' mode, while that underneath is in the 'secretory' mode, for definition of 'pump' and 'leak', see section 2.1

The latter possibility is quite feasible and would depend upon the change being induced by the action of some agent, for example, a hormone such as GIP or a prostaglandin (see the paper by MATUCHANSKY) or a toxin (like *E. coli* or *V. cholera*). If both the brush-border membranes and those of the basolateral region are furnished with pumps and leaks, for example, the direction of the salt pumps being outwards, while the leaks function to cause a flow in the inward direction, then by altering the relative pumpiness and leakiness of the two faces, the direction of transport may be altered (Figure 21.8). Thus agents that induce secretion by activating a cellular route may do so by causing an outwardly directed salt pump to appear in the brush-border membranes, while at the same time the activity of the outwardly directed pump located in the basolateral membranes may be suppressed (see also LAUTERBACH).

The question as to whether agents that induce secretion do so by inducing new enzymes in the brush-border membranes remains to be investigated. Studies of the sort described by EBEL would also be useful. The possible role of the paracellular route in secretion by the intestine has already been mentioned (page 421).

THE ROLE OF DIFFUSION IN INTESTINAL ABSORPTION

In studies of intestinal absorption over the last 25 years there has been great emphasis on the part played by 'active transport', and more recently by membrane transport processes in particular. The role of diffusion has been neglected, yet paradoxically diffusion becomes of increasing importance in cases where membrane transport phenomena occur at high rates. In such cases access to the site of membrane transport may be limited by diffusion through a

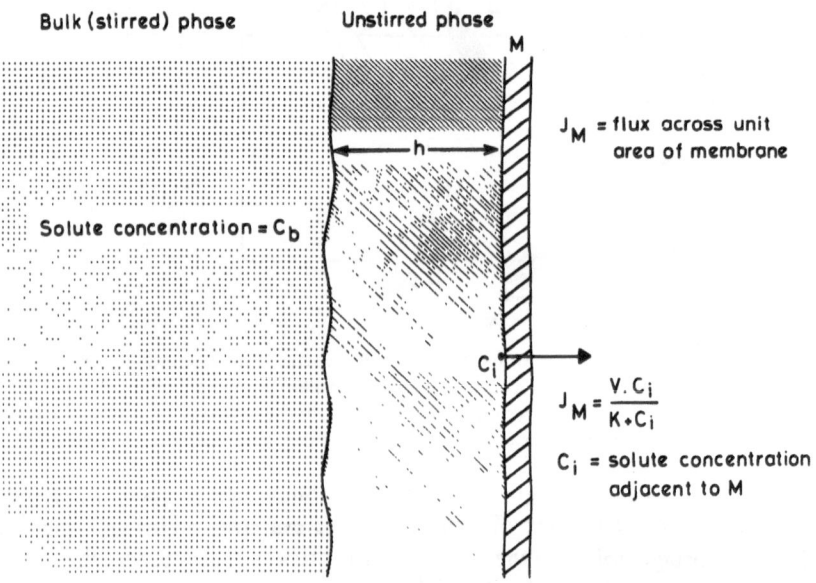

Figure 21.9 Effects of unstirred layer of fluid. The flux across the membrane M is determined by the concentration of solute, c_i, in the region immediately adjacent to M. But, c_i is determined by the flux through the system! Thus, if the layer is h cm thick, and D is the diffusion coefficient of the solute within it then J_M also equals $(c_b-c_i)D/h$ hence $c_i = c_b - J_M h/D$. See also Appendix 2

stationary 'unstirred' layer of fluid adjacent to the membrane (the Nernst[25] diffusion layer).

Generally speaking, as pointed out elsewhere by Winne[26] (see also Fisher[27] and Dietschy and Westergaard[28]), the effect of the Nernst diffusion layer is without influence on the apparent V_{max} of the relevant membrane transport process. However, the layer does have the effect of reducing the apparent affinity of the underlying membrane transport system for the substrate. This is equivalent to the apparent K_t of the membrane transport process being increased by the addition of a term which depends upon the V_{max} of the system. In other words, the effects of the Nernst diffusion layer are most pronounced in cases where the V_{max} is high and the effects are least for substances that are subjected to membrane transport at only low rates.

Table 21.4 Unidirectional fluxes of sodium ions; data of Cereijido and Rotunno[14] recalculated by Parsons[15]

	Na flux (10^3 ions s$^-$ μm^{-2})
Flux across plasma membrane	
Human erythrocyte	<1
Frog skeletal muscle	3–6
Squid nerve axon	20
Flux across epithelia	
Toad urinary bladder	84
Frog skin	330
Rat ileum	800
Guinea-pig caecum	1300
Rabbit ileum	1660

If one writes the equations to deal with the relevant fluxes in the steady state, it is easy to obtain an approximate solution which shows the effects (see Appendix 2 and Figure 21.9). I have calculated the effects of differing activities of membrane transport system on the apparent K_t and the results are given in Table 21.4. Note that the calculations apply to transport occurring across a plane sheet. For a convoluted sheet like the small intestine, the effects must be complicated if the unstirred layer is thick compared with the density of the convolutions.

ALVARADO and MAHMOOD have considered the question of the binding of Na$^+$ in the brush-border region and have discussed the effects of this on favouring the entry of Na$^+$ into the glycocalyx region. This entry could occur by diffusion from the lumen or by recycling from the intercellular spaces via the paracellular route and the zonula occludens.

The effects of binding of substrate on passive movement through a zone where binding can occur are very interesting. If the binding molecule is capable of diffusive movement, then its presence will facilitate the diffusion of the substrate that is bound if certain limiting conditions are met. For example, this is the case for the diffusion of O_2 through solutions that contain haemoglobin. The O_2 is transferred partly as the gas in free solution and partly in combination with the haemoglobin molecules. The same is true for the diffusion of oxygen in muscle in the presence of myoglobin[29,30].

However, the situation is different if the binding sites are stationary. Suppose that diffusion is occurring through a medium containing fixed binding sites which react to bind the diffusing substance at a rate which is very rapid compared with the rate of diffusion.

Then if the concentration of bound substance in the matrix is B where the concentration of the free substance is C, and B = kC, then it is found that the apparent diffusion coefficient for the substance, assumed to be of constant value D in free solution, takes the value $D/(k + 1)$. In other words, the effect of the binding is to slow down the diffusion process[31]. There are evidently both advantages and disadvantages from the physiological point of view in the possession of binding sites.

Relatively few experiments *in vitro* employ techniques that utilise the advantages of vascular perfusion. In most methods tubes, rings or diaphragms of the whole wall, or of the whole wall minus the extrinsic muscle coats are used. Even with the muscle coats removed, the presence of corrugations in the tissue due to the intestinal villi and ridges of the mucosa means that in the tissue there is an unstirred layer, perhaps several millimetres thick across which substrate must pass. It is the role of the mesenteric circulation to reduce the thickness of this layer, the clearance of absorbed substances away from the epithelium being across the basement membrane directly into the epithelium. In this connection the observations made by LOVE concerning human intestinal blood flow and fluid transport are of interest.

The presence of the unstirred layer on the transluminal side of the epithelium makes difficult the application of hormones and transmitters and inhibitors to the epithelium from the serosal side. As a result, interpretation, in physiological terms, of the effects of particular doses of such substances may sometimes be difficult (see page 418).

CONCLUSION

It must be clear to everyone that a major benefit of this meeting has been the fact that it has brought together workers who are interested in very widely differing aspects of intestinal transport. Some are physiologists, others are pharmacologists and biochemists; we have also heard of the experiments of comparative physiologists, of surgeons and of anatomists. It has been very interesting to learn of the adaptations that occur in intestinal function under different conditions including those obtained immediately after birth. We have heard something of the properties of renal tubule cells, and the similarities of the nephron to the intestinal mucosa can in some instances be very striking.

CLOSING SUMMARY

The opportunity to meet and to exchange ideas freely both in formal sessions and informally is of enormous value, and I am convinced we have all benefited greatly. I am sure that the ideas that our deliberations have generated will form the basis of more experiments to answer the new questions that have to be posed as a result of the material presented at Titisee during the last two days.

We are all exceedingly grateful to Dr FALK for making this meeting possible and for seeing that we have been so hospitably entertained. We also thank him for enabling people to come from as far away as Japan and Australia as well as from the United States and Europe to meet and exchange ideas.

We must also thank Dr J. W. L. ROBINSON and his Secretariat for organising this meeting so efficiently and for keeping us all on our toes, not only before the meeting but also during it.

References

1. Glynn, I. M. and Karlish, S. J. D. (1975). The sodium pump. *Ann. Rev. Physiol.*, **37**, 13
2. Macknight, A. D. C., Pilgrim, J. P. and Robinson, B. A. (1974). The regulation of cellular volume in liver slices. *J. Physiol. Lond.*, **238**, 279
3. Oschman, J. L., Wall, B. J. and Gupta, B. L. (1974). Cellular basis of water transport. In: M. A. Sleight and D. H. Jennings (eds). Transport at the Cellular Level; *Symp. Soc. Exp. Biol.* No. 27, p. 305 (London: Cambridge University Press)
4. Rhodin, J. A. G. (1974). *Histology*, Fig. 29–5, 556 (New York: Oxford University Press)
5. Ussing, H. H. (1960). The alkali metal ions in biology. In: O. Eichler and A. Farah (eds). *Handbuch der Experimentellen Pharmakologie*, Vol. 13 (Berlin: Springer Verlag)
6. Ussing, H. H. (1975). Epithelial transport phenomena. In: T. Z. Csáky (ed). *Intestinal Absorption and Malabsorption*, p. 1 (New York: Raven Press)
7. Voûte, C. L., Møllgård, K. and Ussing, H. H. (1975). Quantitative relationship between active sodium transport, expansion of endoplasmic reticulum and specialised vacuoles ('scalloped sacs') in the outermost living cell layer of the frog skin epithelium. *J. Memb. Biol.*, **21**, 273
8. Dick, D. A. T. and Fry, D. J. (1975). Sodium fluxes in single amphibian oocytes: further studies and a new model. *J. Physiol. Lond.*, **247**, 91
9. Parsons, D. S. (1971). Salt transport. In: A. M. Dawson (ed). Intestinal Absorption and its Derangements. *J. Clin. Path.*, **24**, Suppl. (Roy. Coll. Path.) 5, 90
10. Parsons, D. S. (1973). Carbonic anhydrases of the intestinal tract. In L. Bolis, K. Schmidt-Nielsen and S. H. P. Maddrell (eds). *Comparative Physiology*, p. 417. (Amsterdam: North Holland Publishing Co.)
11. Parsons, D. S. and Powis, G. (1971). Some properties of a preparation of rat colon perfused *in vitro* through the vascular bed. *J. Physiol. Lond.*, **217**, 641
12. Florey, H. W., Wright, R. D. and Jennings, M. A. (1941). The secretions of the intestine. *Physiol. Rev.*, **21**, 36
13. Staehelin, L. A. (1974). Structure and function of intercellular junctions. *Int. Rev. Cytol.*, **39**, 191
14. Cereijido, M. and Rotunno, C. A. (1968). Fluxes and distribution of sodium in frog skin. A new model. *J. Gen. Physiol.*, **51**, 280 S
15. Parsons, D. S. (1972). Summary. In: W. L. Burland and P. D. Samuel (eds). *Transport across the Intestine: A Glaxo Symposium* p. 253. (London: Churchill Livingstone)

16. Parsons, D. S. (1968). Methods for investigation of intestinal absorption. *Handbook of Physiology*, Section 6, Vol. 3, Chap. 64, p. 1177 (Washington D.S.: American Physiological Society)

17. Loeschke, K., Bentzel, C. J. and Csáky, T. Z. (1970). Asymmetry of osmotic flow in frog intestine: functional and structural correlation. *Amer. J. Physiol.*, **218**, 1723

18. Anon (1860). Article 'Digestion' in *Chamber's Encyclopaedia* 6, p. 564 (London: L. W. and R. Chambers)

19. Rummel, W. and Stupp, H. F. (1962). The influence of diuretics on the absorption of water from isolated small intestine of the rat. *Experientia*, **18**, 303

20. Forth, W., Rummel, W. and Glasner, H. (1964). Zur resorptionshemmenden Wirkung von Gallensäuren. *Naunyn-Schmiedebergs. Arch Pharmak. Exp. Path.*, **247**, 382

21. Forth, W., Rummel, W. and Glasner, H. (1966). Zur resorptionshemmenden Wirkung von Gallensäuren. *Naunyn-Schmiedebergs. Arch Pharmak. Exp. Path.*, **254**, 364

22. Pope, J. L., Parkinson, T. M. and Olson, J. A. (1966). Action of bile salts on the metabolism and transport of water-soluble nutrients by perfused rat jejunum *in vitro*. *Biochim. Biophys. Acta*, **130**, 218

23. Dietschy, J. M. (1972). (ed) Symposium on bile acids. *Arch. Int. Med.*, **130**, 473

24. Cizek, L. J. (1954). Total water content of laboratory animals with special reference to volume of fluid within the lumen of the gastrointestinal tract. *Amer. J. Physiol.*, **179**, 104

25. Nernst, W. (1904). Theorie der Reaktionsgeschwindigkeit in heterogenen Systemen. *Z. Phys. Chem.*, **47**, 52

26. Winne, D. (1973). Unstirred layer, source of biased Michaelis constant in membrane transport. *Biochim. Biophys. Acta*, **298**, 27

27. Fisher, R. B. (1964). The mutability of K_m. In: F. Dickens and E. Neil (eds). *Oxygen in the Animal Organism* p. 339 (Oxford: Pergamon Press)

28. Dietschy, J. M. and Westergaard, H. (1975). The effect of unstirred water layers on various transport processes in the intestine. In: T. Z. Csáky (ed). *Intestinal Absorption and Malabsorption*, p. 197 (New York: Raven Press)

29. Scholander, P. F. (1960). Oxygen transport through haemoglobin solutions. *Science*, **131**, 585

30. Wittenberg, J. B. (1970). Myoglobin-facilitated oxygen diffusion: role of myoglobin in oxygen entry into muscle. *Physiol. Rev.*, **50**, 559

31. Crank, J. (1964). *The Mathematics of Diffusion*. Chapter 8 (Oxford: Clarendon Press)

32. Woodbury, J. W. (1965). The cell membrane: ionic and potential gradients and active transport. In: T. H. Ruch and H. D. Patton (eds). *Physiology and Biophysics*. (Philadelphia and London: W. B. Saunders)

33. Davies, M. (1973). *Functions of Biological Membranes*. p. 37 and p. 52. (London: Chapman and Hall)

APPENDIX 1

VOLUME REGULATION

GIBBS–DONNAN EFFECTS ON OSMOTIC ACTIVITY OF CELL FLUIDS

Suppose a cell to be enclosed by a membrane that is permeable to water and to small anions and cations. a, small anions; c, small cations. A, 'fixed' anions carrying a net negative charge, z (see Figure 21.1, see also Woodbury[32] and Davies[33]).

428

Σ = sum of concentrations of like ionic species, mmol kg^{-1} water.
Neglecting osmotic coefficients we may write

Osmotic activity of external solution = Π_o mosmol kg^{-1}

$$\Pi_o = (\Sigma a_o + \Sigma c_o) \qquad (1)$$

Osmotic activity of internal solution = Π_i mosmol kg^{-1} water

$$\Pi_i = (\Sigma a_i + \Sigma c_i + A) \qquad (2)$$

The requirements for electrical neutrality put

$$\Sigma c_o = \Sigma a_o \qquad (3)$$

and

$$\Sigma c_i = \Sigma a_i + zA \qquad (4)$$

At equilibrium in a cell that is *not* pumping, the electrochemical potentials of
each species of the mobile ions must be equal on the two sides, hence:

$$\frac{\Sigma a_o}{\Sigma a_i} = \frac{\Sigma c_i}{\Sigma c_o} \qquad (5)$$

Eliminating Σa_i and Σc_i from equations 1 to 5 gives

$$\Pi_i = A + \{z^2 A^2 + \Pi_o^2\}^{0.5}$$

hence

$$\Pi_i > \Pi_o$$

As an approximation we may write

$$\Pi_i = A + \Pi_o + (zA)^2/2\Pi_o$$

In a cell that *is* pumping, equation (5) does not hold, the values of Σa_i and Σc_i
being adjusted so that

$$\Pi_i = \Pi_o$$

APPENDIX 2

UNSTIRRED LAYER

Influence of unstirred layers of fluid (Nernst[25] diffusion layers) on kinetics of
membrane transport (see Figure 21.6). Suppose the concentration of substrate
in the bulk phase is c_b and that in the fluid adjacent to the membrane is c_i.
Then flux across unit area of the membrane is given by

$$J_m = V_{c_i}/(K + c_i)$$

where K and V are constants.

For an unstirred layer of thickness h, the flux from the bulk phase across unit area is

$$\mathcal{J}_h = D(c_b - c_i)/h$$

where D is the diffusion coefficient within the unstirred layer.

In the steady state of transfer $\mathcal{J}_h = \mathcal{J}_m$.

By eliminating c_i from the equations we have as an approximation (see, for example, Fisher[27])

$$\mathcal{J}_m = V_{c_b}/(K' + c_b) \text{ where } K' = K + Vh/D$$

In other words, the effect of the presence of an unstirred layer is to increase the value of the apparent 'half-saturation' constant K of the membrane transport process, by the addition of a term that is proportional to the magnitude of *maximum* capacity of the transport system (see Table 21.5).

Table 21.5 Effects of unstirred layer of fluid (Nernst diffusion layer) on transport. Influence of magnitude of maximum capacity, V_{max} on the apparent 'half saturation' constant K of membrane transport system

V_{max} (μmol cm^{-2} h^{-1})	Vh/D (μmol ml^{-1})
1	0.6
5	2.8
10	5.6
50	28
100	56

Assumptions. (i) thickness of unstirred layer 100 μm = 10^{-2} cm; (ii) diffusion coefficient = 5×10^{-6} cm^2 s^{-1}, that is, approximately that of glucose in free solution; (iii) V is in the range 1–100 μmol cm^{-2} h^{-1}; Note $K' = K + Vh/D$ (see Appendix 2), so that Vh/D is the amount by which the 'half saturation' constant (K) is increased. Note if the unstirred layer of fluid is 500 μm thick, then the values should be multiplied by 5, and so on.